THE YEARBOOK

OF

OBSTETRICS AND GYNAECOLOGY

VOLUME 9

The Yearbook of
OBSTETRICS
and
GYNAECOLOGY

Volume 9

Edited by
David Sturdee, Karl Oláh and Declan Keane

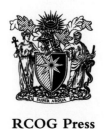

RCOG Press

First published 2001

© Royal College of Obstetricians and Gynaecologists 2001

All rights reserved. No part of this publication may be reproduced, stored in a retrieval system, or transmitted in any form or by any means, electronic, mechanical, photocopying, recording or otherwise, without the prior written permission of the Royal College of Obstetricians and Gynaecologists.

ISBN 1 900364 48 4

Published by the **RCOG Press** at the
Royal College of Obstetricians and Gynaecologists
27 Sussex Place, Regent's Park
London NW1 4RG
Registered Charity No. 213280

RCOG Press Editor: Jane Moody
Cover designed by Geoffrey Wadsley
Produced by FiSH Books Ltd.
Printed in Great Britain

Contents

List of contributors		vii
Foreword		xv
1	Of violent floodings in pregnancy: evolution of the management of placenta praevia *Thomas F. Baskett*	1
2	The influence of folate catabolism on the dietary requirement for folate in pregnancy *John R.J. Higgins*	15
3	Looking backwards: a gynaecologist's view of the anorectum *Christopher N. Hudson*	25
4	The consultant-based service *Patrick B. Forbes*	35
5	Regulations, standards, guidelines – is there any room for freedom of thought? *Robert W. Shaw*	45
6	The consumer's right to evidence-based health care *Marcia Kelson*	53
7	Anterior vaginal-wall prolapse – an historical and anatomical perspective *Elizabeth J. Adams and Mark Slack*	61
8	Understanding health economic terms with reference to infertility *Bolarinde Ola and Masoud Afnan*	71
9	Cost effectiveness and infertility *Masoud Afnan and Bolarinde Ola*	77
10	Does minimal access surgery have a role in ovarian cancer? *Alberto de Barros Lopes*	89
11	Period-free HRT *Timothy C. Hillard*	98
12	Glandular abnormalities: difficult situations in colposcopy *Susan J. Houghton*	119
13	Hormones and cancer of the cervix, vulva, vagina and ovary *Allan B. MacLean*	137
14	Congenital urogenital anomalies for the gynaecologist *Kalpana Patil and Padraig S. Malone*	144
15	Gynaecological malignancy in childhood and adolescence *Khalil Razvi and John H. Shepherd*	157

16	Anal incontinence – the role of the obstetrician and gynaecologist *Abdul H. Sultan and A. Muti Abulafi*	170
17	Minimal access urogynaecology *Andrew J. S. Tapp*	188
18	HRT forever *William Thompson and Karen A. McKinney*	196
19	Bilateral uterine artery embolisation for fibroids *Woodruff J. Walker*	209
20	Vault prolapse *Patrick Hogston*	215
21	Rectovaginal endometriosis *Jeremy T. Wright, David B. Redwine and Norman Ratcliffe*	226
22	Surrogate pregnancy *David D. Boyle*	239
23	What do we do with the pregnant athlete? *Michael M. Dooley*	247
24	Trial of scar? *Harold Gee*	263
25	Maternal suicide *Carol A. Henshaw*	270
26	Fetal hydrops *David James*	277
27	The edge of viability *B. Garth McClure and Angela H. Bell*	288
28	Invasive diagnosis of fetal abnormalities and therapeutic methods *Deirdre J. Murphy and Peter W. Soothill*	295
29	Minimally invasive prenatal diagnosis: fantasy or reality? *Timothy G. Overton*	310
30	Shoulder dystocia *Eric Watson and Khaldoun Sharif*	324
31	Reducing teenage pregnancy *Kate Weaver and Anna Glasier*	338
32	Maternal death and anaesthesia – a perspective *Sheila M. Willatts*	349
Index		361

List of contributors

A. Muti Abulafi MS FRCS
Consultant Colorectal Surgeon
Mayday University Hospital
London Road
Croydon
Surrey CR7 7YE

Elizabeth J. Adams MD MRCOG
Subspecialty Trainee Urogynaecology
Department of Urodynamics
Liverpool Women's Hospital
Crown Street
Liverpool L8 7SS

Masoud A.M. Afnan FRCOG
Consultant Obstetrician and Gynaecologist
 and Director of Infertility
Birmingham Women's Hospital
Metchley Park Road
Edgbaston
Birmingham B15 2TG

**Alberto de Barros Lopes MBChB
 MRCOG**
Consultant Gynaecological Oncologist
Northern Gynaecological Oncology Centre
Queen Elizabeth Hospital
Sheriff Hill
Gateshead NE11 0HQ

**Thomas F. Baskett MB FRCS DHMSA
 FRCOG**
Professor
Department of Obstetrics and Gynaecology
Dalhousie University
5980 University Avenue
Halifax
Nova Scotia
Canada B3J 3G9

Angela H. Bell MD FRCP FRCPCH
Consultant Paediatrician
Neonatal Unit
The Ulster Hospital
Dundonald
Belfast BT16 0RH

David D. Boyle FRCOG
Consultant Obstetrician and Gynaecologist
The Royal Maternity Hospital
Grosvenor Road
Belfast BT12 6BB

Michael M. Dooley MMs FRCOG
Consultant Obstetrician and Gynaecologist
Director of Sports Science and Medicine,
 British Equestrian Federation
Dorset County Hospital
Williams Avenue
Dorchester DT1 2JY

Patrick B. Forbes FRCOG
Consultant Obstetrician and Gynaecologist
168 Hartford Road
Huntingdon
Cambridgeshire PE18 7XQ

Harold Gee MD FRCOG
Consultant Obstetrician
Director of Postgraduate Education
Department of Postgraduate Education
Education Resource Centre
Birmingham Women's Hospital
Edgbaston
Birmingham B15 2TG

Anna Glasier BSc MD FRCOG
Director
Family Planning and Well Woman Services for
 Lothian
18 Dean Terrace
Edinburgh EH4 1NL

Carol A. Henshaw MBChB MRCPsych
Senior Lecturer in Psychiatry
School of Postgraduate Medicine
Keele University
Thornburrow Drive
Hartshill
Stoke-on-Trent ST4 7QB

John R.J. Higgins MD MRCPI MRCOG
Senior Lecturer
Department of Obstetrics and Gynaecology
University of Melbourne
Mercy Hospital for Women
East Melbourne
VIC 3002
Australia

Timothy C. Hillard BM DM MFFP FRCOG
Consultant Obstetrician and Gynaecologist
Department of Obstetrics and Gynaecology
Poole Hospital NHS Trust
Longfleet Road
Poole BH15 2JB

Patrick Hogston FRCS FRCOG
Consultant Gynaecologist
Department of Gynaecology
Saint Mary's Hospital
Milton Road
Portsmouth PO3 6AD

Susan J. Houghton MB ChB MRCOG
Specialist Registrar, Obstetrics and Gynaecology
New Cross Hospital
Wednesfield Road
Wolverhampton WV10 0QP

Christopher N. Hudson MChir FRCS FRANZCOG FRCOG
Emeritus Professor
St. Bartholomew's and Royal London School of Medicine and Dentistry
West Smithfield
London EC1A 7BE

David K. James MA MD DCH FRCOG
Professor
Division of Fetomaternal Medicine
University of Nottingham
Queen's Medical Centre
Nottingham NG7 2UH

Marcia Kelson PhD
Senior Research Fellow
College of Health
St. Margaret's House
21 Old Ford Road
London E2 9PL

Allan B. MacLean MD FRCOG
Professor of Obstetrics and Gynaecology
Royal Free Hospital
Rowland Hill Street
Hampstead
London NW3 2PF

B.Garth McClure MB FRCP FRCPCH
Professor of Neonatal Medicine
Department of Child Health
Institute of Clinical Science
Royal Group of Hospitals
Grosvenor Road
Belfast BT12 6BJ

Karen A. McKinney MD MRCOG
Lecturer in Obstetrics and Gynaecology
Queen's University Belfast
Department of Obstetrics and Gynaecology
Institute of Clinical Science
Grosvenor Road
Belfast BT12 6BJ

Padraig S.J. Malone MB MCh FRCSI FRCS
Consultant Paediatric Urologist
Department of Paediatric Urology
Southampton University Hospitals NHS Trust
Tremona Road
Southampton SO16 6YD

Dierdre J. Murphy MD MRCOG
Consultant Senior Lecturer in Maternal
 Medicine
Division of Obstetrics and Gynaecology
University of Bristol
St Michael's Hospital
Southwell Street
Bristol BS2 8EG

Bolarinde Ola FWACS MRCOG
Clinical Research Fellow in Infertility
Assisted Conception Unit
Birmingham Women's Hospital
Metchley Park Road
Edgbaston
Birmingham B15 2TG

Timothy G. Overton MD MRCGP MRCOG
Consultant Obstetrician and Gynaecologist,
Subspecialist in Maternal and Fetal Medicine
Department of Obstetrics and Gynaecology
Norfolk and Norwich Hospital
Brunswick Road
Norwich NR1 3SR

Kalpana Patil FRCS
Specialist Registrar Paediatric Surgery
Wessex Regional Centre for Paediatric
 Surgery
Southampton General Hospital
East Wing
Tremona Road
Southampton SO16 6YD

Norman Ratcliffe FRCPath
Consultant Pathologist
Ashford and St Peters NHS Trust
St Peter's Hospital
Guildford Road
Chertsey KT16 0PZ

Khalil Razvi FAMS MRACOG MRCOG
Gynaecological Oncology Fellow
The Gynaecological Cancer Centre
St Bartholomew's Hospital
The Royal Hospitals NHS Trust
London EC1A 7BE

David B. Redwine MD
Consultant Gynaecologist
2190 NE Professional Court
Bend
Oregon 97701
USA

Khaldoun Sharif MD MBBCh MFFP MRCOG
Consultant Obstetrician and Gynaecologist
Birmingham Women's Hospital
Metchley Park Road
Edgbaston
Birmingham B15 2TG

Robert W. Shaw MD FRCS(Ed) FRCOG
Professor of Obstetrics and Gynaecology
University Hospital of Wales
Heath Park
Cardiff CF14 4XW

John H. Shepherd FRCS FRCOG
Professor of Surgical Gynaecology and
 Consultant Gynaecological Oncologist
The Gynaecological Cancer Centre
St Bartholomew's Hospital
The Royal Hospitals NHS Trust
London EC1A 7BE

Mark Slack MMed FCOG(SA) MRCOG
Consultant Obstetrician and Gynaecologist
Department of Obstetrics and Gynaecology
Peterborough District Hospital
Thorpe Road
Peterborough PE3 6DA

Peter W. Soothill MRCOG
Professor of Maternal and Fetal Medicine
Fetal Medicine Research Unit
St. Michael's Hospital
Southwell Street
Bristol BS2 8EG

Abdul H. Sultan MB ChB MD MRCOG
Consultant Obstetrician and Gynaecologist
Mayday University Hospital
London Road
Croydon Surrey CR7 7YE

Andrew J.S. Tapp MRCOG
Consultant Obstetrician and Gynaecologist
Royal Shrewsbury Hospital NHS Trust
Mytton Oak Road
Shrewsbury SY3 8XQ

William Thompson MD FRCOG
Professor of Obstetrics and Gynaecology
Queen's University Belfast
Department of Obstetrics and Gynaecology
Institute of Clinical Science
Grosvenor Road
Belfast BT12 6BJ

Woodruff J. Walker FRCR FFR(SA)
Consultant Interventional Radiologist
Royal Surrey County Hospital
Egerton Road
Guildford GU2 7XX

Eric A.J. Watson MRCOG
Specialist Registrar Obstetrics and
    Gynaecology
Walsgrave Hospital
Clifford Bridge Road
Coventry CV2 2DX

Kate Weaver MBChB
Clinical Research Fellow
Family Planning and Well Woman Services for
    Lothian
18 Dean Terrace
Edinburgh EH4 1NL

Sheila M. Willatts MD FRCP FRCA
Consultant in Charge
Intensive Care Unit
Bristol Royal Infirmary
Marlborough Street
Bristol BS2 8HW

Jeremy T. Wright FRCOG
Consultant Obstetrician and Gynaecologist
The Woking Nuffield Hospital
Shores Road
Woking
Surrey GU21 4BY

Foreword

In this volume, we aim to provide an update on the current view of issues and management of obstetric and gynaecological problems, predominantly from Fellows and Members of the College. Many of the chapters are based on presentations given at College or other prestigious meetings. In addition, many of the College's eponymous lectures are included. These are given by eminent authorities in their field and are often the culmination of much research. It is regrettable when such lectures are heard by a limited number of people. In future years, all such speakers will be invited to contribute a chapter to the *Yearbook*, so that these special lectures can be appreciated by a wider audience and recorded for posterity.

We have tried to produce a wide cross-section of the increasingly diverse subjects in our specialty, including new looks at old problems – such as trial of scar, vault prolapse, fetal hydrops, maternal suicide and deaths, rectovaginal endometriosis and prolapse.

Newer techniques and issues presented include minimal access surgery in ovarian cancer and urogynaecology, prenatal diagnosis, uterine artery embolisation for the treatment of fibroids, should period-free HRT be given forever, and what to do with the pregnant athlete.

Practical clinical problems are also addressed in chapters on the difficult colposcopic situation of glandular abnormalities, the much-underestimated prevalence of anal incontinence and the increasingly litigious problem of shoulder dystocia. There are also some non-clinical issues, such as consumer's rights, health economics and our President's thoughts on regulations, standards and guidelines.

We are sure that there are many contributions of interest for both MRCOG trainees and trainers, and we thank and congratulate the authors for their diligence and support in producing such a worthwhile publication.

The title Yearbook remains unsatisfactory and misleading, however, and for several years there have been attempts to produce an alternative, more representative title. Unfortunately, most of those titles that might be suitable are already used for other publications. Suggestions are welcome, and the supplier of a title that is used will be suitably rewarded.

David Sturdee
Publications Officer, 1999–2002

1

Of violent floodings in pregnancy: evolution of the management of placenta praevia

Thomas F. Baskett

Based on the Royal College of Obstetricians and Gynaecologists Historical Lecture, given on 27 April 1999 at the Maritime Museum, Liverpool.

INTRODUCTION

There is scant reference to placenta praevia in the ancient medical literature, perhaps because the male physicians who wrote the texts had little or no involvement in the management of labour, which was carried out by female midwives. In the works of Hippocrates there is only one reference which might describe placenta praevia, albeit in a nonspecific manner: 'When there is a copious discharge of blood before labour, there is a risk that the child may be dead or at least not viable'.[1] Obviously, this reference could be to any of the causes of antepartum haemorrhage. The oldest published work in obstetrics and gynaecology is attributed to Soranus (98–138 AD). Writing in his text *Gynaecology*, Soranus brought together the knowledge of obstetrics, gynaecology and paediatrics of that era. One passage in that work might be interpreted as a description of placenta praevia, although it could be placental abruption, the other common cause of antepartum haemorrhage: 'Moreover, difficult labour occurs, if in consequence of the pain the woman stretches violently or the chorion is torn away from the uterus, or compresses part of the uterus or falls forward entirely'.[2] Soranus did give detailed instructions for the performance of internal version and breech extraction, which was later to be used as part of the management of placenta praevia. However, in his description it is clearly to be used for abnormal fetal lie and there was no mention of its use in cases of haemorrhage.

Moving into the Renaissance era, the first English publication on obstetrics, *The Byrth of Mankynde*, was produced in 1540. This was a translation of an earlier (1513) German text by Eucharius Rösslin entitled *The Garden of Roses for Pregnant Women and Midwives*. There was no mention of placenta praevia, direct or otherwise, in this text.[3] According to Radcliffe, the illustrious Italian anatomist Gabriel Fallopius (1523–62) dissected the bodies of many women who had died in labour and always found the placenta near the uterine fundus.[4] Jacob Rueff (1500–58), a city physician of Zurich, wrote one of the earlier texts on midwifery, *The Expert Midwife*, which was published in 1554. There is one scant reference to placenta praevia: 'But if the secundine or afterbirth come forth before the child, and hinder and let the passage of the infant, that shall be cut-off, but the navell must be bound up, and this pessary following must be conveyed into the necke or privie passage of the matrix'.[5] The English book, *A Directory for Midwives*, written by Nicholas Culpeper (1616–54) and published in 1651, does not mention placenta praevia.[6]

UNDERSTANDING THE PATHOPHYSIOLOGY OF PLACENTA PRAEVIA: MYTH AND FACT

It was Paul Portal (1630–1703), a physician at the Hôtel Dieu in Paris, who first clearly described the attachment of the placenta to the lower uterine segment in cases of placenta praevia. Before his description it was thought that the placenta had fallen down from its fundal attachment.[7] Portal clearly delineated the adherence of the placenta to the lower uterine segment. In his case observation number 41, *The Delivery of a Woman Troubled with a Violent Flux of Blood*, he wrote: 'I put my whole hand into the womb, where the first thing I felt was the after-burthen, I separated it gently from the inner orifice into which it adhered'.[8]

Polycarb Gottlieb Schacher (1674–1737), of Leipzig, is said to have been the first to demonstrate the insertion of placenta praevia at autopsy in 1709.[9] William Hunter (1718–83) provided the first illustration of the true position of placenta praevia in Plates 11 and 12 of his *Anatomy of the Human Gravid Uterus*, published in 1774. He illustrates the case of 'A woman who died of a flooding in the ninth month of pregnancy ... the situation of the large vessels, which were injected, shows, that the placenta was attached forwards, and to the lower part of the womb'.[10] William Giffard, a surgeon and man-midwife working in London, was one of the earliest to describe the anatomical site and pathology of placenta praevia in an English text. In case 224 of his 1734 book, *Cases in Midwifery*, he confirmed that most authors believed the placenta was always attached to the upper part of the uterus, but that he had not always found this to be the case: 'in this case the placenta adhered and was fixed close to and round about the cervix uteri, as I have found it in many other cases'. He went on to explain the cause of bleeding: 'so that upon a dilatation of the os uteri, a separation has always followed, and hence a flooding naturally ensues'.[11] André Levret (1703–80), one of the most influential French obstetricians after Mauriceau, clearly recognised that the placenta was attached to the lower uterine segment in his monograph *Art des Accouchements*, in 1753.[12]

While it was generally agreed that the cause of bleeding was separation of the placenta from the uterine wall, the source of the bleeding was controversial. No less an authority than James Young Simpson (1811–70), of Edinburgh, erroneously believed that the bleeding came from the placental surface, as had Levret before him.[13,14] He reasoned that the connection of the maternal and placental circulations and the fact that haemorrhage in placenta praevia increased during uterine contractions supported his claim. He argued that if the source of haemorrhage was the uterine wall it should be diminished during contractions 'as the orifices will necessarily be temporarily diminished under the contraction of the uterine fibres'.[13] It was later pointed out that bleeding from the uterine wall might decrease during contractions but that the bloodflow during uterine relaxation would be expelled from the vagina at the time of the uterine contractions and therefore appear to be associated.[15,16] Among those to later discount Simpson's theory was his pupil Matthews Duncan (1826–90). He pointed out: 'Were the bleeding through the placenta, having for its source the open utero-placental vessels in the placenta surface, then the bleeding should always be arrested by complete separation'.[17] Manual separation of the placenta from the uterine wall to stem the bleeding had been advocated by Simpson. However, Duncan noted that, even in Simpson's own series, the bleeding continued in half of the cases in which the placenta was completely separated.[17] Thus, by the latter part of the 19th century it was established that the bleeding was due to separation of the placenta and the source of bleeding was the uterine wall.

THE ERA OF DELIVERY BY THE ART AND ACCOUCHEMENT FORCÉ

In the 17th and 18th centuries obstetricians increasingly acknowledged the danger of placenta praevia to the mother. This was so even when the obstetrician did not recognise the true nature of placenta praevia. Even those who felt that when the placenta presented at the cervix it was because it had fallen down from the fundus realised that the bleeding would continue until delivery occurred. Thus, it was advised that the obstetrician should forcibly dilate the cervix if necessary, separate the edge of the placenta until the examining hand reached and ruptured the membranes, grasp the leg of the infant, and deliver it by breech extraction. If necessary, the infant was turned inside the uterus so that the feet could be grasped – internal version. This method of delivery, namely internal version and breech extraction, was known as 'delivery by the art'. When the cervix had to be forcibly dilated to achieve this, it became known as '*accouchement forcé*' – a term first introduced by André Levret. The technique of internal version and breech extraction was reintroduced to obstetrics by the Parisian surgeon Ambroise Paré (1510–90). In his writings, he used this method to deal with transverse lie and shoulder presentation but also taught it to hasten delivery in cases of antepartum haemorrhage.[18] One of his pupils, Jacques Guillemeau (1546–1612), was an early proponent of this technique for delivering patients with placenta praevia. Indeed, in 1599 he saved the life of Paré's daughter, Ann Simon, and later described this encounter in his book.

'Madam Simon ... being near term was surprised by a great haemorrhage. Finding her nearly pulseless, with feeble voice and blanched lips, I made the prognosis to her mother and her husband that her life was in great danger. The way to save her was to deliver her immediately, the which I had seen practised by the late Monsieur Paré, her father who caused me to do the like unto a gentle woman of Madame de Senneterre. The mother and husband entreated me to save her and put the case in our hands. Thus, promptly, following the advice of Messieurs the Physicians, she was happily delivered of a lively infant'.[19]

Other obstetric texts of the 17th and 18th centuries also advocated *accouchement forcé* in cases of placenta praevia, including Astruc,[20] Baudelocque,[21] Deventer,[7] Giffard,[11] Levret,[12] Ould[22] and Portal.[8] Two prominent midwives, Louise Bourgeois[23] in France and Sarah Stone[24] in England, both advised internal version and breech extraction in cases of placenta praevia. The dominant French obstetrician of the 17th century, Francois Mauriceau (1637–1709), has been credited with advocating artificial rupture of the membranes for placenta praevia.[25] However, he also acknowledged that delivery by the art was necessary if bleeding was heavy or sustained: '... that a woman in this condition, for the reasons alleged, must necessarily be delivered, that the floodings may be stopt'.[26] Mauriceau had strong personal reasons to support this as his sister had died from antepartum haemorrhage due to delay in her delivery: '... the sad story of one of my sisters, which I shall not again repeat, being too sadly affected with it'.[26]

It should be noted that because of the heavy bleeding associated with placenta praevia and the lack of clinical differentiation between praevia and other causes of haemorrhage, *accouchement forcé* was often applied to all patients with antepartum haemorrhage. As most cases were not due to placenta praevia this was neither necessary nor desirable. Indeed, Noble, in his 1888 review, noted a maternal mortality of 33% with no interference, compared with 48% with accouchement forcé.[27] Furthermore, the perinatal loss was 58% and 63%, respectively. To this confusion Edward Rigby applied clinical observation and common sense.

ENLIGHTENMENT BY EDWARD RIGBY

In 1775, Edward Rigby (1747–1821) of Norwich published the first of six editions entitled *An Essay on the Uterine Haemorrhage: Which Precedes the Delivery of the Full Grown Foetus; Illustrated with Cases*. Early in his career he noted: 'A case of haemorrhage in which I found the placenta attached to the os uteri ... I considered it, at first merely as a casual and rare deviation from nature. In a few years, however, so many similar instances fell under my notice, as to convince me that it was a circumstance necessary to inquire after'.[28] By careful observation and record Rigby noticed a pattern in cases of antepartum haemorrhage. He observed that in cases of placenta praevia it was inevitable that haemorrhage would occur before the infant was delivered. He wrote: 'The placenta ... must, of necessity, be separated from it in proportion as the uterus opens, and, by that means, an haemorrhage must unavoidably be produced'. Furthermore, he noted that, in cases of bleeding in which the placenta could not be felt attached to the cervix or lower uterine segment, 'it is obvious that the separation of the placenta must be owing to some accidental circumstance'. He thus clearly differentiated between the two main causes of antepartum haemorrhage: one 'unavoidable' and due to placenta praevia and the other 'accidental' due to premature separation of the normally situated placenta – abruptio placentae. Thus, the terms 'unavoidable' and 'accidental' haemorrhage were introduced and remain in the obstetric literature more than two centuries later. At this time, before the clear clinical differentiation between placenta praevia and placental abruption, many obstetricians advocated delivery by the art or *accouchement forcé* in all cases of marked antepartum haemorrhage. Rigby reasoned that the sometimes difficult and dangerous *accouchement forcé* was only necessary in those cases of placenta praevia. He found that patients with placental abruption were best managed by more conservative treatment, including artificial rupture of the membranes. In such cases he found that this conservative management was rarely associated with maternal death. However, in patients with placenta praevia *accouchement forcé* was justified as the bleeding 'cannot possibly be supported by any other method whatever than the timely removal of the contents of the womb'.

Rigby continued to collect cases and his book went into six editions. In the final edition his experience with 106 cases of antepartum haemorrhage is recorded.[29] Towards the end of his text he summarised his principles: 'From what has been said it appears, then, the placenta is fixed to the os uteri much more frequently than has hitherto been supposed: that when it is so situated nothing but turning the child will put a stop to the flooding; then when it is not so situated, nature will, for the most part, expel it safely herself'.

Rigby's book was published in Britain and the USA and also translated into French, German and Russian. It had a profound influence, leading to the more logical management of cases of antepartum haemorrhage and was acknowledged and commended by several of the standard obstetrical texts of the early 19th century.[30–33]

VAGINAL AND UTERINE TAMPONADE

Justus Henrich Wigand (1769–1817), from Hamburg, is credited with being the first to use vaginal packing specifically for placenta praevia.[25] Although vaginal packs with astringent medications had been used since ancient times for uterine haemorrhage, both in the pregnant and nonpregnant woman, others packed the cervical canal in an attempt both to arrest the haemorrhage and induce labour. This really only served to hide the haemorrhage and, as the source of the bleeding became understood, its illogical basis was recognised. As Marshall put it: 'Vaginal plugging is rarely necessary, always undesirable, and only in a few cases really pardonable'.[34]

The use of bags placed in the vagina (colpeurynter) or uterus (metreurynter, Figure 1) and filled with either fluid or air to provide tamponade, was originally tried to induce labour. These bags were adapted and used in Britain to provide tamponade of the lower uterine segment in placenta praevia after placement through the cervix.[35–37] Robert Barnes (1817–1907) of London, in particular promoted the use of his 'Barnes' bag', as opposed to the more traumatic *accouchement forcé*. He argued that this method arrested haemorrhage and allowed more gentle dilatation of the cervix, thereby increasing the chances of survival for both mother and fetus. As he later wrote:

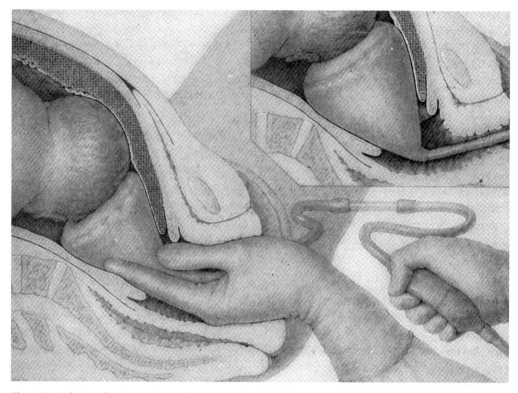

Figure 1 *Application of metreurynter to provide tamponade of the placenta and lower uterine segment (reproduced from* Williams Obstetrics, *10th edition by N.J. Eastman, Appleton-Century-Crofts, 1950)*

'Countless infants have been sacrificed on the altar of false theories ... it is no longer permitted to us, without ample proof of clear necessity, to sacrifice the child in order to save the mother'.[38] The use of Barnes' bag for management of placenta praevia was also advocated in Australia in the mid-19th century.[39] Champetier de Ribes in Paris[40] and James Voorhees of New York[41] improved upon the design of the original cumbersome bags.

THE FETUS AS TAMPON: BRAXTON HICKS' BIPOLAR VERSION AND WILLETT'S SCALP FORCEPS

The potentially traumatic nature of *accouchement forcé* has already been mentioned. The real problem was in cases with little or no cervical dilatation in which the cervix had to be forcibly dilated sufficiently for the operator's hand to reach into the uterus, turn the fetus if necessary, grasp the leg and then proceed with delivery by breech extraction. Once the operator started, he or she was committed to continue until delivery. In 1860, John Braxton Hicks (1823–97), the London obstetrician of Guy's Hospital, published his description of a combined method using both external and internal hands to turn the fetus – bipolar version.[42] With this technique, much less manipulation and force was required from the internal hand. The external hand guided the fetus into position and, if the cervix was only slightly dilated, one or two fingers were placed through it, just enough to grasp the foot and bring the leg down through the cervix. Thus, it was the buttock of the fetus that provided tamponade against the placenta and lower uterine segment (Figure 2). This form of tamponade was extremely effective in reducing blood loss, as Braxton Hicks described: 'Turn, and if you employ the child as a plug the danger is over. Then wait for the pains, rally the powers in the interval and let nature, gently assisted, complete the delivery'.[42] The key element here was that, once tamponade had been applied, the accoucheur was not forced to continue with delivery until the cervix dilated. Gentle traction was placed on the fetal leg either by the hand or a light weight attached to the leg by a bandage. In this way, over the succeeding minutes or hours, blood loss was stopped or greatly reduced, while the cervix dilated by uterine contractions rather than accouchement forcé. Braxton Hicks' technique of bipolar version in placenta praevia was widely adopted and remarkably effective, leading to a reduction in maternal mortality. However, the fetus was often sacrificed in its role as the plug for tamponade to save the mother. Significant improvement in the survival of the infant would await the safe development of caesarean section.

In the early part of the 20th century, most cases of placenta praevia were still delivered vaginally. Braxton Hicks' method of bipolar version and the use of the metreurynter were still common. John Abernethy Willett (1872–1932), working at the City of London Maternity Hospital, felt that in cases of cephalic presentation it would be advisable to use the fetal head for tamponade and devised scalp forceps to apply traction for this purpose. He presented his idea and early results to the Royal Society of Medicine in 1925: 'I had for some time thought that, could the requisite pressure be exerted by the fore coming head, the disadvantage of version and of de Ribes' bag might be obviated; and with the possible advantages of earlier treatment, less interference and so

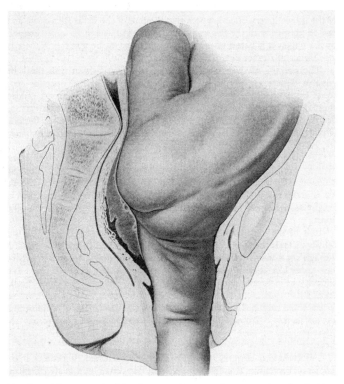

Figure 2 *The fetal breech used for tamponade of the placenta and lower uterine segment (reproduced with permission from Munro Kerr's Operative Obstetrics, 7th edition by J. Chasser Moir, Baillière Tindall and Cox, 1964)*

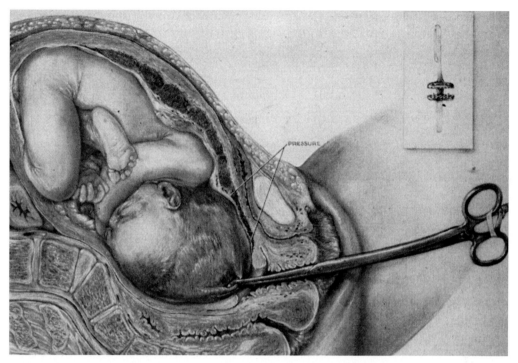

Figure 3 *Willett's forceps (reproduced from* Williams Obstetrics, *10th edition by N.J. Eastman, Appleton-Century-Crofts, 1950)*

diminished risk of sepsis'.[43] His T-shaped forceps had horizontal holding bars approximately half an inch long and could therefore be passed through a marginally dilated cervix (Figure 3). Small rounded holding teeth on the bars ensured a secure grasp of the fetal scalp. A small weight was then suspended over the end of the bed from the handles of the forceps and the patient allowed to deliver as the cervix dilated. This technique proved effective in reducing blood loss and accelerating delivery. However, as the safety of caesarean section increased and fetal viability became a greater consideration, Willett's scalp forceps were used only for the dead or pre-viable fetus.

THE EMERGENCE OF CAESAREAN SECTION

Towards the end of the 19th century, abdominal surgery had become feasible and safer, with the introduction of anaesthesia and the emerging principles of antisepsis and asepsis. However, caesarean section, which was usually performed on women after a prolonged, obstructed labour with established intrauterine sepsis, still had a high mortality. Hence, all methods of treating placenta praevia aimed to achieve vaginal delivery. Working in Birmingham, it was the Scottish gynaecological surgeon, Robert Lawson Tait (1845–99), who first suggested caesarean section for placenta praevia. He did this in an address given in 1890 entitled *The Surgical Treatment of Impacted Labour* and published that same year in the *British Medical Journal*. He noted the high maternal mortality from haemorrhage and sepsis with operative vaginal delivery for placenta praevia and said: 'If I had to deal with a case of placental praevia from the beginning of labour, and could carry out what I believe would be the ideal surgical treatment of this condition, I should amputate the pregnant uterus'.[44] Tait was the most audacious, talented and innovative gynaecological surgeon of his era. He was articulate, opinionated, successful and often right – a combination guaranteed to make him enemies. His suggestion that caesarean section might be appropriate in placenta praevia was ignored in Britain. However, it was performed unsuccessfully twice in the USA in 1891. The first caesarean section for complete placenta praevia with survival of the mother was carried out by Dr A.C. Bernays of St. Louis in 1893.[45] It was not until 21 December 1898 that Tait had his opportunity, when he was consulted in the case of a young pregnant woman in her fourth pregnancy: 'she had been bleeding with alarming profusion for five hours, in spite of many other and orthodox points of treatment'.[46] Having confirmed that the fetus was alive, Tait proceeded to carry out a Porro caesarean hysterectomy. This entailed delivering the infant by caesarean section and then removing the uterus and bringing the cervical stump out through the lower end of the abdominal incision to reduce the risk of sepsis. The mother made a good recovery and the child was born alive, but later died at the age of one month from 'bronchitis'. In a typically cryptic addendum to his paper, Tait wrote: 'The whole thing is over in five minutes, being about the easiest and simplest operation in surgery'.[46] In the ensuing years, others on the European continent and in North America promoted caesarean section for placenta praevia in selected cases.[47,48] With the development of blood transfusion following World War One, caesarean section became the treatment of choice for major degrees of placenta praevia. In the USA, Arthur Bill of Cleveland did much to ensure its acceptance.[49]

Some idea of the slow acceptance of caesarean section in the management of placenta praevia can be gained from studying the different editions of two standard obstetrical texts published throughout the 20th century: John Whitridge Williams' *Obstetrics in the United States*[50] and Munro Kerr's *Operative Obstetrics* in Britain.[51] In the first edition of Williams' *Obstetrics* in 1903, he stated that 'pregnancy or labour should be terminated in the most conservative manner as soon as possible after a placenta praevia has been positively diagnosed'. He added: 'it seems doubtful whether caesarean section will come into general use'. He advocated the metreurynter and Braxton Hicks' method of delivery. This is continued through the second (1908), third (1912) and fourth (1917) editions. By the fifth edition in 1920, Williams acknowledged that more authorities were advocating caesarean section in selected cases. However, he still spoke against it except for rare cases. In the sixth edition in 1930, the last from Williams' pen, he remained opposed to the widespread use of caesarean section but advocated it for selected cases, such as 'women nearing the end of childbearing period, who are especially desirous of a living child.' It was not until the eighth edition in 1941, edited by Henricus Stander of New York and the tenth edition in 1950, by Nicholas Eastman of Johns Hopkins University, Baltimore, that caesarean section came to be widely recommended for placenta praevia.

In Munro Kerr's first edition, entitled *Operative Midwifery*, in 1908, he noted that caesarean section had been performed but felt it was rarely indicated. It was not until the fourth edition in 1937, now entitled *Operative Obstetrics*, that Munro Kerr acknowledged the increasing role of caesarean section in the management of placenta praevia. In the fifth edition, published in 1949, Munro Kerr was joined by Chassar Moir as co-author and they advised that most cases should be delivered by caesarean section.

EXPECTANT MANAGEMENT OF PLACENTA PRAEVIA

In 1945, two independent reports were published advocating a more conservative approach to placenta praevia. One of these was from Houston, Texas, by Herman Johnson[52] and the other from Belfast, Northern Ireland, by Charles Macafee.[53] By this time, the standard management of antepartum haemorrhage was to examine the patient and, if placenta praevia was confirmed, to deliver the fetus. If viable, caesarean section might be performed and if not, vaginal delivery, often using the fetus for tamponade with either Willett's scalp forceps or Braxton Hicks' bipolar version. The rationale behind immediate delivery of patients with placenta praevia, once diagnosed, was the prevailing view that the first bleed could be fatal to the mother. Both Johnson and Macafee, working independently, showed that this was almost never the case provided no attempt at interference or delivery was undertaken. Johnson advocated vaginal examination to confirm the diagnosis and then no further interference until induction or spontaneous labour.

The most comprehensive of the two reports was that of Macafee, involving an eight-year review of 174 cases of placenta praevia. He observed: 'One of the main causes of foetal mortality in placenta praevia is prematurity. This mortality can be reduced only be carrying the pregnancy to as near term as possible'.[53] After years of careful clinical observation and experience, Macafee concluded: 'placenta praevia is not an obstetrical emergency which must necessarily be dealt with at the first haemorrhage, and that a vaginal examination must not be made until the appropriate subsequent treatment can be carried out'. His principles of management involved withholding early digital pelvic examination, expectant hospital management until labour or fetal viability, then pelvic examination in the operating theatre with preparations for caesarean section or amniotomy, depending on the presence and degree of placenta praevia. Most other reports of this era quoted maternal death rates of 5–7% and fetal mortality of 50–60%. Macafee lost one mother of the 174 and the fetal mortality was 23%. In the last three years of his study, the fetal loss was 6% – a remarkable achievement at that time. For the first time it was shown that it was safe from a maternal point of view to direct attention to the infant's survival by gaining time for fetal maturation. This work revolutionised the approach to antepartum haemorrhage in general and placenta praevia in particular, resulting in considerable improvement in both maternal and fetal mortality rates. With minor modifications due to the modern availability of ultrasound, Macafee's principles, which in essence allow safe fetal maturation, remain intact.

PLACENTAL LOCALISATION

The principles of expectant management of placenta praevia involved admitting the patient to hospital and, provided the bleeding settled, which it usually did, a digital pelvic examination was not performed for fear of disturbing the placenta and causing further haemorrhage. This meant that all cases of antepartum haemorrhage had to be admitted with the presumed diagnosis of placenta praevia. As this was only the case in 30–40% of all patients with antepartum haemorrhage, many women were needlessly incarcerated in hospital for several weeks until they bled again, came into labour, or reached fetal viability. An accurate method of placental localisation, excluding direct digital examination, was therefore needed in order to select those women with antepartum bleeding who had placenta praevia and needed to stay in hospital. Attempts to visualise the placenta by X-ray began in the 1930s.[54-56] This depended on the rather inaccurate identification of the soft-tissue placental shadow and inference of the position of the placenta by displacement of the fetal presenting part. Attempts to more clearly differentiate between amniotic fluid and the edge of placenta involved amniography, with the injection of iodine solutions into the uterine cavity to increase the radio-opacity of the amniotic fluid.[57] In 1935, Ude advocated cystography to help delineate the position of a low-lying placenta without having to inject contrast material into the amniotic fluid.[58] In the 1950s and 1960s, radioisotope localisation of the placenta began to supplant X-ray placentography. This initially involved radioactive sodium[59] and, later, radioactive iodine.[60] The technique took account of the exceptional vascularity of the placental bed in which a disproportionately large amount of radioactivity could be detected by a scintillation counter after intravenous injection of the isotope.

The ease, safety and accuracy of placental localisation changed forever in 1966 with the landmark publication by Gottesfeld and his colleagues from Denver.[61] They used B scan ultrasound to localise the placenta and correlated these findings with stringent criteria for placental site definition at the time of delivery. The accuracy was 97%. With the advent and wide availability of real-time ultrasound equipment, placental localisation could be undertaken repeatedly and in a non-invasive manner without radiation. Through the 1970s and 1980s, refinement of the definition of the placental edge along with the development of the lower uterine segment has improved the accuracy.[62] The application of transvaginal ultrasound has further improved the technique.[63,64]

CURRENT CONTROVERSIES

Due to a combination of early recourse to hospital admission, accurate diagnosis, blood transfusion, safe anaesthesia and improved caesarean section techniques, the risk of placenta praevia to the mother in developed countries has been reduced to low levels – almost to that of the general obstetric population. In the last five triennial reports on *Confidential Enquiries into Maternal Deaths in the United Kingdom*, covering the 15 years 1982–96, there have been 11 325 119 births with 15 maternal deaths from placenta praevia – an average of one per year.[65-69] On average there were 755 088 births per annum and, if we accept an incidence of placenta praevia of one in 250 births, 3020 cases of placenta praevia each year. This maternal death rate of approximately one per 3000 cases of placenta praevia represents a 50- to 100-fold reduction in maternal mortality over the past 50 years.

Conservative management, bed rest, fetal assessment and improved neonatal care have also led to a considerable reduction in perinatal mortality. In a recent five-year (1988–92) population-based study in the Canadian province of Nova Scotia, involving 62 226 births with 211 cases of placenta praevia (0.34%), there were no maternal deaths. The caesarean section rate was 99% and the perinatal mortality 33 per 1000, compared with 12 per 1000 for the rest of the population.[70] A USA study of 64 000 cases with placenta praevia from the 1980s found that this condition complicated 0.48% of deliveries and resulted in a maternal death rate of three per 10 000 births.[71]

In the modern era, hospitals and health services are demanding cost-effective health care. Although they represent a small group, women with placenta praevia may spend several weeks in hospital after their initial bleed before they deliver. In recent years, the necessity of this expensive hospital stay has been questioned and the possibility of management at home has been raised. A number of groups have compared inpatient and outpatient management of these women, with inconclusive results.[72-76] The essence of the debate centres on the risk of sudden and life-threatening haemorrhage in the woman with a known placenta praevia who is sent home. The reported studies on home management are not large enough to answer this question and the randomised controlled trial to properly evaluate the maternal and perinatal implications has not been carried out. Until then, perhaps the cautionary words of Rigby should be heeded. He recalls a case in which he and another surgeon were called to a woman's home for a mild haemorrhage, which settled. Nonetheless, they both remained in the house with the patient and he described the frightening rapidity and severity with which haemorrhage can recur: 'but about five in the morning there was a sudden accession of labour pain, and with it an excessive gush of blood. Although the other surgeon and I were under the same roof with the patient, and of course were soon with her, yet in that short time such a loss had been sustained as sunk the patient instantly, and induced a most formidable state of faintness ... This is a striking instance of the rapidity with which this haemorrhage sometimes returns after the beginning of it has been trifling and unalarming'.

It seems appropriate to conclude a chapter on placenta praevia with his words.

Acknowledgement

I am grateful to Miss Patricia Want, Librarian, RCOG, for considerable assistance in tracing and obtaining many original sources. This chapter is based on the dissertation submitted by the author to the Worshipful Society of Apothecaries of London, Postgraduate Diploma Course in the History of Medicine in 1997.

References

1. *The Genuine Works of Hippocrates*, Vol. I (translated by Francis Adams 1849). London: Sydenham Society. p. 114
2. Soranus' *Gynaecology* (translated by Owsei Tenskin 1956). Baltimore: Johns Hopkins University Press (Softshell Books edition; 1991. p. 182)
3. Raynold, T. *The Byrth of Mankynde*. London; 1540. Also published in *The Classics of Obstetrics and Gynecology Library*. New York: Gryphon Editions; 1994
4. Radcliffe, W. *Milestones in Midwifery*. Bristol: John Wright; 1967. p. 15
5. Rueff, J. *The Expert Midwife*. Zurich: C. Froschauer; 1554 (English translation, London; 1637. p. 67)
6. Culpeper, N. *A Directory of Midwives*. London: Cole; 1651
7. Deventer, H. van. *The Art of Midwifery Improved* (English translation). London: Curll; 1716. p. 154-5
8. Portal, P. *The Compleat Practice of Men and Women Midwives: or, the True Manner of Assisting a Woman in Child-bearing*. 1685 (English translation, London: J. Johnson; 1763. p. 143-4)
9. Schacher, P.G. *De Placentae Uterinae Morbis*. Leipzig; 1709. Cited by Ricci, J.V. *The Genealogy of Gynaecology: History of the Development of Gynaecology Throughout the Ages 2000 BC – 1800 AD*. Philadelphia: Blakistan; 1950. p. 348
10. Hunter, W. *The Anatomy of the Human Gravid Uterus*. Birmingham: John Baskerville; 1774. plates 11 and 12
11. Giffard, A.W. *Cases in Midwifery*. London: Motte; 1734. p. 513 (revised and published by Edward Hody)
12. Levret, A. *Art des Accouchements*. Paris: Le Prieur; 1753. p. 29-35
13. Simpson, J.Y. Some remarks on the treatment of unavoidable haemorrhage by extraction of the placenta before the child. *London Medical Gazette* 1845;**5**:1009–16
14. Simpson, J.Y. Additional observations on unavoidable haemorrhage in cases of placental separation. *London Medical Gazette* 1845;**5**:1193–5
15. Read, W. The influence of the placenta upon the development of the uterus during pregnancy. *Am J Med Sci* 1858;**35**:309–22
16. Read, W. *Placenta Praevia: Its History and Treatment*. Philadelphia: J.B. Lippincott; 1861
17. Duncan, J.M. *Contributions to the Mechanism of Natural and Morbid Parturition, Including that of Placenta Praevia*. Edinburgh: A. & C. Black; 1875. p. 305-422
18. Paré, A. *The Works of Ambroise Parey* (translated by T.H. Johnston). London: Clark; 1678
19. Guillemeau, J. *Childbirth or the Happie Deliverie of Women* (English translation). London: Norton; 1635. p. 125-30
20. Astruc, J. *Elements of Midwifery* (translated by S. Ryley). London: Crowder and Coote; 1766. p. 112-14
21. Baudelocque, J.L. *A System of Midwifery*, Vol. 2 (translated by John Heath). London: Parkinson and Murray; 1760. p. 90

22   Ould, F. *A Treatise of Midwifery in Three Parts.* Dublin: Nelson and Connor; 1742. p. 76-8
23   Bourgeois, L. *Observatiais Diverse, sur la Stérilité, Perte de Fruict, Foecondité, Accouchements, et Maladie des Femmes, et Enfants Nouveaux-naiz.* Paris: Saugrain; 1609
24   Stone, S. *A Complete Practice of Midwifery*, pp. 5-7. London: A. Morley; 1737
25   Marr, J.P. Historical background of the treatment of placenta praevia. *Bull Hist Med* 1941;**9**:258–93
26   Mauriceau, F. *The Disease of Women with Child and in Child-bed*, 2nd ed. (translated by Hugh Chamberlen). London: John Darby; 1683. p. 104-16, 261
27   Noble, C.P. Treatment of placenta previa: a historical and critical sketch. *The Medical and Surgical Reporter* 1888;**58**:625–31
28   Rigby, E. *An Essay on the Uterine Haemorrhage, which Precedes the Delivery of the Full Grown Foetus: Illustrated with Cases.* London: J. Johnson; 1775
29   Rigby, E. *An Essay on the Uterine Haemorrhage, which Precedes the Delivery of the Full Grown Foetus: Illustrated With Cases*, 6th ed. London: Hunter; 1822
30   Bard, S.A. *A Compendium of the Theory and Practice of Midwifery.* New York: Collins and Perkins; 1807. p. 154-61
31   Dewees, W.P. *A Compendious System of Midwifery*, 2nd ed. Philadelphia: Casey and Lea; 1826. p. 422-56
32   Collins, R. *A Practical Treatise on Midwifery.* London: Longman; 1835. p. 89-177
33   Blundell, J. *The Principles and Practice of Obstetricy.* London: E. Cox; 1834. p. 335-58
34   Marshall, C.M. Placenta praevia and the lower segment operation. In: Marshall, C.M., editor. *Caesarean Section: Lower Segment Operation.* Bristol: John Wright; 1939. p. 142-63
35   Barnes, R. On flooding before delivery arising from adhesion of placenta to the os and cervix uteri. *Lancet* 1847;**i**:326–30
36   Barnes, R. On flooding before delivery and especially on a new principle and method of treatment of placenta praevia. *Lancet* 1856;**i**:14–15
37   Murray, J.J. Placenta praevia air pessary used to plug and dilate the os uteri. *Medical Times and Gazette* 1859;**18**:596–7
38   Barnes, R. Placenta praevia. *BMJ* 1888;**i**:458–61
39   Tracey, R.T. On the use of Barne's dilators in placenta praevia. *Aust Med J* 1864;**9**:307–12
40   Champetier de Ribes, C.L.A. De l'accouchement provoqué. Dilatation du canal genital (col de l'uterus, vagin et vulve) a l'aide de ballons introduit dans la cavité utérine pendant la grossesse. *Annales de Gynécologie* 1888;**30**:401–38
41   Voorhees, J.A. Dilatation of the cervix by means of a modified Champetier de Ribes balloon. *Medical Record* 1900;**58**:361–6
42   Hicks, J.B. On a new method of version in abnormal labour. *Lancet* 1860;**ii**:28–30
43   Willett, J.A. The treatment of placenta praevia by continuous weight traction – a report of seven cases. *Proc R Soc Med* 1925;**18**:90–4
44   Tait, L. The surgical treatment of impacted labour. *BMJ* 1890;**i**:657–9
45   Young, J.H. Caesarean section in cases of placenta praevia. In: *Caesarean Section: the History and Development of the Operation from Earliest Times.* London: H.K. Lewis; 1944. p. 171-82
46   Tait, L. On the treatment of 'unavoidable haemorrhage' by removal of the uterus. *Lancet* 1899;**i**:364–5
47   Dudley, A.P. Modern caesarean section, an ideal method of treatment of placenta praevia. *N Y Med J* 1900;**72**:754–60
48   Krönig, B. Metreuryse bei placenta praevia. *Zentralbl Gynakol* 1909;**33**:1177–82
49   Bill, A. Treatment of placenta previa by prophylactic blood transfusion and cesarean section. *Am J Obstet Gynecol* 1927;**14**:523–9

50 Williams, J.W. *Obstetrics: a Textbook for the Use of Students and Practitioners.* New York: Appleton; 1st ed. 1903. p. 723–5; 2nd ed. 1908. p. 816–9; 3rd ed. 1912. p. 839–42; 4th ed. 1917. p. 889–92; 5th ed. 1920. p. 891–2; 6th ed. 1930. p. 938; 8th ed. (H. Stander) 1941. p. 1067; 10th ed. (N. Eastman) 1950. p. 571

51 Kerr, J.M.M. *Operative Midwifery.* London: Baillière Tindall; 1st ed. 1908. p. 586–91; 2nd ed. 1911. p. 594. *Operative Obstetrics*, 4th ed. (co-authors D. McIntyre and F. Anderson) 1937; 5th ed. (co-author C. Moir) 1949

52 Johnson, H.W. The conservative management of some varieties of placenta previa. *Am J Obstet Gynecol* 1945;**52**:313–24

53 Macafee, C.G. Placenta praevia – a study of 174 cases. *J Obstet Gynaecol Br Emp* 1945;**52**:313–24

54 Kerr, J.M.M. The diagnosis of placenta praevia, with special reference to the employment of X-rays for this purpose. *Edinb Med J* 1933;**40**:21–32

55 Snow, W., Powell, C.B. Roentgen visualization of the placenta. *Am J Roentgenol* 1934;**31**:37–40

56 Reid, F. Joint discussion on X-rays and their value in the localisation of the placenta. *Proc R Soc Med* 1951;**44**:703–14

57 Menees, T.O., Miller, J.D., Holly, L.E. Amniography: preliminary report. *Am J Roentgenol* 1930;**24**:363–6

58 Ude, W.H., Weum, T.W., Urner, J.A. Roentgenologic diagnosis of placenta previa: report of a case. *Am J Roentgenol* 1934;**31**:231–3

59 Browne, J.C.Mc.C. Localisation of the placenta by means of radioactive sodium. *Proc R Soc Med* 1951;**44**:715–18

60 Hibbard, B.M. The diagnosis of placenta praevia with radioactive isotopes. *Proc R Soc Med* 1962;**55**:640–2

61 Gottesfeld, K.R., Thompson, H.E., Holmes, J.H., Taylor, E.S. Ultrasonic placentography – a new method for placental localization. *Am J Obstet Gynecol* 1966;**96**:538–47

62 King, D.L. Placental migration demonstrated by ultrasonography. *Radiology* 1973;**109**:67–70

63 Oppenheimer, L.W., Farine, D., Ritchie, J.W.K., Lewinsky, R.M., Telford, J., Fairbanks, L.A. What is a low-lying placenta? *Am J Obstet Gynecol* 1991;**165**:1036–8

64 Pauzner, D., Barrett, J. and Farine, D. Transvaginal scanning in the management of placenta praevia. *J Soc Obstet Gynaecol Can* 1995;**17**:231–5

65 Turnbull, A., Tindall, V.R., Beard, R.W., Robson, G., Dawson, M.P., Cloake, E.P. et al. *Report on Confidential Enquiries into Maternal Deaths in the UK 1982–1984.* London: HMSO; 1989 (Department of Health Report on Health and Social Subjects **34**)

66 Department of Health. *Report on Confidential Enquiries into Maternal Deaths in the UK 1985–1987.* London: HMSO; 1991

67 Hibbard, B.M., Anderson, M.M., Drife, J.O., Tighe, J.R., Sykes, K., Gordon, G. et al. *Report on Confidential Enquiries into Maternal Deaths in the UK 1988–1990.* London: HMSO; 1994

68 Hibbard, B.M., Anderson, M.M., Drife, J.O., Tighe, J.R., Gordon, G., Willatts, S. et al. *Report on Confidential Enquiries into Maternal Deaths in the UK 1991–1993.* London: HMSO; 1996

69 Drife, J., Lewis, G. (Eds) *Why Mothers Die. Report on Confidential Enquiries into Maternal Deaths in the UK 1994–1996.* London: The Stationery Office; 1998

70 Crane, J., Armson, B.A., Dodds, L., Liston, R.M., Van den Hof, M. Maternal complications and neonatal risks with placenta praevia. *Proceedings of the Society of Obstetricians and Gynaecologists of Canada* 1996:111–12

71 Iyasu, S., Softlas, A.K., Rowley, D.L., Koonin, L.M., Lawson, H.W., Atrash, H.K. The epidemiology of placenta previa in the United States, 1979 through 1987. *Am J Obstet*

Gynecol 1993;**168**:1424–9
72 D'Angelo, L.J., Irwin, L.F. Conservative management of placenta previa: a cost-benefit analysis. *Am J Obstet Gynecol* 1984;**149**:320–6
73 Droste, S., Keil, K. Expectant management of placenta previa: cost-benefit analysis of outpatient treatment. *Am J Obstet Gynecol* 1994;**170**:1254–7
74 Love, C.D.B., Wallace, E.M. Pregnancies complicated by placenta praevia: what is appropriate management? *Br J Obstet Gynaecol* 1996;**103**:864–7
75 Mouer, J.R. Placenta previa: antepartum conservative management, inpatient versus outpatient. *Am J Obstet Gynecol* 1994;**170**:1683–6
76 Rosen, D.M.B., Peek, M.J. Do women with placenta praevia without antepartum haemorrhage require hospitalisation? *Aust N Z J Obstet Gynaecol* 1994;**34**:130–4

2

The influence of folate catabolism on the dietary requirement for folate in pregnancy

John R.J. Higgins

Based on the Royal College of Obstetricians and Gynaecologists William Blair-Bell Memorial lecture, given at the Belfast Waterfront Hall on 25 May 1999.

INTRODUCTION

William Blair-Bell was the founding president of the Royal College of Obstetricians and Gynaecologists. From very early in his career he appears to have had an almost visionary zeal to develop and improve the specialty of obstetrics and gynaecology. Unlike most visionaries, he had the personal energy, the drive and the steely determination to fulfil his ambitions. This chapter, dedicated to his memory, discusses the important role that the vitamin folate plays in human pregnancy, with particular reference to our efforts at the Rotunda Hospital in Dublin to accurately calculate the increased dietary requirement for folate during pregnancy.

Over the 1990s, there has been an explosion of research interest in folate and its metabolism. This interest in folate spans many disciplines including nutrition, cardiology, vascular biology, haematology and obstetrics. Like an ancient elixir, folate appears to cure all ills. Folate is a water-soluble B vitamin, the major dietary sources of which are green leafy vegetables, liver, kidney, asparagus and legumes. It has a complex chemical structure consisting of a pteridine group linked to an aminobenzoic group which is, in turn, linked to a variable number of glutamate side chains (Figure 1). It is important to note that naturally occurring folate is a polyglutamate, whereas folic

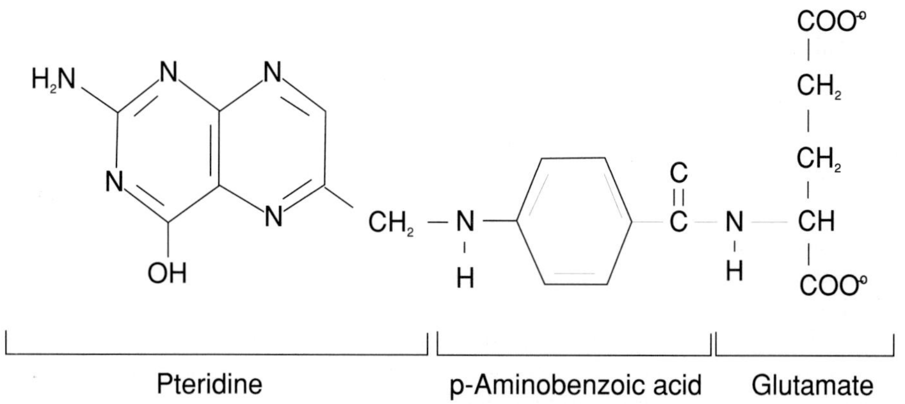

Figure 1 *The biochemical structure of folate*

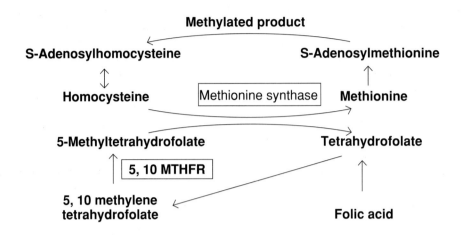

Figure 2 *A schematic representation of folate metabolism*

acid, the synthetic form, is a monoglutamate. Compared with folate, folic acid has significantly greater bioavailability.[1] Folate is involved in two key interlocked biochemical cycles (Figure 2). The first of these involves the conversion of tetrahydrofolate (THF) to 5,10-methylene THF and then to 5-methyl THF. This latter conversion is catalysed by the enzyme methylenetetrahydrofolate reductase (MTHFR). This enzyme is critical to allowing adequate production of 5-methyl THF. In turn, it can be acted upon by the enzyme methionine synthase to be converted to THF with the methyl group being transferred to homocysteine, which is thus converted to methionine. The interconversions of this cycle are linked to DNA biosynthesis (guanine, adenine and thymine). Methionine can then enter the methylation cycle, being initially converted to S-adenosylmethionine, which is a reactive methyl-group donor. The methylation cycle is involved in the methylation of a large range of substances including proteins, lipids, DNA and RNA.[2]

FOLATE AND PREGNANCY – AN HISTORICAL PERSPECTIVE

Almost 70 years ago, Wills reported from Bombay that she had successfully treated macrocytic anaemia of pregnancy with yeast extract.[3] The treatment was administered in the form of one drachm of Marmite taken two to four times a day. Later, the active agent was found to be the vitamin folate. Hibbard, in the 1964 Blair-Bell Memorial Lecture, suggested a more widespread role for folate in pregnancy.[4] He observed that, in addition to maternal anaemia, there were important associations between folate deficiency and placental abruption, miscarriage and fetal malformation. The main focus of his paper was the relationship between folate deficiency and placental abruption. He reported that of 163 patients who were found to have megaloblastic erythropoiesis antenatally, 8% subsequently developed placental abruption compared with the hospital incidence of 1.3%. While these observations had been supported by the earlier work of Hourihane et al.,[5] subsequent research did not appear to confirm these findings. In particular, Hall[6] performed a large prospective trial of routine folic acid supplementation compared with no treatment and found that folic acid therapy did not reduce the incidence of placental abruption. Hall also observed no association between low maternal folate levels and placental abruption either in the index pregnancy or in previous pregnancies.

However, in assessing the potential benefits of folic acid supplementation during pregnancy, it is difficult to allow completely for differences between study populations. Hibbard's subjects were mainly recruited from some of the most socially deprived areas of Liverpool. As he put it, 'This population was poor financially, poor gastronomically and poor obstetrically'. This difficulty is further illustrated when reviewing the relationship between maternal folate intake or status and birth weight. Scholl et al.[7] found that the adjusted odds ratios for having a low-birth-weight infant was 3.56 in mothers taking over 400 μg per day of folate compared with a group of mothers with a folate intake of less than 240 μg per day. Tamura et al.[8] found that maternal serum folate concentration at 30 weeks of gestation correlated positively with birth weight. The most recent Cochrane review[9] on the effect of routine folic acid supplementation in pregnancy observed that the reduction in the number of low-birth-weight infants did not reach statistical significance. The largest study[10] included in their analysis was performed on an Australian population likely to be folate replete. In contrast, Baumslag et al.[11] assessed the benefit of folic acid supplementation in a pregnant Bantu population compared with a white South African population and showed that supplementation in Bantu 'was associated with a significant reduction in the incidence of prematurity (birth weight). No such effect could be demonstrated in white patients subsisting on an average western diet'.[11]

FOLATE AND NEURAL-TUBE DEFECTS

While Hibbard's work[4] on placental abruption has been challenged, his assertion that folate deficiency and defective folate metabolism are responsible for a certain number of abortions and fetal malformations has proved prophetic. In 1976, Smithells et al.[12] reported that women who had a child affected with a neural-tube defect (NTD) had significantly lower folate levels than control mothers. Following on from this observation, several small clinical trials reported a significant protective effect of periconceptual maternal folic acid supplementation in preventing the recurrence of NTDs. To assess this issue definitively, the Medical Research Council undertook a randomised, double-blind, multicentre prevention trial.[13] A group of 1817 women who previously had a pregnancy affected by an NTD were randomly allocated to receive either folic acid (4 mg), other vitamins, both folic acid and other vitamins or neither folic acid or other vitamins. Folic acid was taken for at least one month before conception up to the twelfth week of pregnancy. Six NTDs occurred in the folic acid groups and 21 in the two other groups. Thus, there was a 72% protective effect (relative risk 0.28; 95% CI 0.12–0.71). Czeizel and Dudas[14] assessed the benefit of periconceptual folic acid supplementation in preventing the occurrence of NTDs. A total of 4753 women who were planning pregnancy were randomised to receive either a multivitamin supplement containing 0.8 mg of folic acid or a trace-element supplement (copper, manganese, zinc, vitamin C). None of the women who had been randomised to receive folic acid and other vitamins had a pregnancy complicated by an NTD. There were six cases of NTD in the control group ($P = 0.03$). These two benchmark papers form the basis of public-health policies on periconceptual folic acid supplementation in most developed countries.

DEFECTS IN FOLATE METABOLISM AND NTD

Kirke et al.[15] recruited more than 56 000 gravidae from three Dublin maternity hospitals to have blood samples taken and stored on their first antenatal visit. Subsequent analysis of those mothers, who had pregnancies complicated by an NTD, showed significantly lower levels of plasma folate in mothers whose pregnancies were complicated by an NTD compared with controls. However, most cases of NTDs occurred in women with folate levels in the normal range. Research from the same group has further defined the levels of maternal folate required to give reasonable protection from NTDs. There appears to be a continuous inverse relationship across the full normal range between maternal red-cell folate levels and the risk of having a child with an NTD. First-trimester maternal red-cell folate levels of greater than 400 μg per litre are associated with an eight-times less risk of having a child affected by an NTD compared with maternal levels of less than 150 μg per litre.[16] These studies also observed that maternal serum B_{12} levels were an additional independent risk factor for the development of NTDs. This observation is important because it suggests that methionine synthase (the only known enzyme which requires both folate and B_{12} for normal function) could be an important enzymatic defect linking abnormal folate metabolism with NTDs. Methionine synthase (Figure 2) catalyses the conversion of homocysteine to methionine. A defect in methionine synthase activity could lead to an accumulation of homocysteine.

HOMOCYSTEINE – A TOXIC METABOLITE

Steegers-Theunissen et al.[17] reported that women who had given birth to infants with an NTD had significantly higher fasting plasma homocysteine concentrations compared with controls. Mothers of babies with NTDs also appear to have higher blood levels of homocysteine during pregnancy compared with control women.[18] When homocysteine levels were stratified for B_{12} levels, those women with B_{12} levels below the median (even allowing for folate) still had higher homocysteine levels, suggesting that an abnormality in homocysteine metabolism may contribute to the increased risk of NTDs.

The most common enzyme defect leading to increased levels of homocysteine is homozygosity for the mutation of cytosine to thymidine at nucleotide 667 in the gene encoding for MTHFR (the 'thermolabile variant'). This genetic defect occurs in approximately 12% of the Caucasian population.[19] Whitehead et al.[20] reported that the frequency of homozygosity for this abnormal thermolabile form of MTHFR among subjects with NTDs was 18.3%, whereas the rate in the their control population was 6.1% ($P = 0.01$) giving an odds ratio of 3.5 (95% CI 1.3–9.4). This was the first specific genetic defect associated with NTDs to be identified and the authors estimated that it would account for approximately 13% of NTDs if the findings were extrapolated to the population in general. Similar findings were observed by Van der Put et al.,[21] who studied the frequency of homozygosity for the thermolabile variant of MTHFR in both patients with spina bifida and in their parents. The calculated odds ratio for the homozygous mutation was 2.7 (95% CI 1.0–7.9) for the patients, 3.7 (95% CI 1.5–9.1) for the mothers and 2.2 (95% CI 0.8–6.3) for the fathers compared with controls.

The clinical importance of abnormal homocysteine metabolism and, indeed, defects in the MTHFR enzyme has not been confined to pregnancy. Hyperhomocysteinaemia is now accepted as a common independent risk factor for cardiovascular disease. In the Framingham study,[22] more than 50% of subjects over 65 years of age had raised homocysteine levels. In a Swedish study,[23] 40% of middle-aged and elderly adults had raised homocysteine levels. Many studies have reported that patients with various forms of atheromatous disease, including cardiovascular disease, stroke and peripheral vascular disease, have significantly increased levels of homocysteine compared with controls. These associations may be mediated by toxic effects of homocysteine on the endothelium leading to impaired nitric oxide-mediated vasodilatation, increased endothelial factor V activity and altered thrombomodulin expression.[24] The relationship between homozygosity for the thermolabile variant of MTHFR enzyme, homocysteine and folate levels is now being better defined. Homozygous carriers of this mutation appear only to develop increased homocysteine levels in the presence of folate deficiency.[25]

THROMBOPHILIAS, HOMOCYSTEINE, MTHFR AND PREGNANCY

The toxic effects of increased levels of homocysteine on the endothelium are thrombogenic and, not surprisingly, hyperhomocysteinaemia appears to increase the risk of venous thromboembolism. This defect is now considered part of that group of inherited conditions associated with increased risk of developing thromboembolism collectively referred to as the inherited thrombophilias. The significance of the inherited thrombophilias for obstetric care extends well beyond an increased risk for venous thromboembolism. As with the other inherited thrombophilias, defects in homocysteine metabolism have recently been reported to be associated with a number of important obstetric complications. Dekker et al.[26] reported that 18% of women with a history of severe early-onset pre-eclampsia (tested after pregnancy) had hyperhomocysteinaemia, compared with the control population rate of 2–3%. Nelen et al.[27] reported that 16% of women with recurrent miscarriage were homozygous for the thermolabile variant of MTHFR compared with a control group incidence of 5%, giving an odds ratio of 3.3 (95% CI 1.3–10.1). In a widely quoted paper, Kupferminc et al.[28] reported a case–control study comparing 110 consecutive women who presented to their hospital with pregnancies complicated by either severe pre-eclampsia, severe fetal growth restriction, stillbirth or placental abruption. They found that 22% of these women were homozygous for the thermolabile MTHFR defect compared with 8% of the control population ($P = 0.005$), odds ratio 3.7 (95% CI 1.5–9.0). The suggested common pathophysiological pathway linking these different obstetric complications with hyperhomocysteinaemia is microthrombi deposition within the uteroplacental circulation. However, examination of placental pathology in pregnancies complicated by maternal hyperhomocysteinaemia has revealed changes that are quite nonspecific and inconsistent.[29]

In nonpregnant populations several major intervention trials are under way to assess the benefit of correcting raised homocysteine levels with folic acid supplementation. Recently, Leeda et al.[30] reported that 27 women with a past history of fetal growth restriction or pre-eclampsia were shown to have hyperhomocysteinaemia and were treated with folic acid supplements. All 27 women had normal homocysteine levels after folic acid supplementation. This raises the important question as to whether women with significant obstetric complications who are found to have a raised level of homocysteine will have improved obstetric outcome if they are subsequently treated with folic acid supplements.

DIETARY REQUIREMENT FOR FOLATE

In spite of the vital role that folate plays during pregnancy a fundamental piece of information remains unknown – how much extra dietary folate is required during normal pregnancy? The recommended dietary allowance (RDA) for folate is still based on crude estimates of the effects of differing levels of folate supplementation on populations with folate deficiency. This imprecision is reflected in the wide variation in the dietary recommendations for folate of the different regulatory bodies. The current recommendations in the UK for nonpregnant and pregnant women are 200 μg and 300 μg,[31] from the World Health Organization, 170 μg and 370–470 μg[32] and in the USA, 400 μg and 600 μg,[33] respectively. The increased folate requirement cannot be explained by transfer to the fetoplacental unit as the total calculated folate content at term would only approximate to 800 μg, which is an equivalent maternal additional requirement of less than 5 μg per day.[34]

The early observations by Jukes, in 1947,[35] demonstrated that folate excretion is much less than folate intake. This suggests that folate must undergo some regular catabolic process. Fleming[36] reported a similar finding in pregnancy. Measurement of the rate of catabolism should provide an estimation of the daily requirement. Early animal studies suggested that folate catabolism occurred in mammals as a result of cleavage of the C9–N10 bond producing para-aminobenzoylglutamate (pABGlu) and its acetamido derivative (apABGlu) as well as a mixture of folate-derived pteridines.[37] Krumdieck et al.[38] reported detecting radio-labelled pterin and isoxanthopterin in the urine of human volunteers several weeks after administration of [2–^{14}C]folate, an observation consistent with a C9–N10 cleavage. The description by McPartlin et al., in 1992,[39] of an accurate quantitative assay of folate catabolites in human urine meant that it was now possible to estimate the RDA of folate. Using this technique, we performed a pilot study of folate catabolism in normal pregnancy. Six healthy gravidae had their fluid catabolism assessed once in each trimester and postpartum. Folate catabolism was significantly increased in the second trimester as compared with the first trimester ($P = 0.003$) or postpartum ($P = 0.03$). The rate of folate catabolism in the third trimester was significantly greater than the first trimester or postpartum but was less than excretion in the second trimester ($P = 0.04$). The limitations of this study were that the small numbers made accurate quantitative recommendations difficult, the nonpregnant control group was not taking folic acid and there was a wide spread of gestations within the groups. We undertook a much larger study[40] to measure the rate of folate catabolism throughout pregnancy and in a nonpregnant control group, and thereby to derive the RDA for folate for pregnant and nonpregnant women.

Twenty-four healthy gravidae, recruited from the antenatal clinic of the Rotunda Hospital in Dublin, were followed during pregnancy and compared with 25 healthy nonpregnant controls. The pregnant group was admitted to a specially supervised metabolic ward once in each trimester and on day three postpartum. At 1700 hours on the day of admission their normal diet was replaced with a nutritionally complete, catabolite-free liquid enteral feed (Fortisip®, Cow and Gate). A 24-hour urine collection was commenced at 9 a.m. on day two and the patients were discharged on the morning of day three when this had been completed. The first 16 hours of each admission was a wash-out period to ensure that any folate catabolites excreted in the urine were not due to dietary ingestion but rather due to catabolism of endogenous folate. Owing to our policy of routine supplementation with iron and folic acid (500 µg) during pregnancy, the nonpregnant control group had their rate of folic metabolism measured twice, before and after four months of the same iron/folate supplementation. Urinary apABGlu and pABGlu were measured by high-pressure liquid chromatography. Urinary folate levels were measured by microbiological methods. A detailed dietary assessment performed by a dietician showed that there were no significant differences in folate intake between the control and the pregnancy group.

The daily rate of folate catabolism is calculated on the basis that the catabolites are approximately half the molecular weight of folate. Thus, by doubling the amount of apABGlu and pABGlu excreted and adding the small amount of urinary folate, excreted unchanged, the total rate of catabolism can be calculated in folate equivalents. The mean dietary requirement is then calculated on the generally held assumption that dietary folate is approximately 50% available. The RDA, by convention, is taken as being two standard deviations above the mean. The RDA is, therefore, the average daily intake level that is sufficient to meet the nutrient requirement of nearly all (97–98%) healthy individuals in the population (Table 1).

Table 1 *Explanation for calculating the recommended dietary allowance (RDA)*

Allowance	Definition
Estimated average requirement (EAR)	A nutrient value that is estimated to meet the requirements of half the healthy individuals in a group. It is used to assess adequacy of intakes of population groups and, along with knowledge of the distribution of requirements, to develop RDAs
Recommended dietary allowance (RDA)	The average daily dietary intake level that is sufficient to meet the nutrient requirement of nearly all (97-98%) healthy individuals in a group

If the standard deviation (SD) of the EAR is available, the RDA is set at two SDs above the EAR; $RDA = EAR + 2SD_{EAR}$

Table 2 *Recommended dietary allowances for folate*

Group	Folate intake (μg per day)
Nonpregnant	
Pre-supplementation	250
After supplementation	320
Pregnant	
1st trimester	340
2nd trimester	430
3rd trimester	540
Postpartum	380

The estimated rate of folate catabolism was significantly higher in the third trimester than in the first trimester ($P<0.001$), second trimester ($P<0.03$) or postpartum ($P<0.001$) (Figure 3). In the control group, supplementation significantly increased levels of red-cell folate ($P<0.001$) and serum folate ($P=0.001$) and also increased the mean rate of catabolism ($P=0.002$). RDAs for folate derived from these results are shown in Table 2. The changes in RDA in the control group after supplementation suggest that the effects of supplementation may also have confounded our estimation of catabolism in pregnancy but this is unlikely to be of clinical significance. The increase in calculated RDA in the control group after supplementation was only 70 μg (14% of the 500 μg supplement taken). There are several reasons for suspecting that the effect of supplementation measured in the nonpregnant control group represents a maximum value for the effect of supplementation in the pregnancy group. Firstly, as the requirement in the pregnancy group increased, the imbalance between the total folate intake and folate requirement fell. Secondly, unlike the findings in the nonpregnant control group, levels of red-cell folate and serum folate did not change significantly during pregnancy. Thirdly, despite continued supplementation, there was a profound and precipitous drop in folate catabolism on delivery.

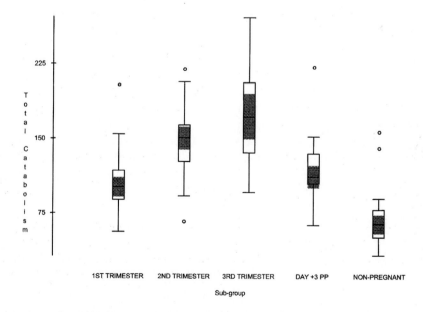

Figure 3 *Mean total rate of folate catabolism during pregnancy and postpartum and in nonpregnant control group in folate equivalents (mg per day); bars are 95th and 5th centiles, boxes the interquartile ranges; the mid-line bar represents the median and the stipple the 95% CI around the median; PP = postpartum*

SUMMARY

In summary, there is a growing body of observational data linking abnormalities in folate metabolism to poor pregnancy outcome. Folic acid supplementation may, therefore, impact potentially on a wide range of obstetric complications such as fetal growth restriction, pre-eclampsia, placental abruption and stillbirth. This chapter demonstrates that the increased requirement for folate in pregnancy is due to increased folate catabolism. The accurate calculation of the increased dietary requirement for folate during pregnancy provides the foundation upon which policies of folic acid supplementation should be built.

Acknowledgements

I would like to thank Dr Michael Darling, Rotunda Hospital (project director), our research colleagues from Trinity College Dublin – Eoin Quinlivan, Dr Joseph McPartlin, Professor John Scott and Professor Donald Weir. I acknowledge the generosity and fortitude of the women who took part in the study and the assistance of research midwife Anna O'Sullivan. The Wellcome Trust and the Friends of the Rotunda provided financial support for this research.

References

1. Gregory, J.F. The bioavailability of folate. In: Bailey, L.B., editor. *Folate in Health and Disease.* New York: Marcel Dekker; 1995. p. 195–235
2. Jaenisch, R., Jahner, D. Methylation, expression and chromosomal position of genes in mammals. *Biochim Biophys Acta* 1984;**782**:1–9
3. Wills, L. Treatment of 'pernicious anaemia of pregnancy' and 'tropical anaemia' with special reference to yeast extract as curative agent. *BMJ* 1931;**i**:1059–64
4. Hibbard, B.M. The role of folic acid in pregnancy with particular reference to anaemia, abruption and abortion. *J Obstet Gynaecol Br Cwlth* 1964;**71**:529–42
5. Hourihane, B., Doyle, C.V., Drury, M.I. Megaloblastic anaemia of pregnancy. *Journal of the Irish Medical Association* 1960;**47**:1–6.
6. Hall, M.H. Folic acid deficiency and abruptio placentae *J Obstet Gynaecol Br Cwlth* 1972;**79**:222–5
7. Scholl, T.O., Hediger, M.L., Schall, J.L., Khoo, C.S., Fischer, R.L. Dietary and serum folate: their influence on outcome of pregnancy. *Am J Clin Nutr* 1996;**63**:520–5
8. Tamura, T., Goldenberg, R.L., Freeberg, L.E., Cliver, S.P., Cutter, G.R., Hoffman, H.J. Maternal serum folate and zinc concentrations and their relationships to pregnancy outcome. *Am J Clin Nutr* 1992;**56**:365–70
9. Mahomed, K. Routine folate supplementation in pregnancy (Cochrane Review). *The Cochrane Library*, Issue 4, Oxford: Update Software; 1998
10. Giles, P.F., Harcourt, A.G., Whiteside, M.G. The effect of prescribing folic acid during pregnancy on birth weight and duration of pregnancy: a double-blind study. *Med J Aust* 1971;**2**:17–21
11. Baumslag, N., Edelstein, T., Metz, J. Reduction of incidence of prematurity by folic acid supplementation in pregnancy *BMJ* 1970;**i**:16–17
12. Smithells, R.W., Sheppard, S., Schorach C.J. Vitamin deficiencies and neural tube defects. *Arch Dis Child* 1976;**51**:944–50
13. MRC Vitamin Study Research Group. Prevention of neural tube defects: results of the

Medical Research Council Vitamin Study. *Lancet* 1991;**338**:131–7
14 Czeizel, A.E., Dudas, I. Prevention of the first occurrence of neural-tube defects by periconceptual vitamin supplementation. *N Engl J Med* 1992;**327**:1832–5
15 Kirke, P.N., Molloy, A.M., Daly L.E., Burke, H., Weir, D.G., Scott, J.M. Maternal plasma folate and vitamin B-12 are independent risk factors for neural tube defects. *QJM* 1993;**86**:703–8
16 Daly, L.E., Kirke, P.N., Molloy, A., Weir, D.G., Scott, J.M. Folate levels and neural tube defects. *JAMA* 1995;**247**:1698–702
17 Steegers-Theunissen, R.P., Boers, G.H., Trijbels, F.J., Finkelstein, J.D., Blom, H.J., Thomas, C.M. *et al*. Maternal hyperhomocysteinemia: a risk factor for neural tube defects? *Metabolism* 1994;**43**:1475–80
18 Mills, J.L., McPartlin, J.M., Kirke, P.N., Lee, Y.J., Conley, M.R., Weir, D.G. *et al*. Homocysteine metabolism in pregnancies complicated by neural-tube defects. *Lancet* 1995;**345**:149–51
19 Frosst, P., Blom, H.J., Milos, R., Goyette, P., Sheppard, C.A., Matthews, R.G. *et al*. A candidate risk factor for cardiovascular disease: a common mutation in methylenetetrahydrofolate reductase. *Nat Genet* 1995;**10**:111–13
20 Whitehead, A.S., Gallagher, P., Mills, J.L., Kirke, P.N., Burke, H., Molloy, A.M. *et al*. A genetic defect in 5, 10 methylenetetrahydrofolate reductase in neural tube defects. *QJM* 1995;**88**:763–6
21 Van der Put, N.M.J., Steegers-Theunissen, R.P.M., Frosst, P., Trijbels, F.J., Eskes, T.K., van den Heuvel, L.P. *et al*. Mutated methylenetetrahydrofolate reductase as a risk factor for spina bifida. *Lancet* 1995;**346**:1070–1
22 Selhub, J., Jacques, P.F., Wilson, P.W.F., Rush, D., Rosenberg, I.H. Vitamin status and intake as primary determinants of homocysteinemia in an elderly population. *JAMA* 1993;**270**:2693–8
23 Brattstrom, L., Lindgren, A., Israelsson, B., Andersson, A., Hultberg, B. Homocysteine and cysteine: determinants of plasma levels in middle-aged and elderly subjects. *J Intern Med* 1994;**236**:633–41
24 De Stefano, V., Finazzi, G., Mannucci, P.M. Inherited thrombophilia: pathogenesis, clinical syndromes, and management. *Blood* 1996;**87**:3531–44
25 Jacques, P.F., Bostom, A.G., Williams, R.R., Ellison, R.C., Eckfeldt, J.H., Rosenberg, I.H. *et al*. Relation between folate status, a common mutation in methylenetetrahydrofolate reductase, and plasma homocysteine concentrations. *Circulation* 1996;**93**:7–9
26 Dekker, G.A., deVries, J.I., Doelitzsch, P.M., Huijgens, P.C., von Blomberg, B.M., Jakobs, C. *et al*. Underlying disorders associated with severe early-onset pre-eclampsia. *Am J Obstet Gynecol* 1995;**173**:1042–8
27 Nelen, W.L., Steegers, E.A., Eskes, T.K., Blom H.J. Genetic risk factor for unexplained recurrent early pregnancy loss. *Lancet* 1997;**350**:861
28 Kupferminc, M.J., Eldor, A., Steinman, N., Many, A., Bar-Am, A., Jaffa, A. *et al*. Increased frequency of genetic thrombophilia in women with complications of pregnancy. *N Engl J Med* 1999;**340**:9–13
29 Khong, T.Y., Hague, W.M. The placenta in maternal hyperhomocysteinaemia. *Br J Obstet Gynaecol* 1999;**106**:273–8
30 Leeda, M., Riyazi, N., de Vries, J.I., Jakobs, C., van Geijn, H.P., Dekker, G.A. Effects of folic acid and vitamin B6 supplementation on women with hyperhomocysteinemia and a history of preeclampsia or fetal growth restriction. *Am J Obstet Gynecol* 1998;**179**:135–9
31 COMA. *Dietary Reference Values for Food, Energy and Nutrients for the United Kingdom*. London: HMSO; 1991 (Report No. 41)
32 Food and Agricultural Organization of the United Nations. *Requirements of Vitamin A, Iron Folate and Vitamin B12*. Rome; 1988

33   Food and Nutrition Board, Institute of Medicine, National Academy of Sciences. *Dietary Reference Intakes: Folate, Other B Vitamins and Choline.* Washington DC; 1998
34   Iyengar, L., Apte, S.V. Nutrient stores in human fetal livers *Br J Nutr* 1972;**27**:313–17
35   Jukes, T.H., Franklin, A.L., Stokstad, E.L.R., Boehne, J.W. The urinary excretion of pteroylglutamic acid and certain related compounds. *J Lab Clin Med* 1947;**32**:1350–5
36   Fleming, A.F. Urinary excretion of folates in pregnancy. *Br J Nutr* 1972;**79**:916–920.
37   Murphy, M., Keating, P., Boyle, P., Weir, D.G., Scot, J.M. The elucidation of the mechanism of folate catabolism in the rat. *Biochem Biophys Res Commun* 1976;**71**:1017–24
38   Krumdieck, C.L., Fukushima, T., Shiota, T., Butterworth, C.E. A long-term study of the excretion of folate and pterins in a human subject after injection of 14C-folic, with observations on the effect of diphenlyhydantoin. *Am J Clin Nutr* 1978;**31**:88–93
39   McPartlin, J., Courtney, G., McNulty, H., Weir, D.G., Scott, J.M. The quantitative analysis of endogenous catabolites in human urine. *Anal Biochem* 1992;**206**:256–61
40   McPartlin, J., Halligan, A., Scott, J.M., Darling, M., Weir, D.G. Accelerated folate breakdown in pregnancy. *Lancet* 1993;**341**:148–9
41   Higgins, J.R., Quinlivan, E., McPartlin, J., Scott, J.M., Weir, D.G., Darling, M.R.N. The relationship between increased folate catabolism and the increased requirement for folate in pregnancy. *BJOG* 2000;**107**:1149–54

3

Looking backwards: a gynaecologist's view of the anorectum

Christopher N. Hudson

Based on the William Meredith Fletcher Shaw Memorial Lecture, given on 26 May 1999 at the Belfast Waterfront Hall.

After gynaecology broke away from general surgery and joined with obstetrics it was the only specialty to take a specific interest in the female pelvis. The non-gynaecological pelvic compartments were within the province of general surgery, albeit with local special interests. When urology began to develop as a specialty, its focus was on the male; prostatic disease is exclusively male and it happens that bladder cancer is rare in females. Incontinence remained within the realm of the gynaecologist. In the posterior compartment, rectal cancer was managed by combined excision with permanent colostomy and rectal prolapse by rectosigmoidectomy. Faecal incontinence was nobody's special interest, except for those gynaecologists who had been responsible for perineal reconstruction following damage during childbirth, including complete division of the perineal body involving the anal sphincters. The perineal conditions treated by general surgeons included ischiorectal abscess, haemorrhoids and fistula-in-ano.

In the 1950s, urology emerged as a definite subspecialty rather than merely a special interest. It was then that urologists began to develop an interest in female incontinence. In 1969 at St Bartholomew's Hospital, London, Brown and Wickham pioneered electronic urethral pressure measurement.[1] It was in response to increasing sophistication and interest in this area that urogynaecology came to be recognised as a subspecialty within our discipline. World-wide, gynaecologists have held, and continue to hold, centre stage in the management of urogenital fistula of childbirth origin. Lack of opportunity in the developed world means that subspecialists in urogynaecology need specific experience and training in this field. It is equally true that, although locally trained urologists have useful expertise, they may lack the versatility and experience of transvaginal surgery.

The development of subspecialty interest in the posterior pelvic compartment has been somewhat different. The abdomen remains one of the last bastions of general surgery and, within it, compartmentalisation has been slow to develop. St Mark's Hospital, Harrow, Middlesex, has long been the 'Mecca' of colorectal surgeons and, until quite recently, all St Mark's surgeons had, indeed were required to have, a general surgical appointment elsewhere. It was, however, one of the great part-time subspecialty surgeons of St Mark's, the late Sir Alan Parks, who pioneered the study of faecal incontinence, a problem long neglected by gynaecologists, in spite of female predominance of the symptom. Faecal incontinence is a secret problem not volunteered in history nor sought out by interrogation. It has, however, emerged as an area of common interest to both our specialties now that occult obstetric injury to the anal sphincters has been recognised as a clinical entity.

The writer's personal interest in the proctological fringe of gynaecology came after training in general surgery and a serendipitous encounter with the gynaecological manifestations of Crohn's disease.[2] Because of the transmural nature of the inflammatory process and ulceration in regional enteritis, Crohn's disease has a particular propensity for intestinal adhesion to other viscera and, hence, to fistula formation. The overall fistula rate is of the order of 40% and the genital tract is involved in 7% of female cases. Diagnostic confusion in this condition is surprisingly common.

Figure 1 shows barium studies in a case of terminal regional ileitis for which the sole presenting symptom was green vaginal discharge. The cause was a small ileovaginal fistula in the posterior fornix, overlooked on various occasions on vaginal examination. The lack of obvious and specific symptoms of an alimentary nature in some cases of Crohn's disease is the basis of the diagnostic confusion. It is also a minefield for the surgically unwary. Even operating in the vicinity of diseased bowel without any apparent direct injury can result in fistula formation. In a subsequent study of inflammatory bowel fistula at St Mark's Hospital, it became apparent that the occurrence of a totally unexpected intestinal fistula following gynaecological surgery should at least raise the possibility that there may have been associated, but undiscovered, Crohn's disease. The Crohn's inflammatory process can involve the female genital tract by direct extension, notably to the fallopian tubes and the vulva.

Fistula is obviously a major feature of the proctological-gynaecological interface. Some data from University College Hospital Ibadan, in Nigeria, from the unit headed by John Lawson and Paul Hendrickse, are pertinent. Ibadan was a tertiary referral unit for fistula in West Africa and nearly all of those seen were of obstetric origin. Among these, rectal fistulae were only about one tenth as common as urinary fistulae. Many were low fistulae commonly associated with an incompletely healed perineal tear and, as such, associated with anal sphincter division and separation. These are almost certainly under-represented, as, in an unsophisticated community, this injury is of limited social disability. There was, however, a minority group of high-fistula cases that were compression slough injuries just like the obstetric vesicovaginal fistulae with which they are almost always associated. A high fistula presents a formidable surgical challenge whether treated by

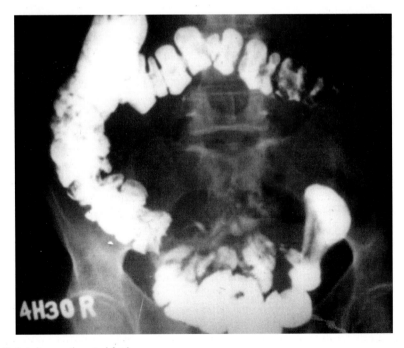

Figure 1 *Crohn's disease – ileovaginal fistula*

the vaginal route or abdominally. Lawson himself made an important original contribution by the technique of transabdominal repair associated with subtotal hysterectomy and median split of the cervix to expose the posterior fornix.[3]

A retrospective review of the data concerning Ibadan rectal fistulae provided an audit on faecal diversion by colostomy before rectovaginal fistula repair.[4] This review was not randomised nor stratified but, *prima facie*, there was no obvious difference in the success rate for fistula closure. However, it was an 'article of faith' that major fistula repair should be covered by a diverting preliminary colostomy and repaired in three stages. When, however, the audit was extended to closure of concomitant urinary fistula with or without prior faecal diversion, there was an apparent difference, but this, of course, has not been tested in an evidential manner. Lawson himself was opposed to simultaneous repair of double fistulae on the grounds that the main problem when there has been tissue loss is repair without tension, and simultaneous repairs may pull in opposite directions, except perhaps when the anal fistula is low and small. Others are more sanguine about double repair.

Successful closure of rectal fistulae depends upon the same principles that govern the management of vesicovaginal fistulae, namely removal of the epithelial-lined tract, excision of scar and other unhealthy tissue, closure without tension and, where possible, separation of adjacent suture lines. Non-reactive sutures are preferred to catgut, colorectal surgeons being more sanguine about non-absorbable suture material than gynaecologists. Certainly non-absorbable sutures in the vagina should always be removed. Closure may be difficult when there has been serious tissue loss from pressure necrosis and one of the most important measures for high fistula advocated by Mahfouz[5] was to open the pouch of Douglas and bring down peritoneal-covered bowel to close the fistula (Figure 2). It does not seem to matter that the vagina at the vault cannot be closed, as the exposed serosa will undergo squamous metaplasia.[6]

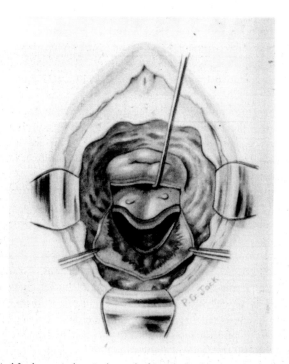

Figure 2 *High rectovaginal fistula – vaginal repair; the pouch of Douglas has been opened and peritoneal covered rectum brought down for closure*

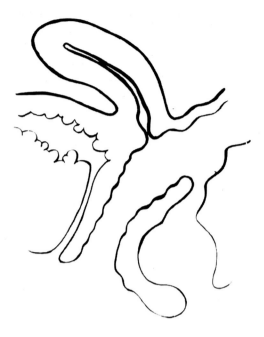

Figure 3 *High rectovaginal fistula – virtually complete segmental loss of rectum*

Anteriorly, the concept of circumferential or segmental urethrovesical loss (complete destruction of the bladder neck) is well recognised. A similar problem can occasionally be found in the posterior compartment. After segmental loss of the lower rectum, the anal canal terminates blindly and the proximal rectum discharges completely into the posterior fornix. In such cases an abdominoperineal approach is required with a colo-anal anastomosis (Figure 3).[7]

The desirability of separating suture lines in the adjacent viscera led to the development of the operation of colpocleisis, which involves denuding all or part of a cylinder of vagina.[8]

Upper partial colpocleisis denudes the vaginal vault and is commonly used for posthysterectomy fistula. A note of caution should be sounded when the fistula is intestinal because access to the vagina may have been through an intervening abscess cavity; it is important then that the bowel defect be identified and closed separately.

Lower partial colpocleisis, in which a distal cylinder of vaginal wall is removed, leaves a cavity at the vault that is effectively a diverticulum of the adjacent viscus. In cases where there is a double vaginal fistula this then becomes a vesicorectal fistula. This type of procedure is particularly suitable for post-irradiation fistula, especially if there is suspicion that disease activity may not have been controlled. Under these circumstances, the distal cylindrical dead space should be filled with a pedicle graft of non-irradiated tissue,[9] either a Martius bulbospongiosus fat pad graft or the gracilis muscle. Once again, it is important to identify the segment of bowel involved; if the intestinal aperture cannot be reached by digital rectal examination the fistula is likely to be colovaginal. In such a case, colpocleisis is likely to fail, as there is almost certainly an associated stricture. It is necessary then to fenestrate the anterior rectal wall into the upper compartment. Effectively, this makes an end-to-side anastomosis of the fistulated vagina into the mid-rectum.[6] Such a procedure needs to be considered as a serious alternative to colostomy for terminal palliation. Colostomy will do little to alleviate the discharge and aroma from necrotic tissue at the vaginal vault, nor does it help with the urinary fistula, which all too often is associated.

The next point of interest is the proctogynaecological interface along the posterior vaginal wall and the perineal body. There is an expanding and multidisciplinary interest in total pelvic floor deficiency. There are two points of anorectal interest to which gynaecological surgery can make a useful contribution. Rectal prolapse, or rectal procidentia, a process that is more common in women, begins as an intussusception at the fundus of a deep pouch of Douglas, the apex of which passes through the anus as a full-thickness rectal prolapse. There is, coincidentally, major inhibition of the pelvic floor muscles, as shown by Parks et al.,[10] associated with the chronic straining of constipation. This in turn leads to traction neuropathy involving the puborectalis, pubococcygeus and external anal sphincter muscles and so, to the problem of chronic constipation is added faecal incontinence. The deep pouch of Douglas may also protrude into the posterior vaginal fornix as a pulsion enterocele.[11] Thus, there is thus the occasional combination of genital and rectal prolapse, which may be synchronous or sequential (Figure 4). The problem for gynaecologists is to avoid overlooking this possibility; the importance of taking an adequate defecation history cannot be over-emphasised. Because rectal prolapse and vaginal pulsion enterocele have a common aetiological factor of deep pouch of Douglas, a properly executed full colpoperineorrhaphy[12] may prevent, at least for a while, the rectal intussusception by removing the redundant pouch of Douglas and plicating the prerectal fascia. Pubococcygeus (levator ani) approximation was at one time used in the abdominal treatment of rectal prolapse but is largely redundant now that rectopexy with a synthetic mesh wrap-round is used.[13] Puborectalis approximation can, however, help to support a defective external anal sphincter. The transvaginal approach is much less of a major undertaking in the frail, obese or elderly than is any form of abdominal rectopexy with prosthetic insertion. A recent addition to Shaw's procedure is to add an endo-anal sphincteroplasty to reduce the patulous anus and displace it posteriorly as part of the protective realignment.[14]

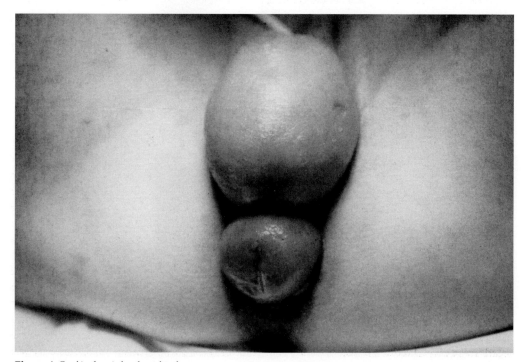

Figure 4 *Combined genital and rectal prolapse*

Somewhat similar considerations apply to the surgical correction of rectocele for defecatory symptoms rather than just for a complaint of genital prolapse. Mere reduction of gaping introitus by perineorrhaphy will not alleviate such symptoms and, after such an operation, an anorectal pouch can balloon down to the level of the perineal skin in front of an intact external anal sphincter. This sacculation, which can be responsible for incomplete defecation, is not visible on vaginal examination as a recognisable rectocele.

It was actually abdominal surgery for combined rectal and genital prolapse (rectopexy and sacrocolpopexy) that gave the idea for an extension to the hitherto standard approach to ovarian cancer. Rectal mobilisation in these prolapse cases succeeded in elevating the base of the pouch of Douglas to the level of the anterior abdominal wall (Figure 5). This manoeuvre also facilitates the clean removal of ovarian malignancy with local adherence or spread, on the working hypothesis that complete macroscopic removal must be better than subtotal debulking.[15]

The retroperitoneal operation for ovarian malignancy, also known as radical oophorectomy, has become accepted as part of the armamentarium of the gynaecological oncologist. In some cases, dissection in the muscle plane of the rectal wall is feasible but this is liable to lead to mucosal button-holing if extensive. Initially, simple wedge excision and repair was tried but, perhaps because of tension over the inversion of the 'dog's ears' at the end of the stitch line, there was an unacceptable leak rate. It was necessary to proceed to limited rectosigmoid resection and anastomosis in some 20% of cases in which there was intimate involvement of the bowel wall.[16] This is actually a relatively easy colorectal anastomosis carried out at the peritoneal reflection and may be contrasted with a difficult low anastomosis in the cramped inaccessible conditions of a male pelvis and without the mesenteric shortening or thickening associated with diverticular disease.

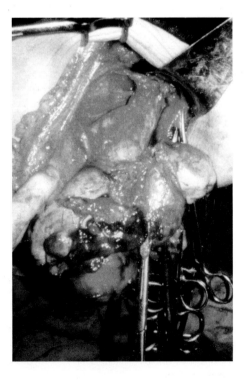

Figure 5 *Radical oophorectomy – elevation of the pouch of Douglas with the uterus and malignant ovarian cyst still adherent* in situ; *the uterus has been freed from the vagina in a retrograde manner*

Every gynaecologist operating on ovarian neoplasia must decide for themselves the extent of personal involvement in such procedures. There is a great temptation to use the term 'debulking' as an excuse to downgrade the completeness of pelvic surgery because of reluctance to cross tissue and organ boundaries. Perhaps clinical guidelines should suggest that a generalist gynaecological surgeon should biopsy, close and pass the patient with adherent or extended ovarian cancer to a gynaecological oncologist to perform a complete operation, rather than attempt to justify incomplete surgery in this way.

The important message for the generalist is that the potential for macroscopically complete surgery in ovarian cancer is actually determined in the upper abdomen. If extra-pelvic disease is completely resectable or reducible to residual disease no greater than 0.5 cm in diameter, then radical pelvic surgery is worthwhile. Such surgery would be made more difficult, even as an interval procedure, if hysterectomy and bilateral oophorectomy are carried out leaving visible pelvic disease. Colorectal surgeons and urologists both, on occasions, need to remove the uterus in the course of surgery for extensive pelvic malignancy arising in their respective fields. The need for a gynaecological oncologist to undertake equivalent adjacent tissue resections is beyond dispute.

Most recently, attention has been focused on the most distal segment of the anogenital passage. This concerns the perineal body, whose anatomy is both ill-understood and disputed, including the alterations brought about by childbirth. For many years there was a happy collaboration between St Marks Hospital and the gynaecological department at St Bartholomew's Hospital, London. Collaborative studies by serial dissection on fresh abdominoperineal rectal excisions have revised the anatomy as demonstrated by endo-anal ultrasound.[17] Damage to the anorectal continence mechanisms by vaginal delivery was well documented. Much of the damage is recoverable or compensatable.[18] However, in a small number of women early or late impairment of continence ensues. There has been some difficulty in quantitating the physical damage because of the anatomical fact that the anal sphincter in women is not a symmetrical cylinder but quite oblique with a much shorter anterior (vaginal) wall, which can lead to over-reporting of asymptomatic sphincter defects.

One of the surprising features was the demonstration of internal sphincter damage without a documented complete (third or fourth degree) perineal tear. Perineal damage at childbirth is usually thought of as being radial and on this basis it would be difficult to account for a torn internal sphincter without complete division of the external sphincter. Posterolateral episiotomy has been alleged to protect the anal sphincter by making the radial introital extension pass to one side. It is a common experience, however, that even a large posterolateral episiotomy will not prevent third degree anal sphincter tears.[19] Childbirth injury is clearly more complex. Less well recognised, and generally not taught to midwives, are circumferential tears of the introitus, which begin at 6 o'clock in the navicular fossa and extend laterally on each side around the vestibule. A third mechanism for childbirth genital trauma has been postulated. This is forcible posterior displacement of the anorectum and its sphincters at the level of the apex of the perineal body, thus tearing the attachment of the sphincter complex and rectum from the posterior free margin of the perineal membrane. The fibrous attachment of the posterior vaginal wall to the apex of the perineal body is familiar to gynaecological surgeons as the last structure to be divided in a posterior repair before entering the loose arcolar tissue of the rectovaginal space. Less obvious are the lateral arms of the perineal membrane, at this level attaching just off-centre to the perineal body and sphincter complex, overlaid by the superficial transverse perineal muscle, which itself decussates with part of the external anal sphincter. These bands may be seen on magnetic resonance imaging and validated by postmortem dissection.

A posterolateral episiotomy will only release the membranous attachment on one side, which would still permit contralateral tearing if there has been posterior displacement. May[20] described an episiotomy variant, which actually increased the available size of the introital space by 10%. It may also protect the anal sphincter mechanisms from the distraction injuries produced by posterior displacement. This variant is a short median episiotomy stopping well short of the anal sphincter, then converted subcutaneously into an inverted 'T' by two additional subcutaneous cuts of 1 cm, which will free the perineal body from its attachment to the perineal membrane. In view of the known risk of occult sphincter damage from midline episiotomy and forceps delivery,[21] there is the potential for a randomised clinical trial to compare this episiotomy with the traditional posterolateral episiotomy, validated with postnatal per-anal ultrasound.

Faecal incontinence is the most secret and occult of symptoms and it is a serious source of embarrassment to the sufferer. It is one of which gynaecologists have been largely ignorant and which they have certainly neglected over the years and to which our colorectal colleagues are now drawing due attention. We must learn from their contributions but must not abdicate our responsibilities as a specialty for the treatment of acute perineal injuries in childbirth. It is important to recognise that the management of chronic unhealed injuries requires different techniques and procedures from those used for repair in the acute situation in the delivery room. There is no doubt that the repair of significant perineal injury should not be left to midwives or junior trainees but should be dealt with by those with adequate training. It is doubtful whether the overlap technique for chronic anal sphincter injuries is also appropriate for the acute management of third- and fourth-degree tears. However, all obstetricians should be aware of the newer high-polymer suture materials in preference to catgut.

In summary, the common interface between the genital tract and the lower bowel has four important facets:

(1) Childbirth perineal injuries, both acute and chronic, which remain within the province of the obstetrician and gynaecologist;

(2) Pelvic floor weakness and herniation of the posterior compartments, to which the gynaecological surgeon can make a significant contribution, provided that surgery is individually tailored and not just a 'cook book' posterior repair;

(3) Genital fistula that is best dealt with according to the specialty concerned with the underlying pathology. Prudent gynaecologists should avoid responsibility for local inflammatory bowel disease but those who are trained and experienced can and should deal with obstetric and traumatic fistulae and perineal body injuries;

(4) Within specialist gynaecological oncology, the retroperitoneal approach to radical oophorectomy, with a periodic need for limited rectosigmoid resection, puts this operation outside the scope of the average general gynaecologist. The justification of locally incomplete and suboptimal pelvic clearance of ovarian cancer implied by misapplication of the term 'debulking' should be 'debunked'. Generalists operating on a locally fixed ovarian tumour, should stage, confirm the diagnosis and refer.

Gynaecological oncologists must be true and complete pelvic surgeons trained and capable of operating on and with the adjacent viscera.

CONCLUSION

In the USA, there is a prestigious multidisciplinary Society of Pelvic Surgeons. In New Zealand, an equivalent body is termed the Cloaca Club. In the UK, however, the importance of the posterior pelvic compartment interface has long been neglected. We do not have a specialty of proctogynaecology but, in view of the functional importance of the subject, perhaps we can all subscribe to the sentiments of the 'Ode to the Goddess Cloacina' (Victorian poem; Anon.):

> 'O Cloacina, Goddess of this place
> Look upon thy servant with a smiling face
> Soft and cohesive let my offering flow
> Not rudely swift nor obstinately slow'.

Acknowledgements

The author acknowledges a personal debt to his mentors John Howkins, Alec Badenoch, Ronald Canney, Ian Todd, John Lawson and Paul Hendrickse, and to colleagues at St Bartholomew's and St Mark's Hospitals in London.

References

1. Brown, M., Wickham, J. Urethral pressure profile. *Br J Urol* 1969;**42**:714–23
2. Hudson, C.N. Gynaecological manifestations of Crohn's disease. *J Obstet Gynaecol Br Cwlth* 1963;**70**:437–42
3. Lawson, J.B. Recto-vaginal fistula following difficult labour. *Proc R Soc Med* 1972;**65**:283–6
4. Hudson, C.N. Acquired fistulae between the intestine and the vagina. *Ann R Coll Surg Engl* 1970;**46**:20–40
5. Mahfouz, N. A new technique in dealing with superior recto-vaginal fistulae. *J Obstet Gynaecol Br Emp* 1934;**41**:579–65
6. Hudson, C.N. Recto-vaginal fistula. In: Fielding, L.P., Goldberg, S.M., editors. *Surgery of the Colon, Rectum and Anus (Rob and Smiths Operative Surgery)*. Oxford: Butterworth; 1993. p. 749–57
7. Bentley, R.J. Abdominal repair of high recto-vaginal fistula. *J Obstet Gynaecol Br Cwlth* 1973;**80**:364–7
8. Blaikley, J.B. Colpocleisis for difficult vaginal fistulae of bladder and rectum. *Proc R Soc Med* 1965;**58**:581–6
9. Lawson, J.B., Hudson, C.N. The management of vesico-vaginal and urethral fistulae. In: Stanton, S., Tanagho, E., editors. *Surgery of Female Incontinence*. Berlin: Springer Verlag; 1980. p. 162–3
10. Parks, A., Swash, M., Urich, M. Sphincter denervation in ano–rectal incontinence. *Gut* 1977;**18**:656–65
11. Zacharin, R.F. (1985) *Pelvic Floor Anatomy and the Surgery of Pulsion Enterocele*. Berlin: Springer Verlag; 1985
12. Shaw, W., O'Sullivan, J.J.F. A perineorrhaphy operation and its use in the treatment of enterocele and rectocele. *J Obstet Gynaecol Br Emp* 1951;**58**:920–5
13. Ripstein, C.B. Surgical care of massive rectal prolapse. *Dis Colon Rectum* 1965;**8**:34–8
14. Hudson, C.N. Female genital prolapse and pelvic floor deficiency. *Int J Colorectal Dis* 1988;**3**:181–5
15. Hudson, C.N. A radical operation for fixed ovarian tumours. *J Obstet Gynaecol Br Cwlth* 1968;**75**:1155–60
16. Hudson, C.N. Surgical treatment of ovarian cancer. *Gynecol Oncol* 1973;**1**:370–8

17. Sultan, A.H., Nichols, R.J., Kamm, M.A., Hudson, C.N., Beynon, J., Bartram, C.I. Anal endosonography and correlation with *in vitro* and *in ano* anatomy. *Br J Surg* 1993;**80**:508–11
18. Snooks, S.J., Swash, M., Henry, M.M., Setchell, M.E. Injury to pelvic floor sphincter musculature in childbirth. *Lancet* 1984;**ii**:546–50
19. Sultan, A.H., Kamm, M.A., Hudson, C.N., Bartram, C.I. Third degree obstetric anal sphincter tears, risk factors and outcome of primary repair. *BMJ* 1994;**308**:887–91
20. May, J.L. Modified median episiotomy minimizes the risk of third degree tears. *Obstet Gynecol* 1996;**83**:151–7
21. Signorello, L.B., Harlow, B.L., Charkos, A.K., Repke, J.T. Midline episiotomy and anal incontinence. *BMJ* 2000;**320**: 86–90

4

The consultant-based service

Patrick B. Forbes

INTRODUCTION

Imagine a National Health Service (NHS) unit where all significant medical care is provided personally by accredited consultants. A unit where 24-hour cover for the delivery suite and emergency gynaecology is provided by consultants who have no other clinical commitments during such cover, and where there is still a throughput of elective work which is on a par with comparably sized hospitals.

This would sound like an ideal arrangement for patients, a double-edged sword for managers and a nightmare for the consultants. However, such a unit exists in Huntingdon, Cambridgeshire, UK. The arrangement is by no means perfect, and this chapter describes its good and bad points, with suggestions as to how such an arrangement might fit into the NHS in the future.

HISTORY

In the 1980s, a decision was made to separate off the Huntingdonshire district from the then Cambridge Health Authority. With a local population of 140 000 and an historical identity, it seemed a reasonable attempt to make NHS care more local. Part of the scheme was a new, 'best-buy' district general hospital. At about this time, the Short report[1] was published, and the higher authority decided that it would be opportune to invest the new district general hospital with a staffing structure that would satisfy the principles of that report. The main thrust was that more care should be provided by consultants, and the message was taken to the extreme by ensuring that the new hospital would not have an intermediate-registrar tier.

In 1983, Hinchingbrooke Hospital opened its doors with, initially, two obstetric consultants and two senior house officers (SHOs). Originally, it was believed that local GPs would continue to provide obstetric cover, as they had for the now-closed GP maternity unit. However, the mix of consultant, GP and midwife was an uncomfortable one and the maternity department quickly settled down as a consultant unit. Gradually, the number of consultants rose to four, while the number of deliveries increased more rapidly than planned.

It soon became clear that women were coming to Hinchingbrooke from outside its catchment area and, by 1991, a third of the 2500 women who delivered at Hinchingbrooke came from outside the Huntingdon Health Authority area. In parallel, the paediatric service grew, and the hospital had three neonatal intensive care spaces and a full special-care-baby service. All degrees of obstetric risk were accepted, except those where some neonatal surgical intervention might be required. However, the perinatal mortality rate was among the lowest in the region, which itself had the lowest rate in the UK.

In the 1990s, several changes took place. The unit expanded to six consultants, with five SHOs. There was a gradual trend for other specialties to introduce a partial intermediate tier; some through compulsion (paediatrics) and some through desire (medicine, surgery). However, 24-hour anaesthetic cover for the maternity unit continued at consultant level.

Despite upheavals in the way the NHS is managed (Hinchingbrooke became a trust in 1993), the service has continued much as it has in the past. However, such a service is subject to strain, as will become clear.

STAFFING STRUCTURE

Medical

There are now six full-time consultants and one associate specialist. There are five SHOs, although the Royal College of Obstetricians and Gynaecologists has given training approval for six. The majority of the SHOs are GP trainees (scheme or independent), but there are regularly one or two who are planning a career in obstetrics and gynaecology. These professional SHOs have varying degrees of experience, but none is considered to have sufficient experience to 'go solo' in any but minor procedures.

Consultants are not compulsorily resident when on call. It is left to individual judgement as to whether they feel that they can get to the delivery suite as quickly as if resident. Some choose to stay in. Generally, the theatre team and anaesthetist could be called while the consultant is coming in, if, on the basis of the grade-G midwife's judgement, the situation is serious enough to warrant this.

Midwives

For historical reasons, the community midwifery staffing levels are high, while the delivery unit has to rely on community input to keep up to safe levels. This came about as a consequence of a combination of the ill-fated *Changing Childbirth* report,[2] and disinvestment (i.e. cuts in funding) by the health authority, which by now had become part, once again, of Cambridgeshire. Midwives at Hinchingbrooke have traditionally been given more clinical freedom than their counterparts elsewhere. For example, they can augment labour in primigravidae, allow the second stage to continue beyond traditional limits, request epidurals and a number of other things which would be regarded as the registrar's role in other, more conventional, hospitals. However, they do not perform operative deliveries or manual removals of placenta and would call a consultant for a difficult perineal repair.

The grade-G midwife has direct access to the consultant on call. Junior midwives must refer to the senior midwife. Medical problems may be seen by the SHOs and midwives are encouraged to involve SHOs in decision making. However, in an urgent or serious case, the consultant may be contacted directly.

CONSULTANT TIMETABLE AND WORKLOAD

The working arrangements are, understandably, complex. First of all, there is the need to ensure continuing cover when a consultant is absent. Second, there is a desire to avoid a heavy clinical load on the day after a night on call. Third, there is a need to fit in the other work of the department, including clinics, theatre, ward work, audit, teaching and administration. No session can take place in the absence of the consultant, although sessions are often run in the absence of the SHO. The workload is planned such that the presence or absence of the SHO is immaterial. Indeed, because of the need for teaching, the SHO's presence is a neutral factor.

Pairs

The six consultants are organised as three pairs. It is axiomatic that if one of the pair is absent, the other must be present. If, in pair A and B, A is away, A's theatre and clinic sessions are cancelled. However, B would see A's postoperative cases or antenatal and postnatal problems.

The most complex thing is the duty roster, which is presently run on a fortnightly basis. Pair A and B are on call on alternate Tuesdays, pair C and D on alternate Wednesdays and pair E and F on alternate Thursdays. Everyone does one Friday, one Monday and one Saturday/Sunday weekend in six. It is arranged so that A or B, for example, would not be on duty on a consecutive Monday and Tuesday. It becomes even more complex when leave has to be taken into account. If A wants to take leave when he or she would be rostered for a weekend, he or she has to exchange with a colleague. This can have repercussions; if A exchanges with E, for example, E might have to cancel sessions on a Monday having been unexpectedly on duty for the weekend.

It is endeavoured that no-one has a clinical session (theatre or clinic) after a 24-hour call. However, it occasionally arises that an unexpected call might be followed by a session. It is up to the individual whether or not this is cancelled, reduced or carried out. A sample timetable for a fortnight is given in Table 1.

The above reflects the current situation. However, there are a number of factors that will result in considerable changes to the current situation, not the least of which is the European Working Hours Directive.

ADVANTAGES AND DISADVANTAGES

Patients

The advantages to the patients seem considerable and include:

(1)   Always seeing an experienced clinician;

(2)   Always seeing the same clinician;

Table 1 *Typical fortnightly timetable for a consultant at Hinchingbrooke Hospital*

Day	Week 1	Week 2
Monday		
am	Gynaecology clinic	Gynaecology clinic
pm	Antenatal clinic	Antenatal clinic
		On call 1 in 6 (1730–0845 hours)
Tuesday		
am	Delivery suite and emergencies	(On call if pair absent)
pm	(on call 24 hours)	No clinical session
Wednesday		
am	No clinical session	No clinical session
pm		
Thursday		
am	Gynaecology special interest clinic	Theatre
pm	Peripheral antenatal clinic X	Peripheral antenatal clinic Y
Friday		
am	Theatre	Theatre
pm	Audit/meetings (on call 1 in 6; 1300–0900 hours)	Audit/Meetings
Saturday/Sunday		On call 1 in 6 (Saturday 0900–Mon 0845 hours)

(3) Definitive treatment plan;

(4) Early discharge from clinic (no six-monthly reviews by a succession of SHOs);

(5) Operation performed by consultant who has been seeing the patient;

(6) Decisions taken at highest levels;

(7) Even in delivery suite, operative intervention by experienced consultant;

(8) If SHO involved, consultant always present;

(9) On-call consultant always immediately available;

(10) Consultant has current experience and practice.

The disadvantages are:

(1) Delay in clinic appointment;

(2) Longer waiting time in clinic;

(3) A possible longer waiting list if operation required;

(4) No other opinion;

(5) Difficulty in establishing common protocols between consultants.

General practitioners

Again, the advantages for GPs are numerous. In addition to the advantages experienced by their patient, the GP benefits from:

(1) Easy contact with consultant;

(2) Familiarity with consultant's practice;

(3) Confidence that the patient will be seen by the consultant in the clinic;

(4) Likelihood that consultant will be familiar with case if further help sought;

(5) Geographical links through peripheral clinics;

(6) Consultant familiar with GP and practice.

The disadvantages are as for the patient, although it is the waiting time that is likely to cause the patient to consult the GP again.

Hospital

The advantages to the hospital result largely from the above-noted points:

(1) Effective use of resources (but see below);

(2) Reduced risk of complaints and litigation;

(3) No locums;

(4) Junior doctors well supervised.

The disadvantages are financial and organisational:

(1) Expensive for minor activity;
(2) Need for reduced sessions due to increased active on-call;
(3) Lack of time for administration and managerial activities;
(4) More consultants (more management difficulties).

Senior house officers

Over the years, the author has come to recognise that what SHOs get from the system is in proportion to what they put in. A relatively indolent junior doctor who wishes to be spoon-fed, or the GP trainee who is only doing the job because it is regarded as necessary, tends to be dissatisfied. The enthusiastic participant, who is intrigued by the arcane and eager for knowledge and experience, finds the system the best they have encountered because of:

(1) One-to-one training by a consultant;
(2) Close support;
(3) Responsibility devolved only to the individual trainee's perceived limits or desires;
(4) Service component limited (the unit still functions);
(5) Small, friendly unit.

The disadvantages relate to the 'sidelining' of juniors by the system of call described above:

(1) Potential lack of direct input into obstetric decision making;
(2) Five SHOs make a roster difficult to run;
(3) Junior doctors' hours directives mean reduced training opportunities;
(4) Possibility of 'personality clash' with consultant.

Consultants

It might be felt that consultants have little to gain from a system which requires so much input from them. However, there are definite bonuses, although these may only be appreciated by some consultants. Indeed, the advantages cannot simply be detailed by a series of points. The crux of the matter is a philosophical one related to responsibility and delegation.

Consultants are ultimately responsible for what happens to their patients, except in emergencies when another consultant is responsible. The advantage of the 'hands-on' approach is that if something does not go well, then it is absolutely clear who is responsible. This may strike some as an appalling situation. The author's view is that it is much easier to discuss an adverse outcome or unfortunate incident if one has been directly involved, rather than to try to explain the actions or inactions of a junior. The patient will be much more likely to accept that everything possible was done if the senior person was involved. I have no desire to spend hours on ward rounds trying to defend indefensible decisions which have been made about patients by well-intentioned but poorly supervised junior doctors. Moreover, I am familiar with my cases. Of course, I do not know every woman on sight, or recall her particular problem. But a brief flick through one's own notes makes everything clear. Provided one is consistent, there is no problem in picking up from where one left off. If, however, the patient has been seen by someone else, it is like starting all over again.

However, the disadvantages may be listed as:

(1) Out-of-hours workload;

(2) Workload during normal working hours;

(3) Frequency of disturbed nights on call;

(4) Calls for relatively trivial matters;

(5) Cancelled clinics mean busier ones earlier or later;

(6) Cover for colleagues' absence;

(7) Need to swap duties for leave (locums are less easy to absorb);

(8) Difficulty in accommodating study leave;

(9) No leeway to accommodate ever-increasing demand;

(10) Timing of necessary but less pressing activities (for example, ward rounds);

(11) Difficulty in reaching consensus on protocols (see below);

(12) Difficulty in management of other consultants' patients.

Some of the above requires further discussion. For example, the employment of a locum consultant in a conventional hospital is unlikely to be a major problem. However, since the system at Hinchingbrooke is critically dependent on the performance of the consultant, and most locum consultants will find it difficult suddenly to take over in such a situation, it is, paradoxically, easier to cancel everything possible and then catch up than to employ a locum and catch up. However, some locums are excellent; it is not their fault, it is the fault of the system.

Protocols

It might be imagined that it would be easier to establish protocols when only six consultants and no juniors are involved. However, this is not the case, for a number of reasons:

(1) As experienced people, consultants are more likely to have firm views on management, based on their own experience.

(2) Consultants have varying views on the strength of evidence-based medicine. Protocols based on evidence-based medicine are only as good as the evidence base, and some evidence-based medicine is based on grade II evidence or worse. Because of our proximity to the clinical shop floor, we can often envisage the trial that needs to be done, but lack the time and resources to perform it.

(3) Consultants have the final responsibility and are unwilling to be bound by written protocols. What we have are guidelines. Some of these are for general guidance. Some are there to remind us of dosage regimens, etc. Some are there to ensure that a standard response is mounted until the consultant is involved. However, as we are ultimately taking decisions and taking responsibility, we need the ability to deviate from what is written.

(4) Such problems do not arise for units where the bulk of the care is provided by registrars. Consultants in such units may be much more likely to agree to a common protocol, when they know they will rarely be in a position to have to deviate from it.

(5) There is also a need to involve other professions, particularly midwives. In the Hinchingbrooke type of unit, where the SHO is not part of the obstetric decision-making hierarchy, the midwives will be less willing to be bound to strict protocols, with some of which they are uncomfortable. Accordingly, it is much more difficult for the consultants to compose protocols for the slavish obedience of all, and so it should be.

THE FUTURE

A brief analysis of the timetable in Table 1 suggests that we are working well over the contracted hours. The workload stems from traditional referral patterns, which evolved before the health reforms and the purchaser-provider split, partly due to the popularity of the unit and the founding staff. When the hospital became a Trust, we were contracted to provide a throughput which was already at that time beyond the capacity of the unit.

Further strains have been put on the unit. Outpatient referrals are rising at 12% per year. Outpatient procedures are replacing some which used to take place in theatre. Women, quite rightly, expect more time and explanation. Clinical irrelevancies such as the *Patients' Charter* put added pressure on the system. NHS managers outside the trust are obsessed with numbers rather than quality. Trust managers have to provide endless statistics of questionable accuracy and value to higher authorities, which respond with new and counterproductive targets. Clinicians are then pressed to achieve these.

Primary care groups or trusts are the new budget-setters. As groups of GPs, their commitment to a growing secondary-care system may be constrained by their perceptions of deficiencies in primary care. New consultant appointments must be 'approved' by primary care trusts. Each new appointment means over £60,000 less for the primary-care budget.

It is against this background of increasing demand and restricted resources that we must deal with the four main professional imperatives:

(1) Working time;

(2) Consultant input;

(3) Patient waiting times;

(4) Training.

European Working Hours Directive

The European Working Hours Directive has been in force since April 1999. It restricts the numbers of total hours and continuous hours of work, and stipulates the number and duration of rest-free periods:

(1) A maximum 48-hour working week averaged over a reference period;

(2) A minimum daily rest period of 11 consecutive hours per day;

(3) A rest break where the working day is longer than six hours;

(4) A minimum rest period of one day per week.

The maximum number of hours per week takes no account of the contracted 38.5 hours per week or the absence of overtime payments.

Table 2 *Average working hours per week*

Task	A	B	C	D
Antenatal clinics	7.0	3.5	3.5	3.5
Gynaecology clinics	3.5	3.5	1.75	3.5
Specialist clinics	1.75	1.75	1.75	1.75
Theatre	5.25	3.5	3.5	3.5
Weekday call[a]	12.0	12.0	12.0	12.0
Friday call[a]	3.5	3.5	3.5	2.5
Monday call[a]	2.7	2.7	2.7	0
Weekend[a]	8.0	8.0	8.0	6.0
Ward rounds	2.5	2.5	1.8	2.5
Audit	2.0	1.0	1.0	1.0
Teaching	2.0	2.0	0	1.0
Administration, meetings	7.0	4.0	0	3.0
Total per week	57.2	47.95	39.5	40.25

A is the current average, counting on-call[a] as hours worked, which they are if resident; the true figure is greater because of leave and cover for leave (by about 12%); B is the reduction in clinical work to get hours down to 48 per week on average with six consultants; C is the reduction in work to get hours down to contracted hours (full-time) with six consultants; D is the possible workload with eight consultants; in fact, 60% of nights on call (2300–0800 hours) are disturbed and almost 100% of evenings (1700–2300 hours) and weekend days

One of the main problems of this directive will be the unpredictability of the workload at night. A single telephone call at home will constitute work and will interrupt a period of consecutive hours' rest. At units like Hinchingbrooke, where there are likely to be interrupted nights, a compensatory two-day rest period is ordered.

There is a danger that this could lead to a shift system, with a breakdown in continuity and quality of care. Shift systems may be suitable for specialties such as A&E or anaesthetics, but not for acute specialties with a continuing caseload. Accordingly, consultant obstetricians and gynaecologists will have to plan their working week to ensure adequate rest periods. If consultant cover of whatever sort is to continue, as it must, all units will have to employ more staff.

Calculations of working hours are given in Table 2.

Consultant input

It might seem from the above that the drive for increased consultant input is irrelevant for Hinchingbrooke. This is far from the case. Other more conventional units are subject to this pressure but will not move towards a consultant-based service without a considerable injection of funds. This is understandable. The problem for Hinchingbrooke is that we are seen already to be there and are, therefore, seen by others to require no such injection of resources. Recent attempts to establish a minimal intermediate presence (rather than a full tier one) have failed because of the decline in specialist registrar numbers. The last thing that is needed is more SHOs.

Do we need more consultants? The answer would seem to be 'yes,' but this is not necessarily the best solution in a unit such as Hinchingbrooke. The establishment of new associate specialist posts is blocked by the Royal College. So, why is an increase in the consultant numbers a double-edged sword?

(1)   Cost;

(2)   More people to disagree about guidelines;

(3)   Reduced continuity of care;

(4) No extra lists or clinic time available;

(5) Therefore, reduction in established consultants' hours means that the total throughput will drop, not rise;

(6) More, not fewer, sessions lost through leave, etc.

The most neutral solution would be the appointment of additional consultants coupled with a reduction in total workload, but one can imagine the enthusiasm with which such a proposal would be welcomed in management circles. Indeed, the continued existence of the unit appears to depend on an increase in referrals.

Waiting times

The present Government is obsessed with numbers. Quality is more complex and difficult to measure. At present, each consultant-only firm here has a caseload that is, on average, equivalent to that dealt with by a full consultant-led firm in a conventional unit. If we reduce numbers seen in clinic to a reasonable level, the time patients wait to get an appointment will rise exponentially.

Increased clinic throughput will put pressure on operation waiting lists. We already do a higher proportion of our surgery as day cases than almost any other unit. Moving procedures to outpatient clinics moves pressure from the operation waiting list to clinic waiting times.

One advantage of our service should be that women attending the gynaecology clinics are less likely to have unnecessary investigation, treatment and follow-up. However, examination of the statistics reveals wide variation between consultants, even allowing for personal special interests. So-called 'one-stop' clinics will inevitably result in increased and unnecessary investigation, unless the referral protocols are tight and rigorously enforced.

Frequency of antenatal-clinic attendance is falling but the clinics appear just as busy, as more time is spent on difficult problems. Many women ask to be booked at Hinchingbrooke because of its reputation. Many of these women will have complex past histories and, sometimes, demands that are difficult to accommodate. Our caesarean section rate of 24% is above the average, partly because of our desire to involve women in decisions regarding their care (Table 3). Moving care out to the community puts further pressures on the budget, as this does not release useful resources in hospital.

Table 3 *Clinical workload (1999)*

	Number	Percent
Women delivered	2298	
Caesarean sections	544	24
Instrumental vaginal	185	8
Perinatal deaths	16	7 per 1000
Stillbirths	12	
Epidural in labour	322	
Inductions	536	
New gynaecology referrals	3056	
Colposcopy referrals	530	
Inpatient FCEs	1306[a]	
Day case FCEs	1516[a]	

[a] Includes admissions without procedures

Training

Hinchingbrooke is ideally placed to provide professional specialist training for specialist registrars, particularly towards the end of their Calman years. We already have such men and women attending for one-to-one surgical tuition, for example in urogynaecology. This, however, would put further pressure on waiting lists, because the proper training of a junior doctor slows down the surgical throughput. Such people must not be left to 'get on with it' on their own until they are demonstrably fit to do so.

CONCLUSIONS

Our model of service provision is not regarded as one to which district general hospitals should aspire. Indeed, there is evidence, from applications for our posts, that newly accredited obstetricians and gynaecologists do not wish to work in such a way, although there is also evidence (from a recent manpower meeting at the Royal College) that younger doctors see residency on-call duty as inevitable when they become consultants. A recent consultant survey (circulated with a letter from the President of the College) suggests that 74% of respondents thought that specialists/consultants should be immediately available on call, 24 hours a day.

It would seem, therefore, that future consultants are willing to be resident on call, but not without intermediate support.

Our long-term aim is to maintain the viability of the trust as a provider of acute services, including obstetrics. This can only be achieved by a reduction in workload, with or without the establishment of a limited intermediate tier. Such a tier would not be vital to service provision, however, but would provide extra interest for those of us who are keen to teach, and the occasional luxury of a further pair of competent, yet well-supervised, hands.

Finally, consultants who work in this type of service should have some compensation. The most ideal in the author's view would be the right to retire at 58 years of age with full pension rights. Otherwise, there will be a need to have two tiers of consultants, with senior people ceasing to be first on call after the age of 55 years.

Acknowledgement

The opinions stated in this article are my own, may not reflect those of others working in the trust, and are not an expression of trust policy.

References

1. *Fourth Report from the Social Services Committee of the House of Commons*, Vol. I. London: HMSO; 1981
2. Department of Health. *Changing Childbirth: Report of the Expert Maternity Group* (Chairman: Baroness Cumberlege). London: HMSO, 1993

5

Regulations, standards, guidelines – is there any room for freedom of thought?

Robert W. Shaw

INTRODUCTION

As we enter a new millennium, there can be no doubt that we enter a new climate for medical practice. This applies across the whole spectrum of medicine, where the levels of standards and personal performance that are meant to be achieved and maintained are higher than they have ever been. In addition, changes within hospital services in terms of finance and transfer of the work traditionally carried out by specialists in hospitals to general practice and primary health care will result in tremendous changes to the way obstetricians and gynaecologists practise within hospitals.

These changes will inevitably force management to consider reconfiguration and amalgamation of hospital units in an endeavour to provide the standards and first-class service which we would wish to achieve and which patients now expect as a right, but which are limited by the willingness of Government to fund the service to these levels. The quality of care across the UK shows many variations and there is a desire to lessen such variations and achieve more uniform outcomes. How then are these issues being addressed?

OBSTETRICS AND GYNAECOLOGY – A CHANGING SPECIALTY

It was at the beginning of the 20th century that the specialty of obstetrics and gynaecology began to evolve, with the establishment of the first specialty College, separate from that of medicine and surgery, which previously had encompassed all aspects of medical practice and directed its training. In 1929, the British College of Obstetricians and Gynaecologists was established and received its Royal Charter in 1948. Since that time, the College and our specialty have grown from strength to strength, contributing to the development of obstetrics and gynaecology not only within the British Isles but worldwide, through the College's links with its overseas Fellows and Members, who have become consultants and specialists practising in all parts of the globe. During the 20th century, as the specialty has developed, great progress in disease treatment and survival has been seen, confirming the importance that contributions from doctors with high levels of expertise in specific areas of medicine can achieve. These are perhaps most easily demonstrated through changes in perinatal mortality rates and maternal mortality rates from the beginning to the end of the 20th century, where there has been a ten-fold reduction in perinatal mortality rates and a 50-fold reduction in the maternal mortality rate within the UK (Table 1). Clearly, these dramatic improvements have resulted not only from the establishment of the specialty of obstetrics and gynaecology but from improvements in the general health of the population and in the workplace environment. Contributions made by specialists in other highly developed areas of medicine (neonatal, paediatric

Table 1 *Progress in reducing perinatal and maternal mortality rates in the 20th century in the UK*

	1900	1999
Perinatal mortality rate	100/1000	8/1000
Maternal mortality rate	50/10 000	1/10 000

and intensive care, anaesthetics and oncology) have contributed towards improved outcomes of obstetric and gynaecological patients, to the development and access to a nation-wide hospital service and to antibiotic therapy, blood transfusion and radio- and chemotherapy.

Advances have also been achieved in gynaecological surgical procedures, not least in the wide spectrum of operative procedures now available. Huge advances have been made in diagnosing and treating the problems and disorders of reproductive health and the treatment options for women with gynaecological cancers. There exists now, in many instances, a real potential for cure in many of the gynaecological malignancies, particularly when early diagnosis is achieved. There are other major advances that have been achieved in preventative strategies in reproductive health, markedly in areas of fertility control, sexually transmitted diseases and screening programmes for premalignant stages of some gynaecological cancers.

These advances have been achieved due to in-depth training programmes for obstetricians and gynaecologists and through the uptake and application of the advances achieved by the pharmaceutical industry and particular advances that have allowed development of new surgical techniques and development.

With these advances come new concerns and pressures, both on the health services to provide finances to fund them but, more specifically, on doctors, in terms of the wider knowledge-base necessary to provide patients with the most up-to-date information and appropriate treatment option and the continual need to acquire new skills from those that would have been appropriate at the time when our own training commenced. Only a minority of specialists has failed to respond appropriately and to learn new techniques effectively before widely applying them but these cases have resulted in the increased public concern regarding the competence of doctors. These have been the driving force behind a series of regulatory and assessment processes currently being introduced.

PROFESSIONAL REGULATIONS

In the UK, following qualification from medical school and satisfactory completion of a pre-registration house-officer year, doctors become fully registered with the General Medical Council (GMC). This gives them significant rights and privileges and, in return, they are required to observe standards of competence, care and conduct set by the profession. Standards of competence, care and conduct will, of course, change with time and our profession has been privileged to have regulation of these standards granted by society through Parliament. That self-regulation is not a right. A series of high-profile cases across many specialties has raised questions about the continued relevance of the medical profession and the GMC in exercising such professional self-regulation. In addition, the medical Royal Colleges have a major role in contributing to standard setting by supervising the training of specialists (examinations and assessments), providing the means by which specialists can remain updated (education and continuing medical education) and to provide the basis to acquire new skills (continuing professional development). To continue effectively with the process of self-regulation, patients must be able to trust doctors not only for their well-being but on many occasions with their lives. To justify that trust, the profession has a duty to maintain a good standard of practice and care while showing respect for human life. In 1995,[1] the GMC reviewed many of these aspects and stated that, with relevance to performance, a doctor must:

(1) Keep their professional knowledge and skills up to date;

(2) Recognise the limits of their professional competence;

(3) Act promptly to protect patients from risk;

(4) Report to the GMC individuals whom they have reason to believe may be unfit to practise.

The latter statement was a major change in emphasis of the role of the GMC. This resulted in the establishment of the Poor Performance Procedures, which became law following an amendment to the Medical Act in July 1997. These performance procedures were developed to achieve two main purposes.

(1) To protect the public;

(2) To rehabilitate a poorly performing doctor.

The changes in emphasis by the GMC resulted in various headlines in tabloid newspapers such as 'shop a doc'. Clearly, we would all accept that it is appropriate that, when a doctor is aware that a colleague's practice is resulting in inadequate care outcome, they should seek means of helping that doctor improve their standards of care to protect patients. How that is achieved is perhaps the question. In many instances it can be achieved through discussion with the individual and direction towards correcting those deficiencies at an early stage. If, for whatever reason, these individuals fail to take such advice or prove unable to correct their deficiencies then referral to the GMC is essential. However, providing the means to prevent such deficiencies occurring is a far better option than letting poor performance become established. The Royal College of Obstetricians and Gynaecologists has spent considerable time and effort providing means for specialists to maintain and develop their clinical skills, as will be outlined below, to help reduce the number of instances when referral to the GMC or indeed suspension from practice would become necessary.

CONTINUING MEDICAL EDUCATION

Continuing medical education (CME) is an important component of maintaining knowledge base and clinical effectiveness. The College has established a mandatory CME programme extending over a five-year cycle and encompassing all consultants and individuals not in training-grade posts. The initial programme aimed to accrue 200 points (one per hour spent on activity) over a five-year period. This has now been increased to 250 points in a five-year cycle. The first five-year cycle ended in January 1999, when the names of individuals who had satisfactorily completed the cycle were published. This represented the vast majority of those who were initially registered. Further lists will now be published on an annual basis of those who have satisfactorily completed their five-year cycle. As the CME programme has developed so the variety of methods of self-education has expanded, giving a more flexible and relevant CME programme for each individual to cover relevant specific areas of their practice and across the specialty of obstetrics and gynaecology.

CONTINUED PROFESSIONAL DEVELOPMENT

Continued professional development (CPD) is a process of continuing learning and skills development to implement changes in the clinical management of patients. It is well recognised that there are ongoing new developments within the specialty and that it is essential that obstetricians and gynaecologists continue to encompass and develop those skills needed to match the service needs of patients and the hospitals within which they work. For CPD to be effective requires a mechanism by which those new skills can be identified and an agreement with each individual who wants to undertake acquisition of these skills as to mechanisms by which time can be allocated to acquire them. To achieve this it may be necessary to train outwith the hospital in which they work. To close the cycle it is then essential that a further assessment is undertaken to ensure that the new skills are effectively being applied within hospital practice – some form of accreditation and assessment would be required, together with an audit of outcomes.

ANNUAL APPRAISAL OF PERFORMANCE

A key component of the CPD cycle is the annual appraisal. This should:

(1) Be professionally led;

(2) Be repeated at yearly intervals;

(3) Include a summary of the outcome agreed by both parties;

(4) Be a remedial process that is not confrontational.

Such an appraisal process has not been part of the National Health Service (NHS), although it has for some years been part of many university administrations. For simplicity and direct relevance to hospitals, these appraisals are likely to be undertaken by the immediate line manager. For clinicians, this would be the clinical director and for the clinical director this would be the medical director. Training of individuals undertaking this role would be required to ensure that appraisals were undertaken appropriately using the reasons and methods for which they were developed.

The value of appraisals, as correctly undertaken in assessing poor performance, may not be robust. To evaluate poor performance would require a formal assessment process, best performed by clinicians from outside the trust. Issues exist regarding the appropriate assessment process and the standards against which the doctor will be compared (recognising the complex issues of varying case mix). These are strong arguments, therefore that, where there are issues of concern regarding performance, an outside external review team, organised through the relevant Royal College, would be a much more appropriate way in which to undertake such a full assessment. The RCOG may assist trusts in these areas and has produced a policy document giving guidance in this area.[2]

MENTORING AND SUPPORT OF DOCTORS

A doctor will feel particularly isolated and vulnerable whenever there is a question about their competence and even more if they are deemed a potential risk to patients such that they are also suspended from practice while an enquiry is undertaken. At these times, the RCOG recommends that a mentor be appointed to advise the doctor in a purely supportive role. This arrangement should be one of absolute confidentiality and the mentor should have the mutual respect of the doctor for whom they are providing mentorship. They should have an ability to discuss and agree the boundaries, purpose and duration of the mentoring process, which may well extend beyond the time of the enquiry and provide further benefits during the difficult period of return to work. To be a mentor can be particularly emotionally and physically demanding and it needs special individuals to fulfil this role.

REVALIDATION

In 1999, the GMC intimated that they wished to develop a process by which doctors on the Medical Register would undergo periodic assessment to confirm that they should remain on the Register. This process has been termed revalidation. The final format and the means by which revalidation will be carried out are being developed by a working party established by the GMC. It has been stated that the final model for the process of revalidation will be agreed by the summer of 2001.

The RCOG has spent considerable time debating this issue and produced its own draft document,[3] which was circulated to all Fellows and Members and submitted to the GMC in January 2000. In essence, the document indicated that it is hoped that evidence of:

(1) Participation in a CME programme;

(2) Active participation in CPD;

(3) The use of the clinical effectiveness programme developed by the Royal College;

(4) Being involved in audit and evaluation of the outcome of individuals case notes; should provide an adequate basis for recommending revalidation of an individual.

The College deems it inappropriate to undertake examinations involving multiple-choice questions or objective structured clinical examinations equivalent to the MRCOG examination. Such components already exist within the Poor Performance Procedures of the GMC for the small group of individuals about which there are major concerns and for whom revalidation could not be immediately recommended. The College clearly supports the ethos of revalidation, to reassure patients of a doctor's continuing competence, and would wish to see a robust and relatively simple mechanism developed. This should not be too cumbersome or the process would be impossible to administer and would become administratively costly and unwieldly. The College awaits with interest the final published and agreed mechanisms to be recommended by the GMC in 2001.

CLINICAL GUIDELINES

Without doubt, inequalities in health are linked to inequalities in life circumstances. It is also true that there are differences throughout the UK in the availability of specific healthcare services. In some instances, these differences are a reflection of the historic and *ad hoc* manner in which healthcare provision has developed since the inception of the NHS. One method by which the most appropriate health care can be determined for an individual is through the development and use of guidelines. These are systematically developed statements aiming to assist decisions about appropriate care in specific clinical circumstances. It would not be appropriate to have guidelines to cover all areas of practice. In the first instance, guideline development should be in areas of practice and treatment where:

(1) There is excessive morbidity, disability or mortality;

(2) Treatment offers good potential for reducing these;

(3) There is a wide variation in clinical practice around the country;

(4) The services involved are resource intensive;

(5) Management involves both primary and secondary care sectors.

The RCOG has been involved in producing guidelines for some considerable time. In 1993, the

RCOG Scientific Advisory Committee began to produce what have become known as the 'greentop' Clinical Guidelines. These began as a consensus view of statements from a panel of experts concentrating on a small area of clinical practice. They have been developed in recent years to contain the levels of evidence from which the guidelines have been developed.

More robust national 'evidence-based clinical guidelines' have been developed since 1996, with the first appearing in October 1998. The development of such evidence-based guidelines is complex and time consuming for the multidisciplinary group involved in their production and costly, because of the need to undertake an extensive literature search for the pertinent evidence. Recommendations are linked to the evidence available in the literature and are graded according to the level of evidence on which they are based:

Level A   Randomised controlled trials;

Level B   Other robust experimental observational studies;

Level C   More limited evidence but the advice has expert opinion and the endorsement of relevant authorities.

The clinical and national evidence-based guidelines have proved to be highly successful. The list of topics covered to date is given in Table 2.

Table 2 *Clinical 'greentop' and national evidence-based guidelines published to date (April 2001)*

Number	Title
1(A)	Beta-agonists for the Care of Women in Preterm Labour
6	Working with Visual Display Units in Pregnancy
7	Antenatal Corticosteroids to Prevent Respiratory Distress Syndrome
8	Amniocentesis
9	Alcohol Consumption in Pregnancy
10	Management of Eclampsia
12	Pregnancy after Breast Cancer
13	Chickenpox in Pregnancy
14	Pelvimetry – Clinical Indications
15	Peritoneal Closure
16	Induction of Labour
17	The Management of Recurrent Miscarriage
18	The Management of Gestational Trophoblastic Disease
19	Hormone Replacement Therapy/Venous Thromboembolism
20	The Management of Breech Presentation
21	Management of Tubal Pregnancies
22	Use of Anti-D Immunoglobulin for Rh Prophylaxis
23	Methods and Materials used in Perineal Repair
24	The Investigation and Management of Endometriosis
25	Management of Early Pregnancy Loss
26	Instrumental Vaginal Delivery
27	Placenta Praevia: Diagnosis and Management
28	Thromboembolic Disease in Pregnancy and the Puerperium: Acute Management
National evidence-based guidelines	
Number	**Title**
1	The Initial Management of Menorrhagia
2	The Initial Investigation and Management of the Infertile Couple
3	The Management of Infertility in Secondary Care
4	Male and Female Sterilisation
5	The Management of Menorrhagia in Secondary Care
6	The Management of Infertility in Tertiary Care
7	The Care of Women Requesting Induced Abortion

AUDIT OF CHANGE

A guideline programme is only as good and effective as the take-up and implementation at local level of such guidelines, to achieve changes and improvements in practice. How best to implement such programmes is currently being reviewed. It is known that patients and clinicians will not always follow guidelines and when this happens it is important to analyse variations in practice from the guidelines. These variations in practice are helpful in updating and amending the guidelines and should always be reviewed at set intervals. The main questions regarding guidelines is whether the introduction of a wider range inhibits or prohibits the right of clinicians and patients to alternative approaches to management. There is always concern that persistent and dogmatic adherence to guidelines will result in moves towards a managed care approach, dictating care to be given rather than allowing clinicians to make their own decisions.

In addition, guideline recommendations could be used as the basis for setting standards by reviewing authorities, such as the Commission for Health Improvement, the Audit Commission and the King's Fund. It is essential then that those standards are set at an appropriate level. An inability to reach those standards may be beneficial to clinicians in improving their service if they are unable to meet these standards through lack of facilities, equipment or staff, rather than through failure to implement the recommendations or through poor performance. Guidelines can be of great help if they are used wisely as guidance and not as rules or directives.

CLINICAL EFFECTIVENESS

Clinical effectiveness programmes aim to link together a number of incentives. The role of a clinical effectiveness programme is to:

(1)   Invest an increasing proportion of resources in interventions that are known to be effective;

(2)   Systematically monitor changes achieved;

(3)   Reduce investment in interventions that have been shown to be less effective.

The RCOG has been involved in many aspects of clinical effectiveness but there has been little concerted effort to co-ordinate activities to achieve effective standards of care. The establishment of the Clinical Effectiveness and Standards Unit within the College has the purpose of setting standards to improve women's health by co-ordination and development of the College's programmes in relation to quality improvement, guidelines, risk management, accreditation of services and consumer issues.

The Clinical Effectiveness Unit now exists to achieve those aims. It is involved in the guideline production programme, linking the development of guidelines with new national audit programmes and linking the launch of guidelines with the educational programmes most likely to achieve implementation. Some may argue that clinical audit has been undertaken for many years, but has it made any difference? In many instances, audits have been undertaken in isolation to guideline and directed-resource initiatives. It is hoped that this new co-ordinated approach will succeed where other initiatives have failed. If nothing else, the clinical effectiveness programme should provide the basis for obstetricians and gynaecologists to achieve local clinical governance, judged against nationally set and agreed targets.

Only time will reveal how successful these initiatives will be. Whether we want it or not, our specialty and the ways in which we provide services to our patients are undergoing unprecedented change. If we want to play an active role in this process of change we have to act both speedily and decisively or else accept what others will implement for us.

References

1. General Medical Council. *Maintaining Good Medical Practice*. London; 1995
2. Royal College of Obstetricians and Gynaecologists. *Policy for Assisting Trusts and Doctors in Cases of Concern or Suspension Related to Standards of Practice*. London; July 2000
3. Royal College of Obstetricians and Gynaecologists. *Discussion Document on Revalidation in Obstetrics and Gynaecology. Report of a Working Party*. London; 2000

6

The consumer's right to evidence-based health care

Marcia Kelson

INTRODUCTION

In recent years, National Health Service policy has placed increasing emphasis on evidence-based health care, the aim being to ensure that all decisions relating to patient care are based, as far as possible, on the findings of up-to-date, rigorously conducted research studies. Within obstetrics, summarised research findings were compiled in a single source in 1989,[1] followed by the Cochrane Collaboration's Pregnancy and Childbirth Database, a twice-yearly updated computer database and a paperback version of the original guide in 1995.[2] However, some clinicians have voiced resistance to this approach, preferring to base their practice on tradition and experience.[3]

Parallel policy developments have focused on involving 'consumers' (patients, service users, carers, patient representatives and the public) in a range of areas within the NHS. Consumer involvement encompasses both the involvement of individuals (for example, the central role of patients in decisions about their own health and care) and involvement at a more collective level (patient representatives, for example, actively contributing to NHS policy and planning decisions). Within the field of maternity care, government policy endorses the right of the childbearing woman to be at the centre of her care and to have her individual needs met by health professionals and health services.[4]

This chapter considers the impact of policy developments in both consumer involvement and evidence-based health care on the provision of care to patients. Divided into three sections, it considers:

(1) The policy context within which consumer involvement operates;

(2) Issues relating to consumer access to evidence-based health care;

(3) Issues relating to consumer access to evidence-based information.

CONSUMER INVOLVEMENT: THE POLICY CONTEXT

The Department of Health is engaged in a widespread programme of reforms to modernise NHS services, with a commitment to building a health service that is responsive to the needs of patients and the wider public. Recent policy documents, including the White Paper *The New NHS*,[5] together with *A First Class Service*[6] and *Clinical Governance*,[7] all discuss the importance of involving consumers across the range of NHS activities with the expectation that consumer involvement should become integral to work in every part of the NHS. The most recent version of the Department of Health's planning and priorities guidance[8] identifies the need to involve and respond to patients and the public as part of NHS strategies for ensuring equity of access to high-quality services.

Attempts to translate the policy into reality have resulted in the publication of a number of documents that seek to provide guidance on consumer involvement in a number of areas:

(1) Encouraging partnerships between the NHS, patients and the public;[9]

(2) Suggesting practical ways for involving patients in clinical audit;[10]

(3) Advising on how best to secure patient involvement in the NHS;[11]

(4) Securing public involvement in a range of NHS activities.[12]

Within maternity care, many of these policy directives were pre-dated and pre-empted by the publication in 1994 of *Changing Childbirth*.[4] Consumer involvement was a central feature, both in terms of the involvement of childbearing women, and their representatives, in the process of developing the document and in terms of placing individual women at the centre of their care.

From a consumer perspective, *Changing Childbirth* represented a watershed for health-service provision in general and for maternity services in particular, because it drew directly on the views of consumer representatives as well as those of policy makers, health professionals and managers. Providing a clear response to an earlier House of Commons enquiry into maternity care, *Changing Childbirth* reiterated many of the Health Committee's recommendations,[13] especially those advocating choice and continuity of care and those questioning the routine use of clinical interventions. Drawing on these recommendations and driven by the three principals of choice, continuity and control, *Changing Childbirth* set out its own recommendations and guidelines, summarised in its first principle of maternity care: 'The woman must be the focus of maternity care. She should be able to feel that she is in control of what is happening to her and able to make decisions about her care, based on her needs, having discussed matters fully with the professionals involved'.

Despite the innovative way in which *Changing Childbirth* placed consumers firmly at the centre of care, six years on there is growing concern among consumer organisations that the early impetus is being lost, particularly in regard to the implementation of its recommendations.

In March 1999, the National Childbirth Trust (NCT) convened a meeting of the Maternity Forum at the House of Lords. Participants complained of a 'falling apart' of *Changing Childbirth*. It was described as 'having no teeth', with considerable variation between obstetric units in terms of the extent to which recommendations were implemented. With no statutory requirements for the recommendations to be achieved, the feeling was that many key targets have not been met. To give just one example: while *Changing Childbirth* advocated that more than 70% of women should know their midwife in labour, a national NCT survey of user representatives on maternity services liaison committees reported that in practice this was happening in only 23% of cases. Participants at the Maternity Forum were concerned that, while *Changing Childbirth* had produced some innovative pilot projects, inadequate resources and lack of official audit of changes that were implemented had led to it 'quietly fading away'.

One possible reason for perceived failures in the implementation of *Changing Childbirth* lies in the fact that it has been superseded by a wealth of new programmes. The setting up of the National Institute for Clinical Excellence and the Commission for Health Improvement, the development of clinical governance initiatives, health improvement programmes and national service frameworks are all recent innovations aimed at improving the quality of health-service provision. However, current initiatives are focusing on specific topics (for example, cancers and coronary heart disease) and specific patient groups (for example, the elderly) and not on maternity care. In terms of a policy framework for maternity services, the lack of profile currently afforded maternity services poses a number of key questions, not only for government and the Department of Health, but also for organisations such as the Royal College of Obstetricians and Gynaecologists and for consumer representative organisations.

(1) Where do *Changing Childbirth* recommendations stand alongside all the new policy initiatives aimed at monitoring and improving the quality of clinical care?

(2) Where do *Changing Childbirth* initiatives fit into new commissioning arrangements? For example, what opportunities, if any, will there be for local maternity users, either through their own user organisations or via maternity services liaison committees, to inform and influence the work of bodies such as primary care groups?

(3) Where are the resources to allow providers to meet targets for maternity services that have cost implications? With the increasing shortage of trained midwives in particular, it becomes difficult to see how targets relating, for example, to choice of place of birth or to continuity of carer are likely to improve in the foreseeable future.

(4) If the apparent decline in the impact of *Changing Childbirth* is substantiated, what alternative framework is being adopted to ensure consistency in the quality of clinical care available to maternity service users around the country?

(5) To what extent is the clinical care provided to maternity patients governed by nationally agreed frameworks based on the best evidence currently available?

CONSUMER ACCESS TO EVIDENCE-BASED HEALTH CARE

NHS policy has established that health service consumers should have access to a quality service regardless of where they live. Resources should be spent on treatments that give the best possible outcomes for patients and not wasted on ineffective procedures.

In practice, however, published evidence suggests that not all women are receiving care based on the best evidence currently available.

The pocket guide version of *Effective Care in Pregnancy*,[2] used not only by health professionals but also by many pregnant women, gives direct access to information on what care to expect in the light of currently available evidence. Appendix 4 of the document lists 60 items described as 'forms of care that should be abandoned in the light of the available evidence'. These include:

(1) Regimens which fail to involve women in decisions about their care;

(2) Regimens which fail to provide continuity of care during pregnancy and childbirth;

(3) Management that involves doctors and obstetricians in the care of all women during pregnancy;

(4) Limiting the duration of second stage of labour arbitrarily;

(5) Repeating caesarean section routinely after previous caesarean section;

(6) Providing additional fluids and formula supplements to breastfed infants routinely;

(7) Scheduling duration of postnatal hospital stay inflexibly.

It is of some concern to those with an enthusiasm for providing, or wishing to receive, evidence-based care, that the Audit Commission's survey of maternity services, published in 1997,[14] revealed variations in the extent to which routine provision of these forms of care had been abandoned. The Audit Commission report specifically highlighted a need to 'pay more attention to bringing the evidence that does exist into clinical practice'.

Page notes that many labour and delivery wards still resemble intensive care units rather than places to give birth.[15] 'They are' she says, 'anxious places'. She argues that the wholesale use of technology, for example, routine electronic fetal monitoring and ultrasound scans, has been introduced without adequate evaluation and its use has not been reversed by evidence which raises questions about its benefits. At the same time, forms of care which have been shown to have considerable benefit (for example, the presence of a trained care-giver) have been largely ignored. Burr et al.,[16] in a survey of obstetricians' attitudes to the management of term breech, concluded that, in the specific health authority where the survey took place, the research on external cephalic version had not been translated fully into clinical practice. Iqbal et al.[17] surveyed doctors and midwives working in two teaching hospital maternity units. They found that, for most areas of clinical care, a majority of professionals agreed with the research-based evidence but practice appeared to be inconsistent with the evidence in more than half of these areas. These published studies are corroborated by consumer organisations' concerns about various aspects of childbirth.

(1) Lack of choice available to women in decisions about their care (women not getting choice about place of birth or about some of the treatment options available during pregnancy and labour; staff shortages leading to some options not being available);

(2) Lack of access to continuity of carer (in a focus group run by one maternity service liaison committee, 10 of the 12 women taking part did not know who was their named midwife);

(3) Scheduling of interventions according to consultant preferences rather than individual clinical circumstances (the 'I don't let my women go over 11 days so we'll induce you on Monday' scenario);

(4) Time limits placed on the second stage of labour, with women feeling unable to negotiate over what they sometimes perceived as arbitrary cut-off points;

(5) Concerns about rising caesarean rates, especially after previous caesarean section;

(6) Lack of support for breastfeeding and poor experiences of postnatal care.

Unfortunately, there is a tendency sometimes to criticise reports, whether from individual patients or from consumer organisations, as anecdotal or 'unrepresentative' experiences and to negate the need to actively engage consumer views.

Two quotes from a survey reported in the *British Journal of Midwifery*[18] perhaps illustrate ways in which the need to engage the views of service users, or the views themselves, can sometimes be marginalised or dismissed. Firstly, a midwife, when asked about what providing high-quality care meant replied: 'Knowing we are right when the patients tell us that we are wrong'. Secondly, a GP who did not consider formal monitoring of consumer views to be necessary because: 'If women were not happy, we would have heard about it by now'. However, adopting an evidence-based approach surely involves drawing on issues raised, for example by small numbers of women or their representatives, and testing them out on larger samples? This would provide one means of obtaining evidence-based information firmly grounded in the experiences of those on the receiving end of care rather than, as sometimes happens, their being dismissed on the basis of subjective assumptions attributed to such reports.

What seems clear, from published research and the concerns of consumer organisations, is that having an evidence base is not in itself sufficient to ensure that research findings are translated into routine clinical practice. If women are to have access to evidence-based care there is arguably a need for improved mechanisms both to support the dissemination of evidence and to audit practice with a view to improving adherence to the evidence.

Perhaps one starting point lies in suggestions made by the NCT. Focusing specifically on the rising number of caesarean sections, the NCT has voiced concerns about the continuing increase in caesarean section rates, coupled with considerable variations between hospitals and regions that cannot be attributed to clinical need. Data suggesting that caesarean sections carry higher mortality and morbidity rates than vaginal births have fuelled these concerns. In the light of these concerns, the NCT has provided two suggestions for addressing such variations:[19]

(1) Evidence-based, hospital-based protocols, made available in every hospital with a maternity unit and not just in those where availability depends upon local enthusiasms and leadership;

(2) Routine audit and re-audit, not only of caesarean sections but also of the management of factors which may predispose to caesarean section (for example previous caesarean, failure to progress and breech presentation).

Such approaches could be adopted, not only for caesarean sections but also for many other aspects of maternity care, to improve the way in which research evidence is taken up in clinical practice.

Potential improvements in encouraging the uptake of evidence-based practice are not, of course, the sole remit of NHS providers. Commissioners also have a role to play, for example in encouraging local adoption and implementation of evidence-based guidelines and using contracts to develop local services that deliver high quality, clinically-effective care.

With the increasing emphasis on consumer involvement described earlier in this chapter, both commissioners and providers have a responsibility actively to involve women who use local maternity services in monitoring the quality and effectiveness of local service provision. Women, and society in general, also have to take some responsibility for decisions about the ways in which patient choice is exercised, particularly where certain choices may conflict with what, in the light of currently available evidence, is known to be clinically effective.

Finally, there must also be responsibility at national level to commission research where there continue to be gaps in knowledge regarding the clinical effectiveness (or otherwise) of the treatment and management of certain conditions or circumstances. If this research is to be relevant to those who use maternity services, then women's views and priorities need to be taken into account when decisions about research priorities are taken.

CONSUMER ACCESS TO EVIDENCE-BASED INFORMATION

One of the common themes that emerges when talking to patients is that the overwhelming majority would like access to as much unbiased information as possible. You only need to look at the range of titles available in high-street bookshops to judge the apparently insatiable demand for literature on all aspects of pregnancy and childbirth. Quotes from the Audit Commission's report on maternity services,[14] however, demonstrate differences in how information can be communicated during pregnancy.

> 'The midwife I had was absolutely brilliant. She answered all questions asked by myself and my husband and if she didn't know or wasn't sure she would find out in time for my next visit.'

> 'I went to see my GP before I was pregnant for advice – he vaguely mentioned folic acid but that was it. I found more advice in Sainsbury's on what to eat, etc.'

As a previous Audit Commission report on communication with patients demonstrated,[20] there are still too many examples of poor communication, information being withheld from patients, poor access to information and poor quality information.

It is not only patient demand for information that drives the production of patient information materials, but also a recognition that patients cannot make informed choices in a vacuum of knowledge. It can be an interesting exercise in its own right to spend an hour in a GP's surgery or hospital outpatient department looking at exactly what patient information is provided in the racks or on notice boards and the quality of that information. To what extent, for example, do leaflets cite the sources used in drawing together the information contained in them and to what extent are such leaflets in any way evidence-based? Good quality patient information comprises three key elements. It should:

(1) Be clearly communicated;

(2) Involve patients;

(3) Be evidence-based.

Changing Childbirth made no less than 15 direct references to the need and desirability for women to be able to make informed choices about their own care. Compared with some other specialties, maternity service users have been relatively spoilt in terms of access to information leaflets that are evidence-based. Of particular note are the MIDIRS 'Informed Choice' leaflets for maternity service users. These provide a good example of how individual users, user representatives and professionals were able to collaborate to produce clear, non-technical, evidence-based patient information, which complemented professional versions. In all, ten leaflets were produced, covering issues from place of birth to fetal monitoring in labour, from alcohol in pregnancy to management of breech presentation. The concept behind the leaflets was that women could access full, unbiased, evidence-based information to enable them, in partnership with their clinicians, to weigh up the pros and cons of all effective treatment options and to express their preference for the one they favour most. What seems to be a pity is that this initiative, like so many others arising from *Changing Childbirth*, has 'faded away'. While the leaflets are still produced, no new topics have been added to the original list. (In the light of current concerns about rising caesarean section rates, perhaps information on the pros and cons of alternative modes of delivery might be an appropriate topic to consider at the moment.) For those leaflets that were produced and continue to be available, it is disappointing that many maternity units do not make them routinely available to women because of cost considerations.

CONCLUSIONS

Consumer rights to evidence-based health care need to be considered within the context of the opportunities that consumers have to:

(1) Participate in decisions on their own care;

(2) Participate in decisions about how services are delivered;

(3) Access evidence-based services;

(4) Access evidence-based information on which to base their choices.

In the context of maternity service provision, *Changing Childbirth* emphasised the involvement of maternity service users in decisions relating both to their own care and to the ways in which maternity services are delivered. Six years on, however, it appears that some women continue to have problems in availing themselves of the three key principles of *Changing Childbirth*, namely choice, continuity and control.

Since the publication of *Changing Childbirth*, health policy has focused increasingly on encouraging evidence-based practice. However, there continue to be variations in the extent to which research evidence is translated into clinical practice, thereby raising questions about the extent to which all women have access to truly clinically effective services.

If women are to participate fully in decisions relating to their own care or relating to how maternity services are delivered, they need access to evidence-based information to inform those decisions. While maternity service users are possibly better served than many other patient groups, the amount of evidence-based information available to them is at present restricted, either in terms of the topics covered or in terms of the availability of published information materials.

While NHS policy rhetoric implies that consumers do have a right to expect high quality, clinically effective care, the reality is that inequalities continue to exist. Future discussions about consumer access to evidence-based care need to be tempered with an understanding that access is only possible where opportunities to exercise informed choice exist. The reality is that there is a pressing need for policy makers, health service professionals and consumers to engage in a far more open debate about what choices are available in reality to patients, rather than to focus on emotively charged discussions about patient or consumer 'rights'.

References

1. Chalmers, I., Enkin, M., Keirse, M.J.N.C. *Effective Care in Pregnancy and Childbirth*. Oxford: Oxford University Press; 1989
2. Enkin, M., Keirse, M.J.N.C., Renfrew, M., Neilson, J. *The Guide to Effective Care in Pregnancy and Childbirth*, 2nd ed. Oxford: Oxford University Press; 1995
3. Drife, J. Choice and instrumental delivery (commentary). *Br J Obstet Gynaecol* 1996;**103**:132–3
4. Department of Health. *Changing Childbirth: Report of the Expert Maternity Group* (Chairman: Baroness Cumberlege). London: HMSO; 1993
5. Department of Health. *The New NHS*. London: HMSO; 1997
6. Department of Health. *A First Class Service: Quality in the New NHS*. Wetherby: DoH; 1998
7. NHS Executive. *Clinical Governance: Quality in the New NHS*. Wetherby: DoH; 1999
8. Department of Health. *Modernising Health and Social Services: National Priorities Guidance 2000/01–2002/03*. Wetherby: DoH; 1999
9. Department of Health. *Patient and Public Involvement in the New NHS*. Wetherby: DoH; 1999
10. Kelson, M. *Promoting Patient Involvement in Clinical Audit: Practical Guidance on Achieving Effective Involvement*. London: College of Health; 1998
11. Kelson, M. *User Involvement: A Guide to Developing Effective User Involvement Strategies in the NHS*. London: College of Health; 1997
12. Barker, J., Bullen, M., de Ville, J. *Reference Manual for Public Involvement*, 2nd ed. Bromley: Bromley Health; 1999
13. House of Commons Health Committee. *Second Report – Maternity Services, Volume I*. London: HMSO; 1992
14. Audit Commission. *First Class Delivery: Improving Maternity Services in England and Wales*. London; 1997
15. Page, L. Evidence-based practice in midwifery: a virtual revolution? *Journal of Clinical Effectiveness* 1997;**2**:10–13
16. Burr, R., Johanson, R., Watt, I., Wyatt, J., Jones, P. A survey of obstetricians' attitudes to the management of term breech. *Journal of Clinical Excellence* 1999;**1**:35–40

17 Iqbal, Z., Clarke, M., Taylor, D. Clinical effectiveness: the potential for change in maternity care. *Journal of Clinical Effectiveness* 1998;**3**:67–71
18 Pope, R., Cooney, M., Graham, L., Holliday, M., Patel, S. Aspects of Care. 4: Views of professionals and mothers. *British Journal of Midwifery* 1998;**6**:144–7
19 National Childbirth Trust. *Caesarean Section: A National Childbirth Trust Briefing for MPs.* London; 1999
20 Audit Commission. *What Seems to be the Matter?* London; 1993

7

Anterior vaginal-wall prolapse – an historical and anatomical perspective

Elisabeth J. Adams and Mark Slack

INTRODUCTION

Anterior vaginal-wall prolapse is a common problem that is poorly understood and provides many challenges for gynaecological surgeons. There is an impression that the results of surgical repair are not as good as previously believed and that surgery may fail to relieve symptoms. In England in 1995/96, 22 000 procedures were performed, either alone or in combination, for the management of anterior wall prolapse (Department of Health statistics). This is an increase from 11 706 in 1989/90.

HISTORICAL ASPECTS

A wide range of techniques has been attempted to repair the prolapsing anterior vaginal wall. Geradin tried denudation of vaginal mucosa for the management of prolapse in 1823 on a cadaver. It was first performed on a living patient in 1830. By 1866, Simm had performed a series of denudation operations similar to a modern anterior colporrhaphy.[1] The majority of historical papers describing the aetiology of, and treatment for, the cystocele regard the condition as analogous to a herniation of the anterior abdominal wall. Consequently, all the surgical techniques concentrate on excision of the redundant vaginal tissue with plication of the cut ends of the fascia in the midline.[2,3] In 1909, White[4] wrote of his frustration with the suboptimal outcome of operations for the repair of the cystocele. White believed that the practice of removing part of the anterior wall before suturing the cut ends together was irrational and destined for failure. In his paper[4] he made the first reference to the lateral supports of the anterior wall. He proposed that injuries at parturition produced tears in the fibres of the white line, allowing the anterior wall to dislocate from its attachments and present as a cystocele.

His solution was a vaginal technique allowing attachment of the lateral sulci of the vagina to the white line using absorbable sutures. The technique described is not dissimilar to the current paravaginal repair described by Richardson.[5] Nineteen cases with no recurrence were described. White appreciated that the operation, in addition to correcting the prolapse, did not compromise the capacity of the vagina. The prevailing belief at the time was that anterior vaginal wall prolapse represented a central herniation of the bladder through the anterior fascia and, therefore, would not be served by an operative procedure that only approached the lateral supports. In consequence, the procedure was largely ignored until its resurrection by Richardson in 1981.[5]

In the interim, surgeons concentrated their efforts on improving the outcome of the midline techniques. Attention was given to correction of midline 'fascial' defects by 'lapping' techniques.[6,7] The abdominal approach was introduced in 1939 and underwent subsequent modifications.[8–11] Macer, in 1978,[12] concluded that the abdominal procedure was superior to the vaginal approach.

Various techniques originally described for the management of genuine stress incontinence were also tried in the management of anterior wall defects.[13,14] These have failed to make any real impact on the management of the condition which continues to be managed by vaginal plication by most surgeons.

With the reintroduction of the paravaginal repair by Richardson[5] and Shull[15] it seems as if the management of the problem has gone full circle.

ANATOMY OF THE ANTERIOR VAGINAL WALL

In order to understand the various operations that have been proposed to correct cystocele, it is necessary to have a three-dimensional understanding of the anatomy of the anterior vaginal wall. The mechanisms by which the uterus and vagina are supported have been investigated in cadaveric dissections and our knowledge in this area is mainly due to the work of Delancey,[16] which has brought a mechanical framework to the landmarks described in anatomy textbooks. These concepts are relatively new and have altered surgical approaches in prolapse as a result. The following paragraphs attempt to summarise Delancey's ideas about supporting structures in the pelvis. It is necessary to have prior knowledge of the anatomical landmarks referred to below.

Delancey introduced the concept of three levels, or forms, of support that can be analysed for any organ in the pelvis. Support is provided mainly by the endopelvic fascia which invests each organ and which forms condensations or named ligaments. In addition to endopelvic fascia, the muscles of levator ani provide indirect support by closing the genital hiatus and providing a platform against which rises in abdominal pressure compress the pelvic organs. Delancey described level-I support as vertical suspension of the organ, level-II support as lateral attachment to the sidewalls of the pelvis and level-III support as the fusion of the lower end of the organ to the cloacal area. Failure of any of these supports can lead to organ prolapse and incontinence.

In the case of the uterus and vagina, the suspensory supports (level I) are provided by the cardinal and uterosacral ligaments, while level-II support of the vagina is provided by connective tissue (called paracolpium by Delancey) which connects the vagina to the arcus tendineus fascia pelvis or 'white line', a fibrous condensation running along the pelvic side-wall from about 1 cm lateral to the pubic symphysis to the ischial spine, which forms part of the origin of the levator ani muscles. As well as fixing the vagina laterally, the paracolpium forms a supportive layer under the bladder anteriorly, which is called the pubocervical fascia. The posterior aspect of the paracolpium is similarly attached to the superior fascia of the levator ani muscles, forming the rectovaginal septum or Denonvilliers fascia. Level-III support of the lower third of the vagina is provided by fusion of the vaginal connective tissue posteriorly to the perineal body and anteriorly to the urethra (Figure 1).

The main support of the bladder and bladder neck is the hammock-like anterior vaginal wall and the condensation of pubocervical fascia around the vagina, which extends laterally to the arcus tendineus fascia pelvis and fuses to the levator ani muscles beneath. As the distal urethra passes through the perineal membrane the fascia surrounding it fuses densely with the pubic bone. The indirect lateral attachments to the levator ani muscles (specifically the pubococcygeus portion) provide a base against which the urethra is compressed during rises in intra-abdominal pressure, closing the urethral lumen. When the levator ani muscles are voluntarily contracted, they are able to provide compression which can interrupt the urinary stream.

Anterior vaginal prolapse can arise in a number of different ways. Defects in the endopelvic fascia in the midline lead to a central cystocele while detachment of the pubocervical fascia from the white line gives rise to lateral prolapse of the anterior vaginal wall. In addition, superior transverse defects have been described in the endopelvic fascia where the pubocervical fascia

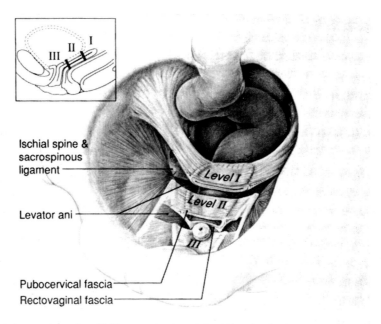

Figure 1 *Levels of vaginal support in a cadaver, bladder removed at the vesical neck (reproduced with permission from Delancy[16])*

attaches to the cervix, merging with the uterosacral and cardinal ligament complex, leading to a high central cystocele.[17] At the bladder neck, failure of the supporting structures will give rise to genuine stress incontinence. The types of fascial defects present need to be carefully assessed in the individual patient in order to repair and support the different structures that have failed. In addition, at least 35% of women will have occult genuine stress incontinence, which needs to be assessed by urodynamic investigations with and without reduction of the prolapse, prior to any surgery.[18]

DIAGNOSIS OF DEFECTS AND EXAMINATION OF THE ANTERIOR VAGINAL WALL

It is important to remember that a cystocele can remain asymptomatic in which case repair is seldom indicated. Symptoms include feelings of pressure and 'falling out' sensations. The patient may be aware of a bulge that protrudes beyond the hymeneal margin. Occasionally, in severe cases, it may be associated with alterations in the urinary stream and symptoms of incomplete emptying.

In diagnosing the type and degree of pelvic organ prolapse, it is important to carry out an examination of the anterior wall that identifies all the sites where loss of support has occurred. This is best achieved with the patient in the left lateral position, using a Sim's speculum and sponge holders, as well as an assistant to help lift the patient's right buttock. Good lighting is essential. The full International Continence Scoring system for prolapse should be performed, with the patient maximally straining (with an empty bladder).[19] The Sim's single-bladed speculum is initially placed along the posterior vaginal wall, in order to evaluate the anterior vaginal segment. The loss of the lateral sulci is evaluated, along with the degree of any central anterior defect and the mobility of the urethra and bladder during straining. In the case of lateral wall defects, open sponge forceps are used to support the lateral sulci and return the vagina to its normal position, then the presence of

Table 1 *Surgical options for the management of anterior vaginal-wall prolapse*

Approach	Procedure
Vaginal	Anterior colporrhaphy
	Vaginal paravaginal repair
Abdominal	Abdominal (Macer) colporrhaphy
	Abdominal paravaginal repair
Abdominoperineal	Four-corner repair

central defects is assessed with the patient straining. If there is no further descent with the lateral walls supported, then paravaginal defects exist and paravaginal repair will be required. A central defect may coexist with lateral defects. If the sponge forceps supporting the midline at the bladder base reduce the prolapse completely, then only a central defect exists (suitable for an anterior colporrhaphy). Many authors recommend that the patient is also examined in the standing position in order to evaluate the maximum degree of prolapse.

SURGICAL APPROACHES TO ANTERIOR VAGINAL-WALL PROLAPSE

In this chapter, only operations designed to correct anterior vaginal prolapse are described. In the case of bladder-neck descent leading to stress incontinence or combined prolapse and stress incontinence, the various operations may be combined with procedures to support the bladder neck, such as a Burch colposuspension or sling procedure, which are outside the scope of this chapter. The various surgical options are shown in Table 1.

Anterior colporrhaphy

A large number of variations have been described. In the main, the operation involves a midline incision of the vaginal mucosa with dissection of mucosal flaps to expose the bladder and proximal urethra. Absorbable mattress sutures are placed into paravesical tissues and fascia laterally in order to support the bladder in the midline. The excess vaginal mucosa is excised and closed in the midline with further absorbable sutures.

As a result of the anatomical concepts described above, it is now felt that only a central fascial defect will respond to anterior colporrhaphy. Any evidence of displacement of the vaginal wall from the white line laterally will require attachment of the prolapsed tissue back on to the white line (a paravaginal repair).

Weber and Walters[20] have reviewed the numerous retrospective studies of anterior colporrhaphy as a treatment for prolapse. No randomised trials of different variations in repair method have been performed. The majority of studies had recurrent cystocele rates of 3-20% after two- to eight-year follow-up but, as these were all retrospective studies, it is unclear what assessment of lateral defects was carried out prior to surgery. Porges and Smilen[21] carried out a retrospective analysis of their caseload of 486 prolapse procedures over a period of 23 years. For primary anterior repairs they had a recurrence rate of 1.4% for mild prolapse and 3.8% for severe prolapse. In the recurrent surgery group, recurrences of 2.9–4.5% are quoted.[21] No complications of the surgery are reported but there were two deaths; one due to medical problems and the other due to pelvic sepsis in a diabetic. Stanton et al.[22] noted a recurrence rate of 15% after two years for anterior colporrhaphy performed for prolapse, although the study concentrated on the pre- and postoperative urodynamic findings.

Synthetic prostheses

Dissatisfaction with the outcome of operations for the management of anterior wall prolapse has encouraged surgeons to experiment with a variety of natural and synthetic grafts. A report of the use of tantalum mesh was published in 1955.[23] Ten patients had tantalum-mesh grafts inserted for the repair of large symptomatic cystoceles. Follow-up was short (6–18 months) and was completed on nine of the patients. Five had a complete resolution of the symptoms but in four the mesh was exposed and required trimming.

Friedman and Meltzer reported in 1970[24] on the use of a collagen-mesh prosthesis in the management of four patients with a variety of pelvic floor defects. In one patient with a uterine and anterior wall prolapse the mesh was placed below the epithelium of the anterior wall. No objective or long-term (greater than ten years) results are available.[24] Rosing et al.[25] described fibrin sealant placed in the cave of Retzius. In a group of nine patients with anterior-wall defects and a high body mass index, Rosing et al. successfully corrected the prolapse. No details of type or length of follow-up are available.[25] Zacharin[26] produced a descriptive paper on the use of a free full-thickness epithelial graft for the correction of prolapse. Again, no results are available. More recently, Julian[27] used Marlex™ mesh to address this problem in a randomised prospective study. Twenty-four patients were randomised into control and treatment groups. All patients underwent an anterior colporrhaphy, paravaginal repair and urethral suspension. In the treatment group, a Marlex™ polypropylene mesh was placed under the anterior vaginal wall before closure. There were only four failures, which all occurred in the control group. Three patients suffered vaginal erosions but these were successfully treated conservatively.[27] Data on the use of synthetic prostheses are limited but, following the success of the tension-free vaginal tape for the treatment of urinary incontinence, there will no doubt be renewed interest.[28] Polypropylene is probably one of the ideal bio-compatible materials. It is strong and both chemically and physically inert; it is not carcinogenic and is easy to produce. It is possible that the characteristics of the weave impart specific properties to the mesh and thus not all forms of polypropylene are identical.[29] The behaviour of different forms of mesh in the suburethral position may be due as much to tissue reactivity as to operative technique.

Experience with the complications of artificial slings in the suburethral position should act as a warning to surgeons planning to use mesh for cystocele repair.[30] Although the use of mesh is tempting, its widespread introduction should be preceded by careful clinical trials.

Abdominal cystocele repair

Several techniques of abdominal repair of cystocele at the time of hysterectomy have been described, although these have fallen out of favour.[8-12] The basis of these techniques is to dissect the bladder at abdominal hysterectomy much more fully than usual, exposing vaginal mucosa at the level of the urethra and removing a diamond-shaped portion of vaginal mucosa in the midline. The repair is oversewn using absorbable sutures.

In 1978, Macer[12] published his 20-year experience of the technique. Subjective assessment of 76 patients showed an overall recurrence of cystocele in 7.9% of cases, which Macer compared with a recurrence rate of 22% in his anterior colporrhaphy cases over the same period. There was no objective assessment of the patients or any indication of any complications resulting from the surgery.

Abdominal paravaginal repair

Paravaginal repair of lateral wall defects aims to reapproximate the vaginal wall to the arcus tendineus fascia pelvis or white line. The most widely used surgical approach has been abdominal, via the retropubic space, although the same structures can also be approached vaginally.

The procedure is similar to that employed in a Burch colposuspension. After exposure of the lateral vagina by medial dissection of the bladder base, between four and six permanent sutures are placed through the vagina along its length and then via the arcus tendineus fascia pelvis (white line) rather than the iliopectineal ligament, in order to restore lateral vaginal support. A modification described by Shull and Baden[31] is to anchor the majority of the sutures through the arcus tendineus fascia pelvis but place the middle sutures via the iliopectineal ligament, without elevation, as an additional support in case the sutures in the white line fail.

Vaginal paravaginal repair

Initially described by White in 1909[3] and rediscovered by Richardson in 1976,[5] this operation can be performed through a midline vaginal incision or through bilateral vaginal incisions. The bladder is dissected medially from the vagina and the pelvic sidewalls, exposing the ischial spines. Permanent sutures are placed from the iliococcygeus fascia anterior to the ischial spine and then through the vagina (leaving the epithelium intact), suspending the vagina bilaterally in the same technique as sacrospinous fixation. Further sutures are then placed through the arcus tendineus fascia and through the lateral vaginal wall to reattach the vagina on both sides to the white line. Any central defects can be repaired by an anterior colporrhaphy: the lateral wall sutures are only tied to elevate the anterior wall after the vaginal mucosa has been closed.

A modification of the technique, described by Scotti *et al.*,[32] is the use of ischial periosteum anterior to the ischial spine or the obturator membrane as an anchoring tissue rather than the arcus tendineus fascia. In a prospective study of 40 patients, 75% of whom also had genuine stress incontinence, only one patient had a recurrent paravaginal defect during the follow-up period (mean 39 months, range 7–52 months). However, a high proportion of patients had other procedures performed concomitantly, which ranged from abdominal sacral colpopexy to suburethral sling procedures, so the results are difficult to interpret.

Results of abdominal and vaginal paravaginal repair

Shull *et al.*[15] reported on 62 women with bilateral paravaginal defects, leading to severe cystocele (87% beyond hymen) operated on vaginally and followed up for a mean of 1.6 years. Sixty-nine percent had undergone previous pelvic surgery, including anterior or posterior repair in 55%. As well as bilateral paravaginal repairs, additional procedures were carried out in a proportion of patients, with 73% having a form of culdoplasty and all patients also having a perineorrhaphy and posterior repair. Thirty-three percent developed recurrent anterior vault prolapse, none of which was as severe as the pre-operative state and none of which had required further surgery, although the follow-up data and method of assessment were unclear.

Benson *et al.*[33] carried out a randomised study of patients with primarily uterine or vault prolapse associated with relaxation of the anterior vaginal wall, up to or beyond the hymen, with a paravaginal defect present. Women with central cystoceles were excluded. Eighty-eight women were operated on after careful assessment, including subtracted dual channel cystometry. Forty-eight women were randomised to a vaginal approach that included bilateral sacrospinous fixation and vaginal paravaginal repair, using permanent monofilament sutures. In addition, however, vaginal hysterectomy, Pereyra urethropexy or sling, McCall culdoplasty or anterior colporrhaphy were also undertaken at the surgeon's discretion. Forty women underwent an abdominal surgical approach, with the main part of the procedure being sacrocolpopexy and abdominal paravaginal repair, also with permanent monofilament sutures. In addition, in this arm of the study patients underwent abdominal hysterectomy, Burch or sling procedures, culdoplasty or a Macer abdominal anterior wedge repair as well. Thirty percent of the abdominal group required a vaginal anterior colporrhaphy and, in 50% of the abdominal group and 67% of the vaginal group, posterior repairs were also performed. Patients were followed up at six months and annually for five years by an independent co-author (not the surgeon). Patients operated on vaginally had significantly shorter operating times and operative costs, but longer duration of catheter use (more than five days in 75% compared with 48% in the abdominal group) and twice the rate of postoperative urinary incontinence. Mean time to recurrence of prolapse was 11.2 months (± 11.5 months) in the vaginal group and 22.2 months (± 16.2 months) in the abdominal group, which was significant. Re-operation for cystocele was required in 29% of the vaginal group and only 10.5% of the abdominal group. Despite the confounding differences in the other surgical procedures performed, this study does indicate some possible advantages for the abdominal route, especially in terms of the longevity of the repair.

Monga[34] described the results of paravaginal repair for cystourethrocele as 'cure' in between 76% and 97% of patients. However, he noted that the patient groups were often mixed and definitions of 'cure' varied.

Abdominoperineal procedures: four-corner repair

Raz et al.[35] suggested an abdominoperineal procedure for the correction of anterior vaginal-wall laxity. The initial description was for a group of patients with grade II to III cystocele and a significant number of these patients had coexistent stress incontinence.[35] The procedure is based on the same principles as the Raz long-needle colposuspension. In addition to two para-urethral sutures, two further sutures are placed more proximally, through the entire vaginal wall. The four sets of sutures are transferred to the abdomen with a double-pronged needle through a suprapubic incision. The degree of elevation of the bladder neck is estimated cystoscopically, then the prolene sutures are tied abdominally across the rectus sheath.

Both in this series and in a second series of patients with grade IV cystocele[14] a cure rate of greater than 90% was reported for cystocele. A more modest success rate was achieved for the cure of genuine stress incontinence.

Using the same technique in a smaller series, Miyazaki and Miyazaki[36] had excellent results at six weeks but this had dropped to 59% at four years. The failures had all occurred at the vagina.

Kohli et al.[37] retrospectively compared two groups of patients, 27 who had undergone anterior colporrhaphy alone and 40 who underwent four-corner repair for anterior wall prolapse and concomitant genuine stress incontinence. The patients were a mixed group, with 28 of the 67 patients having undergone previous pelvic-floor surgery, including seven who had undergone previous bladder-neck surgery. The authors aimed to assess the degree of anterior-wall descent in the two groups postoperatively. After mean follow-up in both groups of 13 months (range 4-38 months), 7% of the anterior repair group had a recurrent cystocele compared with 33% of the four-corner repair group. This was a statistically significant difference and indicated that needle suspension did not add further support to the anterior repair. It does not appear that this procedure has any real advantages over a standard anterior colporrhaphy.

COMPLICATIONS OF ANTERIOR WALL SURGERY

Direct complications with these procedures remain rare. An injury rate of 0.5–2.0% of cases has been reported.[38] Obviously, damage to the bladder and urethra at the time of operation has been described. These are easily corrected surgically and, apart from the need for continuous urinary drainage for ten days, are unlikely to have any long-term consequences. The use of non-absorbable suture material is uncommon and should minimise complications secondary to suture placement into the lumen of the bladder. Recurrent urinary tract infections secondary to penetration of the bladder wall with chromic suture material have been reported. Diagnosis with the help of ultrasound or at the time of cystoscopy is easily achieved. Removal at the time of cystoscopy should be straightforward.[39]

In an assessment of urinary function after colporrhaphy, Stanton et al.[22] demonstrated a reduction in the symptoms of urge and stress and a resolution of the presenting symptoms. These patients had no alteration in flow rate, maximum voiding pressure or residual urine and no increase in detrusor instability.[22] However, in an earlier report from a tertiary practice, Delaere et al.[40] reviewed a series of 85 women referred after having developed complications as a result of anterior vaginal repair. Iatrogenic or persistent urinary stress incontinence occurred in 72% of the women. In addition, 40% had bladder-outlet obstruction and 25% had detrusor instability. Of this entire group, 23% were troubled by recurrent urinary tract infections.[40] One can assume that the paravaginal repairs will mirror the complications of their abdominal and vaginal counterparts. On purely theoretical grounds the abdominal approach could cause a denervation injury to the bladder,[41] which could produce detrusor instability.

It would seem that because of a paucity of information about the true complication rates and reluctance on the part of the patients to complain, the size of the problem might be underestimated.

SUMMARY

The anatomical alterations that lead to vaginal prolapse are starting to be better understood and applied by surgeons. A number of different operations have been described in the past to repair the anterior vaginal wall, the most common of which is still the anterior colporrhaphy. As a result of the anatomical studies described above, the role of the paravaginal repair has increased in prominence in the last 15 years. Unfortunately, the patient groups included in most of the available reports are so diverse in terms of previous surgery, the presence or absence of incontinence and the number of repair procedures performed concurrently, that any comparison of different surgical approaches is impossible. There is a need for a properly randomised study of anterior repair alone versus anterior repair with paravaginal repair and paravaginal repair alone. With the advent of the International Continence Society scoring system for prolapse[19] there is an opportunity to objectify the follow-up of prolapse surgery for the first time.

References

1. Emge, L.A., Durfee, R.B. Pelvic organ prolapse: four thousand years of treatment. *Clin Obstet Gynecol* 1966;**9**:997–1032
2. Kreutzmann, H.J. The uniform principle in performing operations for lacerated perineum, cystocele, rectocele and prolapse. *Am J Obstet Gynecol* 1902;**45**:359–65

3   Hurd, R.A. Observations and conclusions on plastic operations in gynaecology. *Am J Obstet Gynecol* 1929;**19**:633–40
4   White, G.R. Cystocele, a radical cure by suturing lateral sulci of vagina to white line of pelvic fascia. *JAMA* 1909;**53**:1707–10
5   Richardson, A.C., Edmonds, P.B., Williams, N.L. Treatment of stress urinary incontinence due to paravaginal fascial defect. *Obstet Gynecol* 1981;**57**:357–63
6   Bissell, D. A vaginal hysterectomy technique for the cure of prolapse of the uterus when the removal of the uterus is necessitated. *Surg Gynecol Obstet* 1918;**28**:138–45
7   Weinstein, M., Roberts, M. Simultaneous repair of cystocoele and high rectal prolapse during total hysterectomy. *West J Surg Obstet Gynecol* 1949;Jan:34–7
8   Masters, W.H. The abdominal approach to cystourethrocele repair. *Am J Obstet Gynecol* 1954;**67**:85–91
9   Spiers, R.E. The abdominal approach for repair of a cystocele. *Surg Obstet Gynecol* 1956;**102**:245–7
10 Macer, G.A. Transabdominal repair of cystocele. *West J Surg Obstet Gynecol* 1961;**69**:182–4
11 Weinberg, M.S., Stone, M.L. Abdominal cystocele repair. *Obstet Gynecol* 1963;**21**:117–21
12 Macer, G.A. Transabdominal repair of cystocele, a 20-year experience, compared with the traditional vaginal approach. *Am J Obstet Gynecol* 1978;**131**:203–7
13 Goetsch, C. Suprapubic vesicourethral suspension as a primary means of correcting stress incontinence and cystocele. *West J Surg Obstet Gynecol* 1954;**62**:201–4
14 Raz, S., Little, N.A., Juma, S., Sussmen, E.M. Repair of severe anterior vaginal wall prolapse. *J Urol* 1991;**146**:988–92
15 Shull, R.L., Benn, S.J., Kuehl, T.J. Surgical management of prolapse of the anterior vaginal segment: an analysis of support defects, operative morbidity and anatomic outcome. *Am J Obstet Gynecol* 1994;**171**:1429–39
16 Delancey, J.O.L. Anatomic aspects of vaginal eversion after hysterectomy. *Am J Obstet Gynecol* 1992;**166**:1717–28
17 Richardson, A.C., Lyons, J.B., Williams, N.L. A new look at pelvic relaxation. *Am J Obstet Gynecol* 1976;**126**:568–73
18 Bergman, A., Koonings, P.P., Ballard, C.A. Predicting postoperative urinary incontinence development in women undergoing operation for genitourinary prolapse. *Am J Obstet Gynecol* 1988;**158**:1171–5
19 Bump, R.C., Mattiasson, B.K., Brubaker, L.P., Delancey, J.O.L., Klarskov, P., Shull, B.L. et al. The standardization of terminology of female pelvic organ prolapse and pelvic floor dysfunction. *Am J Obstet Gynecol* 1996;**175**:10–17
20 Weber, A.M., Walters, M.D. Anterior vaginal prolapse: review of anatomy and techniques of surgical repair. *Obstet Gynecol* 1997;**89**:311–18
21 Porges, R.F., Smilen, S.W. Long-term analysis of the surgical management of pelvic support defects. *Am J Obstet Gynecol* 1994;**171**:1518–28
22 Stanton, S.L., Norton, C., Cardozo, L. Clinical and urodynamic effects of anterior colporrhaphy and vaginal hysterectomy for prolapse with and without incontinence. *Br J Obstet Gynaecol* 1982;**89**:459–63
23 Moore, J., Armstrong, J.T., Wills, S.H. The use of tantalum mesh in cystocele with critical report of ten cases. *Am J Obstet Gynecol* 1955;**69**:1127–35
24 Friedman, E.A., Meltzer, R.M. Collagen mesh prosthesis for repair of endopelvic fascial defects. *Am J Obstet Gynecol* 1970;**106**:430–3
25 Rosing, U., Fianu, S., Larsson, B. A new surgical technique for repairing cystocoele in hysterectomised women. *J Gynecol Surg* 1990;**6**:281–5

26   Zacharin, R.F. Free full-thickness vaginal epithelium graft in correction of recurrent genital prolapse. *Aust N Z J Obstet Gynaecol* 1992;**32**:146–8
27   Julian, T.M. The efficacy of Marlex mesh in the repair of severe recurrent vaginal prolapse of the anterior midvaginal wall. *Am J Obstet Gynecol* 1996;**175**:1472–5
28   Ulmsten, U., Falconer, C., Johnson, P., Jomaa, M., Lanner, L., Nilsson, C.G. *et al.* A multicenter study of tension-free vaginal tape for surgical treatment of stress urinary incontinence. *Int Urogynecol J Pelvic Floor Dysfunct* 1998;**9**:210–13
29   Iglesia, C.B., Fenner, D.E., Brubaker, L. The use of mesh in gynecologic surgery. *Int Urogynecol J Pelvic Floor Dysfunct* 1997;**8**:105–15
30   Morgan, J.E., Farrow, G.A., Stewart, F.E. The Marlex sling operation for the treatment of recurrent stress urinary incontinence: a 16-year review. *Am J Obstet Gynecol* 1985;**151**:224–6
31   Shull, B.L., Baden, W.F. A six year experience with paravaginal defect repair for stress urinary incontinence. *Am J Obstet Gynecol* 1989;**160**:1432–40
32   Scotti, R.J., Garely, A.D., Greston, W.M., Flora, R.F., Olson, T.R. Paravaginal repair of lateral vaginal wall defects by fixation to the ischial periosteum and obturator membrane. *Am J Obstet Gynecol* 1998;**179**:1436–45
33   Benson, J.T., Lucente, V., McClellan, E. Vaginal versus abdominal reconstructive surgery for the treatment of pelvic support defects: a prospective randomised study with long-term outcome evaluation. *Am J Obstet Gynecol* 1996;**175**:1418–22
34   Monga, A. Fascia: defects and repair. *Curr Opin Obstet Gynecol* 1996;**8**:366–71
35   Raz, S., Klutke, C.G., Golomb, J. Four-corner bladder and urethral suspension for moderate cystocoele. *J Urol* 1989;**142**:712–15
36   Miyazaki, F.S., Miyazaki, D.W. Raz four-corner suspension for severe cystocoele: poor results. *Int Urogynaecol J* 1994;**5**:94–7
37   Kohli, N., Sze, E.H.M., Todd, W.R., Karram, M.M. Incidence of recurrent cystocoele after anterior colporrhaphy with and without concomitant transvaginal needle suspension. *Am J Obstet Gynecol* 1996;**175**:1476–82
38   Spirnak, J.P., Resnick, M.I. Intraoperative consultation for the bladder. *Urol Clin North Am* 1985;**12**:439–46
39   Neuman, M., Alon, H., Langer, R., Golan, A., Bukovsky, I., Caspi, E. *et al.* Recurrent urinary tract infections in the presence of intravesical suture material after vaginal hysterectomy and anterior colporrhaphy. *Aust N Z J Obstet Gynaecol* 1990;**30**:184–5
40   Delaere, K.P.J., Moonen, W.A., Debruyne, F.M.J., Michiels, H.G., Renders, G.A. Anterior vaginal repair: cause of troublesome voiding disorders? *Eur Urol* 1979;**5**:190–4
41   Brading, A.F., Turner, W.H. The unstable bladder: towards a common mechanism. *Br J Urol* 1994;**73**:3–8

8

Understanding health economic terms with reference to infertility

Bolarinde Ola and Masoud Afnan

Health economics is the study of how to prioritise the allocation of scarce resources in health care. This definition generally implies the choice between or among alternative treatments in order to gain the most benefit. However, it may at other times imply the choice of the next best outcome, in order to make the most rational use of scarce resources. For other conditions still, economic analyses may dictate a little more of treatment A in favour of a little less of treatment B. Economic analyses in health care can be considered from many points of view, including those of the patient, the physician or surgeon, pharmaceutical companies, taxpayers and the Government. Cost evaluation can be complex and some might even argue that it is unending, especially when total disease burden, disability life year adjustments and other external factors are included in the equations. It is therefore important, for whatever method used, to define the scope and state at the onset, from whose point of view the economic analysis is being performed.

COSTS AND DEFINITIONS

Cost is the focal point of all economic analyses. Costs of interventions can be fixed or variable, real or intangible. Real costs can be direct or indirect.

(1) Fixed costs are incurred irrespective of the outcome in the short term (in the long term, fixed costs can change with, for example, the prevailing rate of inflation or general improvement in services provided).

(2) Variable costs depend upon factors such as the type and duration of treatment and outcome. For example, with *in vitro* fertilisation (IVF), variable costs are less when no pregnancy results than when a pregnancy is achieved. Similarly, costs incurred may be greater when complication arises.

(3) Direct costs are expenditures made in precise monetary terms, for example, bus or taxi fares to hospital, drugs and appliances, lodging and catering.

(4) Indirect costs are monetary expenditures incurred due to absence from work or for part-time replacements.

(5) Intangible costs are subjective measures of suffering, disability, family feuds and social stigma. In many ethnic groups, infertility can disrupt the family. A childless woman is exposed to ridicule by in-laws.

(6) The total cost is the sum of the fixed and variable costs.

(7) The average cost is the total cost divided by the number of interventions or by the number of outcomes. The choice of denominator depends on the type and dimension of clinical outcome (see below).

QUALITY OF LIFE

Many indices have been described to measure the economics of the social burden and intangible costs of disease. Questionnaires are popular methods of assessing suffering from disease.[1-3] The Short Form (SF-36) general health questionnaire is an adequately validated example. Another method of assessing quality of life places health preference values on disease conditions. This can be done by several methods. One method is the 'time trade-off assessment' whereby patients are asked how many health-years they wish to trade off for being cured of their disease. An alternative method is the 'rating scale', with death at one end and perfect health at the other. The patient is asked to mark where their condition (for example infertility) is located on the scale. The 'standard gamble method'[4] has some similarities to the rating scale. The difference is that the patient is given varying probabilities of cure and asked to rate the strength of his decision to undertake treatment that would kill him if it failed or restore him to perfect health if successful.

A commonly used measure is the disability-adjusted life year (DALY), a World Bank tool used in estimating and comparing healthy life years lost due to the disability of various diseases.[5-7] Infertility is not given deserved prominence on these indices, being relegated to the bottom of the list of priorities and funding. It is therefore not surprising that most governmental and non-governmental organisations regard infertility as a disease without physical suffering or disability.

BENEFITS

Benefits can be categorised as economic, clinical, disability adjustment or improvement in the quality of life. Clinical benefit may be considered as either incremental or absolute. Examples of clinical benefit in infertility include induced ovulation rate, fertilisation and implantation rates, pregnancy and live-birth rates. Economic benefits would include a reduction in hospital visits, an early return to paid work and avoidance of hospitalisation. Quality of life is improved by a reduction in pain and suffering, improved mobility and, for infertility, eradication of social stigma.

Increments in benefit are useful when the effectiveness of two or more outcomes is being compared. Assuming that a randomised controlled trial shows that intervention A leads to a pregnancy rate of 25% and intervention B to 30%, the absolute treatment effect (ATE) is 5% or 0.05 or 1 in 20. This clinical 'bottom line' means that for every 20 interventions, one extra pregnancy is gained by using intervention B in preference to intervention A. This is referred to as number needed to treat (NNT), derived by inverting ATE.

AVERAGE COST EQUATIONS

The most appropriate average cost equation (whether cost minimisation, cost utility, cost benefit or cost consequence analyses) for a clinical scenario is chosen depending on whether the important outcome is one-dimensional or multidimensional or whether two or more interventions produced identical outcomes or whether the outcomes are disputed or subject to probability of change.

Cost minimisation

When all interventions produce exactly the same important outcome, this is an appropriate economic equation. This equation converts all interventions into the same monetary terms and compares the direct cost per intervention in one condition with another, in order to determine how to minimise costs. In clinical practice, however, this equation is seldom useful because no two conditions produce identical outcomes, especially when adverse effects and complications are taken into consideration. To illustrate, two procedures for treating proximal fallopian tubal blockage are compared. Assume that selective salpingography and tubal catheterisation (SS), an outpatient two-in-one procedure, costs £500 and has a success rate of 15%. This is the same as hysteroscopic tubal catheterisation (HC), a day-case operative procedure costing £700 but requiring a preliminary diagnostic hysterosalpingography (HSG), which costs £300. Cost minimisation shows not only that SS is cheaper but also that it involves fewer visits to hospital or procedures.

Cost benefit analysis

This is an economic analysis that converts clinical effects into the same monetary terms as the cost and compares total cost of achieving an outcome event in one condition with another. Cost benefit analyses in infertility, for example, help in comparing the total costs of achieving a pregnancy (or other stated event) by one method (tubal surgery) with another (IVF).

Cost utility

When interventions produced a multidimensional important outcome, cost utility equation converts effects into some health preferences (or utility) and describes the costs for some additional health gain.[8] Health preferences are usually estimated using any of the methods described above for quality-of-life assessment.[9] Therefore:

(1) Cost utility = Net cost of treatment/DALYs gained, where DALYs = number of health years, free from disability gained following treatment;

(2) Net cost = Total cost of treatment, including complications − cost saved from averting diseased state

To illustrate, assume that a study carried out in Asian communities in the UK, using time trade-off questionnaires, shows that azoospermic men would trade, on average, five healthy years for the cure of their condition by intracytoplasmic sperm injection (ICSI), but only 0.5 years to be cured by donor insemination (assuming that donor insemination has an overall clinical pregnancy rate of 15% and major complication rate of 2% and ICSI a success rate of 27% and major complication rate of 10%). If 100 patients each undergo donor insemination, at a cost of £400 per cycle, and ICSI at £3000, Table 1 shows a hypothetical cost utility analysis. The social stigma attached to the use of donor sperm is responsible for the high cost utility of donor insemination shown in this example. Therefore, when social and other intangible factors surrounding the use of donor gametes are considered, ICSI is clearly preferred despite its exorbitant monetary cost.

Table 1 *Comparison of cost utility between donor insemination (DI) and intracytoplasmic sperm injection (ICSI) in 100 men with azoospermia*

Gain/loss	DI	ICSI
Gain (preventing adverse outcomes)	£400 × 15 = £6000	£3000 × 27 = £81 000
Losses (from failed outcomes)	£400 × 85 = £34 000	£3000 × 73 = £219 000
Losses (treating direct major complications, e.g. ectopic, ovarian hyperstimulation syndrome at an average cost of £200 per case)	£2000 × 2 = £4000	£2000 × 10 = £20 000
Disability adjusted life years gained from successful outcome	0.5 × 15 = 7.5 years	5 × 27 = 135 years
Cost utility (net cost/disability adjusted life years gained)	£38 000/7.5 = £5067	£239 000/135 = £1770

Cost consequence analysis (decision analysis)

When outcome events are subject to variable influences or are not clear-cut, a cost benefit equation is applied at every stage, following sensitivity analysis to build an algorithm depicting different 'what-if scenarios'. For example, assume that using drug C will induce ovulation in 60% of patients and cost benefit analysis shows that each induced ovulation costs £200. If, however, in obese patients, drug C is combined with agent M at £60 per course, the success rate (based on evidence from published literature), may improve to 75% and, in one-third of those who still fail to respond to medical option 2, surgical intervention D, which costs £850, will be likely to succeed (based on local experience). A cost consequence analysis will be aimed at showing decision pathways and whether they are associated with increased or decreased spending per induced ovulation. Cost consequence analysis is frequently incorporated into the Markov's model.[10]

The Markov's model is used to describe a hypothetical cohort of patients moving from one state of health to another, in time frames referred to as Markov's cycles. In infertility, the Markov's cycle can be conveniently considered as the average duration of one menstrual cycle, set within a time limit of, for example 18 months. This should be described at the onset of a study. At the junction of each cycle, sensitivity followed by cost benefit or cost effectiveness analyses are performed, based on reasonable variations in important outcome events or, better still, variations previously defined in robust peer-reviewed studies.

Cost effectiveness analysis

Cost effectiveness analysis or incremental cost effectiveness ratio (ICER) is strictly not an average cost equation because the numerator is incremental rather than total cost and the denominator is the difference in, rather than total, health gain (or losses). It is an equation that converts clinical effects into health gains (or losses) and compares the incremental costs between interventions for achieving one additional health gain (or loss). This is the most appropriate equation when necessary to compare the effects of two different interventions where the important outcome is one-dimensional. It helps planners determine the best compromise in the use of scarce resources, within the boundaries of acceptable event rates. The most effective intervention may therefore not necessarily be the most cost effective.

Cost needed to treat

Cost needed to treat (CNT) is the cost needed to gain one additional health benefit. It is easily derived from NNT, the number needed to prevent one additional adverse outcome. Conversely, cost needed to harm can be derived from number needed to harm (NNH). NNT and NNH are common output measurements of randomised controlled trials. Numerically, CNT is equal to ICER, as demonstrated below.

ATE = Event rate from control intervention A (CER) minus event rate from experimental intervention B (EER), which can be expressed as

$$ATE = CER - EER$$

Number Needed to Treat (NNT) = The number of people needed to be treated with an intervention A to prevent one additional adverse outcome over that from use of an intervention B, which can be expressed as

$$NNT = 1/(CER - EER) = 1/ATE$$

As
Cost Needed to Treat (CNT)

= (Difference in total costs between two interventions) × NNT
= (Difference in total costs between two interventions) ÷ ATE

And
Incremental Cost Effectiveness Ratio (ICER)

= (Difference in total costs between two interventions) ÷ (CER − EER)
= (Difference in total costs between two interventions) ÷ ATE

Therefore, CNT = ICER

COST BENEFIT OR COST EFFECTIVENESS?

Cost benefit has occasionally been used synonymously with cost effectiveness, without due consideration for the essential criteria in the definition of the latter.[11-13] To illustrate the difference between cost benefit and cost effectiveness equations, refer back to the hypothetical clinical scenario above, where intervention A leads to a pregnancy rate of 25% and intervention B to 30%. The absolute treatment effect is 5% or 0.05. This means that for every 20 interventions, one extra benefit is gained by using intervention B in preference to intervention A. Assuming that intervention A costs £2000 and intervention B £2200 per cycle of treatment, it will cost £200,000/25 (or £8000) and £220,000/30 (or £7333), respectively, per pregnancy produced. This is cost benefit analysis, showing that costs are less per pregnancy produced by the more effective intervention B. An incremental cost effectiveness analysis will, however, show that for every additional pregnancy gained by intervention B, £200 × 20 (or £4000) has been spent over what would have been expended on a choice of intervention A. In a political scenario, where resources are scarce and there is pressure for as many as possible to get a slice of the cake, intervention A is clearly going to be better favoured, because the pregnancy rate of 25% is within the expected event range for the condition described.

CONCLUSION

Cost evaluation can be complex and such analysis may vary depending on the point of view when it was performed. Valid health economic equations can be seen from different points of view. For example, one drug company might use cost per pregnancy achieved (a cost-benefit equation) in order to advertise intervention B; whereas another would emphasise incremental cost effectiveness ratio to promote intervention A. A surgeon vastly experienced in procedure SS may present his budget to the hospital board using simple cost utility to show its advantage per finished consultant episode, whereas another surgeon might deliver a superb decision analysis that favours procedure HC in the long term.

References

1   Gill, T.M., Feinstein, A.R. A critical appraisal of the quality of quality of life measurements. *JAMA* 1994;**272**:619–26

2. Hickey, A.M., Bury, G., O'Boyle, C.A, Bradley, F., O'Kelly, F.D., Shannon, A. A new short-form individual quality of life measure (SEIQoL-DW): application in a cohort of individuals with HIV/AIDS. *BMJ* 1996;**313**:29–33
3. Cairns, J. Measuring health outcomes. *BMJ* 1996;**313**:6
4. Krabbe, P.F.M., Essink-Bot, M-L., Bonsel, G.K. On the equivalence of collectively and individually collected responses: standard-gamble and time trade-off judgements of health status. *Med Decis Making* 1996;**16**:120–32
5. Barker, C., Green, A. Opening the debate on DALYs. *Health Policy Plan* 1996;**11**:179–83
6. Hyder, A.A., Rotllant, G., Morrow, R.H. Measuring the burden of disease: healthy life years. *Am J Public Health* 1998;**88**:196–202
7. Bowie, C., Beck, S., Bevan, G., Raftery, J., Silverton, F., Steven, A. Estimating the burden of disease in an English region. *J Public Health Med* 1997;**19**:687–92
8. Cochrane glossary. *The Cochrane Library*, Issue 2. Oxford: Update Software; 1998
9. Forbes, R.B., Lees, A., Waugh, N., Swingler, R.J. Population based cost utility study of interferon beta-1b in secondary progressive multiple sclerosis *BMJ* 1999;**319**:1529–33
10. Beck, J.R., Pauker, S.G. The Markov process in medical prognoses. *Med Decis Making* 1983;**3**:419–58
11. Ola, B., Afnan, M., Hammadieh, N, Daya, S., Gunby, J. Recombinant versus urinary FSH for ovarian stimulation in assisted reproduction. *Hum Reprod* 2000;15:1208–9
12. Goldfarb, J.M., Austin, C., Lisbona, H., Peskin, B., Clapp, M. Cost-effectiveness of *in-vitro* fertilisation. *Obstet Gynecol* 1996;**87**:18–21
13. Greenhalgh, T. How to read a paper: papers that tell you what things cost (economic analyses). *BMJ* 1997;**315**:596–9

9

Cost effectiveness and infertility

Masoud Afnan and Bolarinde Ola

INTRODUCTION

The aim of this chapter is to propose principles by which an infertility programme can be most efficiently organised. It is hoped that this will be useful to purchasers and providers alike.

The chapter is written from the perspective of the National Health Service (NHS) in the UK. The goal of the NHS is 'to secure through the resources available, the greatest improvement in the physical and mental health of people in England'.[1] One of the motivations behind Professor Archie Cochrane's treatise was concern over the spiralling costs of medical inflation that he foresaw. Cochrane wrote: 'the development of effective health care needs hard evidence, preferably from randomised trials, that the use of each technology either alters the natural history of disease or otherwise benefits many patients at a reasonable cost'.[2] In the UK, the NHS is, by statute, free at the point of delivery to all. This is not the case for infertility in the year 2000. Techniques are used to circumvent this statutory obligation, all of which serve to dissimulate this fact. It is the duty of purchasers and providers alike to rise above expediency, to ensure that patients receive the best possible service available. This is the cornerstone of clinical governance and the basis for using economic evaluations in clinical practice.

THE IMPACT OF NEW TECHNOLOGIES

The treatment of infertility has made phenomenal progress over the past 25 years. New techniques have been introduced (*in vitro* fertilisation, IVF, in 1978;[3] intrauterine insemination, IUI, in 1986;[4] and intracytoplasmic sperm injection, ICSI, in 1992[5]). These techniques have revolutionised the opportunity for intervention and offered successful treatment where none was previously available. As a result of the success associated with the treatment of specific patient groups, the new technologies have often been applied to other patients indiscriminately. An analysis of the economic benefits is helpful in identifying which techniques should be applied to which patients.

Additionally, as new treatment options have become available through new technologies or more accessible through cost reductions, so there has had to be a drastic re-evaluation of the diagnostic process. This has taken place in a haphazard and inconsistent way. Two studies have highlighted the inconsistencies in the diagnostic process. In a survey from the USA,[6] anomalies were found such as female physicians ordering two to three times more cervical cultures than their male colleagues, serum hormone estimations more commonly ordered by younger physicians and more investigations ordered in private practice. A similar survey of teaching hospitals in Europe also revealed considerable inconsistencies.[7] Of specific interest in this survey, given the costs and the invasiveness of the procedures, is the range of investigators who performed routine hysterosalpingography (14-100%) and routine laparoscopy (14-100%) in the investigation of the infertile couple.

Similar variations exist among clinicians when determining the treatment of choice for a couple within a diagnostic category. For example, tubal disease can be treated either by tubal surgery or IVF. Superficially, the choice of treatment depends on the severity of the disease and the likely chance of achieving a pregnancy with either treatment. However, availability and access to treatment depends on a number of other factors. First is the pattern of reimbursement (in the UK, tubal surgery is invariably funded, whereas IVF is not) and second is the expertise of the operator. As training focuses increasingly on assisted conception, fewer specialists are trained in tubal surgery.[8,9] The same variation can be found in treating male factor, anovulation, uterine disease, etc. The patient, therefore, receives a service based upon their postal code, a fact for which politicians are often criticised but not clinicians.

BENEFITS OF USING HEALTH ECONOMIC EVALUATIONS IN CLINICAL PRACTICE

Health economic evaluations are:

(1) Stating explicit measurable aims and outcomes (effectiveness);

(2) Having an understanding of the costs of the process;

(3) Keeping abreast of developments;

(4) Leading to sensible treatment paradigms;

(5) Able to implement change;

(6) Monitor the effects of that change.

DETERMINING THE OUTCOME MEASURES (THE NUMERATOR)

The most important outcome must be that which the patients, the group whom we serve, seek. As a secondary and tertiary referral centre we surveyed 100 consecutive couples who attended an infertility clinic and asked them to identify, out of four options, what was the most important reason for them attending the infertility clinic (Table 1). The implications of this are that, while other outcomes are considered, for the vast majority the main outcome should be a baby.

There are a number of additional measures that can be considered as part of the process. The following have been determined in consultation with a number of local stakeholders in Birmingham – the health authority, GP representatives, patient representatives, clinicians and hospital managers.

(1) All patients should have access to GPs for primary-care provision of infertility services as defined by the Royal College of Obstetricians and Gynaecologists;

Table 1 *Choice of options for attending an infertility clinic*

Option	% chosen
Become pregnant and have a baby	83
Find out what is wrong	7
Be given a prognosis	8
Screen for other potential problems	2

(2) All patients should have access to secondary care to establish a working diagnosis and to be offered counselling. This should include an understanding of what is wrong, the treatment options available, the chances of conceiving with and without treatment, and whether there are any other conditions (non-infertility) to be diagnosed, prevented or treated (e.g. long-term risk of endometrial hyperplasia in patients with polycystic ovaries);

(3) All patients in the appropriate diagnostic categories should be offered treatment for anovulation (without recourse to assisted conception); for example clomiphene, insulin-sensitising agents[10] and laparoscopic ovarian diathermy;

(4) Patients within certain specific social, demographic and clinical criteria should be allowed access to tertiary care, including tubal surgery, artificial insemination and IVF;

(5) Although the funding available for infertility is capped, the outcome measures should be achievable, sustainable and allow for further development if funds are forthcoming;

(6) A waiting list, which is clearly untenable, should not develop. It is recognised that fecundity declines with advancing age, and so to have a waiting list of over two years, for example, is clearly detrimental;

(7) Within the above political and financial parameters the most efficient (the cheapest) and effective (the most number of live births) service should be provided;

(8) A system of primary, secondary and tertiary care that is co-ordinated to carry out the above paradigm and capable of being audited both internally and by external agencies should be established.

In addition, the following have been agreed, due to limiting financial factors, even though there is some merit in them and they would otherwise have been desirable outcomes:

(1) Not to offer treatment unless there is a reasonable (realistic) chance of success. It is recognised, however, that many couples feel better after having had 'a go' at treatment, even if they understand that the chances of conception are extremely low. Counselling is obviously crucial with these couples;

(2) Not to offer couples an equal chance of getting pregnant. Thus, a patient with hydrosalpinges who is undergoing IVF is known to have a reduced chance of conceiving by approximately 50% compared with one who does not have hydrosalpinges but is not offered double the number of treatments.[11]

EVALUATING OUTCOMES – THE IMPORTANCE OF THE DENOMINATOR

If we accept that a live birth is the appropriate outcome or numerator, what is the denominator? It is often presented as the number of treatment cycles (such as the number of IVF cycles). However, this is to ignore a number of confounding variables. The denominator should be a clearly defined population.

Background pregnancy rates

There is a significant background pregnancy rate[12-15] of approximately 1–2% per month or 12–15% per annum. The most important factors that affect the background pregnancy rate[16] are the female partner and duration of infertility.

The implications are two-fold. First, any intervention has to have significantly higher pregnancy rates than the background rate. Second, if patients are going to get pregnant anyway, why treat them? It is not an explicit outcome measure to expedite the time to pregnancy, which is the usual benefit of treating patients who have a high background chance of conceiving.

Dropout rates

In most disease states, there will be patients who commence the management process but who do not complete it. They are an important group to identify as they represent a significant use of resource which, if not accounted for, would be misleading as it would underestimate the costs. It also affords an opportunity to save money by reducing dropout rates if the factors that predispose to dropout can be identified. It is evidently important for the purposes of feedback to know why a couple does not complete the process (possibly dissatisfaction with the clinic). The final issue is one of wastage of resource and implications for the management paradigm. If there is a large dropout rate, say within three months of initial referral and before treatment can be offered, it does not make sense to perform expensive diagnostic tests which add only a little, if anything, to the diagnosis and the treatment paradigm. Dropout rates vary between 20-40%[17] and depend on a number of factors, including whether the patient is seen in a specialist or a general clinic. It is for this reason that it has been decided that infertility care should only be carried out in specialist infertility clinics, in line with the recommendation from the RCOG guidelines.[18]

The importance of assessing pregnancy rates by population and not by technique

The pregnancy rates quoted for a technique will vary according to the diagnostic category as well as the therapeutic options exercised prior to commencement of treatment.

For example, for 100 couples in whom the woman is under the age of 35 years, with unexplained infertility after one year of trying, the options available are to wait for a natural conception, consider clomiphene for six months, artificial (intrauterine) insemination (IUI) with the partner's sperm or IVF. The only controversial treatment would be clomiphene, for which the evidence is not convincing, although it is still advocated by many as an appropriate treatment. Assuming that the population to be treated has a high fertility potential – for example 80% of couples would be expected to conceive within two years of treatment and to go on to have a live birth – there are two treatment options.

Option 1: Treat all couples with IVF without waiting – say three cycles to achieve a cumulative live birth rate of 80% for three IVF cycles.

Option 2: Wait one year and perhaps 20 women will conceive naturally. Without considering clomiphene, offer three cycles of IUI and say another 30 couples conceive with this treatment – leaving 50 couples. If three cycles of IVF are now offered to the remaining 50 couples and if the fertility potential of the population (maximum 80) remains the same, the live-birth rate for three cycles of IVF has decreased from 80% to 30 of 50 or 60%. For the same overall pregnancy rate, the total cost of treatment for the population has decreased, even though the cumulative pregnancy rate for IVF as a technique appears lower.

This example demonstrates the pitfalls of looking at live-birth rates per technique without characterising the inclusion criteria of the population being treated. This is a concept that is common when performing studies. The inclusion criteria must be clearly defined.

Over treatment

There is a tendency to over treat couples complaining of infertility. The drivers behind this unusual situation are many and include:

(1) Increasing pressure from desperate infertile couples for whom each passing month without a pregnancy is a source of grief;

(2) Fear of the clinician that the treatment might fail, for example failed fertilisation at IVF (out of concern for the patient or out of concern for litigation);

(3) The need for clinics to demonstrate superior pregnancy rates to other clinics in a market that is competitive, both in the NHS and the private sector;

(4) The financial cost of failure in the private sector.

The restraints, on the other hand, are fewer and of less immediate importance: the increased costs overall and the risks of treatment (generally more with the more sophisticated expensive procedures). An interesting study by Karande et al.[19] compared the two treatment paradigms of moving straight to IVF or following the standard approach of artificial insemination prior to IVF in a well-defined population. In their study, the standard approach was the most cost effective.

OTHER COST CONSIDERATIONS

Population screening

Health economic evaluations can also be used for example to assess cost effectiveness of screening for chlamydia infection in an asymptomatic population to prevent future infertility or ectopic pregnancies.[20] Screening for high-risk populations and treatment of infertile couples is justified in some populations.[21] The costs of screening can be compared with the costs of a repeat intervention in the event of the first cycle of treatment failing. Thus, by using numbers needed to treat analysis, the cost of screening for sperm antibodies in an IVF programme to prevent one failure to fertilise was estimated. This was found to be less than a repeat cycle using ICSI and it was therefore not cost effective to screen for sperm antibodies.[22]

Type of clinic which should offer infertility services

Much of the whole process of infertility care (except for those few cases needing surgical intervention), can be offered in an exclusively outpatient setting, including IVF and ICSI, with access to inpatient care elsewhere. There will be occasional need for egg collection to be carried out in a hospital theatre to avoid complications of the procedure but happily these are rare. It may appear that to offer infertility services in a purely outpatient facility would be cheaper than offering it in a hospital setting with the attendant general overheads of inpatient care. There are three reasons why this is a false economy if treatment is transferred to a non-NHS facility. First, while the treatment takes place in a non-NHS facility, there is little or no control over the practices of that clinic, leaving the NHS to pick up the complications of treatment, such as multiple pregnancies etc. Second, essential to the future is responsible, supervised and monitored training of future infertility specialists. The infrastructure in the UK means this is best carried out in NHS trusts. Finally, moving the service out of an NHS facility only serves to drive up overhead and indirect costs for the other services. It may be that, in the future, the NHS will move towards outpatient specialist services in a managed way, of which infertility could be one.

UNDERSTANDING THE COSTS OF THE PROCESS

Cost effectiveness analysis is an important means of improving quality of care while controlling costs.[23] Costs can be reduced by altering work practices within a specific technique, such as IVF.[24–26] Monitoring of IVF cycles by ultrasound alone compared with ultrasound and hormonal measurements has been evaluated. Ultrasound monitoring alone proved to be cheaper, more convenient and less time consuming with no difference in the pregnancy rate.[27]

At the Birmingham Women's Hospital, clinicians have taken responsibility for understanding the costs (and income) of the infertility service. The benefits of this approach have been considerable and it is recommended. Some of the advantages of this approach are:

(1) Identifying areas in which the service is poorly run;

(2) Having hard financial data to correct injustices in the provision of services;

(3) Knowing if the service is a net gain or loss for the trust. If the service makes a loss, it is not sustainable and needs to be reorganised or discussions held with the stakeholders. With hard financial data, people are not only sympathetic, but also helpful. It is in no-one's interest to have a service that is not sustainable. If the service makes a 'profit', discussions can be held with the trust management as to how these profits can be best used;

(4) It will also encourage service developments, as it is easier to make the 'business case' for them. Some service developments will save money, which can be freed up to spend in other areas;

(5) It also allows a prioritisation based at least in part on the economic benefits of new developments.

While there must be a team approach to the management and financial control of the service, it is essential that the infertility specialist has a thorough grasp of principles and practice as a tool for good clinical care.

Keeping abreast of developments leading to sensible treatment paradigms

Clinical guidelines

Clinical guidelines are the systematically developed statements which assist the individual clinician and patient in making decisions about appropriate health care for specific conditions.[28]

Clinical guidelines are not new. There are numerous examples from history, from Hippocrates to Osler, of leading clinicians of the day who have put in writing specified clinical actions that follow as a result of the prevailing knowledge. What has changed is the explosion of medical knowledge and the need for a systematic approach to formalise these attempts to shape and alter behaviour. In addition, with the development of publicly funded health programmes, there has been a demand to ensure that all patients receive the best available care within specified constraints, such as finance. The benefits of clinical guidelines can be summarised as:

(1) To inform: synthesis and dissemination of knowledge;

(2) To bring about change: implementation of actions as a result of that knowledge.

The benefits of this simple paradigm are enormous. The process of health care can now be monitored. Effectiveness (of an intervention within a population) and efficiency (demonstrating a health benefit compared with other interventions) can be assessed and the process can be audited. Research can be directed and carried out within a strategic plan.

As a result, patient care is improved by either changing existing practices or developing new ones. There is an important caveat to these statements. Guidelines have a limited life, and are relevant only within a local setting. This fact acts as a reminder that even guidelines have to be justified and brought into local practice based on local conditions using the expertise available locally. Sir Miles Irvine has defined health technology as the 'method used by health professionals to promote health' and encompasses 'the evaluation of the benefits and costs (clinical, social, economic and system-wide) of transferring the technology of interest into clinical practice'.[29] Guidelines are themselves a technology and therefore need to be subjected to rigorous assessment.

The Royal College of Obstetricians and Gynaecologists has published detailed guidelines for the primary, secondary and tertiary care of the infertile couple. It is not within the scope of this review to list the recommendations, but Members and Fellows can access these guidelines through the RCOG or online at www.rcog.org.uk.

It now behoves each local provider of infertility services to determine how they are going to use these guidelines and to what end. It is inevitable that some members of the profession will have different views from those contained within the guidelines. However, the guidelines represent the views of some of the most respected and knowledgeable infertility experts and it would be inappropriate for any Member (or Fellow) of the RCOG to consider themselves above these guidelines. The question is not, 'should the guidelines be implemented' but how? Any variations should be predetermined with an explicit statement explaining the reason for the difference, such as local expertise or even as 'not cost effective'. The whole service, that within the guidelines and that without, then needs to be assessed. An example of how these guidelines have been used persuasively can be seen in an excellent report from Scotland (the EAGISS report), which can be found online at www.show.scot.nhs.uk/Publications/ME/eagiss.pdf.

Implementing and monitoring change: clinical audit

Clearly, clinical audit is critical.[30] As we wish to assess cost effectiveness, at the very minimum we need to monitor activity, the costs associated with that activity and achievment of the explicitly stated outcome measures (the standards). Other events we may wish to measure are adherence to pre-agreed protocols, variations from the protocol with indications and, if there have been differences from the guidelines, some sort of comparison of outcome.

The next step is the most difficult: effecting a change in clinical behaviour.[31] This is the step which usually does not happen. There are two main reasons for this: lack of input from the clinican and fear of change. Clinicians clearly have to be involved in the process at an early stage.[32] The clinicians should really be driving the process, although lack of trust and fear of change are perhaps some reasons why they do not. It is always tempting to preserve the *status quo* to keep stability and spend energies on maintaining the strongest defensive structure possible, instead of moving forward.[33] Organisations that grow acknowledge that growth involves disequilibrium rather than solidity. Organisational equilibrium is a sure path to institutional death.[34] While change is essential, so too is audit, to ensure that when mistakes are made they are recognised, lessons learned, and more changes made.

COST EFFECTIVENESS STUDIES

Diagnostic tests

There is much debate and variation as to what diagnostic tests should be carried out.[6,7]

Semen analyses have a poor positive predictive value but a strong negative predictive value; that is to say that a normal semen analysis is not a good predictor of fertility but azoospermia is a strong predictor of infertility.[35] Normal sperm morphology of less than 5% is associated with a significant failure to fertilise at IVF.[36] The routine measurement of sperm antibodies is not recommended by the RCOG, as there is little conclusive evidence of their predictive value.[37] However, fertilisation rates do seem to be impaired in IVF if the antibodies are present in significant amounts.[38] Advanced sperm function tests are not advocated in routine use but do have a place in the hands of specialists.[39,40] The post-coital test is a poorly carried out and reproducible test, with poor predictive value,[41,42] and is not recommended by the RCOG in its guidelines. However, a recent study has suggested its usefulness in those couples with less than three years duration of infertility as a predictor of natural conception.[43]

In women with irregular cycles there clearly needs to be a full endocrine investigation as advocated in the RCOG guidelines to determine the cause. In women with regular cycles, advanced testing over and above a single midluteal-phase progesterone level is of no value.[44]

The assessment of uterine disease is not advocated routinely in the RCOG guidelines. Despite the self-evident need for a uterus with an intact uterine cavity and the relative ease by which it is assessed, either by hysterosalpingogram (HSG), hysteroscopy or hysterosonogram at the same time as assessing tubal patency, the prevalence of uterine abnormalities in women with no prior significant history or abnormal examination findings is low.[45,46]

Controversy still exists about the most cost-effective test of assessing tubal patency. In the absence of an abnormality in the history or the examination, it would appear that an HSG is a useful cost-effective screening procedure.[47] In the event of a normal HSG, the likelihood of finding significant abnormalities at laparoscopy are low.[48] Selective salpingography is probably the best method of diagnosing proximal tubal patency.[49] In practice, other factors such as expertise and the facilities available to the infertility specialist will determine the method of investigation.

Treatment

Anovulation is treated successfully according to the cause.[50] For patients with polycystic ovaries, treatment with insulin-sensitising agents such as metformin and clomiphene are cost effective.[51] In clomiphene-resistant patients, laparoscopic ovarian diathermy is also useful, especially in patients with a good prognosis, such as those in which the luteinising hormone level is raised.[52] It is also associated with a lower miscarriage rate than with gonadotrophins. Various gonadotrophin induction regimens have been proposed[53] but all are associated with high miscarriage rates. One study compared ovulation induction with IVF[54] in clomiphene-resistant patients. IVF was found to be more cost effective.

Severe endometriosis and tubal disease are best treated by IVF, whereas mild and possibly moderate disease should be treated with surgery.[14,51,55] Considered overall, IVF is at least as cost effective as surgery.[23,56]

Mild or moderate sperm dysfunction can be treated effectively with stimulated intrauterine insemination[51,56,57] and is more cost effective than IVF. Severe male factor is treated by donor insemination or ICSI.[51,58] Donor insemination is more cost effective than ICSI, although it is not as acceptable.[58] Reversal of vasectomy is a cost-effective option compared with ICSI in vasectomised males.[59]

Perhaps the treatment of unexplained infertility has been the most scrutinised of all the infertility diagnostic categories. This is because there is no specific pathology to treat and treatment is aimed at increasing fecundity. In addition, there are a number of treatment options available. It is also difficult to consider cost effectiveness in isolation. Thus a couple in which the woman is 38 years of age will have different priorities than one in which the woman is 28 years of age, especially if they wish to have more than one child. However, cost-effectiveness analysis is helpful to inform choice and allows health purchasers and providers alike to determine appropriate care pathways. In a retrospective study of the 45 reports in the literature by Guzick and colleagues, clomiphene citrate combined with intrauterine insemination was found to be the most cost effective option, even though it had the lowest pregnancy rate per cycle and was not significantly different from the background pregnancy rate. Conversely, IVF was found to have the highest pregnancy rate per cycle but to be the least cost effective.[60]

Perinatal costs of treatment

These are significant and pale into insignificance the costs of infertility treatment itself.[61] Many of the costs are associated with multiple pregnancy and every effort must be made to prevent triplets and higher-order births.[62,63]

CONCLUSION

The cost-effective approach is a useful tool in the purchase and provision of infertility services, leading to sensible treatment paradigms and making the best use of limited available resources.

References

1   Lakhani, A. The role of outcomes assessment in improving clinical effectiveness. In: Deighan, M., Hitch, S., editors. *Clinical Effectiveness: From Guidelines to Cost-effective Practice*. Manchester: Earlybrave Publications; 1995. p. 39–44
2   Cochrane, A. *Effectiveness and Efficiency. Random Reflections on Health Services*. London: Nuffield Provincial Hospitals Trust; 1972
3   Steptoe, P.C., Edwards, R.G. Birth after the reimplantation of a human embryo. *Lancet* 1978;**ii**:366
4   Lalich, R.A., Marut, E.L., Prins, G.S., Scommegna, A. Life table analysis of intrauterine insemination pregnancy rates. *Am J Obstet Gynecol* 1988;**158**:980–4
5   Palermo, G., Joris, H., Devroey, P., Van Steirteghem, A.C. Pregnancies after intracytoplasmic injection of single spermatozoon into an oocyte. *Lancet* 1992;**340**:17–18
6   Glatstein, I.Z., Harlow, B.L., Hornstein, M.D. Practice patterns among reproductive endocrinologists: the infertility evaluation. *Fertil Steril* 1997;**67**:443–51
7   Helmerhorst, F.M., Oei, S.G., Bloemenkamp, K.W., Keirse, M.J. Consistency and variation in fertility investigations in Europe. *Hum Reprod* 1995;**10**:2027–30
8   Lilford, R.J., Watson, A.J. Has *in vitro* fertilization made salpingostomy obsolete? *Br J Obstet Gynaecol* 1990;**97**:557–60
9   Winston, R.M., Margara. R.A. Microsurgical salpingostomy is not an obsolete procedure. *Br J Obstet Gynaecol* 1991;**98**:637–42
10 Mitwally, M.F., Kuscu, N.K., Yalcinkaya, T.M. High ovulatory rates with use of troglitazone in clomiphene-resistant women with polycystic ovary syndrome. *Hum Reprod* 1999;**14**:2700–3
11 Strandell, A., Waldenstrom, U., Nilsson, L., Hamberger, L. Hydrosalpinx reduces *in-vitro* fertilization/embryo transfer pregnancy rates. *Hum Reprod* 1994;**9**:861–3
12 Collins, J.A., Burrows, E.A., Wilan, A.R. The prognosis for live birth among untreated infertile couples. *Fertil Steril* 1995;**64**:22–8

13 Snick, H.K., Snick, T.S., Evers, J.L., Collins, J.A. The spontaneous pregnancy prognosis in untreated subfertile couples: the Walcheren primary care study. Hum Reprod 1997;**12**:1582–8
14 Tulandi, T., Collins, J.A., Burrows, E., Jarrell, J.F., McInnes, R.A., Wrixon, W. et al. Treatment-dependent and treatment-independent pregnancy among women with periadnexal adhesions. Am J Obstet Gynecol 1990;**162**:354–7
15 Gleicher, N., VanderLaan, B., Pratt, D., Karande, V. Background pregnancy rates in an infertile population. Hum Reprod 1996;**11**:1011–12
16 Collins, J.A., Rowe, T.C. Age of the female partner is a prognostic factor in prolonged unexplained infertility: a multicenter study. Fertil Steril 1989;**52**:15–20
17 Gleicher, N., Vanderlaan, B., Karande, V., Morris, R., Nadherney, K., Pratt, D. Infertility treatment dropout and insurance coverage. Obstet Gynecol 1996;**88**:289–93
18 VanderLaan, B., Karande, V., Krohm, C., Morris, R., Pratt, D., Gleicher, N. Cost considerations with infertility therapy: outcome and cost comparison between health maintenance organization and preferred provider organization care based on physician and facility cost. Hum Reprod 1998;**13**:1200–5
19 Karande, V.C., Korn, A., Morris, R., Rao, R., Balin, M., Rinehart, J. et al. Prospective randomized trial comparing the outcome and cost of in vitro fertilization with that of a traditional treatment algorithm as first-line therapy for couples with infertility. Fertil Steril 1999;**71**:468–75
20 Buhaug, H., Skjeldestad, F.E., Backe, B., Dalen, A. Cost effectiveness of testing for chlamydial infections in asymptomatic women. Med Care 1989;**27**:833–41
21 Wessels, P.H., Viljoen, G.J., Marais, N.F., de Beer, J.A., Smith, M., Gericke, A. The prevalence, risks, and management of *Chlamydia trachomatis* infections in fertile and infertile patients from the high socioeconomic bracket of the South African population. Fertil Steril 1991;**56**:485–8
22 Culligan, P.J., Crane, M.M., Boone, W.R., Allen, T.C., Price, T.M., Blauer, K.L. Validity and cost-effectiveness of antisperm antibody testing before *in vitro* fertilization. Fertil Steril 1998;**69**:894–8
23 Van Voorhis, B.J., Stovall, D.W., Allen, B.D., Syrop, C.H. Cost-effective treatment of the infertile couple. Fertil Steril 1998;**70**:995–1005
24 Belaisch-Allart, J., Dufetre, C., Allart, J.P., De Mouzon, J. Comparison of transvaginal and transabdominal ultrasound for monitoring follicular development in an *in-vitro* fertilization programme. Hum Reprod 1991;**6**:68–9
25 Belaisch-Allart, J., Briot, P., Allart, J.P., Dufetre, C., Mussy, M.A., Adle, F. et al. Delayed embryo transfer in an *in-vitro* fertilization programme: how to avoid working on Sunday. Hum Reprod 1991;**6**:541–3
26 Rutherford, A.J., Subak-Sharpe, R.J., Dawson, K.J., Margara, R.A., Franks, S., Winston, R.M. Improvement of *in vitro* fertilisation after treatment with buserelin, an agonist of luteinising hormone releasing hormone. BMJ 1988;**296**:1765–8
27 Murad, N.M. Ultrasound or ultrasound and hormonal determinations for *in-vitro* fertilization monitoring. Int J Gynaecol Obstet 1998;**63**:271–6
28 Executive, N. Priorities and planning guidance for the NHS: 1997/8. London: Department of Health; 1996
29 Irvine, M. Health technology assessment. In: Deighan, M., Hitch, S., editors. *Clinical Effectiveness: From Guidelines to Cost-Effective Practice*. Manchester: Earlybrave Publications; 1995. p. 7–10
30 Department of Health. *Working for Patients. Medical Audit*. London: HMSO; 1989
31 Humphris, D., Machell, S. It's good to talk: clinical guidelines as a stimulus for purchaser/provider negotiation on improving clinical effectiveness. In: Deighan, M., Hitch,

S., editors. *Clinical Effectiveness: From Guidelines to Cost-Effective Practice*. Manchester: Earlybrave Publications; 1995. p. 105–10

32 Grimshaw, J.M., Russell, I.T. Achieving health gain through clinical guidelines II. Ensuring guidelines change clinical practice. *Qual Health Care* 1994;**3**:45–52

33 Wheatley, M.J. *Leadership and the New Science: Learning about Organisations from an Orderly Universe*. San Francisco: Berrett Koehler; 1994

34 Winyard, G. Improving clinical effectiveness; a co-ordinated approach. In: Deighan, M., Hitch, S., editors. *Clinical Effectiveness: From Guidelines to Cost-Effective Practice*. Manchester: Earlybrave Publications; 1995. p. 1–5

35 Crosignani, P.G., Rubin, B.L. Optimal use of infertility diagnostic tests and treatments. The ESHRE Capri Workshop Group. *Hum Reprod* 2000;**15**:723–32

36 Coetzee, K., Kruge, T.F., Lombard, C.J. Predictive value of normal sperm morphology: a structured literature review. *Hum Reprod Update* 1998;**4**:73–82

37 Collins, J.A., Burrows, E.A., Yeo, J., YoungLai, E.V. Frequency and predictive value of antisperm antibodies among infertile couples. *Hum Reprod* 1993;**8**:592–8

38 Ford, W.C., Williams, K.M., McLaughlin, E.A., Harrison, S., Ray, B., Hull, M.G. The indirect immunobead test for seminal antisperm antibodies and fertilization rates at *in-vitro* fertilization. *Hum Reprod* 1996;**11**:1418–22

39 Gwatkin, R.B., Collins, J.A., Jarrell, J.F., Kohut, J., Milner, R.A. The value of semen analysis and sperm function assays in predicting pregnancy among infertile couples. *Fertil Steril* 1990;**53**:693–9

40 Whittington, K., Harrison, S.C., Williams, K.M., Day, J.L., McLaughlin, E.A., Hull, M.G. et al. Reactive oxygen species (ROS) production and the outcome of diagnostic tests of sperm function. *Int J Androl* 1999;**22**:236–42

41 Oei, S.G., Helmerhorst, F.M., Keirse, M.J. When is the post-coital test normal? A critical appraisal. *Hum Reprod* 1995;**10**:1711–14

42 Collins, J.A., So, Y., Wilson, E.H., Wrixon, W., Casper, R.F. The postcoital test as a predictor of pregnancy among 355 infertile couples. *Fertil Steril* 1984;**41**:703–8

43 Glazener, C.M., Ford, W.C., Hull, M.G. The prognostic power of the post-coital test for natural conception depends on duration of infertility. *Hum Reprod* 2000;**15**:1953–7

44 van Zonneveld, P., Koppeschaar, H.P., Habbema, J.D., Fauser, B.C., te Velde, E.R. Diagnosis of subtle ovulation disorders in subfertile women with regular menstrual cycles: cost-effective clinical practice? *Gynecol Endocrinol* 1999;**13**:42–7

45 Maneschi, F., Zupi, E., Marconi, D., Valli, E., Romanini, C., Mancuso, S. Hysteroscopically detected asymptomatic Müllerian anomalies. Prevalence and reproductive implications. *J Reprod Med* 1995;**40**:684–8

46 Woolcott, R., Petchpud, A. The efficacy of hysteroscopy: a comparison of women presenting with infertility versus other gynaecological symptoms. *Aust N Z J Obstet Gynaecol* 1995;**35**:310–13

47 Mol, B.W., Swart, P., Bossuyt, P.M., van Beurden, M., van der Veen, F. Reproducibility of the interpretation of hysterosalpingography in the diagnosis of tubal pathology. *Hum Reprod* 1996;**11**:1204–8

48 Mol, B.W., Collins, J.A., Burrows, E.A., van der Veen, F., Bossuyt, P.M. Comparison of hysterosalpingography and laparoscopy in predicting fertility outcome. *Hum Reprod* 1999;**14**:1237–42

49 Woolcott, R., Fisher, S., Thomas, J., Kable, W. A randomized, prospective, controlled study of laparoscopic dye studies and selective salpingography as diagnostic tests of fallopian tube patency. *Fertil Steril* 1999;**72**:879–84

50 Collins, J.A., Hughes, E.G. Pharmacological interventions for the induction of ovulation. *Drugs* 1995;**50**:480–94
51 Philips, Z., Barraza-Llorens, M., Posnett, J. Evaluation of the relative cost-effectiveness of treatments for infertility in the UK. *Hum Reprod* 2000;**15**:95–106
52 Li, T.C., Saravelos, H., Chow, M.S., Chisabingo, R., Cooke, I.D. Factors affecting the outcome of laparoscopic ovarian drilling for polycystic ovarian syndrome in women with anovulatory infertility. *Br J Obstet Gynaecol* 1998;**105**:338–44
53 Hugues, J.N., Cedrin-Durnerin, I., Avril, C., Bulwa, S., Herve, F., Uzan, M. Sequential step-up and step-down dose regimen: an alternative method for ovulation induction with follicle-stimulating hormone in polycystic ovarian syndrome. *Hum Reprod* 1996;**11**:2581–4
54 Fridstrom, M., Sjoblom, P., Granberg, M., Hillensjo, T. A cost comparison of infertility treatment for clomiphene resistant polycystic ovary syndrome. *Acta Obstet Gynecol Scand* 1999;**78**:212–16
55 Marcoux, S., Maheux, R., Berube, S. Laparoscopic surgery in infertile women with minimal or mild endometriosis. Canadian Collaborative Group on Endometriosis. *N Engl J Med* 1997;**337**:217–22
56 Van Voorhis, B.J., Sparks, A.E., Allen, B.D., Stovall, D.W., Syrop, C.H., Chapler. F.K. Cost-effectiveness of infertility treatments: a cohort study. *Fertil Steril* 1997;**67**:830–6
57 Goverde, A.J., McDonnell, J., Vermeiden, J.P., Schats, R., Rutten, F.F., Schoemaker, J. Intrauterine insemination or *in-vitro* fertilisation in idiopathic subfertility and male subfertility: a randomised trial and cost-effectiveness analysis. *Lancet* 2000;**355**:13–18
58 Granberg, M., Wikland, M., Hamberger, L. Cost-effectiveness of intracytoplasmic sperm injection in comparison with donor insemination. *Acta Obstet Gynecol Scand* 1996;**75**:734–7
59 Pavlovich, C.P., Schlegel, P.N. Fertility options after vasectomy: a cost-effectiveness analysis. *Fertil Steril* 1997;**67**:133–41
60 Guzick, D.S., Sullivan, M.W., Adamson, G.D., Cedars, M.I., Falk, R.J., Peterson, E.P. *et al.* Efficacy of treatment for unexplained infertility. *Fertil Steril* 1998;**70**:207–13
61 Porreco, R.P. Perinatal costs of assisted reproductive technology. *Obstet Gynecol Surv* 1998;**53**:393–4
62 Hu, Y., Maxson, W.S., Hoffman, D.I., Ory, S.J., Eager, S., Dupre, J. *et al.* Maximizing pregnancy rates and limiting higher-order multiple conceptions by determining the optimal number of embryos to transfer based on quality. *Fertil Steril* 1998;**69**:650–7
63 Roest, J., van Heusden, A.M., Verhoeff, A., Mous, H.V., Zeilmaker, G.H. A triplet pregnancy after *in-vitro* fertilization is a procedure-related complication that should be prevented by replacement of two embryos only. *Fertil Steril* 1997;**67**:290–5

10

Does minimal access surgery have a role in ovarian cancer?

Alberto de Barros Lopes

INTRODUCTION

Ovarian cancer is the fourth most common cancer in women in the UK, predominantly affecting women in their postmenopausal years. It is generally asymptomatic in the early stages of the disease, with over 60% of cases only being diagnosed at an advanced stage with spread beyond the pelvis. As a result, cure rates remain low with an overall five-year survival of less than 40%.

Over the last 20 years, the standard management for ovarian cancer has been cytoreductive surgery followed in advanced cases by chemotherapy. Surgery involves a thorough staging procedure followed by the removal of as much of the tumour as possible. This invariably includes a hysterectomy, bilateral salpingo-oophorectomy and an infracolic omentectomy. Surgery can often be complex, involving extensive retroperitoneal dissection and, on occasion, can include resection of bowel. Minimal access surgery is not the ideal approach for this type of surgery and one can appreciate why many feel that laparoscopy has little role to play in the management of ovarian cancer. I hope that by the end of this chapter the reader may consider otherwise.

Patrick Steptoe introduced laparoscopy to gynaecologists in England in the 1960s and for the next 20 years the laparoscope was used almost exclusively for diagnostic purposes or sterilisation. However, in the last ten years of the 20th century there has been an explosion in its use for therapeutic procedures. This has occurred mainly due to dramatic improvements in the technology and instrumentation required for laparoscopic surgery.

Harry Reich, in 1989, was the first to perform a laparoscopic hysterectomy. Since then, many centres have made a major shift from the abdominal to the laparoscopic and vaginal approach for performing hysterectomies.

In gynaecological oncology, laparoscopy has an increasing and, possibly in the future, a major role in the management of gynaecological malignancies. Women with endometrial cancer, who are often medically unfit, are benefiting by having their hysterectomies, with or without lymphadenectomy, performed laparoscopically. Early cervical cancers are increasingly being managed by a combination of a laparoscopic and vaginal approach, with preservation of the uterus being performed on occasion for those wishing to retain fertility.

BENEFITS

The main benefit of laparoscopic surgery is that major intra-abdominal surgery can be performed without the need for a large incision. This in turn reduces the postoperative pain and morbidity resulting in a shorter postoperative recovery and convalescence. Furthermore, surgically induced adhesions are less common following laparoscopic surgery, probably due to reduced tissue handling and maintenance of a closed, and hence moist, environment.

The clarity and magnification of the operative field produced by the laparoscope is also superior and fine structures rarely noted during open procedures are often immediately obvious to the surgeon. Taking advantage of this magnification can lead to improved surgical technique.

The principal reasons for considering the laparoscopic approach to gynaecological cancers are similar to those for benign disease. The ability to visualise areas such as the diaphragmatic surfaces is an added bonus. Another potential major advantage is that the combination of laparoscopic surgery with postoperative adjuvant therapy in the form of radiotherapy or chemotherapy, may result in a lower complication rate than when following conventional open surgery.

It is also becoming apparent that laparoscopic surgery allows for greater individualisation in treatment. An example of this is laparoscopic lymphadenectomy with trachelectomy for women with early cervical cancer and who wish to preserve their fertility.

CONCERNS

As a rule, laparoscopic procedures are more time-consuming than conventional open surgery, although with increasing experience and skill operative time will fall. Any prolonged operating time as a result of the laparoscopic approach is more than compensated by the reduction in morbidity experienced by the patient.

The instrumentation used for laparoscopic procedures results in comparatively higher costs compared with open procedures, although these can be reduced to a degree by the use of nondisposable instruments. This cost is again offset by savings to the hospital due to reduction in postoperative stay and to the patient and community by an early return to normality.

In oncology, a major concern with laparoscopic surgery is whether it compromises survival for the patients. For this reason, clinicians using minimal access surgery techniques in gynaecological oncology should maintain long-term survival data on their patients. To date, there are no data to show that women with ovarian cancer who have undergone a laparoscopic procedure have a poorer outcome. There are, however, concerns regarding tumour spillage, port site metastases and the potential of laparoscopy to increase tumour growth.

Tumour spillage and spread

One of the main concerns is the risk of tumour spillage and subsequent spread that may arise from laparoscopic management of an ovarian cancer thought to be benign. A damning report by Kindermann et al.[1] described a questionnaire regarding laparoscopic surgery in ovarian cancer that had been mailed to 273 German gynaecological departments with a response rate of 46%. The report found that 16% of Stage Ia borderline tumours and 39% of Stage Ia ovarian cancers had evidence of spread discovered at early follow-up. In 92.4% of these cases, capsule rupture, morcellation, ovarian cystectomy or salpingo-oophorectomy had been the technique of choice for removal of the tumour. This was thought to be harmful for the majority of patients if subsequent laparotomy was delayed for more than eight days. Early progression to Stage Ic was reported in 20% of cases and to Stages II and III in 53% of cases. An 'endo-bag' was only used in the laparoscopic management of 7.4% of cases of Stage Ia ovarian cancer. In ovarian cancer Stages Ic to III, early seeding in the laparoscopic tract was reported in 52% of cases if laparotomy was delayed more than eight days. The conclusions of Kindermann et al.[1] were that basic oncological standards were not maintained in the laparoscopic management of ovarian malignancy. Capsule rupture, morcellation and delay to laparotomy were considered to be the main pitfalls of the laparoscopic approach.

Port site metastases

Concern regarding port site implantations following laparoscopy is not new. In 1978, Dobronte et al.[2] reported that, in women with ovarian cancer and ascites assessed laparoscopically, metastases developed at the place of penetration of the needle and trocar as early as the second week after surgery. Kruitwagen et al.[3] reported an incidence of port site metastases in 16% of laparoscopic procedures performed in 43 patients with advanced ovarian cancer. As mentioned above, in the review by Kindermann et al.,[1] seeding of the tracts was seen in 52% of cases when laparotomy was delayed more than eight days.

In contrast, Childers et al.[4] reported in 1994 only one case of port site metastasis in their series of 70 patients with ovarian cancer and this was as a result of a second-look procedure with microscopic disease only.

The discrepancy may in part be explained by a recent study that looked at 83 women with primary advanced ovarian cancer and 21 women with recurrent disease who underwent laparoscopy.[5] This study found that recurrence developed at the trocar sites in 7 (58%) of 12 patients undergoing a laparoscopy in which only the skin was closed at the end of the procedure and in 2 (2%) of 92 patients with closure of all layers. The patients with implantation metastasis also had significantly more ascites and a longer interval prior to commencement of chemotherapy or cytoreductive surgery. Van Dam et al.[5] concluded that laparoscopy with layered closure of the port sites followed by chemotherapy or cytoreductive surgery (with excision of the trocar tracts) within one week was safe in patients with disseminated ovarian cancer.

In summary, the main adverse effects of laparoscopic surgery in ovarian cancer appear to be tumour spread and port site metastases. In early disease this may be due to inappropriate surgery such as aspiration, cystectomy or morcellation. The evidence suggests that definitive treatment either by chemotherapy or further surgery should take place within one week to reduce the risk of these complications occurring.

ROLE OF MINIMAL ACCESS SURGERY IN OVARIAN CANCER

Surgical procedures for cancer can be divided into the following categories:

(1) Preventative;

(2) Diagnostic;

(3) Staging;

(4) Therapeutic;

(5) Reconstructive;

(6) Palliative;

(7) Supportive.

With regard to the role of laparoscopic surgery, this chapter will concentrate on the first four categories only.

PREVENTATIVE – PROPHYLACTIC OOPHORECTOMY

Approximately 5–10% of ovarian cancers are caused by the inheritance of a germ-line mutation in a cancer-predisposing gene. The *BRCA1* gene is thought to be responsible for the majority of cases of familial ovarian cancers. Other genes involved are *BRCA2* and the mismatch repair genes associated with Lynch-type syndromes such as hereditary nonpolyposis colon cancer. It is estimated that women with a confirmed *BRCA1* abnormality may have a life-time (by 80 years of age) risk of developing ovarian cancer of up to 60%.[6] Where possible, sequencing of the genes associated with ovarian cancer should be performed in high-risk families, although this is not yet routine in the NHS. Women thought to have a familial risk of ovarian cancer should be referred to a clinical geneticist for assessment of that risk.

Prophylactic oophorectomy is an option in those women thought to be at high risk of developing ovarian cancer. However, it must be stressed to these women that it does not remove the risk completely as cases of peritoneal carcinomatosis have been reported. Despite this, early reports do suggest a major reduction in the risk of developing ovarian cancer.[7]

The laparoscopic procedure is the ideal approach for prophylactic oophorectomy. An exploration of the upper abdomen should be performed initially followed by oophorectomy. Practice at the Northern Gynaecological Oncology Group is to use staples to the infundibulopelvic and ovarian ligaments followed by removal of the ovaries in an 'endo-bag' through one of the port sites.

It is not our routine practice to perform a hysterectomy at the same time for women only at risk of ovarian cancer, due to the increased morbidity associated with this added procedure. However, it is performed in women who specifically request it and for those at increased risk of endometrial cancer, such as women from families at risk of hereditary nonpolyposis colon cancer and those patients taking tamoxifen for breast cancer. When surgery is restricted to oophorectomy the majority of patients are discharged home within 24 hours of surgery.

DIAGNOSTIC PROCEDURES – AS PART OF A SCREENING PROGRAMME

The ovarian tumour is ideal for use in trying to develop a screening strategy. It is a 'silent' tumour, with the majority presenting at an advanced stage, and as a result has a high mortality. In contrast, the few cases presenting with early Stage I disease have five-year survival rates in excess of 90%.

Efforts in developing a screening test have concentrated on ultrasound imaging, currently by transvaginal scan, and serum markers, mainly CA125 levels. Both of these techniques have been assessed in large prospective studies and will shortly be investigated further in a large multicentre randomised trial (the UK Collaborative Trial of Ovarian Cancer Screening). To date, both tests, used either individually or in combination, have resulted in a false-positive rate up to ten times greater than the true positive rate. This inevitably results in a large number of operative procedures being performed to confirm or refute the screen-detected abnormalities. The laparoscopic approach would appear to be the ideal operative technique for the assessment and removal of the screen-detected abnormal ovary or ovaries. In the minority of cases found to be ovarian cancer, definitive treatment should be undertaken within seven days to reduce the complications mentioned earlier. Because of these risks, the role of laparoscopy as part of a screening strategy for ovarian cancer should be carefully assessed as part of any large trial in the future.

STAGING

When ovarian cancer is confined to the ovaries, the majority of patients are cured by surgery alone and current practice is not to give adjuvant chemotherapy. Unfortunately, the diagnosis is often unsuspected at the time of surgery and a thorough staging may not have been performed. In these situations there are three potential management options.

The first is to presume that the disease is confined to the ovaries, with no adjuvant chemotherapy being given. The problem with this approach is that up to 30% of cases thought to be confined to the ovaries are known to be upstaged if a thorough staging procedure is performed. The main sites for this subclinical spread are omentum, diaphragm, pelvic and para-aortic lymph nodes and peritoneal fluid. Therefore, in this situation, up to one-third of patients with metastatic disease would be deprived of adjuvant chemotherapy.

The second option is to 'play safe' and administer chemotherapy even though there is no evidence of metastatic disease. Adopting this practice would result in 70% of women with true Stage I disease receiving unnecessary cytotoxic drugs, with their potential toxicity.

The third option is to reoperate and perform a thorough staging to allow an informed decision on further management to be made. There is often a reluctance to do this as it involves a further laparotomy and associated morbidity.

The concept of using the laparoscopic approach for restaging in this situation is not new. In 1975, Rosenoff et al.[8] reported on the role of laparoscopy in restaging within one month of laparotomy in 30 patients as part of their pretreatment evaluation. Six of the seven patients who were thought to have ovarian carcinoma localised to the pelvis were found to have Stage III disease. Diaphragmatic disease was found in 77% of the patients studied.[8] Piver et al.,[9] in 1977, performed a laparoscopy on 14 consecutive patients referred with the diagnosis of Stage I or II ovarian cancer. Of the 14 women, none was demonstrated to have diaphragmatic metastases but 35% were found to have peritoneal washings demonstrating malignant cells.[9]

Neither of these early studies attempted laparoscopic lymphadenectomy as part of the staging procedure, the technology not being available at the time. In 1994, Querleu and LeBlanc[10] reported the feasibility of performing a laparoscopic para-aortic lymphadenectomy as part of the restaging of ovarian carcinomas. Eight patients with ovarian carcinoma and one with a fallopian-tube carcinoma, who had experienced substandard staging during a previous procedure, underwent laparoscopic restaging. This involved para-aortic lymphadenectomy, peritoneal fluid sampling and multiple staging biopsies. Omentectomy, appendectomy, pelvic lymphadenectomy, contralateral salpingo-oophorectomy, salpingectomy or laparoscopically assisted vaginal hysterectomy was performed as and when necessary. The postoperative periods were uneventful, with an average postoperative hospital stay of 2.8 days. Querleu and LeBlanc concluded that laparoscopic surgery was an acceptable procedure for restaging, including performing a para-aortic lymph node sampling, sparing the patient a laparotomy.[10]

It is clear that expertise is required to perform this extensive surgery laparoscopically but the reduction in postoperative morbidity is marked. The Gynaecological Oncology Group is currently undertaking a trial to assess the role of laparoscopy in this situation.

THERAPEUTIC SURGERY

Early ovarian cancer

A discussion on laparoscopic surgery for adnexal masses is not within the remit of this chapter, although the laparoscope appears an ideal approach for the management of benign adnexal lesions. However, careful preoperative assessment and selection is required to avoid operating on malignant ovarian lesions. Despite this, the incidence of unexpected cancers is quoted at between 0.04 and 3.7%.[11] For this reason, the possibility of malignancy should always be considered during the procedure. A thorough assessment of the peritoneal cavity should be undertaken. Aspiration of a cyst should be performed with an effective aspiration device to avoid spillage, followed by cystectomy or examination of the inside of the cyst wall. If a suspicious lesion or obvious cancer is identified, a gynaecological oncologist should be contacted and an immediate laparotomy considered. If definitive surgery has to be delayed, the data presented earlier would suggest that surgery should be done within one week of the laparoscopic procedure.

Childers et al.[12] reported on their experience of laparoscopy in the management of suspicious adnexal masses. Of the 138 cases described, 28% had serum CA125 values greater than 35 iu/ml, 92% had abnormal ultrasound features and in 32% the lesions were larger than 10 cm. Eleven (8%) of the procedures were converted to laparotomy, six because of the inability to dissect the mass laparoscopically and five for staging or debulking of carcinomas. Three major complications were encountered, an enterotomy and a lacerated vena cava, both of which were repaired laparoscopically, and a small bowel herniation through a lateral port site that required further surgery. There were 19 cancers in the series and, in two patients with apparent Stage I disease, recurrence was diagnosed 6 and 38 months after surgery.[12] Although the authors felt that the laparoscopic approach was feasible there is some concern that the incidence of recurrence may be higher than with an open approach.

In another report, Darai et al.[13] suggested that the laparoscopic approach to borderline ovarian tumours, although possible in early-stage disease, was associated with a high risk of recurrence after cystectomy.

Because of the concerns regarding laparoscopic management of early ovarian cancer highlighted above, operations on suspicious adnexal masses should be performed under the auspices of a gynaecological oncology service. When an early cancer is identified, staging and definitive surgery should be undertaken immediately. If this is performed laparoscopically, chemotherapy if indicated should be commenced within seven days of surgery.

Advanced ovarian cancers

Primary cytoreductive surgery

Standard management for advanced ovarian cancer is primary cytoreductive surgery followed by chemotherapy. The evidence for this is based on retrospective studies, which have shown that prognosis is poorest when residual tumour volume is greatest. In 1975, Griffiths[14] reported that survival was poor if the diameter of the largest residual mass exceeded 1.5 cm, irrespective of the total tumour volume.[14] Subsequently, superior survival has been shown with even smaller volume residual disease and the ideal aim of cytoreductive surgery today should be to remove all intra-abdominal macroscopic disease.

The rationale for attempting maximal cytoreductive surgery is to remove pharmacological sanctuaries of poorly perfused large tumour masses, which may harbour clones of resistant cells, as well as to enhance host immunocompetence by removal of these masses.

In the majority of advanced cases, cytoreductive surgery using the laparoscope would be impossible or, if possible, would be impractical because of the time that would be required. Despite this, debulking of advanced ovarian cancers laparoscopically has been performed and Amara et al.[15] reported three patients who underwent initial laparoscopic staging and therapeutic debulking procedures.

Intervention debulking surgery

In 1995, the European Organization for Research and Treatment of Cancer (EORTC)[16] published their study on the role of intervention debulking in women with residual disease of greater than 1 cm after primary cytoreductive surgery. In this study, women responding to chemotherapy were randomised to a repeat laparotomy or not after three cycles followed by a further three cycles. They showed that debulking surgery significantly lengthened progression free and overall survival. Median survival increased by six months with survival at two years improved by 10% (56% versus 46%).[16]

However, at the time of intervention surgery, 35% of patients had lesions less than 1 cm in size with half of these (17%) having no macroscopic disease. Of the remaining cases, 29% of the total were debulked to less than 1 cm but in 36% lesions greater than 1 cm were left. This suggests that the surgery may have been of little benefit in up to 55% of cases, that is the 36% of cases suboptimally debulked and the 17% with no residual diseases.

It would seem appropriate to assess the role of laparoscopic surgery in this situation both in a diagnostic and therapeutic role. From a diagnostic perspective, work on second-look laparoscopy has shown it to be fairly accurate at assessing residual disease (see below). With intervention surgery, in cases where no evidence of residual disease is seen, there would be no need to proceed to laparotomy. Likewise, in those thought to be inoperable for whatever reason, laparotomy could be avoided. From a therapeutic perspective it may be that in some cases the residual disease could be removed laparoscopically.

Neoadjuvant chemotherapy

Despite the current practice of primary cytoreductive surgery, there is still controversy regarding its true role. There have been no prospective randomised studies looking at the role of debulking surgery and, furthermore, it is also known that in cases with poor prognostic factors such as the presence of ascites, prognosis remains poorer despite optimal cytoreduction. As a result, it has been suggested that prognosis is based more on the intrinsic sensitivity of the tumour to chemotherapy than on any cytoreductive surgery performed.

The EORTC study has increased interest in the role of neoadjuvant chemotherapy with no prior surgery.[16] In essence, if primary surgery was suboptimal and yet intervention surgery improved survival, what about excluding the primary surgery? Vergote et al.[17] reported a retrospective analysis that included 77 patients with advanced disease who were assessed by laparoscopy to decide on operability. Forty-nine (64%) were deemed inoperable and were treated with neoadjuvant chemotherapy. Debulking surgery was undertaken after three cycles in 31 (63%) of these women and 26 were optimally debulked to less than 1 g residual disease.[17] Both the EORTC and the Medical Research Council have initiated neoadjuvant studies with laparoscopy being used as one of the diagnostic modalities recommended.

In future, depending on the outcome of these trials, laparoscopic assessment and biopsy followed by neoadjuvant chemotherapy and further laparoscopic assessment prior to debulking surgery may become a treatment option.

Second-look laparoscopy

It has been standard practice in some centres worldwide, especially in the USA, to perform a second-look laparotomy after primary surgery and adjuvant chemotherapy. As a diagnostic tool it has been used for pathological assessment of response to chemotherapy. Unfortunately, as up to one-third of women with no evidence of residual disease will eventually have a recurrence, there appears to be no major advantage to second-look procedures over clinical assessment. Because of the morbidity associated with a repeat laparotomy, numerous studies have looked at the role of laparoscopy instead.

In 1980, Piver et al.[18] reported a prospective study to evaluate the use of second-look laparoscopy in patients in complete clinical remission. Twenty-two patients with FIGO Stages IIb,

III and IV ovarian adenocarcinoma underwent second-look laparoscopy after therapy. Eight (36.3%) patients had documented evidence of persistent ovarian cancer at laparoscopy and were thus spared second-look laparotomy.[18]

In a retrospective review of 109 patients, 31 patients underwent laparoscopy, 70 patients underwent laparotomy and eight patients underwent both procedures at the same operation.[19] Persistent ovarian cancer was found in 54.8% evaluated by laparoscopy, 61.4% by laparotomy and 62.5% by both procedures. Blood loss was less in patients undergoing laparoscopy and, in addition, the operating time and hospital stay were significantly shorter. With a median follow-up of 22.0 months, recurrence after negative second-look surgery was noted in 14.8% of patients evaluated by laparotomy and 14.3% evaluated by laparoscopy.

In 1999, Clough *et al.*[20] reported a study looking at laparoscopy followed by immediate laparotomy, each patient therefore acting as their own control. Of 20 patients, laparoscopy identified residual disease in six of eight cases confirmed by laparotomy. They found that the presence of adhesions was the main obstacle to a laparoscopic second look.

These studies suggest that laparoscopy is an acceptable alternative to open surgery for second look procedures.

CONCLUSION

Minimal access surgery does have a role in the management of ovarian cancer ranging from prevention and screening through to staging and therapy. In women with Stage I tumours, staging and curative surgery can be undertaken completely laparoscopically. Unfortunately, in the majority of women presenting with advanced disease, its role is limited with regards to the current practice of primary cytoreductive surgery. However, with prospective trials now looking at the role of neoadjuvant chemotherapy and intervention surgery, laparoscopy may well have an increasing role in the diagnosis and treatment of ovarian cancer.

With the current move to centralisation of care for women with ovarian cancer, laparoscopic surgery for these women should be performed either by gynaecological oncologists with advanced minimal access surgery skills or by laparoscopic surgeons operating with gynaecological oncologists.

Because of the concern that laparoscopic procedures may enhance metastatic spread of ovarian cancer, careful audit and evaluation of survival data is mandatory.

References

1. Kindermann, G., Maassen, V., Kuhn, W. Laparoscopic preliminary surgery of ovarian malignancies: experiences from 127 German gynecologic clinics. *Geburtshilfe und Frauenheilkunde* 1995;**55**:687–94
2. Dobronte, Z., Wittmann, T., Karacsony, G. Rapid development of malignant metastases in the abdominal wall after laparoscopy. *Endoscopy* 1978;**10**:127–30
3. Kruitwagen, R.F., Swinkels, B.M., Keyser, K.G., Doesburg, W.H., Schijf, C.P. Incidence and effect on survival of abdominal wall metastases at trocar or puncture sites following laparoscopy or paracentesis in women with ovarian cancer. *Gynecol Oncol* 1996;**60**:233–7
4. Childers, J.M., Aqua, K.A., Surwit, E.A., Hallum, A.V., Hatch, K.D. Abdominal-wall tumor implantation after laparoscopy for malignant conditions. *Obstet Gynecol* 1994;**84**:765–9

5   van Dam, P.A., DeCloedt, J., Tjalma, W.A., Buytaert, P., Becquart, D., Vergote, I.B. Trocar implantation metastasis after laparoscopy in patients with advanced ovarian cancer: can the risk be reduced? *Am J Obstet Gynecol* 1999;**181**:536–41

6   Ford, D., Easton, D.F., Stratton, M., Narod, S., Goldgar, D., Devilee, P. et al. Genetic heterogeneity and penetrance analysis of the BRCA1 and BRCA2 genes in breast cancer families. The Breast Cancer Linkage Consortium. *Am J Hum Genet* 1998;**62**:676–89

7   Struewing, J.P., Watson, P., Easton, D.F., Ponder, B.A., Lynch, H.T., Tucker, M.A. Prophylactic oophorectomy in inherited breast/ovarian cancer families. *J Natl Cancer Inst Monogr* 1995;**17**:33–5

8   Rosenoff, S.H., Young, R.C., Chabner, B., Hubbard, S., De Vita, V.T. Jr, Schein, P.S. Use of peritoneoscopy for initial staging and post-therapy evaluation of patients with ovarian carcinoma. *J Natl Cancer Inst Monogr* 1975;**42**:81–6

9   Piver, M.S., Lopez, R.G., Xynos, F., Barlow, J.J. The value of pre-therapy peritoneoscopy in localized ovarian cancer. *Am J Obstet Gynecol* 1977;**127**:288–90

10 Querleu, D., LeBlanc, E. Laparoscopic infrarenal paraaortic lymph node dissection for restaging of carcinoma of the ovary or fallopian tube. *Cancer* 1994;**73**:1467–71

11 Crawford, R.A., Gore, M.E., Shepherd, J.H. Ovarian cancers related to minimal access surgery. *Br J Obstet Gynaecol* 1995;**102**:726–30

12 Childers, J.M., Nasseri, A., Surwit, E.A. Laparoscopic management of suspicious adnexal masses. *Am J Obstet Gynecol* 1996;**175**:1451–7

13 Darai, E., Teboul, J., Fauconnier, A., Scoazec, J.Y., Benifla, J.L., Madelenat, P. Management and outcome of borderline ovarian tumors incidentally discovered at or after laparoscopy. *Acta Obstet Gynecol Scand* 1998;**77**:451–7

14 Griffiths, C.T. Surgical resection of tumor bulk in the primary treatment of ovarian carcinoma. *J Natl Cancer Inst Monogr* 1975;**42**:101–4

15 Amara, D.P., Nezhat, C., Teng, N.N., Nezhat, F., Nezhat, C., Rosati, M. Operative laparoscopy in the management of ovarian cancer. *Surg Laparosc Endosc Percutan Tech* 1996;**6**:38–45

16 van der Burg, M.E., van Lent, M., Buyse, M., Kobierska, A., Colombo, N., Favalli, G. et al. The effect of debulking surgery after induction chemotherapy on the prognosis in advanced epithelial ovarian cancer. Gynecological Cancer Co-operative Group of the European Organization for Research and Treatment of Cancer. *N Engl J Med* 1995;**332**:629–34

17 Vergote, I., De Wever, I., Tjalma, W., Van Gramberen, M., Decloedt, J., van Dam, P. Neoadjuvant chemotherapy or primary debulking surgery in advanced ovarian carcinoma: a retrospective analysis of 285 patients. *Gynecol Oncol* 1998;**71**:431–6

18 Piver, M.S., Lele, S.B., Barlow, J.J., Gamarra, M. Second-look laparoscopy prior to proposed second-look laparotomy. *Obstet Gynecol* 1980;**55**:571–3

19 Abu-Rustum, N.R., Barakat, R.R., Siegel, P.L., Venkatraman, E., Curtin, J.P., Hoskins, W.J. Second-look operation for epithelial ovarian cancer: laparoscopy or laparotomy? *Obstet Gynecol* 1996;**88**:549–53

20 Clough, K.B., Ladonne, J.M., Nos, C., Renolleau, C., Validire, P., Durand, J.C. Second look for ovarian cancer: laparoscopy or laparotomy? A prospective comparative study. *Gynecol Oncol* 1999;**72**:411–17

11

Period-free HRT

Timothy C. Hillard

INTRODUCTION

Despite the well-established benefits of hormone replacement therapy (HRT) in the management of postmenopausal women, the uptake of HRT and its continuation worldwide remains erratic. Less than 20% of women in the USA are prepared to take long-term HRT.[1] In a UK feasibility study,[2] 18% of 1640 women deemed to be at high risk of osteoporosis rejected the offer of HRT outright, the majority citing the return of bleeding or fear of adverse effects as the main reason. Of the 1127 women who did start HRT, 30% were no longer taking it at two years, with cycle-related problems by far the most common reason for stopping. Overall, less than 50% of women in this high-risk group were taking the appropriate treatment at two years.[2] In many studies, the dislike of the withdrawal bleed is a major factor in women avoiding or discontinuing HRT.[3] Other factors include the fear of breast cancer and adverse effects such as breast tenderness, weight gain, irritability and other premenstrual-like symptoms.[4]

To overcome some of these problems, continuous combined HRT, 'no bleed' HRT or 'period-free' HRT as it is now commonly called, was first used some 20 years ago in Scandinavia.[5] The concept is simple; the continuous addition of a progestogen opposes any oestrogenic stimulation on the endometrium, so there should be no endometrial proliferation and as a consequence no bleeding. At the endometrial level progestogens induce oestradiol-17-β dehydrogenase, which converts oestradiol to the less active oestrone. They also suppress oestrogen and progesterone receptor formation and DNA synthesis. These actions combined with their anti-mitotic activity in the endometrium should mean that that the endometrium remains atrophic. In addition, because the progestogen is given continuously, a lower dose can be used than in the cyclical combinations and, thus, potentially troublesome progestogenic and metabolic adverse effects may be reduced.

These preparations are now widely used and at the time of writing there are currently nine different preparations (seven oral, including tibolone, and two transdermal) available on the UK market. More than 40 studies on this subject have now been published and there have been several comprehensive reviews to which the interested reader is referred for an exhaustive list of the early studies.[6-8] The most recent studies[9-14] have been characterised by larger numbers and randomised treatment allocation (Table 1). This chapter is not a systematic review of all existing data but rather looks at the key data in relation to clinically relevant parameters.

BLEEDING PATTERNS

Absence of bleeding is clearly the *raison d'être* behind this type of treatment. However, clinical and published experience suggests that unscheduled, often quite persistent bleeding is a significant problem. Interpretation of these studies is complicated by the variable reporting of what constitutes bleeding and the different oestrogen and progestogen preparations and doses used.[6,7] For instance, amenorrhoeic rates presented as a percentage of those still in the study reach 85-100%

Table 1 *Percentage of women reporting amenorrhoea with various combinations of period-free HRT at 3, 6 and 12 months in recent randomised studies. The reporting of amenorrhoea is variable (see text)*

Reference	Women in study (n)	Oestrogen (dose per day, mg)	Progestogen (dose per day, mg)	Amenorrhoea at month (%)		
				3	6	12
Menopause Study Group[9]	1724	CEE (0.625)	MPA (2.5)	52	63	75
		CEE (0.625)	MPA (5.0)	57	72	87
Hammar[10]	437	17-β E_2 (2)	NETA (1)	86	88	96
		Tibolone (2.5)		93	94	95
Endometrial study group[11]	1176	Oestradiol (1)	NETA (0.1)	74	77	80
		Oestradiol (1)	NETA (0.25)	75	79	85
		Oestradiol (1)	NETA (0.5)	73	84	90
Mattsson[12]	441	TTS E_2 (0.025)	NETA (0.125)	64	71	86
		TTS E_2 (0.05)	NETA (0.25)	35	48	65
		Oral E_2	NETA (1)	45	68	79
Al-Azzawi[13]	235	E_2 Val (2)	NETA (0.7)	36	61	65
		Tibolone (2.5)		72	81	70
CombiPatch Study[14]	625	TTS E_2 (0.05)	NETA (0.14)	50		54
		TTS E_2 (0.05)	NETA (0.25)	16		40
		TTS E_2 (0.05)	NETA (0.4)	16		44

CEE = conjugated equine oestrogens; MPA = medroxyprogesterone acetate; 17-β E_2 = 17-β oestradiol; NETA = norethisterone; TTS E_2 = transdermal oestradiol; E_2 Val = oestradiol valerate. The figures in the columns for percent amenorrhoea at each month are the figures to the nearest month available. If the study did not actually report the amenorrhoea rate specifically at that month the nearest month is taken, e.g. cycle two for month three, or in some cases[17] the figure represents the percentage of amenorrhoea in the previous three cycles

relatively quickly (within six months). However, if amenorrhoeic rates are presented as a percentage of women who started the study (i.e. including dropouts), they may be as low as 50%.[9,15]

The occurrence of bleeding in the first six months varies considerably and is dependent on what time point is taken (Table 1). However, it is clear that irregular vaginal bleeding is common in the first few months with amenorrhoea rates at six months varying from 48% to 94%. When interpreting Table 1, the above comments about different reporting of bleeding should be borne in mind. For instance, Hammar's figures[10] represent any bleeding in one cycle, whereas the CombiPatch™ study[14] refers to any bleeding in the previous three cycles. In general, the bleeding is usually light or spotting but is unpredictable and inconvenient. The first publication on continuous combined therapy was that of Staland,[5] who reported on 265 women taking continuous combined oestradiol and norethisterone acetate (NETA) for up to 52 months. Bleeding episodes were common in the first three to four months but rare after four months. He postulated that it was likely to take this time to transform the endometrium to an atrophic state. In this study, the further a woman was from her menopause the less likely she was to bleed. Staland suggested that, in those with an already atrophic endometrium, taking the hormones as two divided doses would reduce the likelihood of endometrial stimulation. The Menopause Study Group[9] included 1724 women in a 12-month double-blind randomised study with five groups. All took conjugated equine oestrogens (CEE) 0.625 mg per day and, in addition, two groups took continuous medroxyprogesterone acetate (MPA) (2.5 mg or 5 mg per day) (Table 1), two groups took cyclical MPA (5 mg or 10 mg for 14-day cycle) and one group was given placebo. The total percentages of amenorrhoeic cycles in the continuous combined groups were 61.4% and 72.8%, respectively. The incidence of bleeding appeared to lessen and shorten the longer the treatment continued. In the last seven cycles, 40% and 50% of the women in the continuous combined groups respectively had amenorrhoea and only 12% of those who bled after cycle six had any further bleeding. They also confirmed Staland's observation that those furthest from the menopause were least likely to bleed.[5]

Hammar[10] randomised 450 women to either tibolone or oestradiol 2 mg per day and norethisterone 1 mg per day continuously (Table 1). There was equal symptom control between the two groups but a significantly higher number of women in the oestradiol group had bleeding in the first six months compared with the tibolone group (Figure 1). After seven months there appeared little difference between the groups. Tibolone is structurally related to 19-nortestosterone derivatives such as norethisterone and norethynodrel. It has three major metabolites, which are active steroids themselves; the δ4-isomer, the 3α- and the 3β-hydroxy metabolites. Tibolone is sometimes referred to as tissue-specific because the conversion to these metabolites occurs in the target tissues, for example in the endometrium. Different metabolites have different activities in different tissues. In the endometrium, tibolone is rapidly metabolised to the δ4-isomer[16] which has a marked affinity for the progestogenic and androgenic receptors in the endometrium but no affinity for the oestrogen receptors.[17] The 3α-hydroxy and 3β-hydroxy metabolites, both of which have affinity for the oestrogen receptors, are not present in endometrial tissue. As a consequence of this, tibolone should cause no endometrial stimulation and thus not be associated with any bleeding.

Many studies of period-free HRT report up to 50% of women bleeding in the first three months. This was unacceptable to many women, borne out by dropout rates of up to 50%.[15,18] In clinical practice, away from the enthusiasm and attention that study patients receive, the fall out is likely to be higher still. However, it should be remembered that placebo is associated with 15-20%

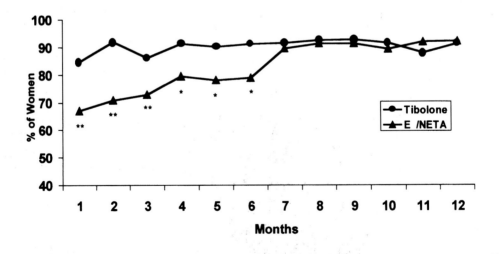

* = p<0.001   ** = p<0.01

Figure 1 Cumulative percentage of postmenopausal women reporting amenorrhoea over 12 months in women taking either tibolone (n = 210) or 17-β oestradiol (2 mg per day) and norethisterone acetate (1 mg per day) E/NETA, n = 213. ** Log rank test: $P < 0.001$; * $P < 0.01$; adapted from Hammar et al.,[10] with permission

bleeding incidence in the first few months.[19,20] The prevalence of bleeding in the first few months seems to be higher among those who have recently been through the menopause[5,9,11] or who have been using sequential therapy.[15,18,19]

In general, all the studies confirm that the rate of amenorrhoea increases with study duration (Table 1)[5-7,9-15,18-35] with 75–100% being amenorrhoeic at 12 months. The few studies that have analysed beyond 12 months report maintenance of this level of amenorrhoea.[5,15,24,26,27,29]

Once a woman becomes amenorrhoeic on period-free HRT there is a good chance she will remain amenorrhoeic. Archer[9] noted that, of those women who were amenorrhoeic between cycles seven, eight and nine, only 12% had any further bleeding. Conversely, of those still bleeding at six months, only 50% eventually achieved amenorrhoea.[9,15] In a later report with lower dose combinations, Archer[11] observed that 50% of women did not bleed at all but others had a propensity to bleed. Nevertheless, late initiation of bleeding was uncommon, just 3% in the NETA 0.25 mg or 0.5 mg group, and when it did occur it was not associated with endometrial abnormalities. Most of the women who reported bleeding in the last three months of the study had suffered bleeding in the first three months. However, a low incidence of late bleeding is not reported in all studies. Prough et al.[22] reported that 12.5% of patients were still bleeding at nine months and Mattsson[21] observed that 31% bled during months 9–12. This latter figure contrasts with the 4% observed by Staland[5] with a virtually identical combination. However, Staland[5] varied the dose according to the bleeding pattern and also split the dose of NETA to try to provide more consistent plasma levels.

Various other strategies have been employed in a number of studies to try to reduce the incidence of bleeding. Some reported lower rates of bleeding with higher doses of progestogen.[9,18,23,30] In Spaulding's study,[33] the majority of women who were bleeding at three months became amenorrhoeic when the dose of progestogen was increased from 2.5 mg to 5 mg per day. Others reported no difference with dose of progestogen.[25,31] In the CombiPatch study group,[14] 625 postmenopausal women were randomised to receive 50 μg transdermal oestradiol per day either alone or with three doses of transdermal norethindrone over 12 months (Table 1). Uterine bleeding was least frequent in the combined group with the lowest dose of NETA. A comparative study of different progestogens suggested that amenorrhoea was achieved faster with NETA than MPA and l-norgestrel but amenorrhoea rates were the same by eight months.[34] Hillard et al.[15] reported no significant differences between NETA and MPA although the numbers were small by the end of the study. NETA induced more marked endometrial atrophy than other progestogen derivatives of progesterone.[35]

Higher oestrogen doses were generally associated with more bleeding,[18,28] although one study claimed the reverse.[30] In Magos' study[18] there were two doses of oestrogen and the dose of NETA was increased by increments until bleeding had stopped. In the lower-dose group (0.625 mg CEE per day) the NETA did not need to go above 1.4 mg per day, whereas in the higher-dose (1.25 mg CEE per day) it had to increase up to 2.1 mg per day.

Recently, attention has focused on reducing the dose of oestrogen and lower-dose period-free preparations have been introduced, for example oestradiol 1 mg per day in combination with norethisterone 0.5 mg per day. These appear to have an improved bleeding profile over the 2-mg preparations.[36] Archer[11] randomised 1176 postmenopausal women to 1 mg oestradiol or oestradiol with three doses of continuous NETA (Table 1). Initial bleeding in the combined groups in the first three months was lower (24–28%) than normally seen with 2 mg preparations and the lowest bleeding incidence was with the highest NETA dose. The dose effect of NETA appeared greatest within three years of menopause (Figure 2) with a smaller dose effect noticeable in women more than three years since menopause. The authors suggested that higher doses of progestogen may be more appropriate for women commencing period-free treatment closer to the menopause.

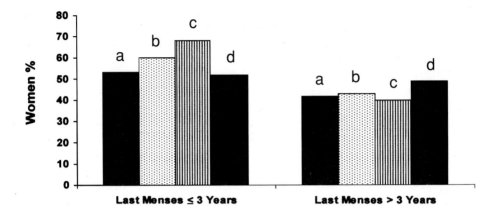

Figure 2 *Percentage of women with at least one bleeding episode during 12 months of treatment, according to time since last menstrual period, with: (a) unopposed 17-β oestradiol; (b) in combination with norethisterone acetate 0.1 mg; (c) 0.25 mg; (d) 0.5 mg; reproduced from Archer et al.,[11] with permission from the American College of Obstetricians and Gynecologists*

Mattsson[12] compared two transdermal and one oral continuous combined preparations over 12 months (Table 1). Both the lower-dose patch combination and oral treatment had similar bleeding profiles and were well accepted but the prevalence of bleeding with the higher-dose patch combination was unacceptably high.

Why women bleed on period-free HRT is often not clear. The potential causes are:

(1) missed tablets;
(2) gastrointestinal upset;
(3) endometrial polyps;
(4) submucous fibroids;
(5) endometrial hyperplasia;
(6) endometrial cancer;
(7) other genital tract lesions;
(8) concomitant medication, for example anti-coagulation;
(9) constitutional, for example continuing ovarian activity;
(10) no identifiable cause.

Bleeding is frequent in the first three months of treatment with these types of preparations and thus it is not usually considered abnormal. Women should be advised of the risk of such bleeding prior to starting treatment. In the absence of clinical signs or other risk factors, bleeding between three and six months is usually considered to be acceptable but persistent bleeding after six months or bleeding commencing after a spell of amenorrhoea should be investigated. In a majority of cases no pathological cause for the bleeding is found and the endometrium is atrophic.[9,37] Why atrophic endometrium should bleed is not known but it may represent a breakdown of the control of angiogenesis.[38] There would appear to be two categories of bleeding. Firstly, the persistent bleeder (bleeding during first year) who may take several months to become amenorrhoeic. In this group, provided there is no previous underlying pathology, a pathological cause is unlikely and it probably represents endometrial adjustment to therapy rather than underlying pathology.[39] Higher dose of progestogen may be helpful but some women clearly have a propensity to bleed and, for them, period-free HRT may not be suitable, at least not for another year or two. The second group are those who bleed after a prolonged period of amenorrhoea. While there is not necessarily a direct correlation with endometrial pathology,[11] this should always be investigated.[40]

The economic cost of abnormal bleeding seen with 'no bleed' HRT should not be overlooked. In a 1998 study, Ettinger et al.[41] compared the number of gynaecological assessments for vaginal bleeding with cyclical and continuous HRT. Thirty-eight percent of women on cyclical HRT and 41% of women on continuous combined HRT re-attended the clinic in one year because of vaginal bleeding. Furthermore, 13% and 20%, respectively, had endometrial biopsies because of abnormal bleeding. While there are undoubtedly differences in clinical practices between the USA and the UK, the potential impact on resources is impressive. Careful patient selection prior to commencing this type of treatment and the adoption of locally agreed care pathways for the management of bleeding on HRT is likely to minimise the cost of this in the UK.

In summary, there are four key practical questions to consider:

(1) How quickly is amenorrhoea achieved with period-free HRT? For the majority of women it is achieved within three to four months. The incidence of bleeding can be reduced by confining its use to clearly postmenopausal women, using low doses of oestrogen and considering a higher dose of progestogen in women within three years of the menopause or those who bleed in the first three months. However, no clear strategy for avoiding bleeding has been devised. Women should be advised of the risk of such bleeding prior to starting treatment.

(2) How well is amenorrhoea maintained? For the majority of women, once amenorrhoea is achieved, it is maintained. Those women who persistently bleed during the first six months may be best advised to revert to sequential therapy.

(3) Is it possible to predict who will bleed? Those within three years of menopause appear to have a higher incidence of bleeding. Period-free HRT should certainly be reserved for women who are clearly postmenopausal. Those who bleed persistently during the first few months are more likely to continue bleeding.

(4) When should the bleeding be investigated? Bleeding in the first three months is not usually considered abnormal. In the absence of clinical signs or other risk factors bleeding between three and six months is usually acceptable but persistent bleeding after six months or bleeding commencing after a spell of amenorrhoea should be investigated. In a majority of cases, no pathological cause for the bleeding is found and the endometrium is atrophic.

ENDOMETRIAL HISTOLOGY

Continuous combined HRT does not appear to stimulate the endometrium. Virtually all studies report endometrial atrophy rates of 90-100% within three months of treatment using lower doses of progestogen than used in sequential treatment.[6-8] Endometrial hyperplasia is uncommon, occurring in less than 1% of the study population in both the Menopause Study Group[42] and the

Postmenopausal Estrogen/Progestin Interventions (PEPI) trial.[43] In many smaller studies hyperplasia is not seen at all.[8,13,36] Two studies of period-free transdermal HRT report hyperplasia rates of 1-2%.[12,14] The UK Kliofem® (Novo Nordisk, Crawley, UK) study[44] (oestradiol 2 mg per day with 1 mg NETA per day) reported no cases of hyperplasia at one year. Tibolone does not appear to cause endometrial stimulation either on histological[19,45] or on ultrasonographic assessment.[45,46] Worldwide, there have been few cases of endometrial hyperplasia or endometrial carcinoma diagnosed while taking tibolone.[47]

These results are in contrast to those with cyclical therapy and unopposed oestrogen. In the PEPI trial the incidence of endometrial hyperplasia after three years was 62% in the oestrogen-only group, 5% in the sequential groups, 1.7% in the placebo group and 0.8% in the continuous combined group.[43] In the Menopause Study Group[42] the hyperplasia rate at 12 months was 20% in the oestrogen-only group but less than 1% in all the combined groups. The only hyperplasia in the combined group occurred with the lowest doses of MPA (2.5 mg per day continuously or 5 mg per day sequentially for 14 days). The authors concluded that the dose of progestogen was probably more important in preventing hyperplasia than whether it was given continuously or sequentially.

However, recent epidemiological evidence has suggested that even cyclical therapy with more than ten days of progestogen addition may be associated with an increased risk of endometrial cancer,[48,49] with more than five years of sequential combined HRT use associated with a three-fold increase in endometrial cancer risk. Continuous combined HRT, on the other hand, was associated with a small decrease in risk (Table 2). Weiderpass[49] noted a slightly greater protective effect against hyperplasia with testosterone-derived progestogens compared with progesterone ones, although the former were prescribed at relatively higher doses. In clinical practice these data suggest that postmenopausal women on cyclical HRT should consider switching to continuous combined therapy after five years. In reality, many will already have done so but there would now appear to be a medical as well as an aesthetic reason for doing so.

Continuous combined HRT appears to be a successful method of converting atypical endometrial hyperplasia to atrophy. In Staland's[5] original series he reported that 16 women had some degree of atypia at the pretreatment biopsy but by three months they had all reverted to endometrial atrophy except one, who was atrophic at six months. All biopsies remained atrophic thereafter. Sturdee[44] also reported that hyperplasia without atypia that occurred while taking sequential HRT reverted to normal with continuous combined treatment. However, Leather et al.[27] reported two cases of early endometrial adenocarcinoma developing after several years of treatment. Both women had undergone a previous biopsy showing atypical hyperplasia. Although both these women had presented with episodes of bleeding, in general there is poor correlation between endometrial histology and bleeding patterns.[39] Endometrial atrophy does not seem to

Table 2 Odds ratio (OR) and 95% confidence intervals (CI) of invasive endometrial cancer in relation to the use of medium potency oestrogens with cyclical or continuous progestogen addition; adapted from Weiderpass et al.,[49] with permission from Oxford University Press

Total use of HRT	Cyclical		Continuous	
	Cases/controls	OR (95% CI)	Cases/controls	OR (95% CI)
Never	597/2963	1.0 (reference)	641/3014	1.0 (reference)
Ever	90/300	2.0 (1.4-2.7)	41/237	0.7 (0.4-1.0)
<5 years' use	38/191	1.5 (1.0-2.2)	32/162	0.8 (0.5-1.3)
>5 years' use	40/78	2.9 (1.8-4.6)	2/53	0.2 (0.1-0.8)

guarantee amenorrhoea and a thin endometrium (less than 4 mm) does not completely exclude endometrial pathology. Women who commence bleeding on period-free HRT having previously established amenorrhoea should be investigated.[40]

SYMPTOM CONTROL

Nearly all studies that look at symptom relief report major improvements in vasomotor symptoms,[6,7] although this is largely based on subjective assessment.[7] This response is to be expected, given that similar doses of oestrogens were being used, as in cyclical treatment. However, the question arises as to whether the addition of continuous progestogen impairs or enhances the symptom-relief profile of standard HRT. Only a few comparative studies have been reported. Some found the continuous combined regimen more effective[34,50] whereas others found no difference.[22,29,31] No study has suggested that the continuous combined combination is worse. The impact on other menopausal symptoms is less clear, although many studies used the Kupperman index, which includes a variety of symptoms. The UK Kliofem® (Novo Nordisk, Crawley, UK) multicentre study[51] assessed quality of life in 2151 women on Kliofem using the Greene climacteric scale. The majority had previously been on sequential therapy. Treatment with the continuous combined therapy was at least as effective as previous sequential therapy in alleviating all menopausal symptoms and over 90% preferred the continuous combined to the previous sequential therapy. Mattsson et al.[12] reported good symptom control as measured by the Women's Health questionnaire. Both transdermal doses were as effective as the 2-mg oral preparation in relieving symptoms but the lower-dose group was associated with fewer adverse experiences. Tibolone appears to be as effective as continuous combined HRT in terms of relief from hot flushes and vaginal dryness.[10] It also has reported beneficial effects on libido[52] and is the only oral HRT preparation with a licence for reduced libido.

Again, studies with lower dose combinations are now being reported; 1 mg oestradiol in combination with 0.5 mg NETA appears to be as effective in relieving vasomotor symptoms as 2 mg in combination with NETA[36] and more effective than 1 mg oestradiol alone[53] suggesting that the continuous progestogen may have an additive effect.

ADVERSE EFFECTS/DISCONTINUATION

Long-term compliance with HRT is essential if its main benefits are to be realised. Results from early studies of period-free HRT indicated continuation rates of around 80% at 12 months, with a range of 35-100%.[7] The lowest continuation rates were in those switching from sequential therapy.[15] However, few of the earlier studies specifically addressed the issue of compliance or continuance. Grey reported 86% compliance at 12 months, although this was assessed retrospectively.[32] In the PEPI study,[43] 81% of women on sequential therapy and 86% on continuous combined therapy were still taking the study medication at three years.

However, participants in such trials are likely to be quite highly motivated and encouraged compared with the general population. Hill[54] has reported adherence data from the Group Health Co-operative at Puget Sound in Washington State. Women enrolled in the health plan were contacted 12–15 months after initiating HRT. Continuation with the originally prescribed HRT was higher in users of continuous combined therapy (69%) than in users of sequential therapy (54%). Users of continuous combined therapy were less likely to switch regimens (10% versus 20%) but the overall discontinuation rate was relatively high in both groups (21% continuous combined versus 25.4% sequential). Ultimately, however, it is long-term compliance that is required. The UK Kliofem study reported that 66% of women were still in the study after five years[55] and the Guy's Hospital group reported 58% adherence to tibolone after eight years.[56]

Generally, irregular bleeding was the most common reason for dropout in most studies. Other reasons included breast tenderness, weight gain, irritability, depression, co-existent medical conditions and personal reasons. Archer[11] reported lower dropout rates in the continuous combined group than in the oestrogen-only group and the lowest dropout rate due to bleeding in the group with the highest progestogen dose. Superior compliance with continuous combined HRT was also reported by Doren.[57] In a comparative study of tibolone and oestradiol 2 mg plus 0.5 mg NETA there was no overall difference between the continuation rates in the two groups.[10] However, the tibolone group was associated with significantly less mastalgia and bleeding-related dropout than the oestradiol plus NETA group. It is anticipated that the introduction of lower dose no-bleed preparations will improve adherence, particularly in the more elderly (over 60 years), for whom this treatment combination seems particularly suitable. Initial studies report continuation rates as good as placebo[20] and, generally, adverse effects were fewer than with 1 mg oestradiol alone, except for breast tenderness.[53] However, Stadberg[36] reported significantly less mastalgia with the 1 mg oestradiol plus NETA combination than with the 2 mg combination.

Overall compliance or adherence to HRT remains a problem. There seems little doubt that persistence with treatment is higher with period-free HRT than sequential therapy, but there remains room for improvement. Lower dose preparations, on the basis of initial reports, appear to provide a way forward.

METABOLIC EFFECTS

There is consistent evidence from over 40 clinical trials that postmenopausal women who take oestrogens have a considerably lower incidence of heart disease than those who do not take oestrogens.[58] Despite initial doubts, these benefits are still seen with the addition of progestogens, both MPA[59] and levonorgestrel.[60] There are no epidemiological data on the use of continuous combined HRT but as cyclical progestogens have no overall adverse effect the assumption is generally made that continuous progestogens will do the same. Is this valid?

The exact mechanisms by which oestrogens reduce cardiovascular disease risk are not known but likely mechanisms have been reviewed.[61,62] Much attention has focused on the effects on lipids and lipoproteins, which are estimated to be responsible for 25–50% of the benefit.[63] Menopause itself is associated with rise in low density lipoprotein (LDL) and total cholesterol and a fall in high density lipoprotein (HDL) cholesterol[64] and oestrogens alone reverse this pattern.[65] The effects of continuous combined HRT on lipid profiles have been extensively reviewed.[6–8] Most of the initial studies were inadequately designed to address this issue[6] but the two largest studies have provided useful comparative data.[66,67] It seems clear that unopposed oestrogens and combined HRT, regardless of type or dose of progestogen, lower total and LDL cholesterol significantly. The effect on HDL is less clear. Oestrogens alone lead to an increase in HDL cholesterol. This increase is not significantly altered by the addition of non-androgenic progestogens such as MPA or micronised progesterone[66,67] but HDL is lowered by the addition of androgenic progestogens such as NETA,[23,68] even in a lower dose combination (1 mg oestradiol and 0.5 mg NETA).[69]

The true significance of all these observations is not known. It has been postulated that for every 1 mg/dl rise in HDL there is a 3% reduction in heart disease risk.[70] On this basis, the addition of androgenic progestogens might be expected to have a reduced impact not observed in epidemiological studies.[60] However, progestogens have a number of other metabolic effects that may be beneficial, such as lowering of triglycerides and lipoprotein-a (Lp-a).[71] These latter effects may be more relevant than the effects on LDL and HDL cholesterol. Furthermore, a fall in HDL *per se* is a crude assessment of a complicated function and may not necessarily indicate an increased tendency to atherogenesis.[72] Tibolone does not change LDL cholesterol and leads to a significant fall in HDL but also large falls in Lp-a and triglycerides.[72]

Clearly, there is still much we do not understand but on the basis of evidence currently available the effect of continuous addition of progestogen is probably more dependent on the type and dose used rather than the fact that it is given continuously. For the vast majority of women the type of progestogen probably has little overall effect but for those with established cardiovascular disease or with underlying dyslipidaemias the type chosen may be of more relevance.

BONE CONSERVATION

The benefits of HRT on osteoporosis and fracture prevention are well established.[73–76] As yet, there are no long-term fracture data on continuous combined HRT but there are plenty of bone density data demonstrating that continuous combined HRT or tibolone at conventional doses has equivalent effects to those seen with oestrogen only or sequential preparations.[7,24,32,77,78]

However, strategies on osteoporosis management are changing.[79,80] The beneficial effects of oestrogen on the skeleton appear to be maintained for as long as treatment is continued but are lost fairly soon after stopping.[81] The concept that ten years of HRT immediately after the menopause will delay bone loss sufficiently to protect against future osteoporotic fractures appears to be no longer valid. Several studies have observed that when women stop HRT there is an accelerated phase of bone loss.[82,83] Less than seven years of HRT did not confer much benefit against fracture prevention[84] and even among those who had taken HRT for longer, by the age of 75 years there was little difference in bone density when compared with those who had never taken oestrogen. Cauley et al.[85] found no decrease in hip, or wrist fractures among past users of HRT (mean duration of use 4.8 years). Michaelsson et al.[81] observed a substantial reduction in risk of fracture with oestrogens, which was increased further by duration of use and the addition of progestogens. However, the risk reduction diminished with time since last use and was virtually lost five years after cessation. Equally, women who start HRT after 60 years of age demonstrate good increases in bone mass.[32,86,87] In the Rancho Bernardo Study[88] the current late users (started HRT at 60 years of age or more with current use) had a similar bone density to those who had been taking it since the menopause (current continuous users). The past early users (started before 60 years of age and taken for an average of ten years but with no current use) had similar bone density to non-users. This concept is represented diagrammatically in Figure 3.[89] Although this model was proposed in 1994, the results of the Rancho Bernardo study[88] would seem to support this hypothesis.

Thus, it appears that for fracture prevention it may be possible to delay starting HRT until just before the time of increased risk. There would also be no need to start HRT purely for fracture prevention around the menopause unless there were strong risk factors, for example premature menopause. However, this approach should not be widely adopted until clear evidence has emerged that late intervention really does reduce fracture risk. All this makes it increasingly likely that the majority of women taking HRT for osteoporosis prevention will be using period-free HRT. Interest has now focused on reducing the dose of oestrogen to minimise possible adverse effects such as breast tenderness and thus improve tolerability and compliance in the older population. While there has been some previous evidence that low doses of oestrogen (less than 2 mg/day) may be sufficient to prevent bone loss at the lumbar spine,[90] data at other sites have been lacking. Recently, Delmas et al.[91] have shown that 1 mg oestradiol plus 0.5 mg NETA prevents bone loss in postmenopausal women at the lumbar spine, hip and distal radius over two years (Figure 4). The increases in bone density observed were greater than those reported for unopposed oestradiol,[90] although the study was not a comparison of the two. The increases in bone density

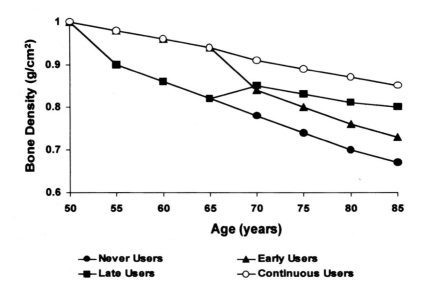

Figure 3 *A diagrammatic representation of estimated changes in bone density after menopause in different scenarios: women who had never used oestrogen (never users); those who used oestrogen continuously beginning at menopause (continuous users); those who began at menopause and stopped at 65 years of age (early users); and those who began at 65 years of age (late users) (assuming a 5% increase in bone density at the time oestrogen was introduced); adapted from Ettinger and Grady,[89] with permission*

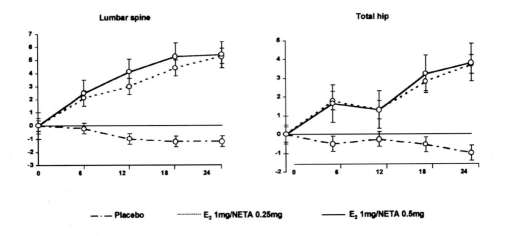

Figure 4 *Mean (± SEM) percentage change in bone density at lumbar spine and total hip in postmenopausal women treated with placebo, 17-β oestradiol 1 mg and 0.25 mg norethisterone acetate/day (-------) or 17-β oestradiol 1 mg and 0.5 mg norethisterone acetate/day (——) for 24 months; adapted from Delmas et al.,[91] with permission*

were similar, regardless of time since menopause, and the nonresponder rate was less than 5%, which is similar to standard-dose studies.[92] One possible conclusion is that NETA had an additive effect allowing lower doses of oestrogen to be used. Whether the same is true for other low dose oestrogen/progestogen combinations remains to be seen. NETA on its own has been shown to have a positive effect on bone[93] and it has been suggested that the combination of oestradiol and norethisterone seems better than other oestrogen/progestogen combinations.[24] However, preliminary 12-month data suggest that 1 mg oestradiol in combination with 5 mg, 10 mg or 20 mg dydrogesterone will also prevent bone loss at the lumbar spine and hip.[94] Tibolone is equally as effective in conserving bone mass as conventional doses of HRT.[95]

RISKS

The principal risks of HRT are an increased risk of venous thromboembolism (VTE), breast cancer and endometrial cancer. The latter has already been addressed. Large-scale epidemiological data on continuous combined HRT and the other two risks are not available. However, does the addition of progestogen continuously rather than cyclically have any overall bearing on these risks?

The addition of progestogen *per se* does not seem to lower the increased risk of breast cancer seen with oestrogen alone,[96–98] indeed it may increase it.[99] Persson *et al*.[100] reported a moderate increase in breast cancer risk with long-term HRT with possible further enhancement with added progestins. Ross *et al*.[101] observed an increased risk of breast cancer with sequential oestrogen/progestogen therapy (OR 1.38; 95% CI 1.13-1.68) when compared with continuous combined oestrogen/progestogen therapy (OR 1.09; 95% CI 0.88-1.35) although the difference was not statistically significant. Mammographic observations in the PEPI study saw a much greater increase in density with combined oestrogen/progestogen therapy than with oestrogen alone but no difference between cyclical and continuous progestogens.[102] However, Lundstrom *et al*.[103] found that increased mammographic density was more common in those on continuous progestogens (52%) than in those on sequential progestogens (13%) or oestrogen alone (18%). As mammographic density may be associated with increased cancer risk[104] these findings are of some concern. Tibolone appears to have different biological effects to HRT on the breast with no apparent stimulatory effect,[105] less reported breast tenderness[10] and no increase in mammographic density.[106] There are no epidemiological data on tibolone and breast cancer risk.

Several studies have now demonstrated a small but significant increased risk of VTE in unselected women going on to HRT.[107] This risk seems to be greatest in the first year of treatment and is probably dose related. In a recent observational study from Norway, 140 women with a past history of VTE were randomised to placebo or HRT (2 mg oestradiol plus 1 mg NETA daily).[108] The study was terminated early with a 2.3% incidence of VTE in the placebo group compared with 10.7% in the HRT group. All events happened within the first eight months of the study. Whether the type or combination of HRT has an impact on the risk of VTE is not clear from available data. Equally, there is no consensus about the mechanisms involved. Oestrogens have a mixed effect on haemostatic parameters, with some of its effects being antithrombotic, e.g. decreased fibrinogen, and some prothrombotic, e.g. decreasing anti-thrombin and protein S.[109] One study has suggested that combined oestrogen/progestogen therapy may have less effect on coagulation factors than oestrogen alone.[110] Transdermal HRT may have a less marked effect on the haemostatic system as it has less impact on liver enzymes.[111] In a recent comparative study, tibolone and, to a lesser extent, continuous combined oral HRT changed haemostatic parameters to a more fibrinolytic profile, which might be expected to actually reduce the risk of VTE.[112] Clearly, further studies in this area are needed but at present it seems reasonable to assume that all HRT products are associated with a small increase in risk. Thus, the lowest appropriate dose should be used and those with a strong personal or family history should be screened for thrombophilias. The transdermal route may be more suitable for those at higher risk. At present there are no data to support the use of prophylactic low-dose aspirin or warfarin in conjunction with HRT.

OTHER CLINICAL SCENARIOS

There are several specific clinical scenarios where period-free HRT may be particularly useful.

Previous endometrial cancer

HRT is generally contraindicated in this situation, although several studies have reported no increased risk of recurrent disease in women with previous endometrial cancer who have been given HRT.[113,114] As progestogens have an antimitotic effect on the endometrium, if there is a strong indication for HRT, it would seem reasonable to prescribe combined HRT rather than oestrogen alone,[115] even though the women will almost certainly have undergone hysterectomy.

Endometriosis

Many women with a history of symptomatic endometriosis will have had both ovaries removed, often at an early age, and thus have strong indications to take HRT. Theoretically, the reintroduction of oestrogens could cause recurrent disease, although it has been reported even in women not on HRT.[116] There are few studies addressing this issue. Henderson and Studd[117] found only one case of recurrent disease among 75 women given unopposed oestrogens immediately after hysterectomy, although they were also given testosterone, which may have had a confounding effect. However, the use of continuous combined HRT or tibolone in these women is probably to be recommended.[118]

Previous breast cancer

The use of HRT in women with a previous history of breast cancer is generally contraindicated. However, many of these women have troublesome menopausal symptoms. Current thinking on the possible use of HRT in this group of women was reviewed in 1998.[119] There are currently no data to indicate which, if any, preparation is most appropriate in this situation. However, two studies did observe a reduction in the risk of recurrent disease with progestogens given continuously.[120,121] In the Eden study[121] the dose of progestogen (MPA 50 mg daily) was much higher than that used in conventional combined regimens.

ALTERNATIVES

Conventional period-free HRT involves the continuous administration of oestrogen and progestogen. However, a number of alternative methods to achieve amenorrhoea have been explored. By far the most successful has been the use of the progestogen-releasing intrauterine system (IUS). Promising results in terms of compliance, bleeding patterns and endometrial response have been reported over five years.[122] Although currently not licensed for this indication in the UK, it is becoming increasingly used as part of HRT, particularly in Scandinavia. Spaulding[33] adopted a rather different approach: if women on conventional period-free HRT bled, the dose of progestogen was doubled. Most stopped bleeding at this stage, although 13% continued bleeding and in these women he carried out a hysteroscopic endometrial ablation with complete cessation of bleeding in all cases. Others have tried intermittent progestogen administration with some success.[123]

SUMMARY

The development of period-free HRT has been a major advance in the management of postmenopausal women. Although its use was first reported nearly 20 years ago it has only become a standard part of HRT in the UK in the last five to six years with the introduction of appropriately licensed products. Current data clearly indicate that period-free HRT is effective at preventing postmenopausal bone loss and protecting the endometrium. However, irregular and sometimes persistent bleeding is a common feature, particularly in the first six months. Careful patient selection and counselling are needed prior to using period-free HRT to maximise its benefits and adherence to therapy. Once amenorrhoea has been established it is usually maintained and further bleeding needs investigating. Period-free HRT is not suitable for women within 12 months of their last menstrual period, whatever their age and for those within three years of their last menses it may be worth considering higher doses of progestogen. A minority of women have persistent bleeding and for them sequential HRT or non-HRT alternatives may be a better option. The continuous addition of a progestogen does not appear to detract from the symptomatic benefits of HRT and in some women may be associated with reduced adverse effects. Long-term data on cardiovascular disease prevention and breast cancer risk are needed but, at present, it seems reasonable to assume a similar impact to sequential combined HRT. The introduction of lower-dose preparations holds promise for the future and would appear to be a particularly suitable option for women who wish to continue HRT long-term or to start it later (over 60 years) for the continuing prevention of osteoporotic fractures. However, more data are required on whether this approach will actually lead to a reduction in fractures before it is widely adopted.

References

1. Cauley, J.A., Cummings, S.R., Black, D.M., Mascioli, S.R., Seeley, D.G. Prevalence and determinants of estrogen replacement therapy in elderly women. *Am J Obstet Gynecol* 1990;**163**:1338–44
2. Purdie, D.W., Steel, S.A., Howey, S., Doherty, S.M. The technical and logistical feasibility of population densitometry using DEXA and directed HRT intervention: a 2-year prospective study. *Osteoporos Int* 1996;**3**:S31–6
3. Hope, S., Rees, M.C.P. Why do British women start and stop hormone replacement therapy? *J Br Meno Soc* 1995;**1**:26–7
4. Marsh, M.S., Whitehead, M.I. The practicalities of hormone replacement. *Baillière's Clin Endocrinol Metab* 1993;**7**:183–202
5. Staland, B. Continuous treatment with natural oestrogens and progestogens: a method to avoid endometrial stimulation. *Maturitas* 1981;**3**:145–56
6. Whitehead, M.I., Hillard, T.C., Crook, D. The role and use of progestogens. *Obstet Gynecol* 1990;**75**:559–76
7. Udoff, L., Langenberg, P., Adashi, E.Y. Combined continuous hormone replacement therapy; a critical review. *Obstet Gynecol* 1995;**8**:306–16
8. Pickar, J.H., Thorneycroft, I., Whitehead, M.I. Effects of hormone replacement therapy on the endometrium and lipid parameters: a review of the randomised clinical trials. *Am J Obstet Gynecol* 1998;**178**:1087–99
9. Archer, D.F., Pickar, J.H., Bottiglioni, F. Bleeding patterns in postmenopausal women taking continuous combined or sequential regimens of conjugated estrogens with medroxy-progesterone acetate. *Obstet Gynecol* 1994;**83**:686–92

10. Hammar, M., Christau, S., Nathorst-Boos, J., Rud, T., Garre, K. A double blind randomised study comparing the effects of tibolone and continuous combined hormone replacement therapy in postmenopausal women with menopausal symptoms. Br J Obstet Gynaecol 1998;**105**:904–11

11. Archer, D.F., Dorin, M.H., Heine, W., Nanavati, N., Arce, J-C. Uterine bleeding in postmenopausal women on continuous therapy with estradiol and norethindrone acetate. Obstet Gynecol 1999;**94**:323–9

12. Mattsson, L.Å., Bohnet, H.G., Gredmark, T., Torhorst, J., Hornig, F., Huls, G. Continuous combined hormone replacement: randomised comparison of transdermal and oral preparations. Obstet Gynecol 1999;**94**:61–5

13. Al-Azzawi, F., Wahab, M., Habiba, M., Akkad, A., Mason, T. Continuous combined hormone replacement therapy compared with tibolone. Obstet Gynecol 1999;**93**:258–64

14. Archer, D.F., Furst, K., Tipping, D., Dain, M.P., Vandepol, C. A randomised comparison of continuous combined transdermal delivery of estradiol-norethindrone acetate and estradiol alone for menopause. CombiPatch Study Group. Obstet Gynecol 1999;**94**:498–503

15. Hillard, T.C., Siddle, N.C., Whitehead, M.I., Fraser, D.I. Continuous combined equine estrogen-progestogen therapy: effects of medroxyprogesterone acetate and norethindrone acetate on bleeding patterns and endometrial histologic diagnosis. Am J Obstet Gynecol 1992;**167**:1–7

16. Tang, B., Markiewicz, L., Kloosterboer, H.J., Gurpide, E. Human endometrial 3β-hydroxy steroid dehydrogenase isomerase can locally reduce intrinsic estrogenic/progestogenic activity ratios of a steroidal drugs. J Steroid Biochem Mol Biol 1993;**45**:345–51

17. Markiewicz, L., Gurpide, E. In vitro evaluation of estrogenic, estrogenic antagonistic and progestogenic effects of a steroid drug (Org OD14) and its metabolites on human endometrium. J Steroid Biochem 1990;**35**:535–41

18. Magos, A.L., Brincat, M., Studd, J.W.W., Wardle, P., Schlesinger, P., O'Dowd, T. Amenorrhea and endometrial atrophy with continuous oral oestrogen and progestogen therapy in postmenopausal women. Obstet Gynecol 1985;**65**:496–9

19. Rymer, J., Fogelman, I., Chapman, M.G. The incidence of vaginal bleeding with tibolone treatment. Br J Obstet Gynaecol 1994;**101**:53–6

20. Baerug, U., Winge, T., Nordland, G., Faber-Swensson, E., Heldaas, K., Larsen, S. et al. Do combinations of 1mg oestradiol and low doses of NETA effectively control menopausal symptoms? Climacteric 1998;**1**:219–28

21. Mattsson, L.Å., Callberg, G., Samsioe, G. Evaluation of a continuous oestrogen-progestogen regimen for climacteric patients. Maturitas 1982;**4**:95–102

22. Prough, S.G., Askel, S., Wiebe, R.H., Shepherd, J. Continuous estrogen/progestin therapy in menopause. Am J Obstet Gynecol 1987;**157**:1449–53

23. Sporrong, T., Hellgren, M., Samsioe, G., Mattsson, L.A. Comparison of four continuously administered progestogen plus oestradiol combinations for climacteric symptoms. Br J Obstet Gynecol 1988;**95**:1042–8

24. Christiansen, C., Riis, B.J. Five years with continuous combined oestrogen/progestogen therapy. Effects on calcium metabolism, lipoproteins and bleeding patterns. Br J Obstet Gynaecol 1990;**9**:1087–92

25. Weinstein, L., Bewtra, C., Gallagher, J.C. Evaluation of a continuous combined low dose regimen of estrogen-progestin for treatment of the menopausal patient. Am J Obstet Gynecol 1990;**162**:153–62

26. Marslew, U., Riis, B.J., Christiansen, C. Bleeding patterns during continuous combined oestrogen progestogen therapy. Am J Obstet Gynecol 1991;**164**:1163–8

27 Leather, A.T., Savvas, M., Studd, J.W. Endometrial histology and bleeding patterns after 8 years of continuous combined estrogen and progestogen therapy in post menopausal women. *Obstet Gynecol* 1991;**78**:1008–10

28 Clisham, P.R., deZeigler, D., Lozano, K., Judd, H.L. Comparison of sequential versus continuous estrogen and progestogen replacement therapy in post menopausal women. *Obstet Gynecol* 1991;**77**:241–6

29 Obel, E.B., Munk-Jensen, N., Svenstrup, B., Bennett, P., Micic, S., Henrik Nielsen, R. et al. A two-year double-blind controlled study of the clinical effect of combined and sequential postmenopausal replacement therapy and steroid metabolism during treatment. *Maturitas* 1993;**16**:13–21

30 Rauch, U., Taubert, H.D. Continuous hormone replacement therapy with oestradiol valerate and chlormadinone acetate in adjustable doses. A preliminary study. *Maturitas* 1993;**17**:123–7

31 Luciano, A.A., De Souza, M.J., Roy, M.P., Schoenfeld, M.J., Nulsen, J.C., Halvorson, C.V. Evaluation of low dose estrogen and progestin therapy in postmenopausal women. A double blind, prospective study of sequential versus continuous therapy. *J Reprod Med* 1993;**38**:207–14

32 Grey, A.B., Candy, T.F., Reid, I.R. Continuous combined oestrogen/progestin therapy is well tolerated and increases bone density at the hip and spine in postmenopausal osteoporosis. *Clin Endocrinol* 1994;**40**:671–7

33 Spaulding, C.B. Endometrial ablation for refractory postmenopausal bleeding with continuous hormone replacement. *Fertil Steril* 1994;**6**:1181–5

34 MacLennan, A.H., MacLennan, A., Wenzel, S., Chambers, H.M., Eckert, K. Continuous low dose oestrogen and progestogen hormone replacement therapy: a randomised trial. *Med J Aust* 1993;**159**:102–6

35 Song, J.Y., Fraser, I.S. Effects of progestogens on human endometrium. *Obstet Gynecol Surv* 1995;**50**:385–94

36 Stadberg, E., Mattsson, L-A., Uvebrant, M. 17-β estradiol and norethisterone acetate in low doses as continuous combined hormone replacement therapy. *Maturitas* 1996;**23**:31–9

37 Ginsburg, J., Prelevic, G.M. Cause of vaginal bleeding in postmenopausal women taking tibolone. *Maturitas* 1996;**24**:107–10

38 Rees, M.C.P. Endometrial bleeding and hormone replacement therapy. *J Br Meno Soc* 1999;**5**:S17–19

39 Pickar, J.H., Archer, D.F. Is bleeding a predictor of endometrial hyperplasia in postmenopausal women receiving hormone replacement therapy? *Am J Obstet Gynecol* 1997;**177**:1178–83

40 Hillard, T.C. Serving without stimulation. *J Br Meno Soc* 1999;**5**:S11–13

41 Ettinger, B., Li, D.K., Klein, R. Unexpected vaginal bleeding and associated gynecological care in postmenopausal women using hormone replacement therapy: comparison cyclic versus continuous combined schedules. *Fertil Stertil* 1998;**69**:865–9

42 Woodruff, J.D., Pickar, J.H. Incidence of endometrial hyperplasia in postmenopausal women taking conjugated estrogens (Premarin) with medroxy-progesterone acetate or conjugated estrogens alone. *Am J Obstet Gynecol* 1994;**170**:1213–23

43 The Writing Group for the PEPI Trial. Effects of hormone replacement therapy on endometrial histology in postmenopausal women: The Post-menopausal Estrogen/Progestin Interventions Trial. *JAMA* 1996;**275**:370–5

44 Sturdee, D.W., Ulrich, L.G., Barlow, D.H., Wells, M. The endometrial response to sequential and continuous combined oestrogen-progestogen replacement therapy. *BJOG* 2000;**107**:1392–400

45 Hanggi, W., Bersinger, N., Altermatt, H.J., Birkhauser, M.H. Comparison of transvaginal ultra

sonography and endometrial biopsy in endometrial surveillance in postmenopausal HRT users. *Maturitas* 1997;**27**:133–43

46 Botsis, D., Kassanos, D., Kalogirou, D., Antoniou, G., Vitoratos, N., Karakitsos, P. Vaginal ultrasound of the endometrium in post-menopausal women with symptoms of urogenital atrophy on low-dose estrogen or tibolone treatment: a comparison. *Maturitas* 1997;**26**:57–62

47 von Dadelszen, P., Gillmer, M.D.G., Gray, M.D., McEwan, H.P., Pyper, R.J., Rollason, T.P. *et al.* Endometrial hyperplasia and adenocarcinoma during tibolone (Livial) therapy. *Br J Obstet Gynaecol* 1994;**101**:158–61

48 Beresford, S.A., Weiss, N.S., Voigt, L.F., McKnight, B. Risk of endometrial cancer in relation to use of oestrogen combined with cyclic progestogen therapy in postmenopausal women. *Lancet* 1997;**349**:458–61

49 Weiderpass, E., Adami, H-O., Baron, J.A., Magnusson, C., Bergstroem, R., Lindgren, A. *et al.* Risk of endometrial cancer following estrogen replacement with and without progestins. *J Natl Cancer Inst* 1999;**91**:1131–7

50 Hargrove, J.T., Maxson, W.S., Wentz, A.L., Barnett, L.S. Menopausal hormone replacement therapy with continuous daily oral micronised estradiol and progesterone. *Obstet Gynecol* 1989;**73**:606–12

51 Ulrich, L.G., Barlow, D.H., Sturdee, D.W., Wells, M., Campbell, M.J., Nielsen, B. *et al.* Quality of life and patient preference for sequential or continuous combined HRT: the UK Kliofem multicenter study experience. *Int J Gynaecol Obstet* 1997;**59**:S11–17

52 Nathorst-Boos, J., Hammar, M. Effect on sexual life: a comparison between tibolone and a continuous estradiol-norethisterone acetate regimen. *Maturitas* 1997;**26**:15–20

53 Notelovitz, M., Arce, J-C., Nanavati, N., Huang, W.C. (1998) Norethindrone acetate at 0.5 mg dose adds to efficacy of 1mg 17-β estradiol on vasomotor symptom relief. *Menopause* 1998;**5**:250–1

54 Hill, D.A., Weiss, N.S., LaCroix, A.Z. Adherence to postmenopausal hormone replacement therapy during the year after initial prescription: a population based study. *Am J Obstet Gynecol* 2000;**182**:270–6

55 David Sturdee, personal communication.

56 Rymer, J., Robinson, J., Fogelman, I. Effects of eight years of tibolone 2.5 mg daily on postmenopausal bone loss. *Osteoporos Int* 2001;in press

57 Doren, M., Reuther, G., Minne, H.W., Schneider, H.P.G. Superior compliance and efficacy of continuous combined oral oestrogen-progestogen replacement therapy in postmenopausal women. *Am J Obstet Gynecol* 1995;**17**:1446–51

58 Grodstein, F., Stampfer, M.J. The epidemiology of coronary heart disease and estrogen replacement in postmenopausal women. *Prog Cardiovasc Dis* 1995;**38**:199–210

59 Grodstein, F., Stampfer, M.J., Manson, J.E., Colditz, G.A., Willett, W.C., Rosner, B. *et al.* Postmenopausal estrogen and progestin use and the risk of cardiovascular disease. *N Engl J Med* 1996;**335**:453–61

60 Falkeborn, M., Persson, I., Adami, H.O., Bergstrom, R., Eaker, E., Lithell, H. *et al.* The risk of acute myocardial infarction after oestrogen and oestrogen-progestogen replacement. *Br J Obstet Gynecol* 1992;**99**:821–8

61 Grodstein, F., Stampfer, M.J. The cardioprotective effects of estrogen. In: Studd, J.W.W., editor. *The Management of the Menopause, Annual Review 1998.* Carnforth: Parthenon; 1998. p. 211–19

62 Mendelsohn, M.E., Karas, R.H. The protective effects of estrogen on the cardiovascular system. *N Engl J Med* 1999;**340**:1801–11

63 Barrett Connor, E., Bush, T.L. Estrogen and coronary heart disease in women. *JAMA* 1991;**265**:1861–7

64 Matthews, K.A., Milan, E., Keller, L.H., Kelsey, S.F., Cagoule, A.W., Wing, R.R. Menopause and risk factors for coronary heart disease. *N Engl J Med* 1989;**32**:641–6
65 Bush, T.L., Miller, V.T. Effects of pharmacologic agents used during menopause. Impact on lipids and lipoproteins. In: Mishell, D., editor. *Menopause: Physiology and Pharmacology*. Chicago: Year Book Medical Publishers; 1986. p. 187–208
66 Lobo, R.A., Pickar, J.H., Wild, R.A., Walsh, B., Hirvonen, E. for the Menopause Study Group. Metabolic impact of adding medroxyprogesterone acetate to conjugated estrogen therapy in postmenopausal women. *Obstet Gynecol* 1994;**84**:987–95
67 Postmenopausal Estrogen/Progestin Interventions Trial. Effects of estrogen or estrogen/progestin regimens on heart disease risk factors in postmenopausal women. *JAMA* 1995;**273**:199–208
68 Farish, E., Fletcher, C.D., Dagen, M.M., Hart, D.M., Al-Azzawi, F., Parkin, D.E. et al. Lipoprotein and apolipoprotein levels in postmenopausal women on continuous combined oestrogen/progestogen therapy. *Br J Obstet Gynecol* 1989;**96**:358–64
69 Samsioe, G., Larsen, S., Arce, J-C. Favourable changes in lipid and lipoproteins associated with continuous combined 1 mg 17-β estradiol and low doses of norethindrone acetate. *Menopause* 1998;**5**:259
70 Gordon, D.J., Probstfield, J.L., Garrison, R.J., Neaton, J.D., Castelli, W.P., Knoke, J.D. et al. High-density lipoprotein cholesterol and cardiovascular disease. Four prospective American studies. *Circulation* 1989;**79**:8–15
71 Crook, D. Effects of estrogens and progestogens on plasma lipids. In: Fraser, I.F., Jansen, R.P.S., Lobo, R.A., Whitehead, M.I., editors. *Estrogens and Progestins in Clinical Practice*. London: Churchill Livingstone; 1998. p. 787–98
72 Crook, D. Tibolone and the risk of arterial disease. *J Br Meno Soc* 1999;**5**:S30–3
73 Ettinger, B., Genant, H.K., Cann, C.E. Long term estrogen replacement therapy prevents bone loss and fractures. *Ann Intern Med* 1985;**102**:319–34
74 Kiel, D.P., Felson, D.T., Anderson, J.J., Wilson, P.W., Moskowitz, M.A. Hip fracture and the use of estrogens in postmenopausal women: the Framingham study. *N Engl J Med* 1987;**317**:1169–74
75 Kreiger, N., Kelsey, J.L., Holford, T.R., O'Connor, T. An epidemiologic study of hip fracture in postmenopausal women. *Am J Epidemiol* 1982;**116**:141–8
76 Maxim, P., Ettinger, B., Spitalny, G.M. Fracture protection provided by long-term estrogen therapy. *Osteoporos Int* 1995;**5**:23–9
77 Lippuner, K., Haenggi, W., Birkhauser, M.J., Jaeger, P. Prevention of postmenopausal bone loss using tibolone, conventional peroral or transdermal replacement therapy. *J Bone Miner Res* 1997;**12**:806–12
78 Eiken, P., Neilsen, S.P., Kolthoff, N. Effects on bone mass after eight years of hormone replacement therapy. *Br J Obstet Gynaecol* 1997;**104**:702–7
79 Schneider, D.L., Morton, D.J. Timing of postmenopausal estrogen for optimal bone mineral density. In: Studd, J.W.W., editor. *The Management of the Menopause, Annual Review 1998*. Carnforth: Parthenon; 1998. p. 135–42
80 Kanis, J. Treatment strategies in osteoporosis. *J Br Meno Soc* 2000;**6**:S17–19
81 Michaelsson, K., Baron, J.A., Fahramand, B.Y., Johnell, O., Magnusson, C., Persson, P.G. et al. Hormone replacement therapy and the risk of hip fracture: population based case-control. *BMJ* 1998;**316**:1858–63
82 Christiansen, C., Christensen, M.S., Transbol, I. Bone mass in postmenopausal women after withdrawal of oestrogen/progestogen replacement therapy. *Lancet* 1981;**i**:459–61
83 Tremollieres, F., Pouilles, J.M., Ribot, C. Cessation of estrogen replacement therapy is

associated with a significant vertebral bone loss: a longitudinal study. *J Bone Miner Res* 1997;**12**:S103
84. Felson, D.T., Zhang, Y., Hannan, M.T., Kiel, D.P., Wilson, P.W., Anderson, J.J. The effect of postmenopausal estrogen therapy on bone density in elderly women. *N Engl J Med* 1993;**329**:1141–6
85. Cauley, J.A., Seeley, D.G., Ensrud, K., Ettinger, B., Black, D., Cummings, S.R. Estrogen replacement therapy and fractures in older women. *Ann Intern Med* 1995;**122**:9–16
86. Lindsay, R., Tohme, J.F. Estrogen treatment of patients with established osteoporosis. *Obstet Gynecol* 1990;**76**:290–5
87. Lufkin, E.G., Wahner, H.W., O'Fallon, W.M., Hodgson, S.F., Kotowicz, M.A., Lane, A.W. et al. Treatment of post menopausal osteoporosis with transdermal estrogen. *Ann Intern Med* 1992;**117**:1–9
88. Schneider, D.L., Barrett-Connor, E.L., Morton, D.J. Timing of post menopausal estrogen for optimal bone mineral density. *JAMA* 1997;**277**:543–7
89. Ettinger, B., Grady, D. Maximising the benefits of estrogen therapy for prevention of osteoporosis. *Menopause* 1994;**1**:19–24
90. Ettinger, B., Genant, H.K., Steiger, P., Madvig, P. Low-dosage micronised 17-β estradiol prevents bone loss in postmenopausal women. *Am J Obstet Gynecol* 1992;**166**,479–88
91. Delmas, P.D., Confavreux, E., Garnero, P., Fardellone, P., de Vernejoul, M-C., Cormier, C., et al. A combination of low doses of 17-β estradiol and norethisterone acetate prevents bone loss and normalises bone turnover in postmenopausal women. *Osteoporos Int* 2000;**11**:177–87
92. Hillard, T.C., Whitcroft, S.J., Marsh, M.S., Lees, B., Whitehead, M.I., Stevenson, J.C. Long-term effects of transdermal and oral hormone replacement therapy on postmenopausal bone loss. *Osteoporos Int* 1994;**4**:341–8
93. Riis, B.J., Christiansen, C., Johansen, J.S., Jacobson, J. Is it possible to prevent bone loss in young women treated with luteinizing hormone releasing hormone agonists? *J Clin Endocrinol Metab* 1990;**70**:920–4
94. Stevenson, J.C. Continuous 17-β-oestradiol (1 mg)/dydrogesterone, (5-20 mg) increases BMD. *Maturitas* 2000;**35**:S78
95. Prelevic, G.M., Bartram, C., Wood, J., Okolo, S., Ginsburg, J. Comparative effects of bone mineral density of tibolone, transdermal oestrogen and oral oestrogen/progestogen therapy in postmenopausal women. *Gynecol Endocrinol* 1996;**10**:413–20
96. Bergkvist, L., Adami, H.O., Persson, I., Hoover, R., Schairer, C. The risk of breast cancer after estrogen and estrogen-progestin replacement. *N Engl J Med* 1989;**321**:293–7
97. Colditz, G.A., Hankinsson, S.E., Hunter, D.J., Willett, W.C., Manson, J.E., Stampfer, M. et al. The use of estrogens and progestins and the risk of breast cancer in postmenopausal women. *N Engl J Med* 1995;**332**:1589–93
98. Persson, I., Yuen, J., Bergkvist, L. Schairer, C. Cancer incidence and mortality in women receiving estrogen and estrogen-progestin replacement therapy. Long-term follow-up of a Swedish cohort. *Int J Cancer* 1996;**67**:327–32
99. Schairer, C., Lubin, J., Troisi, R., Sturgeon, S., Brinton, L., Hoover, R. Menopausal estrogen and estrogen-progestin replacement therapy and breast cancer risk. *JAMA* 2000;**283**:534–5
100. Persson, I., Thurfjell, E., Bergstrom, R., Holmberg, L. Hormone replacement therapy and the risk of breast cancer. Nested case-control study in a cohort of Swedish women attending mammography screening. *Int J Cancer* 1997;**72**:758–61
101. Ross, R.K., Paganini-Hill, A., Wan, P.C., Pike, M.C. Effects of hormone replacement therapy on breast cancer risk: estrogen versus estrogen plus progestin. *J Natl Cancer Inst* 2000;**92**:328–32

102 Greendale, G.A., Reboussin, B.A., Sie, A., Singh, H.R., Olson, L.K., Gatewood, O. et al. Effects of estrogen and estrogen-progestin on mammographic parenchymal density. Postmenopausal Estrogen/Progestin Interventions (PEPI) Investigators. *Ann Intern Med* 1999;**130**:262–9

103 Lundstrom, E., Wilczek, B., von Palffy, Z., Soderqvist, G., von Schoultz, B. Mammographic bone density during hormone replacement therapy: differences according to treatment. *Am J Obstet Gynecol* 1999;**181**:348–52

104 Byrne, C., Schairer, C., Wolfe, J., Parekh, N., Salane, M., Brinton, L.A. et al. Mammographic features and breast cancer risk: effects with time, age and menopause status. *J Natl Cancer Inst* 1995;**87**:1622–9

105 Gompel, A., Kandouz, M., Siromachkova, M., Lombet, A., Thevenin, D., Mimoun, M. et al. The effect of tibolone on proliferation, differentiation and apoptosis in normal breast cells. *Gynecol Endocrinol* 1997;**11** Suppl 1:77–9

106 Erel, C.T., Elter, K., Akman, C., Ersavasti, G., Altug, A., Seyisoglu, H. et al. Mammographic changes in women receiving tibolone therapy. *Fertil Steril* 1998;**69**:870–5

107 Barlow, D. Epidemiology and findings from recent HRT studies. In: Sturdee, D., editor. *HRT and Thromboembolism*. London: Royal Society of Medicine Press; 1997. p. 17–24

108 Hoibraaten, E., Qvigstad, E., Arnesen, H., Larsen, S., Wickstrom, E., Sandset, P.M. Increased risk of recurrent venous thromboembolism (VTE) during hormone replacement therapy (HRT); results of the estrogen in venous thromboembolism trial. *Maturitas* 2000;**35**:S11

109 Lowe, G. Effects of oestrogen on thromboembolism. In: Sturdee, D., editor. *HRT and Thromboembolism*. London: Royal Society of Medicine Press; 1997. p. 3–16

110 Lowe, G. Coagulation, fibrinolysis and hormone replacement therapy. In: Shaw, R.D., editor. *Oestrogen Deficiencies – Causes and Consequences*. Carnforth: Parthenon; 1996. p. 29–44

111 Kroon, U.B., Silverstople, G., Tengborn, L. The effects of transdermal estradiol and conjugated estrogens on haemostasis variables. *Thromb Haemost* 1994;**71**:420–3

112 Winkler, U.H., Altkemper, F., Kwee, B., Helmond, F.A., Coelingh Bennik, H.J.T. Effects of tibolone and continuous combined hormone replacement therapy on parameters in the clotting cascade: a multicenter, double blind, randomised study. *Fertil Steril* 2000;**74**:10–19

113 Creasman, W.T., Henderson, D., Hinshaw, W., Clarke-Pearson, O.C. Estrogen replacement therapy in the patient treated for endometrial cancer. *Obstet Gynecol* 1986;**17**:326–30

114 Lee R.B., Burke R.C., Park R.C. Estrogen replacement therapy following treatment for stage 1 endometrial carcinoma. *Gynecol Oncol* 1990;**36**:189–93

115 Lauritzen, C. Hormone replacement therapy after endometrial cancer. In: Whitehead, M.I., editor. *The Prescribers Guide to Hormone Replacement Therapy*. Carnforth: Parthenon; 1998. p. 79–82

116 Kempers, R.D., Dockerty, M.B., Hunt, A.B., Symmonds R.E. Significant postmenopausal endometriosis. *Surg Gynecol Obstet* 1960;**111**:348–56

117 Henderson, A.F., Studd, J.W.W. The role of definitive surgery and hormone replacement therapy in the treatment of endometriosis. In: Thomas, E.J., Rock, J.A., editors. *Modern Approaches to Endometriosis*. London: Kluwer;1991. p. 275–90

118 Brosens, I.A. Hormone replacement therapy and endometriosis. In: Whitehead, M.I., editors. *The Prescribers Guide to Hormone Replacement Therapy*. Carnforth: Parthenon; 1998. p. 83–93

119 Marsden, J., Sacks, N.P.M. Hormone replacement therapy and breast cancer. In: Whitehead, M.I., editor. *The Prescribers Guide to Hormone Replacement Therapy*. Carnforth: Parthenon; 1998. p. 95–113

120 Stoll, B.A. Hormone replacement therapy in women treated for breast cancer. *Eur J Cancer Clin Oncol* 1989;**25**:1909–13

121 Eden, J.A., Bush, T., Nand, S., Wren, B.G. A case-controlled study of combined continuous oestrogen–progestogen replacement therapy amongst women with a personal history of breast cancer. *Menopause* 1995;**2**:67–72

122 Suvanto-Luukkonen, E., Kauppila, A. The levonorgestrel intrauterine system in menopausal hormone replacement therapy: five year experience. *Fertil Steril* 1999;**72**:161–3

123 Casper, R.F., Chapdelaine, A. Estrogen and interupted progestins: a new concept for menopausal hormone replacement therapy. *Am J Obstet Gynecol* 1993;**168**:1188–94

12

Glandular abnormalities: difficult situations in colposcopy

Susan J. Houghton

INTRODUCTION

Cervical cancer is the second most common female cancer worldwide.[1] The incidence of adenocarcinoma of the cervix is variously quoted as ranging from 5.5%[2] to 34%[3] of all cervical carcinomas and is increasing,[4] most notably in young women (aged less than 35 years).[5-7] Squamous carcinoma of the cervix, which accounts for the vast majority of cervical cancers, has a well-defined preinvasive stage.[8-10] Progression from premalignant cervical intraepithelial neoplasia (CIN) to invasive squamous carcinoma is well documented.[11,12] Cervical cytology screening programmes designed to detect CIN have led to a reduction in the incidence of invasive squamous carcinoma of the cervix.[13,14] Since the introduction of an organised national screening programme in England in 1988, there has been an overall decrease of 35% in the incidence of invasive cervical cancer[15] and an accelerated reduction in mortality of approximately 7% per year.[16]

It has been postulated that preinvasive glandular lesions of the cervix also exist and that these are the precursors of cervical adenocarcinoma.[17] Management of these premalignant glandular lesions is far more contentious than that of CIN. The relative rarity of the condition, lack of understanding of the natural history of the disease and diagnostic difficulties have resulted in a lack of definitive management guidelines. This chapter highlights these difficulties and defines current treatment trends.

HISTOPATHOLOGY

Histological classification of cervical preinvasive glandular lesions

Intraepithelial glandular lesions of the cervix, like their squamous counterparts, form a morphological spectrum that ranges from minor changes to severe abnormalities. A wide variety of terms and classification criteria has been used by different authors to describe these lesions.

The concept of a preinvasive precursor to adenocarcinoma was first introduced by Helper *et al.* in 1952.[18] In 1953, the term adenocarcinoma *in situ* (AIS) of the cervix was described by Friedell and McKay,[19] referring to all intraepithelial glandular lesions of the cervix not classified as invasive adenocarcinomas. The entire spectrum is better described as cervical intraepithelial glandular neoplasia (CIGN).[20] It has been suggested that CIGN should be divided into three grades comparable to the terminology used for CIN.[17] However, the most reproducible classification system divides the spectrum into two grades, low- and high-grade CIGN. Other two-grade classification systems commonly quoted use the terms glandular atypia and AIS[21] or glandular dysplasia and AIS.[22,23]

Histological characteristics of CIGN

Glandular preinvasive lesions are located within the cervical columnar epithelium. This extends from the outer limit of the acquired transformation zone (the line of the original squamocolumnar junction) to the upper limit of the endocervical canal at the level of the internal cervical os. This includes columnar epithelium lying in the crypts and tunnels of the endocervix (Figure 1). Although CIGN may affect any part of the cervical columnar epithelium, most lesions are found adjacent to the squamocolumnar junction.[22,24,25]

Normal endocervical columnar epithelium is characterised by a regular, single layer of tall columnar cells with basal nuclei and abundant mucin-rich cytoplasm. The cellular characteristics of CIGN include loss of nuclear polarity, variation in nuclear size (pleomorphism) and in nuclear shape (anisokaryosis), increased nuclear staining (hyperchromasia), increased mitotic activity, a reduction in cytoplasmic mucin and nuclear stratification (Figures 2 and 3).

CIGN often retains the architectural pattern of normal gland crypts, with abrupt transitions between normal and abnormal epithelium within the same crypt. If disrupted, CIGN may show the architectural characteristics of cellular crowding leading to pseudostratification, variation in size and shape of glands, papillary infoldings and outpouchings ('tunnel clusters') (Figure 4).

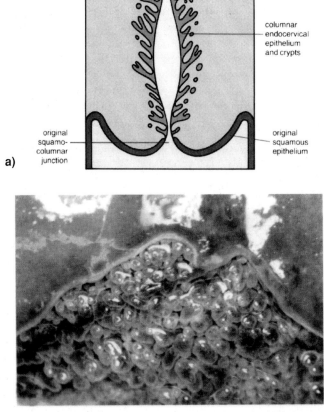

Figure 1 *(a) The original squamocolumnar junction is situated at the external cervical os; the columnar epithelium is situated in the endocervical canal; (b) colposcopic appearances of normal columnar epithelium at the squamocolumnar junction; (reproduced with permission from Anderson et al.[76])*

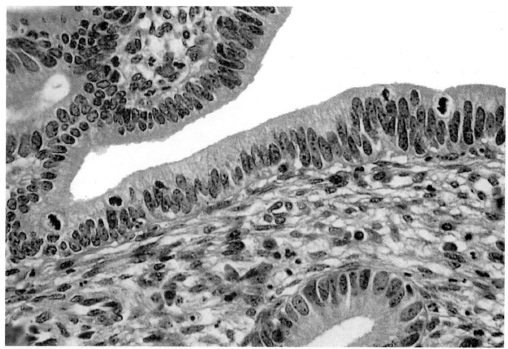

Figure 2 *Low-grade cervical intraepithelial glandular neoplasia showing an increase in nuclear size, nuclear pleomorphism and mitotic figures; polarity is largely maintained and mucin-containing cytoplasm is seen (reproduced with permission from Anderson et al.[76])*

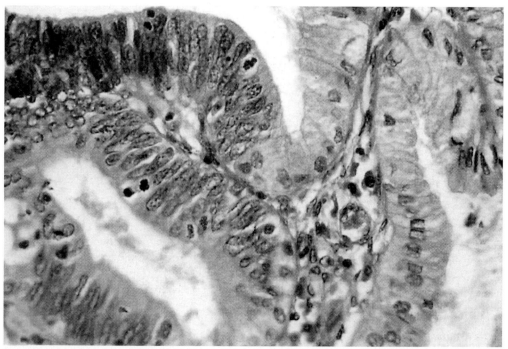

Figure 3 *High-grade cervical intraepithelial glandular neoplasia or adenocarcinoma* in situ *showing numerous mitotic figures (reproduced with permission from Anderson et al.[76])*

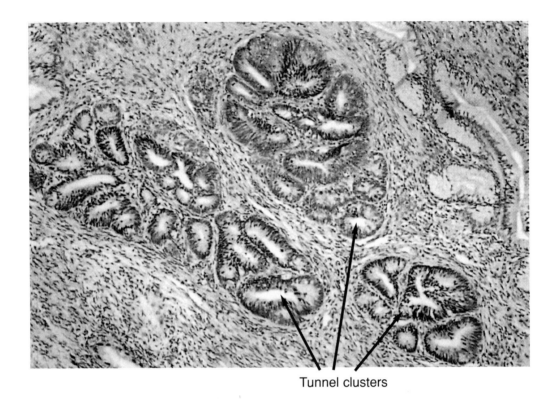

Tunnel clusters

Figure 4 *High-grade cervical intraepithelial glandular neoplasia or adenocarcinoma in situ showing disruption of the architectural pattern, with glandular reduplication and formation of 'tunnel clusters' as shown (reproduced with permission from Anderson et al.[76])*

Histological differential diagnosis of CIGN

A variety of non-neoplastic lesions may be found in the cervix that are difficult to distinguish histologically from CIGN. The differential diagnoses include tubo-endometrial metaplasia and endometriosis, papillary endocervicitis and other inflammatory changes, adenomatoid proliferation, Arias-Stella reaction, mesonephric remnant hyperplasia and microglandular endocervical hyperplasia. It can also be difficult to distinguish CIGN from invasive adenocarcinoma.

Identification of early invasion on histology depends upon the ability to recognise which glandular structures represent CIGN involving pre-existing gland crypts and which are truly invasive. CIGN generally becomes a well-differentiated adenocarcinoma either by budding off well-formed invasive glandular structures, which may be more irregular and crowded than CIGN, or by extending beyond the normal crypt field. Invasion should be suspected in the presence of budding and reduplication of crypts resulting in a cribriform pattern or a stromal inflammatory response.

Immunohistochemical staining with the monoclonal antibody HMFG1 (human milk-fat globule antigen) may help differentiate between CIGN and invasive adenocarcinoma from benign conditions.[26] Staining is cytoplasmic in CIGN and invasive disease and on the luminal surface of the cells in benign lesions.

AETIOLOGY

The aetiology of CIGN is unknown. Co-existent CIN has been found in 48-89% of cases of AIS.[24,25,27-34] It has been postulated that both CIN and AIS have a common cell of origin, the subcolumnar reserve cell.[35,36]

CIGN is associated with low parity, late age of onset of menarche, an early age at first coitus, an increased number of sexual partners and oral contraceptive usage.[37,38] Evidence points to a sexually transmitted factor, probably human papillomavirus (HPV), acting as a carcinogen or co-carcinogen and having a role in the pathogenesis of both squamous and glandular cervical preinvasive and invasive disease.[39,40]

More than 100 types of HPV have been isolated, with HPV 16 and 18 infection most commonly identified in squamous and glandular cervical lesions, respectively.[41,42] Using the highly sensitive polymerase chain reaction, HPV DNA can be detected in up to 85% of adenocarcinomas of the cervix.[43] HPV DNA has also been identified in AIS and low-grade CIGN.[44,45] HPV is thought to target the endocervical reserve cells and infection with the virus could be an early event in oncogenesis. In areas of CIN co-existing with AIS, the same type of HPV, predominantly HPV 18, has been identified.[46] HPV produces two oncoproteins, E6 and E7, which bind to and inactivate the tumour-suppressor proteins produced by *p53* and the retinoblastoma gene, respectively. Expression of the host *p53* gene can normally block entry to the cell cycle until any DNA damage is repaired. Repression of *p53* may allow accumulation of DNA mutations, leading to deregulated cellular proliferation and transformation. Other events such as exposure to chemical or physical carcinogens or the action of oncogenes may act as co-factors in carcinogenesis.

CIGN AS A PRECURSOR OF CERVICAL ADENOCARCINOMA

There is no direct proof that CIGN is a precursor of invasive cervical adenocarcinoma. However, there is much circumstantial evidence supporting the view that a preinvasive phase exists and it is now widely accepted that AIS, or high-grade CIGN, is a premalignant lesion and precedes invasive adenocarcinoma.[34,47]

The mean age of women with high-grade CIGN is 10-20 years younger than those with invasive disease.[35,48] Plaxe and Saltzstein,[49] in a recent epidemiological study of 5845 women with glandular lesions, found that the mean age at diagnosis for AIS was 13 years younger than for adenocarcinoma, supporting the concept of a lengthy preclinical phase of progression to invasion.

High-grade CIGN and adenocarcinoma often co-exist and are found adjacent to each other.[50] Retrospective analysis of histological specimens has confirmed the presence of CIGN several years before the diagnosis of invasive adenocarcinoma. Boon et al.[51] studied 52 cases of adenocarcinoma, 18 of whose previous endocervical biopsies were reported as showing no glandular abnormality, taken between three and seven years prior to the diagnosis of invasive disease. On review, five of the biopsies were found to contain atypical endocervical tissue.

DETECTION OF CIGN

CIGN is an uncommon condition with unknown incidence. Christopherson et al.[52] quote an incidence ratio of AIS to CIN 3 of 1:239, following a large population-based study, compared with a ratio of 1:25 quoted by Boon et al.[53] Due to the relative rarity of the disease, most clinicopathological studies are small and retrospective. CIGN is asymptomatic in the vast majority of cases, although, occasionally, patients may present with abnormal bleeding or discharge. Its detection usually depends upon cytological abnormalities suggestive of a glandular lesion or incidental histologic findings in surgical specimens taken in the treatment of suspected CIN or in hysterectomy specimens.

It is well recognised that preinvasive glandular lesions are frequently underdiagnosed, both on cytology and histology.

Cytology

If the duration of the premalignant phase of cervical adenocarcinoma is lengthy, the opportunity may exist for screening, early treatment and the prevention of invasive disease. The concept of cytological screening for cervical adenocarcinoma was proposed in a retrospective review of the cervical cytology of 13 women diagnosed with invasive adenocarcinoma.[54] Six of these women had abnormal smears between two and eight years prior to the diagnosis of invasion, supporting the theory that a preinvasive glandular lesion existed that could be detected on cervical cytology.

The cytological criteria for the diagnosis of CIGN have been well described.[55] Features include nuclear pleomorphism and hyperchromasia, irregular chromatin distribution, prominent nucleoli and poorly-defined, granular, finely vacuolated cytoplasm with indistinct cell borders. Pseudostratification of cells within the smear is common and, rarely, discrete single cells or small clusters, known as 'rosettes' are seen. The differential diagnosis of CIGN on cervical cytology includes invasive adenocarcinoma (Figure 5), high-grade CIN, reactive endocervical glands, tubal or tuboendometrial metaplasia, inflammation, changes associated with IUCDs and microglandular hyperplasia.

CIGN is underdiagnosed cytologically. The sensitivity of cervical smears for CIGN is much lower than that for CIN, as false-negative smear interpretation is common. This poor sensitivity (illustrated in Table 1) may be related to benign metaplastic or dysplastic change in the surface columnar cells obscuring CIGN lesions of deeper glands.[52] It may also be related to the small size of the lesion.[65] When both a squamous and a glandular intraepithelial abnormality coexist on the same cervix, cytological sensitivity in diagnosing a glandular lesion is reduced.[66,67] The cells shed from CIN tend to have more clearly defined cytoplasm and more marked nuclear changes than those from CIGN. This may result in the associated glandular abnormality being incorrectly graded or even overlooked.[55]

The specificity of cytology in the diagnosis of cervical glandular lesions has also been questioned,[68] with a false-positive rate of 2% being reported by one group.[69]

Accurate interpretation of glandular cytological abnormalities requires experience and expertise, as cytologists are less familiar with the diagnostic features. Lee et al.[70] have identified

Table 1 Cytological sensitivity for cervical glandular abnormality in women with histologically confirmed adenocarcinoma in situ

Reference	Sensitivity (%)[b]
Nguyen and Jeannot[56]	65
Ostor et al.[24]	71
Luesley et al.[57a]	71
Anderson and Arffmann[58]	50
Cullimore et al.[59]	53
Widrich et al.[60]	42
Wolf et al.[61]	50
Houghton et al.[62]	42
Denehy et al.[63]	45
Azodi et al.[64]	73

[a] Included glandular atypia; [b] combined cytological sensitivity = 56%

several major cytological characteristics (feathering, cellular crowding and nuclear/cytoplasmic ratio over 50%) that, together with other features (rosettes, mitotic figures and cellular strips), improve the accuracy of diagnosis of AIS. There is recent evidence of increased recognition by cytologists,[60] which will help reduce screening errors.

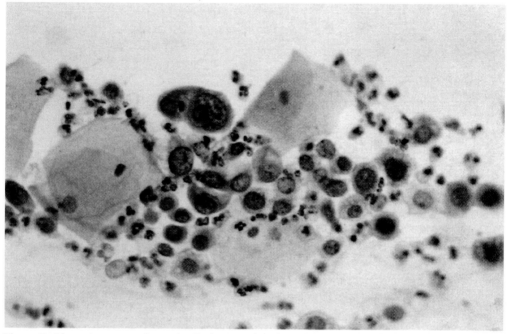

Figure 5 *Adenocarcinoma on cytology with cells showing nuclear pleomorphism and hyperchromasia, with indistinct cytoplasm (reproduced with permission from Anderson et al.[76])*

The lack of cytological sensitivity for CIGN has also been attributed to the use of the Ayre spatula alone.[71] Improved sampling of the transformation zone and endocervix with an endocervical brush smear may offer the opportunity to increase detection of CIGN and limit sampling error.[72,73] Routine sampling of the endocervical canal with a brush smear in high-risk patients has been shown to reduce the rate of inadequate and false-negative smears.[74] Large multicentre prospective studies of the cytological diagnosis of CIGN comparing different sampling techniques are needed to confirm these findings.

Colposcopy

Hinselmann first described the technique of colposcopy in 1925.[75] It is now widely used in the assessment of women with suspected CIN.

The most commonly practised method of colposcopy involves the application of 3% or 5% acetic acid to the cervix, which is then inspected through the colposcope. The colposcope has a stereoscopic microscope providing a three-dimensional image of the cervix or other area of the female lower genital tract, magnified 6–40 times. Schillers's iodine and saline are also used to define and delineate abnormal areas. Squamous lesions of CIN will appear as varying degrees of acetowhiteness and have well-documented colposcopic features that aid diagnosis.

The colposcopist will give a subjective opinion on the grade of CIN present based upon:

(1) The intensity of acetowhitening;
(2) The rapidity of onset and persistence of acetowhitening;
(3) The surface pattern of the lesion;
(4) Lesion size;
(5) Lesion edge definition and regularity;
(6) The degree of punctation and mosaic vessel pattern;
(7) Intercapillary distance;
(8) The presence of abnormal vessels.

Unlike its squamous counterpart, CIGN has no easily detectable colposcopic features.[76] There are no universally accepted criteria for colposcopic diagnosis and most authors believe that it is impossible to reliably diagnose glandular abnormalities of the cervix colposcopically.[24,57,76-78] However, Coppleson[79] suggested that AIS lesions have a 'stark acetowhiteness of either individual or fused villi in discrete patches of varying size'. The lesions are usually within or near the transformation zone and may be surrounded by villi that appear normal. Ferris et al.[80] described a case of AIS diagnosed on colposcopically directed punch biopsy, where the abnormal glandular epithelium was 'a denser, yellow-acetowhite colour compared with the surrounding metaplastic epithelium', with 'several 'root-like' atypical vessels'.

The diagnostic role of cervical punch biopsy in CIGN is limited by the lack of well-established colposcopic characteristics. Luesley et al.[57] demonstrated that 5/17 colposcopically directed punch biopsies correctly diagnosed the glandular abnormality subsequently detected on cervical conisation or hysterectomy, thus confirming previous findings.[24,52]

The anatomical distribution of CIGN may render it inaccessible to colposcopic detection. CIGN may involve any part of the endocervical canal, the abnormality not being confined to a circumscribed transformation zone.[56] The surface epithelium may appear normal and is not always involved when CIGN is present. Jaworski et al.[27] reported 72 cases of AIS and found that the necks of the endocervical glands were involved in 97% of the patients but the surface epithelium was involved additionally only 52% of the time. The surface epithelium also usually shows no abnormal features or vascular changes if CIGN is located on the ectocervix.[24,58] A negative colposcopic examination may indicate missed occult disease and any foci identified may underestimate the severity of the abnormality present.

Despite its lack of sensitivity for detecting CIGN, colposcopic assessment is mandatory in any case where abnormal glandular cells have been detected cytologically and CIGN is suspected. AIS is associated with CIN in approximately 50% of cases and it is essential to identify and define the extent of any co-existing squamous lesion on colposcopy, so that appropriate treatment can be undertaken. Vaginal colposcopy is advised to exclude co-existing vaginal intraepithelial neoplasia. A co-existing vaginal lesion would require a concomitant colpectomy. Colposcopy may also be useful in the detection of invasive adenocarcinoma (Figure 6).

Endocervical curettage

The role of endocervical curettage in the management of squamous intraepithelial neoplasia is strongly debated. It is rarely performed in the UK but is routinely practised by some in the

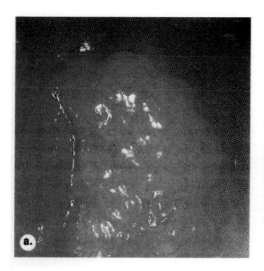 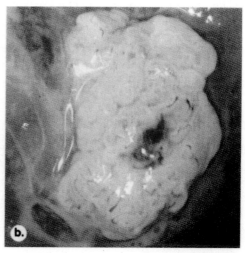

Figure 6 *Colposcopic appearances of adenocarcinoma before (a) and after (b) application of acetic acid; the lesion is raised and shows atypical vessels (reproduced with permission from Anderson et al.[76])*

investigation of an abnormal smear. It has been suggested that endocervical curettage may be useful in the management of AIS, although this has been evaluated in only a few studies. Nguyen and Jeannot[56] reported that endocervical curettage was falsely negative in three of four women with AIS. Poynor et al.[34] found that only 43% of pre-conisation curettage operations were positive for AIS, compared with 35% reported by Wolf et al.[61] It has also been recommended that endocervical curettage should be performed after the conisation to represent true sampling of tissue beyond surgical margins.[63]

Endocervical curettage may have a role if cytology is equivocal and suggestive of a low-grade glandular abnormality. A negative result may justify a 'wait and see' policy and reduce the number of unnecessary cone biopsies performed but this awaits prospective analysis.

MANAGEMENT OF CIGN

The optimal management of CIGN remains controversial. It is a rare condition and thus precludes an extensive clinical experience to determine management based upon the natural history of the disease. Most concern is expressed over the appropriate treatment of high-grade CIGN or AIS, as this is thought to be a preinvasive entity.

Hysterectomy

Hysterectomy has been advocated as treatment of high-grade CIGN or AIS. Early studies recommend extrafascial hysterectomy to ensure excision of 'skip lesions' present high in the endocervical canal in cases of multifocal AIS[52,65] and to exclude invasive disease.[81] Cases of residual disease in hysterectomy specimens following cone biopsy where margins were uninvolved by disease have been reported.[52,65] Concerns have also been expressed about deep glandular involvement and upper endocervical extension leading to recurrent disease if more conservative treatment is undertaken. A recent meta-analysis reviewing the incidence of residual disease following cone biopsy for AIS, with uninvolved margins, found an overall incidence of 10.2%.[82] The authors supported the use of hysterectomy as treatment for AIS.

However, there is no doubt that women with high-grade CIGN or AIS no longer desirous of fertility or who have other co-existent gynaecological pathology, are best treated by hysterectomy.

Cervical conisation

The median age of women with AIS is the fourth decade of life (mid 30s). Many women wish to preserve their fertility and the correct management of these women is of paramount importance. Several studies have shown that AIS involves glands to a depth of 4 mm and in most cases the abnormal glands extend no further than 25 mm from the cervical os.[24,25,56,58] The presence of 'skip lesions' has also been shown to be far less frequent than previously thought, with Ostor et al.[24] reporting multifocal lesions in 3/21 cases and Bertrand et al.[25] in 3/23 cases of AIS. Ostor et al.[24] also reported nine women with AIS who underwent hysterectomy following conisation. In six of these women the margins of the cone biopsy were involved by disease and four of these six had residual disease at hysterectomy. There was no residual disease found at hysterectomy in the three women who had cone biopsy margins with uninvolved excision margins. Qizilbash[35] previously reported that eight women with disease-free margins at conisation (one of whom had a 'microinvasive adenocarcinoma') had no residual disease at hysterectomy.

In the light of this information, the role of conisation as a more conservative treatment of AIS has been evaluated. The status of the excision margins in the diagnostic cone specimen is central to the decision to treat AIS conservatively. Any woman electing to undergo conservative management must be counselled about the risk of invasive disease and the need for intensive and long-term follow-up.

Involvement of the cone biopsy margins with AIS is associated with a significant risk of residual disease. Table 2 illustrates the incidence of residual disease in hysterectomy specimens taken after cone biopsy for AIS. It is universally recommended that further surgery, either a repeat cone biopsy or simple hysterectomy, is required where cone biopsy margins have been involved with disease. This is necessary to exclude any unsuspected, occult invasion and to prevent progression of any residual disease.

Bertrand et al.[25] after an anatomic study of 27 hysterectomy specimens with AIS, recommended that a deep cylindrical conisation, encompassing the transformation zone and extending parallel to the endocervical canal for at least 25 mm, would be therapeutic in most cases, if margins were uninvolved by disease. This recommendation was supported by Luesley et al.[57] who reported a retrospective review of 19 cases of AIS and 12 cases of glandular atypia. Ten women had hysterectomy following cone biopsy, with one of two with disease-free margins and four of eight with involved margins having residual disease at hysterectomy, respectively. Conisation alone was successful in 12/13 cases with a follow-up of 24–36 months.

Other authors have also suggested that there may be a role for conservative management of AIS in younger patients if conisation margins are uninvolved.[29,58,82] Nicklin et al.[82] measured the proximal linear extent from the squamocolumnar junction of 34 cases of AIS and found that this was positively correlated with the age of the woman. In women less than 36 years of age, 13/14 had lesions within 10 mm of the squamocolumnar junction, with the glands involved by AIS extending as far as 6 mm. The authors suggested that this should be taken into account when incising the cervix circumferentially under colposcopic guidance to define the transformation zone.

Table 2 *Residual disease rates in hysterectomy specimens following conisation for adenocarcinoma in situ*

Author	Proportion with residual disease			
	Negative margins		Positive margins	
	n	%	n	%
Ostor et al.[24]	0/3	0	4/6	67
Bertrand et al.[25]	0/4	0	0/1	0
Luesley et al.[57]	1/2	50	4/8	50
Hopkins et al.[83]	1/7	14	4/5	80
Anderson and Arffmann[58]	0/4	0	2/4	50
Nicklin et al.[82]	2/11	18	5/11	46
Muntz et al.[29]a	1/12	8	7/10	70
Cullimore et al.[59]	0/2	0	1/8	13
Poynor et al.[34]b	4/10	40	4/8	50
Im et al.[33]c	4/9	44	4/6	67
Widrich et al.[60]d	0/3	0	5/6	83
Wolf et al.[61]e	6/19	32	8/14	57
Denehy et al.[63]	4/6	67	4/5	80

aIncludes two cases of invasive adenocarcinoma; bincludes one case of invasive adenocarcinoma; c includes one case diagnosed on large loop excision of the transformation zone (LLETZ) (one case with involved margins underwent repeat conisation not hysterectomy); dincludes two cases that underwent reconisation not hysterectomy; eincludes six cases of invasive adenocarcinoma (cases diagnosed on LLETZ were excluded)

studied 18 cases of AIS diagnosed on cervical conisation and found residual disease on hysterectomy in four of nine women with disease-free resection margins and four of six women with involved margins. They concluded that negative margins on conisation did not reliably predict the absence of residual disease and did not consider conisation as definitive management of AIS. However, they suggested that conisation followed by close clinical monitoring with cervical cytology, endocervical curettage and colposcopy may be acceptable to preserve fertility, due to the low incidence of invasive disease following conisation for AIS.[33]

Poynor et al.[34] reported that 7/15 women with AIS, conservatively managed with repeat conisation or follow-up, developed recurrent disease, including two invasive adenocarcinomas. The authors questioned the safety of conisation but, in this study,[34] four of ten women with uninvolved margins had residual disease in a second surgical specimen, raising doubts about the adequacy of the initial surgical specimen and pathological interpretation.

The only prospective trial to date of cervical conisation in the management of CIGN supports the safety and efficacy of cold-knife cone biopsy, with uninvolved surgical margins, as conservative treatment of the disease.[59] Of the 51 women in the study population, 42 had cone-biopsy margins free of disease. Of these, 35 (83%) were managed by cone biopsy alone and had negative follow-up cytology after a median follow-up of 12 months. No residual glandular disease was detected in the seven remaining women who developed abnormal glandular cytology on follow-up, although one case of CIN 1 and one case of CIN 3 was identified. However, further follow-up of this cohort over several years is required to provide stronger evidence about the long-term effectiveness and safety of conisation as conservative treatment of CIGN.

LLETZ

Large loop excision of the transformation zone (LLETZ), as described by Prendiville et al.,[84] has become increasingly popular as an outpatient treatment for CIN.[85] LLETZ combines the advantages of local destructive techniques with those of conisation and allows complete excision of the transformation zone with minimal tissue damage. It is a quick procedure with high patient acceptability[86] and is associated with minimal immediate or long-term morbidity.[87,88] The incidence of cervical stenosis post-LLETZ is significantly less than that related to cone biopsy, which can occur in up to 40% of women, depending upon the length of the cervical canal excised.[89] Several authors have assessed the efficacy of LLETZ as conservative treatment of AIS to determine whether it is adequate management of the disease.

Widrich et al.[60] reviewed 46 cases of AIS and found that cold-knife conisation resulted in a 33% rate of positive margins for AIS compared with 50% for LLETZ. In women treated conservatively, they reported a recurrence rate of AIS of 16% (1/18) in those managed with initial cold-knife cone biopsy, compared with 29% (4/14) in those managed by LLETZ. One woman from this series developed invasive adenocarcinoma of the cervix one year after conservative treatment of AIS by LLETZ.[90] The initial LLETZ specimen had positive margins for AIS, but there was no evidence of residual disease on repeat LLETZ one month later. The authors[90] recommended that a cold-knife cone biopsy should be performed whenever AIS is suspected, a view that was later supported by Muntz.[91]

Azodi et al.[64] reported in 1999 a retrospective review comparing LLETZ with conisation in the management of AIS. LLETZ cones were significantly more likely to have positive endocervical margins than cold-knife cones (24% compared with 75%) and women with positive endocervical margins had a higher incidence of residual disease. One of the study cases developed invasive adenocarcinoma 15 months after a cold-knife cone biopsy with negative cone margins. However, in our retrospective review of 19 cases of AIS diagnosed on LLETZ, there were no confirmed cases of residual disease, with a median follow-up of 19 months.[62]

Cold-knife conisation specimens are of larger volume and more adequate for histologic evaluation than LLETZ specimens.[92] LLETZ also removes significantly less of the endocervix compared with cold-knife conisation.[93] Most clinicians now believe that AIS may be managed conservatively by cold-knife conisation, provided the cone-biopsy margins are free of disease. There is little evidence currently available to support the use of LLETZ as treatment for AIS, while simple hysterectomy or at least repeat cold-knife conisation is advocated where the biopsy margins are involved by disease.

Large prospective cohort studies are required to determine the long-term efficacy of LLETZ as conservative treatment for AIS. If LLETZ proves to be an effective treatment, a multicentre randomised prospective study comparing LLETZ and cold-knife conisation is needed to determine the most effective conservative treatment method.

FOLLOW-UP OF WOMEN TREATED FOR CIGN

All patients treated for CIGN require long-term cytological and colposcopic follow-up. Cytological and colposcopic assessment is necessary post-conisation due to the occurrence of subsequent squamous abnormalities and to detect recurrent glandular disease. Recurrent and invasive glandular disease have been reported following both conservative treatment and after hysterectomy for AIS.[34,60] The need for long-term cytological follow-up and thorough colposcopic assessment of the upper vagina following hysterectomy for CIGN, if follow-up cytology is abnormal, is illustrated in a case report by Cullimore et al.[94] High-grade glandular neoplasia of the left angle of the vaginal-vault suture line was diagnosed five years after hysterectomy for AIS. The smear suggested malignant cells of glandular origin and the area of recurrence had colposcopic features resembling normal columnar epithelium, allowing directed punch biopsy.

The effectiveness of cytological follow-up in detecting residual or recurrent glandular disease has not yet been proven by long-term prospective studies. Muntz et al.[29] expressed doubts about the reliability of post-conisation cervicovaginal cytology, especially in the presence of cervical stenosis. However, Cullimore et al.[59] found in their prospective series that abnormal cytology after conisation was a more sensitive indicator of residual disease than identification of positive cone margins. The authors justified the use of follow-up cytology after conservative management of CIGN, despite the lack of sensitivity of cytology in detecting glandular lesions pretreatment, by recommending the use of both Ayre's spatula and endocervical brush smears. The use of an endocervical brush would ensure specific sampling of the endocervical glandular epithelium and should be mandatory in the follow-up of any woman undergoing conservative treatment for CIGN.

The optimal interval between follow-up smears and desired length of follow-up in women treated for CIGN is unknown. Women in the prospective cone-biopsy study underwent smears at four-monthly intervals for two years and annually thereafter, according to the study protocol.[59] Other authors recommend smears every three to six months following conservative treatment.[63,64] Although there are no definitive guidelines about follow-up cytology interval, all authors advocate long-term follow-up and aggressive investigation of abnormal glandular follow-up cytology with colposcopic assessment and submission of further surgical specimens for pathological evaluation.

CONCLUSION

Adenocarcinoma of the cervix is becoming an increasing problem. The effectiveness of cervical cytology screening in detecting squamous premalignant lesions has resulted in a dramatic decline in the incidence of squamous carcinoma of the cervix. There is evidence to support the existence of premalignant glandular lesions and, therefore, the potential for diagnosis at a preinvasive stage. Further research on the natural history of CIGN is required to determine its malignant potential and resources should also be focused on improving all aspects of detection and diagnosis.

The current trend for treatment of CIGN is towards a more conservative approach. Stronger evidence from large multicentre prospective studies is urgently required to assess conservative treatment modalities and to define treatment guidelines and follow-up protocols. These studies should be co-ordinated by gynaecological oncologists in cancer centres to ensure consensus on study protocols and widespread acceptance of study recommendations.

References

1. Parkin, D.M., Laara, E., Muir, C.S. Estimates of the worldwide frequency of 16 major cancers in 1980. *Int J Cancer* 1998;**41**:184–97
2. Abell, M.R., Gosling, J.R.G. Gland cell carcinoma (adenocarcinoma) of the uterine cervix. *Am J Obstet Gynecol* 1962;**83**:729–55
3. Davis, J.R., Moon, L.B. Increased incidence of adenocarcinoma of the uterine cervix. *Obstet Gynecol* 1975;**45**:79–83
4. Shingleton, H.M., Gore, H., Bradley, D.H., Soong, S-J. Adenocarcinoma of the cervix. I. Clinical evaluation and pathologic features. *Am J Obstet Gynecol* 1981;**139**:799–812
5. Peters, R.K., Chao, A., Mack, T.M., Thomas, D., Bernstein, L., Henderson, B.E. Increased frequency of adenocarcinoma of the uterine cervix in young women in Los Angeles county. *J Natl Cancer Inst* 1986;**76**:423–8
6. Schwartz, S.M., Weiss, N.S. Increased incidence of adenocarcinoma of the cervix in young women in the United States. *Am J Epidemiol* 1986;**124**:1045–7

7   Silocks, P.B., Thornton-Jones, H., Murphy, M. Squamous and adenocarcinoma of the uterine cervix: a comparison using routine data. *Br J Obstet Gynaecol* 1987;**55**:321–5

8   Younge, P.A., Hertig, A.T., Armstrong, D. A study of 135 cases of carcinoma *in situ* of the cervix at the Free Hospital for Women. *Am J Obstet Gynecol* 1949;**58**:867–95

9   Smith, G.V., Pemberton, F.A. The picture of very early carcinoma of the uterine cervix. *Surg Gynecol Obstet* 1934;**59**:1–8

10 Richart, R.M. Natural history of cervical intraepithelial neoplasia. *Clin Obstet Gynecol* 1968;**10**:131–3

11 Koss, L.G. Concept of genesis and development of carcinoma of the cervix. *Obstet Gynecol Surv* 1969;**24**:850–60

12 McIndoe, W.A., McLean, M.R., Jones, R.W., Mullins, P.R. The invasive potential of carcinoma *in situ* of the cervix. *Obstet Gynecol* 1984;**64**:452–8

13 Laara, E., Day, N.E., Hakama, M. Trends in mortality from cervical cancer in the Nordic countries: association with organised screening programmes. *Lancet* 1987;**i**:1247–9

14 Nieminen, P., Kallio, M., Hakama, M. The effect of mass screening on incidence and mortality of squamous and adenocarcinoma of cervix uteri. *Obstet Gynecol* 1995;**85**:1017–21

15 Quinn, M., Babb, P., Jones, J., Allen, E. Effect of mass screening on incidence and mortality from cancer of the cervix in England: evaluation based on routinely collected statistics. *BMJ* 1999;**318**:904–8

16 Sasieni, P., Cuzick, J., Farmery, E. Accelerated decline in cervical cancer mortality in England and Wales. *Lancet* 1995;**346**:1566–7

17 Brown, L.J.R., Wells, M. Cervical glandular atypia associated with squamous intraepithelial neoplasia: a premalignant lesion? *Am J Clin Pathol* 1986;**39**:22–8

18 Helper, T.K., Dockerty, M.B., Randall, L.M. Primary adenocarcinoma of the cervix. *Am J Obstet Gynecol* 1952;**63**:800–8

19 Friedell, G.H., McKay, D.G. Adenocarcinoma *in situ* of the endocervix. *Cancer* 1953;**6**:887–97

20 Gloor, E., Hurlimann, J. Cervical intraepithelial glandular neoplasia (adenocarcinoma *in situ* and glandular dysplasia). *Cancer* 1986;**58**:1272–82

21 Anderson, M.C. Invasive carcinoma of the cervix. In: Symmers, W. St C., editor. *Systemic Pathology*, 3rd ed. Edinburgh: Churchill Livingstone; 1991. p. 105–28

22 Jaworski, R.C. Endocervical glandular dysplasia, adenocarcinoma *in situ* and early invasive (microinvasive) adenocarcinoma of the uterine cervix. *Semin Diagn Pathol* 1990;**7**:190–204

23 Scully, R.E., Bonfiglio, T.A., Kurman, R.J., Silverberg, S.G., Wilkinson, E.J. *Histological Typing of Female Genital Tract Tumours*, 2nd ed. Berlin: Springer-Verlag; 1994

24 Ostor, A.G., Pagano, R., Dvaoren, R.A.M., Fortune, D.W., Chanen, W., Rome, R. Adenocarcinoma *in situ* of the cervix. *Int J Gynecol Pathol* 1984;**3**:179–90

25 Bertrand, E., Lickrish, G.M., Colgan, T.J. The anatomic distribution of cervical adenocarcinoma *in situ*: implications for treatment. *Am J Obstet Gynecol* 1987;**157**:21–5

26 Brown, L.J.R., Griffin, N.R., Wells, M. Cytoplasmic reactivity with monoclonal antibody HMFG1 as a marker of cervical glandular atypia. *J Pathol* 1987;**151**:203–8

27 Jaworski, R., Pacey, N., Greenberg, M., Osborn, R. The histological diagnosis of adenocarcinoma *in situ* of the uterine cervix and related lesions of the cervix uteri. *Cancer* 1988;**61**:1171–81

28 Colgan, T.J., Lickrish, G.M. The topography and invasive potential of cervical adenocarcinoma *in situ*, with and without associated squamous dysplasia. *Gynecol Oncol* 1990;**36**:246–9

29 Muntz, H.G., Bell, D.A., Lage, J.M., Goff, B.A., Feldman, S., Rice, L.W. Adenocarcinoma *in situ* of the uterine cervix. *Obstet Gynecol* 1992;**80**:935–9

30 Higgins, G.D., Phillips, G.E., Smith, L.A., Uzelin, D.M., Burrell, C.J. High prevalence of human papillomavirus transcripts in all grades of cervical intraepithelial glandular neoplasia. *Cancer* 1992;**70**:136–46

31 Duggan, M.A., Benoit, J.L., McGregor, S.E., Inoue, M., Nation, J.G., Stuart, G.C. Adenocarcinoma *in situ* of the endocervix: human papillomavirus determination by dot blot hybridisation and polymerase chain reaction amplification. *Int J Gynecol Pathol* 1994;**13**:143–9

32 Alejo, M., Macado, I., Matias-Guiu, X., Prat, J. Adenocarcinoma *in situ* of the uterine cervix: clinicopathological study of nine cases with detection of human papillomavirus DNA by *in situ* hybridisation and polymerase chain reaction. *Int J Gynecol Pathol* 1993;**12**:219–23

33 Im, D.D., Duska, L.R., Rosenheim, N.B. Adequacy of conization margins in adenocarcinoma *in situ* of the cervix as a predictor of residual disease. *Gynecol Oncol* 1995;**59**:179–82

34 Poynor, E.A., Barakat, R.R., Hoskins, W.J. Management and follow-up of patients with adenocarcinoma *in situ* of the uterine cervix. *Gynecol Oncol* 1995;**57**:158–64

35 Qizilbash, A.H. *In situ* and microinvasive adenocarcinoma of the uterine cervix: a clinical, cytologic and histologic study of 14 cases. *Am J Clin Pathol* 1975;**64**:155–70

36 Rollason, T.P., Cullimore, J., Bradgate, M.G. A suggested columnar cell morphological equivalent of squamous carcinoma *in situ* with early stromal invasion. *Int J Gynecol Pathol* 1989;**8**:230–6

37 Ursin, G., Peters, R.K., Henderson, B.E., d'Ablaing, G., Monroe, R.K. Oral contraceptive use and adenocarcinoma of the cervix. *Lancet* 1994;**344**:1390–1

38 Thomas, D.B., Ray, R.M. Oral contraceptives and invasive adenocarcinomas and adenosquamous carcinomas of the uterine cervix. The World Health Organization Collaborative Study of Neoplasia and Steroid Contraceptives. *Am J Epidemiol* 1996;**144**:281–9

39 zur Hausen, H. Human papillomavirus in the pathogenesis of anogenital cancer. *Virology* 1991;**184**:9–13

40 Schiffmann, M.H., Bauer, H.M., Hoover, R.N., Glass, A.G., Cadell, D.M., Rush, B.B. Epidemiologic evidence showing that human papillomavirus infection causes most cervical intraepithelial neoplasia. *J Natl Cancer Inst* 1993;**85**:958–64

41 Tase, T., Okagaki, T., Clark, B., Manias, D.A., Ostrow, R.S., Twiggs, L.B. et al. Human papillomavirus types and localisation in adenocarcinoma and adenosquamous carcinoma of the uterine cervix: a study by *in situ* DNA hybridisation. *Cancer Res* 1988;**48**:993–8

42 Farnsworth, A., Laverty, C., Stoler, M.H. Human papillomavirus messenger RNA expression in adenocarcinoma *in situ* of the uterine cervix. *Int J Gynecol Pathol* 1989;**8**:321–30

43 Tenti, P., Romsgnoli, S., Silini, E., Zappatore, R., Spinillo, A., Giunta, P., et al. Human papillomavirus types 16 and 18 infection in infiltrating adenocarcinoma of the cervix. PCR analysis of 138 cases and correlation with histologic type and grade. *Am J Clin Pathol* 1996;**106**:52–6

44 Okagaki, T., Tase, T., Twiggs, L.B.L., Carson, L.F. Histogenesis of cervical adenocarcinoma with reference to human papillomavirus-18 as a co-carcinogen. *J Reprod Med* 1989;**34**:639–44

45 Leary, J., Jaworski, R., Houghton, R. *In situ* hybridisation using biotylated DNA probes to human papillomavirus in adenocarcinoma *in situ* and endocervical glandular dysplasia of the uterine cervix. *Pathology* 1991;**23**:85–9

46 Tase, T., Okagaki, T., Clark, B.A., Twiggs, L.B., Ostrow, R.S., Faras, A.J. Human papillomavirus DNA in adenocarcinoma *in situ*, microinvasive adenocarcinoma of the uterine cervix, and coexisting cervical intraepithelial neoplasia. *Int J Gynecol Pathol* 1989;**8**:8–17

47   Hocking, G.R., Hayman, J.J., Ostor, A.G. Adenocarcinoma in situ of the uterine cervix progressing to invasive adenocarcinoma. *Aust N Z J Obstet Gynaecol* 1996;**85**:1017–21
48   Kurian, K., Al-Nafussi, A. Relation of cervical glandular intraepithelial neoplasia to microinvasive and invasive adenocarcinoma of the uterine cervix: a study of 121 cases. *J Clin Pathol* 1999;**52**:112–17
49   Plaxe, S.C., Saltzstein, M.D. Estimation of the duration of the preclinical phase of cervical adenocarcinoma suggests that there is ample opportunity for screening. *Gynecol Oncol* 1999;**75**:55–61
50   Delgidisch, I., Escay-Martinez, E., Cohen, C.J. Endocervical adenocarcinoma: a study of 23 patients with clinical-pathological correlation. *Gynecol Oncol* 1984;**18**:326–33
51   Boon, M.E., Baak, J.P., Kurver, P.J.H., Overdiep, S.H., Verdonk, G.W. Adenocarcinoma *in situ* of the cervix: an underdiagnosed lesion. *Cancer* 1981;**48**:768–73
52   Christopherson, W.M., Nealon, N., Gray, L.A. Non-invasive precursor lesions of adenocarcinoma and mixed adenosquamous carcinoma of the cervix uteri. *Cancer* 1979;**44**:975–83
53   Boon, M.E., Tabbers-Boumeester, M.L. *Gynaecological Cytology, Textbook and Atlas*. London: Macmillan Press; 1980
54   Boddington, M.M., Spriggs, A. I., Cowdell, R.H. Adenocarcinoma of the uterine cervix; cytological evidence of a long pre-clinical evolution. *Br J Obstet Gynaecol* 1976;**83**:900–3
55   Bousfield, L., Pacey, F., Young, Q., Krumins, I., Osborn, R. Expanded cytologic criteria for the diagnosis of adenocarcinoma *in situ* of the cervix and related lesions. *Acta Cytol* 1980;**24**:283–96
56   Nguyen, G., Jeannot, A.B. Exfoliative cytology of *in situ* and microinvasive adenocarcinoma of the uterine cervix. *Acta Cytol* 1984;**28**:461–7
57   Luesley, D.M., Jordan, J.A., Woodman, C.B.J., Watson, N., Williams, D.R., Waddell, C. A retrospective review of adenocarcinoma *in situ* and glandular atypia of the uterine cervix. *Br J Obstet Gynaecol* 1987;**94**:699–703
58   Andersen, E.S., Arffmann, E. Adenocarcinoma *in situ* of the uterine cervix: a clinicopathologic study of 36 cases. *Gynecol Oncol* 1989;**35**:1–7
59   Cullimore, J.E., Luesley, D.M., Rollason, T.P., Byrne, P., Buckley, C.H., Anderson, M., et al. A prospective study of conization of the cervix in the management of cervical intraepithelial glandular neoplasia (CIGN) – a preliminary report. *Br J Obstet Gynaecol* 1992;**99**:314–18
60   Widrich, T., Kennedy, A.W., Myers, T.M., Hart, W.R., Wirth, B.S.N. Adenocarcinoma *in situ* of the uterine cervix: management and outcome. *Gynecol Oncol* 1996;**61**:304–8
61   Wolf, J., Levenback, C., Malpicia, A., Morris, M., Burke, T., Mitchell, M.F. Adenocarcinoma *in situ* of the cervix: significance of cone biopsy margins. *Obstet Gynecol* 1996;**88**:82–6
62   Houghton, S.J., Shafi, M.I., Rollason, T.P., Luesley, D.M. Is loop excision adequate primary management of adenocarcinoma *in situ* of the cervix? *Br J Obstet Gynaecol* 1997;**104**:325–9
63   Denehy, T.R., Gregori, C.A., Breen, J.L. Endocervical curettage, cone margins, and residual adenocarcinoma *in situ* of the cervix. *Obstet Gynecol* 1997;**90**:1–6
64   Azodi, M., Chambers, S.K., Rutherford, T.J., Kohorn, E.I., Schwartz, P.E., Chambers, J.T. Adenocarcinoma *in situ* of the cervix: management and outcome. *Gynecol Oncol* 1999;**73**:348–53
65   Weisbrot, I.M., Stablinsky, C., Davis, A.M. Adenocarcinoma *in situ* of the uterine cervix. *Cancer* 1972;**18**:807–10
66   Ayer, B., Pacey, F., Greenberg, M., Bousfield, L. The cytologic diagnosis of adenocarcinoma *in situ* of the cervix uteri and related lesions. I. Adenocarcinoma *in situ*. *Acta Cytol* 1987;**31**:397–411

67 Keyhani-Rofagha, S., Brewer, J., Prokorym, P. Comparative cytologic findings of in situ and invasive adenocarcinoma of the uterine cervix. *Diagn Cytopathol* 1995;**12**:120–5

68 Lee, K.R. False-positive diagnosis of adenocarcinoma *in situ* of the cervix. *Acta Cytol* 1988;**32**:276–7

69 Pacey, F., Ayer, B., Greenberg, M. The cytologic diagnosis of adenocarcinoma *in situ* of the cervix uteri and related lesions. III. Pitfalls in diagnosis. *Acta Cytol* 1988;**32**:325–33

70 Lee, K.R., Manna, E.A., Jones, M.A. Comparative cytologic features of adenocarcinoma *in situ* of the uterine cervix. *Acta Cytol* 1991;**35**:117–26

71 Boon, M.E., Guilloud, J.C.D., Kok, L.T., Olthof, P.M., Van Erp, E.J.M. Efficacy of screening for cervical squamous and adenocarcinoma: the Dutch experience. *Cancer* 1994;**59**:862–6

72 Boon, M.E., Alons-van Kordelaar, J.J., Rietveld-Scheffers, P.E. Consequences of the introduction of combined spatula and Cytobrush sampling for cervical cytology. *Acta Cytol* 1986;**30**:264–70

73 Laverty, C.R., Farnsworth, A., Thurloe, J., Bowditch, R. The reliability of a cytological prediction of cervical adenocarcinoma *in situ*. *Aust N Z J Obstet Gynaecol* 1998;**28**:307–12

74 Van Erp, E.J., Blachek-Lut, C.H., Arentz, N.P., Trimbos, J.B. Performance of the Cytobrush in patients at risk for cervical pathology: does it add anything to the wooden spatula? *Eur J Gynaecol Oncol* 1998;**9**:456–60

75 Hinselmann, H. Verbesserung der inspektionsmoglichkeit von vulva, vagina und portio. *Munchener Medizinische Wochenschrifte* 1925;**77**:1733

76 Anderson, M.C., Morse, A.R., Jordan, J.A., Sharp, F. *Integrated Colposcopy for Colposcopists, Histopathologists and Cytologists*, 2nd ed. London: Lippincott, Williams and Wilkins; 1996

77 Brand, E., Berek, J.S., Hacker, N.F. Controversies in the management of cervical adenocarcinoma. *Obstet Gynecol* 1988;**71**:261–9

78 Lickrish, G.M., Colgan, T.J., Wright, V.C. Colposcopy of adenocarcinoma *in situ* and invasive adenocarcinoma of the cervix. *Obstet Gynecol Clin North Am* 1993;**20**:111–22

79 Coppleson, M., Atkinson, K.H., Dalrymple, J.C. Cervical squamous and glandular neoplasia: clinical features and review of management. In: Coppleson, M., editor. *Gynecologic Oncology*. Edinburgh: Churchill Livingstone; 1992. p. 571–607

80 Ferris, D.G., Krumholz, B.A., Jester, D.M., Crosby, J.H., Hanly, M.G., Messing, M.J. Atypical glandular cells of undetermined significance and adenocarcinoma *in situ*: summoning colposcopic expertise? *J Fam Pract* 1996;**43**:181–7

81 Buscema, J., Woodruff, J.D. Significance of neoplastic abnormalities in endocervical epithelium. *Gynecol Oncol* 1984;**17**:356–62

82 Nicklin, J.L., Wright, R.G., Bell, J.R., Samaratunga, H., Cox, N.C., Ward, B.G. A clinicopathological study of adenocarcinoma *in situ* of the cervix: the influence of cervical HPV infection and other factors, and the role of conservative surgery. *Aust N Z J Obstet Gynaecol* 1991;**31**:179–83

83 Hopkins, M.P., Roberts, J.A., Schmidt, R.W. Cervical adenocarcinoma *in situ*. *Obstet Gynecol* 1988;**71**:842–4

84 Prendiville, W., Cullimore, J., Norman, S. Large loop excision of the transformation zone (LLETZ): a new method of management for women with cervical intraepithelial neoplasia. *Br J Obstet Gynaecol* 1989;**96**:1054–60

85 Kitchener, H.C. The 1993 British Society for Colposcopy and Cervical Pathology/National Co-ordinating Network United Kingdom Colposcopy Survey. *Br J Obstet Gynaecol* 1995;**102**:549–52

86 Luesley, D.M., Cullimore, J., Redman, C.W.E., Lawton, F.G., Emens, J.M., Rollason, T.P. et al. Loop diathermy excision of the cervical transformation zone in patients with abnormal

cervical smears. *BMJ* 1990;**300**:1690–3
87 Bigrigg, A., Haffenden, D.K., Sheehan, A.L., Colding, W., Read, M.D. Efficacy and safety of large-loop excision of the transformation zone. *Lancet* 1994;**343**:32–4
88 Cruickshank, M.E., Flannelly, G., Campbell, D.M., Kitchener, H.C. Fertility and pregnancy outcome following large loop excision of the cervical transformation zone. *Br J Obstet Gynaecol* 1995;**102**:467–70
89 Luesley, D.M., McCrum, A., Terry, P.B., Wade-Evans, T., Nicholson, H.O., Mylotte, M.J. *et al.* Complications of cone biopsy related to the dimensions of the cone and the influence of prior colposcopic assessment. *Br J Obstet Gynaecol* 1985;**92**:158–64
90 Kennedy, A.W., Eltabbakh, G.H., Biscotti, C.V., Wirth, S. Invasive adenocarcinoma of the cervix following LLETZ (large loop excision of the transformation zone) for adenocarcinoma *in situ*. *Gynecol Oncol* 1995;**58**:274–7
91 Muntz, H. Can cervical adenocarcinoma *in situ* be safely managed by conization alone? *Gynecol Oncol* 1996;**61**:301–3
92 Mathevet, P., Dargent, D., Roy, M., Beau, G. A randomised prospective study comparing three techniques of conization: cold knife, laser and LLEEP. *Gynecol Oncol* 1994;**54**:175–9
93 Girareli, F., Heydarfadi, M., Koroschetz, F., Pickel, H., Winter, R. Cold knife conization versus loop excision: histopathologic and clinical results of a randomized trial. *Gynecol Oncol* 1995;**55**:358–70
94 Cullimore, J.E., Luesley, D.M., Rollason, T.P., Waddell, C., Williams, D.R. A case of glandular intraepithelial neoplasia involving the cervix and vagina. *Gynecol Oncol* 1989;**34**:249–52

13

Hormones and cancer of the cervix, vulva, vagina and ovary

Allan B. MacLean

HORMONES AND CERVICAL CANCER

A significant proportion of squamous-cell carcinoma of the cervix occurs in premenopausal women and the vast majority of abnormal smears and precancers (cervical intraepithelial neoplasia, CIN) occur in women with active ovaries, while on the oral contraceptive pill or sometimes during pregnancy. Although an increasing ratio of cervical adenocarcinoma to squamous-cell carcinoma is acknowledged little attention has been paid to the possible role of hormones in cervical carcinogenesis.

The association of human papillomavirus (HPV) with cervical carcinoma continues to be acknowledged. We know that there are more than 70 types of HPV, half of which are found in the anogenital region, and 15 or so (HPV 16, 18, 31, 33, 35, etc.) are designated as 'high risk' and are found in almost all cases of CIN 3 and cancer.[1] When HPV is latent or replicating the viral DNA is episomal but during neoplastic transformation the DNA becomes integrated. During integration certain fragments of the viral DNA are lost and other sequences become more important. They become responsible for proteins such as E6 and E7, which experimentally can transform mice cells and have important interactions with the protein products of the tumour suppressor genes *p53* and *pRB* (retinoblastoma gene). However, up to 40% of sexually active women will have high-risk types of HPV, as detected by DNA amplification techniques, and yet only a small percentage will develop CIN or cervical cancer. This suggests that other factors must be involved. Some authors have proposed that other viruses such as herpes simplex virus might have a synergistic role.[1,2] Smoking and immunosuppression contribute to the risk for some women.

The contribution of pregnancy to the risk of cervical neoplasia may relate to the effect of hormones on cervical eversion, or ectopy and alteration in the width of the transformation zone. The regeneration of cervical epithelium after vaginal delivery may amplify minor changes or be modified by altered hormone levels in the puerperium compared with late pregnancy. Most authors who describe cervical cancer suggest that pregnancy has no effect. Hacker *et al.*[3] reported a review of 1657 cases of invasive carcinoma of the cervix seen during pregnancy or in the first 12 months postpartum and found that there was no difference in survival for Stages IB or II compared with data from the FIGO Annual Report.[4] However, when patients were seen with Stage III or IV disease the five-year survival was only 16% compared with 28% for FIGO data. It is suggested that the difference may be related to problems with radiation dosimetry in pregnancy and the need to interrupt radiation therapy more frequently because of genital tract sepsis. It is also suggested that pregnancy facilitates a greater proportion of pregnant women having their disease detected at an earlier stage. However, there are insufficient data to exclude the influence of pregnancy hormones on accelerating tumour growth, dissemination and prognosis in advanced disease. Cervical cancer occurring during pregnancy in the UK and the USA is now so uncommon that further data are unlikely to be revealing.

More substantial information is available on the effect of the oral contraceptive pill on the cervix and cervical neoplasia. Vessey et al.[5] reported that for 17 000 women reviewed in the Oxford Family Planning Clinic after ten years use of the pill or the intrauterine contraceptive device, there was an increase in incidence of cervical neoplasia with increasing duration of pill use. A subsequent publication of this study cohort[6] showed that ever-users of the pill had an odds ratio of 4.44 for invasive cancer, and that this was greatest for current or recent use, and an odds ratio of 1.4 for all cervical neoplasia. These risks are similar to those from World Health Organization (WHO) data[7] from the Collaborative Study of Neoplasia and Steroid Contraceptives, where the relative risk of invasive squamous-cell carcinoma in ever-users of combined oral contraceptive pills was 1.3, with the risk increasing significantly after four to five years of use. Thomas et al.[8] published the WHO findings on invasive adenosquamous carcinomas, with a relative risk of 1.5 in women who have first used the pill while under 20 years of age.

The synergistic effects of the oral contraceptive pill and HPV were shown by Bosch et al.[9] If the odds ratio for developing cervical cancer is adjusted to 1.0 for someone who has never used the pill and who is HPV negative, the odds ratio for someone who is HPV positive and has used oral contraception is high at 113.[9]

Sex steroids are not mutagenic, that is they do not modify DNA. Some DNA sequences will contain 'hormone responsive elements' and when steroids bind to their appropriate receptor, the hormone responsive elements will modify subsequent transcription. Sonnendecker and Sonnendecker[10] summarised a series of experiments where HPV-DNA is modified by steroids. There is a DNA sequence in the non-coding or upstream regulatory region of HPV-16 that contains a 'glucocorticoid responsive element'. When dexamethasone is added to HeLa or cervical cancer cells in culture it produces tyrosine kinase promotion. From these experiments Gloss et al.[11] concluded that glucocorticoid or progesterone enhances the transcription of the HPV-16 genome (or DNA). Pater et al.[12] showed that baby rat kidney cells transfected with HPV-16 DNA and activated with rat oncogene plus progesterone or levonorgestrel as ethanol-soluble extract from the combined oral contraceptive pill, were capable of oncogenic transformation. Other experiments could not be repeated if incubation was in the presence of oestrogen and showed that the anti-progesterone mifepristone was inhibitory.[13] Khare et al.[14] used human ectocervical cells plus modified HPV-16 to establish immortalised cells which formed rafts in culture; hormone treatment-induced dysplastic features within these epithelial cells. Auborn et al.[15] showed that the transformation and immortalisation of such epithelial cells with HPV-16 increased 16-hydroxylation of oestradiol and that prolonged oestrogen effect increased HPV expression by upregulation of the hormone receptor to form a positive feedback loop.

If hormones promote events leading to cervical neoplasia, can they be used once cancer has been diagnosed? There is no evidence that hormone replacement therapy (HRT) increases the risk of cervical cancer in otherwise well women and indeed it may decrease the risk.[16] Secondly, in the study by Ploch,[17] 120 patients whose cervical cancer was treated by surgery and radiotherapy were given sequential HRT or nothing (controls). The percentage of women surviving more than five years was 80% in the HRT group and 65% in the controls.[17] However, it is disappointing that there are no UK data to confirm the safety of using HRT after the treatment of cervical cancer and particularly for those cancers that are adeno or adeno-squamous in nature, where there is theoretical concern that hormones might alter residual tumour cell behaviour.

HORMONES AND VULVAL CANCER

The majority of vulval cancers arise in a background of lichen sclerosus or squamous hyperplasia, occur after the menopause and are not influenced by hormones. The minority arise from vulval intraepithelial neoplasia and occur in younger women.[18] This second group of cancers is usually HPV-associated and hormones may influence them as described above for cervical neoplasia. However, there are no clinical and few experimental data to suggest hormones influence vulval cancer.

Paget's disease of the vulva, which is an adenocarcinoma *in situ* of the vulval epidermis, has some similarities with breast carcinoma and Paget's disease of the breast.[19] However, it occurs in postmenopausal women, contains no oestrogen receptors and does not appear to be associated with or contraindicate the use of exogenous hormones.

HORMONES AND VAGINAL CANCER

The majority of vaginal cancers are secondary to primary lesions of the cervix, vulva, endometrium, trophoblast, or from colon, rectum, or pancreas, etc. Primary carcinoma is usually squamous-cell, but Herbst and Scully[20] reported seven cases of clear-cell adenocarcinoma of the vagina seen in young women, aged between 14 and 22 years, at the Massachusetts General Hospital in Boston, USA. The following year they reported the association between this cancer and maternal use of diethylstilboestrol (DES) during pregnancy.[21] DES use was uncommon in the UK, but Emens[22] reminds us of significant use in Europe, for example in the Netherlands. The risk of developing adenocarcinoma in spite of exposure to DES seems small and other factors must be involved. A secondary rise in the incidence with age cannot be excluded and women with known exposure should be kept under long-term follow-up.

The DES story should also prompt us to be wary about using hormones or other drugs to 'support' an early pregnancy unless we can guarantee safety.

HORMONES AND OVARIAN CANCER

A hospital-based case-control study of ovarian cancer conducted in London and Oxford hospitals between 1978 and 1983 found an increased risk with infertility and a late age at menopause. High gravidity and oral contraceptive pill use were associated with a reduced risk of ovarian cancer.[23] Further information on the epidemiology of ovarian cancer is summarised by Leake.[24] Hillier[25] discusses the two aetiological theories of ovarian epithelial surface disruption with repeat ovulation and increased endogenous or exogenous gonadotrophins stimulating granulosa and thecal cells to produce changes in the surface epithelium. A third possibility is that some underlying defect of the ovary is responsible for both impaired fertility and ovarian pathology.[26,27] This defect may be genetic and familial; sisters or first degree relatives of infertile women appear to have an increased prevalence of ovarian cancer.

Whittemore[28] analysed 12 USA case-control studies conducted by the Collaborative Ovarian Cancer Group and including 2197 cases of epithelial ovarian cancer. There is no overall association between physician-diagnosed female infertility and ovarian cancer but if the women had used fertility treatment the relative risk was increased (RR = 2.8) and was even higher (RR = 4.0) for borderline ovarian tumours. There have been anxieties expressed about the study methodology, with possible recall bias leading to overestimates of the magnitude of these associations.

A review of the literature at that time collected ten case reports of ovarian neoplasms during or after ovulation induction therapy. The patients were young, ranging from 22 to 38 years of age, and seven of the ten tumours were borderline or of low malignant potential histological type.[29]

Rossing *et al.*[30] reviewed a cohort of 3837 women from Seattle who had been evaluated for infertility between 1974 and 1985. Eleven were subsequently found to have ovarian tumours but two were granulosa-cell tumours, five were borderline tumours and only four were epithelial ovarian cancers. The authors demonstrated an increased risk of ovarian tumours with clomiphene use, particularly if more than 12 cycles were used (RR = 11.1). However, there was not a linear or dose-dependent risk and, paradoxically, the greatest risk was in parous rather than nulliparous women.

One study to address the association with the use of ovarian stimulation and subsequent cancers was carried out in Melbourne by Venn et al.[31] It included more than 10 000 women referred for *in vitro* fertilisation (IVF). The 'exposed' group had ovarian stimulation to induce multiple follicles, whereas the 'unexposed' were either those who had registered for IVF but had not received any treatment (93.4%) or who had natural cycles without ovarian stimulation (6.6%). There were 34 breast cancers subsequently identified from various cancer registers but no evidence of increased incidence when compared with age-standardised general population rates. There were six ovarian cancers, with an increased incidence in the cohort but no significant difference for the exposed group. There was an increased incidence of endometrial cancers and, for those patients with unexplained infertility in either group, the standardised incidence ratio (SIR) was 8.3 for cancers of the uterus (body) and 6.98 for cancers of the ovary. A subsequent report from the same authors[32] analysed a larger cohort from ten Australian IVF clinics, which consisted of 20 656 who were exposed to fertility drugs and 9044 who were not. The incidence of breast cancers (SIR 0.91) and ovarian cancers (SIR 0.88) was no greater than expected. The incidence of uterine cancer was significantly higher (SIR 2.47) in the unexposed group and for those women with unexplained infertility there was noted again a higher incidence of uterine cancers (SIR 4.59) and ovarian cancers (SIR 2.64) than expected. Borderline tumours were not included in this study. The invasive ovarian tumours were serous (four), mucinous (one), clear-cell (two) and endometrioid (three), and four of the ten uterine tumours were sarcomas and these were found in the unexposed group.

One of the difficulties with this study is that any exposure to fertility drugs given as infertility treatment at centres outside the ten participating centres is not known. Thus, it is less likely that the 'unexposed group' have never taken fertility drugs. Furthermore, many of the exposed group had limited exposure, with 71% having no more than three stimulated IVF cycles; only 2% had ten or more cycles with the maximum number of treatment cycles being 29. Median duration of follow-up was seven years for patients exposed to ovulation induction. It is uncertain whether this is sufficiently long enough to exclude an association with increased cancer incidence. This study comments on the relation between unexplained infertility and ovarian or uterine cancer or sarcoma. It is possible that the infertility is unexplained because of incomplete diagnostic procedures or that the infertility may be due to neoplastic processes previously unrecognised. These two studies provide some reassurance that exogenous gonadotrophin exposure does not increase the risk of ovarian cancer, at least in the short term.

If increased gonadotrophin exposure influences the risk of ovarian carcinoma, does hormone replacement therapy (HRT) at the menopause have a role in reducing that risk? Booth et al.[23] showed that postmenopausal women had a small but not significantly increased risk of ovarian cancer associated by receiving HRT. Among the hormone-treated group with ovarian cancer were 23% with endometrioid or clear-cell tumours (which might be hormone responsive) compared with 38% in the untreated women, that is hormone replacement did not increase the incidence of these histological types.

Whitemore et al.[33] analysed 12 studies from the USA and found no consistent trends with age at menarche, age at menopause or duration of oestrogen replacement therapy. They showed, however, a decreased risk among current users of HRT compared with never-users, which reached statistical significance in the population-based, but not the hospital-based, studies.

Banks et al.[34] reviewed 13 case-control studies where selected publications were based on more than 20 cases and found one with a significant lower risk of ovarian cancer among ever-users of

HRT, seven with risks close to unity and five with non-significantly elevated risks. Rodriguez et al.[35] reported a significantly raised relative risk of 1.71 with more than 11 years use of HRT and a relative risk of 1.72 among current users for six years or more, based on 436 fatal ovarian cancers from a cohort of over 240 000 women.

Garg et al.[36] performed a meta-analysis of nine articles published between 1966 and 1997. Ever-users of HRT had an increased risk of developing invasive epithelial ovarian carcinoma, with an odds ratio (OR) of 1.15 and 95% confidence intervals (CI) of 1.05 and 1.27; if used for more than ten years the OR was 1.27 (95% CI 1.00 and 1.61). A similar effect was noted for invasive as well as borderline tumours, and the risks may be confounded for HRT users who are nulliparous or have been infertile.

If there is an increased risk for HRT users, it must be balanced by other risk factors of precocious parity and oral contraceptive use. It needs to be reviewed in situations where ovarian dysfunction has led to the need for ovulation induction and later to hormone replacement after an early menopause.

Can women who have had bilateral oophorectomy as management for ovarian cancer be given HRT? Wren[37] urges the use of replacement oestrogen following the rapid onset of hormonal deficiency after surgery, chemotherapy or radiotherapy in the treatment of ovarian cancer. Eeles et al.[38] reviewed 373 patients attending the Royal Marsden Hospital, London, between 1972 and 1988; 78 had received HRT. The overall survival and disease-free survival was not compromised by HRT use, although the authors admit a large prospective randomised control trial is needed.

The question is particularly important in young women with early disease where castration will produce severe short-term symptoms but where long-term survival means that cardiovascular and osteoporosis prophylaxis become important. There are anxieties[37] that certain histological types, for example endometrioid, may be adversely influenced by exogenous hormones but there is insufficient evidence to withhold HRT. It is a point that needs clarification from a multicentre audit.

CONCLUSIONS

One of the growing realisations during the Royal College of Obstetricians and Gynaecologists Study Group on hormones and cancer (see below) was that the possible links between hormones and certain cancers seem possible but unproven. A preoccupation with HPV and the cervix has largely ignored a role for steroid hormones but opportunities for molecular, clinical and epidemiological studies should be addressed. The experimental system described by Hillier[25] to study hormonal factors that could influence the ovarian epithelium seems a good starting point. Even vulval lesions, with exposure to topical glucocorticoids and sometimes oestrogens, provides a challenge for further research.[39]

Acknowledgements

This chapter stems from the author's participation in the RCOG Study Group on 'Hormones and Cancer'. As co-organiser of this meeting, I was fortunate in recruiting the help of Professor Ernst Sonnendecker of Johannesburg, Mr Mike Emens of Birmingham and Professor Robin Leake of Glasgow, to present on the subjects of hormones and cervical cancer, hormones and vaginal and vulval cancer and hormones and ovarian cancer, respectively. I refer you to their chapters in the published proceedings of this study group.[10,22,24]

References

1. MacLean, A.B., Macnab, J.C.M. The role of viruses in gynaecological oncology. In: Studd, J., editor. *Progress in Obstetrics and Gynaecology*, **12**. Edinburgh: Churchill Livingstone; 1996. p. 403–19
2. Kitchener, H.C. Infection as an aetiological agent in carcinoma of the lower genital tract. In: MacLean, A.B., editor. *Clinical Infection in Obstetrics and Gynaecology*. Oxford: Blackwell Scientific; 1990. p. 339–56
3. Hacker, N.F., Berek, J.S., Lagasse, L.D., Charles, E.H., Savage, E.W., Moore, J.G. Carcinoma of the cervix associated with pregnancy. *Obstet Gynecol* 1982;**59**:735–46
4. Kottmeier, H.L., editor. *FIGO Annual Report on the Results of Treatment in Carcinoma of the Uterus, Vagina and Ovary*, **15**. Stockholm: Pogo Prints; 1973. p. 370
5. Vessey, M.P., Lawless, M., McPherson, K., Yeates, D. Neoplasia of the cervix uteri and contraception: a possible adverse effect of the pill. *Lancet* 1983;**ii**:930–4
6. Zondervan, K.T., Carpenter, L.M., Painter, R., Vessey, M.P. Oral contraceptives and cervical cancer – further findings from the Oxford Family Planning Association contraceptive study. *Br J Cancer* 1996;**73**:1291–7
7. Ye, Z., Thomas, D.B., Ray, R.M., WHO Collaborative Study of Neoplasia and Steroid Contraceptives. Combined oral contraceptives and risk of cervical carcinoma in situ. *Int J Epidemiol* 1995;**24**:19–26
8. Thomas, D.B., Ray, R.M., WHO Collaborative Study of Neoplasia and Steroid Contraceptives. Oral contraceptives and invasive adenocarcinoma and adenosquamous carcinoma of the uterine cervix. *Am J Epidemiol* 1996;**144**:281–9
9. Bosch, F.X., Munoz, N., de Sanjose, D., Izarzugaza, I., Gili, M., Viladiu, P. et al. Risk factors for cervical cancer in Colombia and Spain. *Int J Cancer* 1992;**52**:750–8
10. Sonnendecker, E.W.W., Sonnendecker, H.E.M. Hormones and cervical cancer. In: O'Brien, P.M.S., MacLean, A.B., editors. *Hormones and Cancer*. London: RCOG Press; 1999. p. 107–23
11. Gloss, B., Bernard, H.U., Seedorf, K., Klock, G. The upstream regulatory region of the human papilloma virus-16 contains an E_2 protein-independent enhancer which is specific for cervical carcinoma cells and regulated by glucocorticoid hormones. *EMBO J* 1987;**6**:3735–43
12. Pater, A., Bayatpour, M., Pater, M.M. Oncogenic transformation by human papillomavirus type 16 deoxyribonucleic acid in the presence of progesterone or progestins from oral contraceptives. *Am J Obstet Gynecol* 1990;**162**:1099–103
13. Mittal, R., Tsutsumi, K., Pater, A., Pater, M.M. Human papillomavirus type 16 expression in cervical keratinocytes: role of progesterone and glucocorticoid hormones. *Obstet Gynecol* 1993;**81**:5–12
14. Khare, S., Pater, M.M., Tang, S-C., Pater, A. Effect of glucocorticoid hormones on viral gene expression, growth and dysplastic differentiation in HPV 16 immortalised ectocervical cells. *Exp Cell Res* 1997;**232**:353–60
15. Auborn, K.J., Woodworth, C., Di Paolo, J.A., Bradlow, H.L. The interaction between HPV infection and estrogen metabolism in cervical carcinogenesis. *Int J Cancer* 1991;**49**:867–9
16. Parazzini, F., La Vecchia, C., Negri, E., Franceschi, S., Moroni, S., Chatenoud, L. et al. Case-control study of oestrogen replacement therapy and risk of cervical cancer. *BMJ* 1997;**315**:85–8
17. Ploch, E. Hormonal replacement therapy in patients after cervical cancer treatment. *Gynecol Oncol* 1987;**26**:169–77

18 MacLean, A.B. Precursors of vulval cancers. *Curr Obstet Gynaecol* 1993;**3**:149–56
19 MacLean, A.B. Paget's disease of the vulva. *J Obstet Gynaecol* 2000;**20**:7–9
20 Herbst, A.L., Scully, R.E. Adenocarcinoma of the vagina in adolescence: a report of 7 cases including 6 clear-cell carcinomas (so-called mesonephromas). *Cancer* 1970;**24**:745–57
21 Herbst, A.L., Ulfelder, H., Poskanzer, D.C. Adenocarcinoma of the vagina – association of maternal stilbestrol therapy with tumor appearance in young women. *N Engl J Med* 1971;**284**:878–81
22 Emens, J.M. Hormones (including diethylstilboestrol) and vaginal and vulval cancer. In: O'Brien, P.M.S., MacLean, A.B., editors. *Hormones and Cancer*. London: RCOG Press; 1999. p. 124–35
23 Booth, M., Beral, V., Smith, P. Risk factors of ovarian cancer: a case-control study. *Br J Cancer* 1989;**60**:592–8
24 Leake, R.E. Hormones and ovarian cancer. In: O'Brien, P.M.S., MacLean, A.B., editors. *Hormones and Cancer*. London: RCOG Press; 1999. p. 55–66
25 Hillier, S.G. Growth factors and ovarian cancer. In: O'Brien, P.M.S., MacLean, A.B., editors. *Hormones and Cancer*. London: RCOG Press; 1999. p. 75–89
26 Nieto, J.J, Rolfe, K.J., MacLean, A.B., Hardiman, P. Ovarian cancer and infertility: a genetic link. *Lancet* 1999;**354**:649
27 Hardiman, P., Nieto, J., MacLean, A.B. Infertility and ovarian cancer. *Gynecol Oncol* 2000;**76**:1–2
28 Whittemore, A.S., Harris, R., Intyre, J., Halpern, J., Collaborative Cancer Group. Characteristics relating to ovarian cancer risks: collaborative analysis of 12 USA case-control studies. *Am J Epidemiol* 1992;**136**:1175–83

29 Land, J.A. Ovulation, ovulation induction and ovarian carcinoma. *Baillière's Clin Obstet Gynecol* 1993;**7**:455–72
30 Rossing, M.A., Daling, J.R., Weiss, N.S., Moore, D.E., Self, S.G. Ovarian tumors in a cohort of infertile women. *N Engl J Med* 1994;**331**:771–6
31 Venn, A., Watson, L., Lumley, J., Giles, G., King, C., Healy, D. Breast and ovarian cancer incidence after infertility and *in vitro* fertilisation. *Lancet* 1995;**346**:995–1000
32 Venn, A., Watson, L., Bruinsma, F., Giles, G., Healy, D. Risk of cancer after use of fertility drugs with *in vitro* fertilisation. *Lancet* 1999;**354**:1586–90
33 Whitemore, A.S., Harris, R., Intyre, J. and the Collaborative Ovarian Cancer Group. Characteristics relating to ovarian cancer risk: collaborative analysis of 12 US case-control studies II. Invasive epithelial ovarian cancers in white women. *Am J Epidemiol* 1992;**136**:1184–203
34 Banks, E., Beral, V., Reeves, G. The epidemiological of epithelial ovarian cancer: a review. *Int J Gynecol Cancer* 1997;**7**:425–38
35 Rodriguez, C., Calle, E.E., Coates, R.J., Miracle-McMahill, H.L., Thun, M.J., Hjeath, C.W. Estrogen replacement therapy and fatal ovarian cancer. *Am J. Epidemiol* 1995;**141**:828–35
36 Garg, P.P., Kerlikowske, K., Subak, L., Grady, D. Hormone replacement therapy and the risk of epithelial ovarian carcinoma. *Obstet Gynecol* 1998;**92**:472–9
37 Wren, B.G. Hormonal therapy following female genital tract cancer. *Int J Gynecol Cancer* 1994;**4**:217–24
38 Eeles, R.A., Tan, S., Wiltshaw, E., Fryatt, I., A'Hern, R.P.A., Shepherd, J.H. et al. Hormone replacement therapy and survival after surgery for ovarian cancer. *BMJ* 1991;**302**:259–62
39 Rolfe, K.J., Crow, J.C., Benjamin, E., Reid, W.M.N., MacLean, A.B., Perrett, C.W. The effects of topical steroids on p53 and KI-67 in lichen sclerosus. Paper presented at the Blair Bell Society meeting, July 1999

14

Congenital urogenital anomalies for the gynaecologist

Kalpana Patil and Padraig S. Malone

Congenital genitourinary and anorectal anomalies form a rare group of complex disorders. Their impact extends beyond childhood, both in terms of cases where diagnosis is delayed and the long-term effects that these conditions and their treatment can have on continence, sexual and reproductive function. Total correction cannot be achieved by a single procedure and treatment will be required throughout adult life. All gynaecologists will encounter these conditions and therefore should be conversant with them. A synopsis of the relevant embryology is helpful in understanding their pathology and treatment.

EMBRYOLOGY

The upper urinary tract

There are two components of renal development, mesoderm (pronephros, mesonephros and metanephros) and the ureteric buds. The pronephros completely involutes, the mesonephros also degenerates but the mesonephric duct persists and ultimately forms the ureter and the wolffian duct. The metanephros develops caudally to the mesonephros and differentiates around the ureteric bud. The ureteric bud induces the formation of nephric units in the metanephros and, in turn, the metanephros induces branching of the ureteric bud to give rise to the ureter, the pelvis and the major and minor calyces. Occasionally, a double ureteric bud arises from the mesonephric duct and this produces a duplex renal system. If the additional upper ureteric bud arises at a high level from the mesonephric duct, it will fail to be incorporated into the lower urinary tract and will remain confluent with the vestiges of the mesonephric duct in the female and thus communicate with the genital tract and produce incontinence.[1]

The gonads and sex ducts

Much of the understanding of the gonads and sex ducts comes from the work of Jost.[2] The primordial germ cells migrate from the yolk sac to the urogenital ridge. There, differentiation of the gonad into testis or ovary is dependent on the presence or absence of the Y chromosome. On the short arm of the Y the *SRY* gene encodes a protein which functions as a transcription factor and therefore influences other genes that result in the development of the testis.[3] In the absence of the *SRY* gene, gonadal development follows the ovarian pathway. In the developing testis the germ cells are surrounded by somatic cells that are the precursors of the Sertoli, Leydig and interstitial cells. The Leydig cells secrete testosterone and the Sertoli cells Müllerian inhibitory hormone. Both exert a controlling influence over the two sex ducts that are developing simultaneously.[4]

The mesonephric (wolffian) and paramesonephric (Müllerian) duct systems are the primordia of the internal genitalia. Under the influence of testosterone the wolffian ducts form the vas deferens, epididymis and seminal vesicles. Müllerian inhibitory hormone causes the Müllerian ducts to involute. In the absence of a testis, the Müllerian ducts persist and fuse with each other in the midline to give rise to the fallopian tubes, uterus and upper vagina. The Müllerian tubercle marks the caudal junction of the Müllerian ducts with the urinary tract. The wolffian ducts involute in the absence of testosterone.

The lower genitourinary tract

The bladder develops by subdivision of the cloaca and, thus, is closely associated with the development of the hindgut and genital tract.[5] Growth of the mesenchyme in the tail end creates the cloaca (sewer), a chamber common to the urinary, gastrointestinal and genital systems (Figure 1). Further growth of the tail end of the embryo flexes it so that the covering cloacal membrane occupies a ventral position. Thickening of the mesenchyme gives rise to the urorectal septum, which is composed of Tourneaux's fold in the coronal plane and Rathke's plicae from the lateral aspects of the hindgut, separating the urogenital sinus anteriorly from the hindgut posteriorly.

In the early part of development the cloaca is separated from the amniotic space by the cloacal membrane, which occupies the anterior abdominal wall below the umbilicus. An ingrowth of the mesenchyme, between the ectodermal and the endodermal layers of the cloacal membrane, results in the formation of the lower abdominal wall and the pubis. Following the confluence of the urorectal septum with the cloacal membrane, the membrane perforates, giving rise to the anal and urogenital openings.

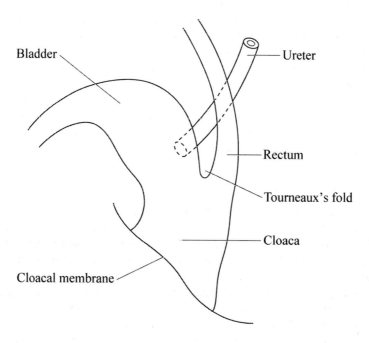

Figure 1 *Diagrammatic representation of the embryology of the cloaca*

Over-development of the cloacal membrane prevents migration of mesenchymal tissue and appropriate development of the anterior portion of the abdominal wall and pubis, giving rise to classic bladder exstrophy.[6] The understanding of cloacal exstrophy is based on the concept that the cloacal membrane ruptures before the urorectal septum completely descends.[7] As a consequence there is a strip of bowel between the two bladder halves.

Cloacal malformations result from abnormal development of the cloacal membrane. The cloacal membrane is too short, resulting in an underdeveloped dorsal aspect of the cloaca leading to impairment of the caudal movement of the urorectal septum. Thus, the hindgut remains in contact with the cloaca, leading to an opening which will develop into a recto-urogenital fistula. Anorectal anomalies with a urorectal or rectogenital communication result from an abnormal division of the cloaca.

The urogenital sinus is the confluence of the urinary and genital tracts and it is a stage of normal embryology in both sexes (Figure 2). In the female, the Müllerian tubercle marks the site of confluence between the urinary and genital tracts. In the absence of androgens, proliferation of endodermal cells gives rise to bilateral invaginations in the area of the Müllerian tubercle, the sinovaginal bulbs. As the sinovaginal bulbs grow, the Müllerian tubercle regresses and the primitive vaginal plate is formed. This contributes to the development of the distal vagina. Canalisation of this cord of cells occurs from the caudal end, separating the vagina completely from the urinary tract. In the male, because of the presence of androgens, a urogenital sinus persists. An arrest in Müllerian duct development gives rise to a persistent urogenital sinus in the female. The confluence of the vagina and urethra may be high or low and is dependent upon an early or late arrest of vaginal differentiation. The most common cause of this anomaly is in congenital adrenal hyperplasia with exposure to excessive androgens but it may rarely occur in isolation. Other abnormalities of vaginal development result from disorders of the vaginal plate and uterovaginal canal leading to agenesis or atresia. Incomplete canalisation of the vaginal plate leads to vaginal obstruction due to an imperforate hymen or a high transverse vaginal septum. Partial or complete failure of union of the Müllerian ducts leads to duplication anomalies of the uterus and vagina.

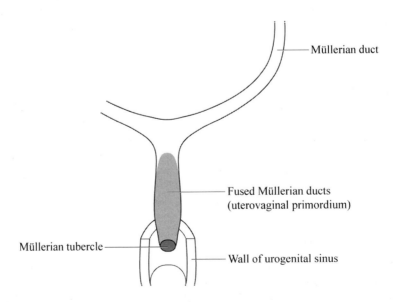

Figure 2 *Diagrammatic representation of the embryology of the Müllerian duct system*

The external genitalia

The common anlagen for the development of the external genitalia are the urogenital sinus, genital tubercle, urethral folds and labioscrotal swellings.

In the male, testosterone is converted to dihydrotestosterone by the action of 5α-reductase. Dihydrotestosterone actively produces virilisation by binding to receptors on the target cells in the genital region.[8] The genital tubercle enlarges to form the penis and the urethral folds fuse ventrally to form the penile urethra. Fusion of the labioscrotal swellings forms the scrotum.

In the female, the genital tubercle forms the clitoris, the unfused genital swellings form the labia majora, the urogenital groove remains open and forms the vestibule and the urethral folds form the labia minora.

If a female fetus is exposed to excessive androgens, as in congenital adrenal hyperplasia, virilisation occurs, producing sexual ambiguity. In 46XY fetuses a state of hormone resistance can occur due to receptor deficiency and is characterised by under-virilisation. This can be partial or complete leading to complete or partial androgen insensitivity syndromes.

URINARY TRACT ANOMALIES THAT MAY PRESENT LATER IN LIFE WITH INCONTINENCE

Renal duplication with ectopic ureter

The ectopic ureter usually inserts into the vagina or, more rarely, into the distal urethra, cervix or uterus. The renal tissue is dysplastic but enough filtrate is produced to cause incontinence. Patients typically present with a history of normal micturition only to become wet shortly afterwards; they have never been dry in the upright position. Genital examination reveals pooling of urine in the vagina. In rare cases an intermittent vaginal discharge, often associated with abdominal pain, may be the only symptom. An ultrasound scan may provide the diagnosis but the most useful investigation is an intravenous urogram. This demonstrates an abnormal axis of the kidney, lateral deviation of the upper ureter and medial deviation of the lower ureter (Figure 3). In the majority of cases, treatment consists of an upper moiety heminephro-ureterectomy.[9]

Primary female epispadias

Primary epispadias is a rare anomaly occurring with a frequency of 1/400 000.[10] Older patients present with urinary incontinence, either continuous dribbling or severe stress incontinence. Genital examination reveals a bifid clitoris with an open urethra and visible bladder neck. Treatment consists of genital and urethral reconstruction and, if this fails to produce continence, further treatment is necessary which may consist of injection of bulking agents around the bladder neck or formal bladder neck reconstruction. If bladder neck reconstruction is required, bladder augmentation may need to be combined with it.[11] These patients are often dependent upon clean intermittent catheterisation for bladder emptying and they may also require a Mitrofanoff procedure.[12]

Congenital short urethra

There is debate as to whether this is a definite entity or part of the spectrum of female epispadias. The clitoris is single and the pubic symphysis is intact. The urethra is extremely short and wide and the patient presents with either dribbling or stress incontinence. Some form of bladder outlet procedure is always required, either a reconstruction or a sling.

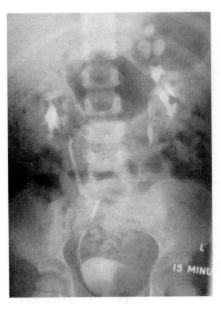 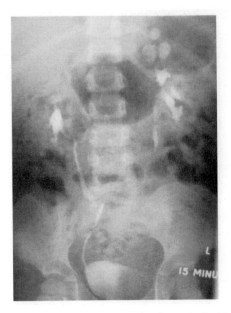

Figure 3 *Intravenous urogram showing bilateral duplex systems with poor function in the left upper moiety and nonfunction in the right*

OBSTETRIC IMPLICATIONS OF LOWER URINARY TRACT RECONSTRUCTION

Patients who have undergone lower urinary tract reconstruction, particularly augmentation cystoplasty, need careful obstetric care. The most common obstetric complication is urinary tract infection, which occurs in 15% of patients and is associated with increased rates of prematurity of 20-50%.[13]

Patients with an augmentation cystoplasty alone may have a vaginal delivery to avoid injury to the augmented bladder during caesarean section. However, those with a bladder neck reconstruction or an artificial urinary sphincter should be delivered by caesarean section to avoid disruption of the continence mechanism. The vascular pedicle should be identified to avoid inadvertent damage and it is probably best if these patients are managed jointly with the reconstructive urologist. The Mitrofanoff procedure was first described in 1980[12] and consists of reimplantation of the appendix or another conduit into the bladder to provide continent abdominal access to the bladder for intermittent catheterisation. Increasing numbers of patients with Mitrofanoff procedures have now successfully completed pregnancy but, if caesarean section is required, great care must be taken.

ANORECTAL ANOMALIES WHOSE TREATMENT MAY AFFECT SEXUAL FUNCTION

Anorectal anomalies are classified as high (supralevator) or low (infralevator). The majority of females have a low anorectal malformation, rectovestibular or rectovaginal fistula. The persistent cloaca will be discussed below.

The rectovestibular/rectovaginal fistula

The newborn presents with an absent anal opening with a fistula from the rectal pouch to the fourchette or vagina (Figure 4). The definitive operation is posterior sagittal anorectoplasty, where the rectum is completely mobilised and placed posteriorly within the sphincter mechanism. Females with anorectal malformations have a high incidence of urogenital anomalies, both acquired and iatrogenic.[14] Up to 32% have anomalies such as vaginal septum, vaginal agenesis, imperforate hymen, distal stenosis, absent lower third of vagina and hymenal band. The upper genital tract anomalies are bicornuate uterus, uterus diadelphys and a hypoplastic uterus. Severe vaginal scarring is seen in up to 29% of patients, a previous vaginoplasty or cloacal abnormality being a predictor of poor vaginal function.

Rintala[15] reported that 57% of patients with low anorectal malformations had offspring compared with 54% of controls. However, only 39% with high malformations had offspring compared with 60% of controls. Twenty percent of patients with high anomalies and 13% of those with low anomalies avoided sexual intercourse due to faecal incontinence.[16] Genital tract function is reported to be impaired in almost half of these patients due to vaginal scarring. This interferes with coitus and future delivery. Caesarean section is recommended for these patients because vaginal delivery may have an impact on faecal continence. All patients require long-term support.

A significant number of patients with high anorectal malformations suffer from long-term faecal incontinence. Many of these are now treated with the ACE (antegrade continence enema) procedure.[17] This is a procedure that provides a continent abdominal conduit for intermittent catheter access to the proximal colon for the administration of enemas. Continence is achieved in approximately 80% of patients.[18] Because of the conduit and pedicle, care must be taken if a caesarean section is required.

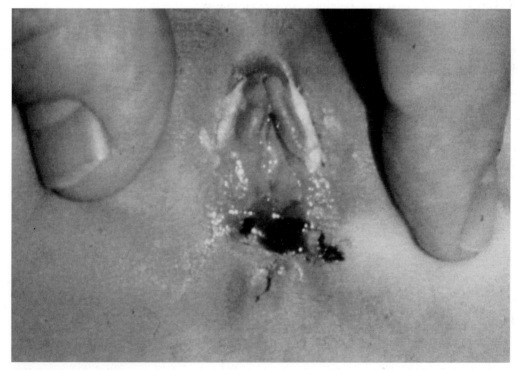

Figure 4 *Rectovestibular fistula*

URINARY OR ANORECTAL ANOMALIES WITH ASSOCIATED GENITAL TRACT ANOMALIES

Classic bladder exstrophy

The incidence of classic exstrophy is 1:50 000. In the adult female, the anus, vagina and introitus are anteriorly displaced and hence appear as structures of the anterior abdominal wall. The vagina is shorter but of normal calibre and the uterus enters superiorly so that the cervix is on the anterior vaginal wall. The ovaries and tubes are normal. The pubic hair lies on either side of the midline and the labia are bifid and rudimentary.

Genital reconstruction is often required and involves introitoplasty, vulvoplasty and monsplasty. The introitoplasty consists of a posterior episiotomy, as vaginal stenosis is seen in most patients. In a number of series the majority of women were satisfied with the cosmetic and functional results.[19,20] Monsplasty involves excision of hairless skin from the midline and rotating hair-bearing skin flaps and underlying fat to cover the midline defect.

Bonnet[21] reported the first pregnancy in an exstrophy patient in 1724. Since then there have been reports of 131 women with exstrophy who have delivered 164 children.[22] Uterine prolapse is one of the main complications after pregnancy and more frequently after introital correction.[23,24] some authors[22] recommend Gortex® (W.L. Gore & Associates, Inc.) wrap repair for procidentia in the exstrophy patient.

Cloacal exstrophy

Cloacal exstrophy of the extreme end of the spectrum of the exstrophy-epispadias complex and occurs with a frequency of 1:400 000 live births. It is a multisystem anomaly involving the gastrointestinal, nervous, musculoskeletal and genitourinary systems. The appearance is that of two hemibladders confluent, superior and inferior, to the central intestinal patch. The penis or clitoris is widely separated and split and the uterus and vagina are frequently duplex (Figure 5).

One of the major controversies in the management of cloacal exstrophy is gender assignment in the male. Males with an inadequate phallus were usually raised as females, with early excision of gonads and immediate reconstruction of the genitalia in the neonatal period. Concern has been expressed about this approach as many patients suffered from gender dysphoria in adult life and reverted to a male role. It is now recommended that males with reasonable corporal tissue are assigned a male gender.[25] Those assigned a female gender will require genital and vaginal reconstruction and thus require long-term gynaecological care.

Cloacal anomaly

Cloacal anomaly is a complex anorectal malformation seen in females. The hindgut, genital and urinary tracts all drain to the perineum via a common channel (Figure 6). Management is similar to the anorectal malformation but, in addition, the vagina needs to be separated from the urinary tract and brought to the perineum. There is a high incidence of duplication of the genital tract and this needs to be dealt with at the same time. As these girls approach puberty and adolescence, a significant proportion suffer unpredicted abdominal problems requiring surgery, such as haematocolpos, haematometra, haematosalpinx and peritoneal pseudocysts. It is important to identify anomalies, specially the asymmetric ones, and to plan their repair in an elective manner. The long-term results in terms of genital function are poorly documented but there seem to be problems with fertility and sexual function.[26]

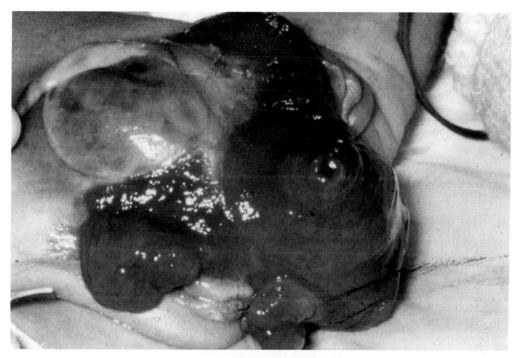

Figure 5 *Cloacal exstrophy; note the hemibladder, the prolapsed bowel and the exomphalos*

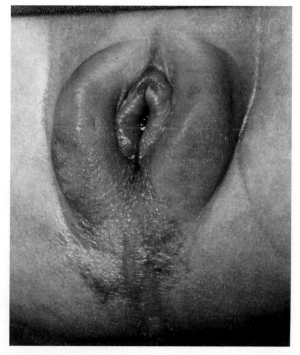

Figure 6 *Single perineal orifice in cloacal anomaly*

ISOLATED GENITAL ANOMALIES

Urogenital sinus

Newborns with this anomaly present with two perineal openings. The most important anatomical consideration is the level of the confluence of the vagina with the urinary tract. Reconstruction aims to separate the vagina from the urethra and to create separate urethral and vaginal openings.[27] The long-term results of these procedures need to be assessed, paying particular attention to continence and sexual function.

Imperforate hymen

This is a common cause of vaginal obstruction leading to hydrocolpos or hydrometrocolpos. In the newborn the presentation is of an abdominal mass usually associated with a bulging hymen (Figure 7). In adolescence, the clinical presentation is amenorrhoea and cyclical abdominal pain and an abdominal mass secondary to haematocolpos. Treatment involves a drainage procedure and vaginal reconstruction after adequately defining the anatomy.

Duplication of the genital tract

Partial or complete failure of the union of the Müllerian ducts gives rise to duplication anomalies. There may be complete duplication with two uteri, cervices and vaginas: uterus didelphys. There may be two uteri fused with a single cervix and a single vagina. On occasions one of the duplicated vaginas may be imperforate. In the newborn period, this may present with an abdominal mass. In pubertal girls the presentation is that of cyclical abdominal pain in spite of regular periods.

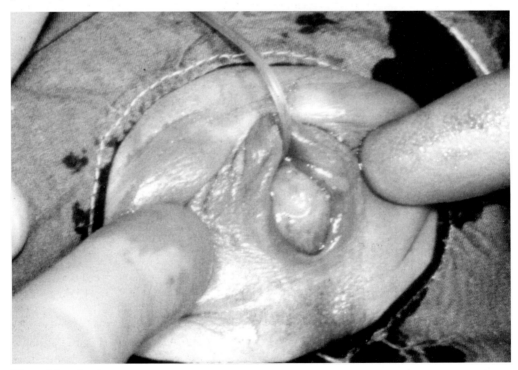

Figure 7 *Imperforate hymen*

Treatment consists of division of the vaginal septum to produce a single common channel. The vagina may also be double due to a complete septum. This may require excision in later life.

Vaginal agenesis

Complete absence of the vagina is the result of a vaginal plate or a uterovaginal canal developmental anomaly. The most common cause is the Mayer-Rokitansky-Kuster-Hauser syndrome which has an incidence of 1/5000.[28] It consists of a spectrum of Müllerian defects which include partial or complete atresia of the Müllerian duct structures and duplication anomalies. The uterus in these patients may develop normally or it can be a rudimentary bicornuate structure without a lumen. Presentation is in the mid-teenage years with failure of onset of menarche. Those with a functional uterus may present earlier with cyclical abdominal pain due to haematometra.

Other causes of vaginal deficiency are:

(1) Vaginal loss secondary to extirpative surgery for rhabdomyosarcoma of the vagina;

(2) Gender reassignment of male to female;

(3) Cloacal anomalies.

Vaginoplasty is usually performed at presentation and at a later date if presentation is in the newborn period.

Vaginoplasty; techniques, timing and long-term outcome

At the present time this is one of the most controversial areas in paediatric urology. Over the past decade there was a trend to perform vaginoplasty in infancy or early childhood when the diagnosis of vaginal agenesis or deficiency was made. The technique that gained most popularity was enterovaginoplasty, using ileum, caecum, transverse or sigmoid colon.[28,29] Good long-term results have been reported by a number of authors but complication rates are high.[30,31] Complications include introital stenosis producing dyspareunia in up to 30% of patients, prolapse of the bowel segment in up to 25% and mucous discharge in up to 16%. These complications have led to an increasing view that surgery should be delayed until adult life when other techniques are available that may have fewer complications.

THE INTERSEX PATIENT

Sexual ambiguity is due to overvirilisation of a genetic female (congenital adrenal hyperplasia) or undervirilisation of a genetic male (androgen insensitivity syndromes) and in very rare cases to true hermaphroditism.

Congenital adrenal hyperplasia

This is an autosomal recessive disorder, accounting for the majority of cases of sexual ambiguity. The pathological anatomy consists of clitoromegaly, labial fusion and persistence of a urogenital sinus. The spectrum may range from mild clitoromegaly or isolated labial fusion to marked clitoromegaly resembling a penis, scrotalisation of the labia and the formation of a phallic urethra.

Antenatal diagnosis and treatment is now possible but remains controversial.[32,33] Dexamethasone, which crosses the placental barrier and supresses the fetal adrenal and consequent virilisation, is administered once the pregnancy has been confirmed. The extent of virilisation is decreased but not prevented. Dexamethasone is continued until chorionic villus sampling (10–11 weeks) or amniotic fluid sampling provides a definitive diagnosis. In congenital adrenal hyperplasia, treatment is continued throughout pregnancy.

The treatment of congenital adrenal hyperplasia involves life-long hormone replacement and surgery. The aim of surgery is to achieve female external genital appearance. The elements of all procedures are to perform clitoral reduction, feminising genitoplasty and vaginoplasty by dividing the urogenital sinus and creating an introitus. It is still recommended that this surgery is performed in infancy but it is now clear that the majority of girls will require revisional surgery in later life to facilitate normal sexual function.[34,35] This usually consists of an introitoplasty. Adult patients have normal female identities but marriage and sexual activity occurs less frequently than in non-affected women.[36,37] About 60% of sexually active patients are fertile. These patients require long-term support from a multidisciplinary team, which should always include a gynaecologist.

Androgen insensitivity syndromes

Patients with complete androgen insensitivity have a 46XY karyotype but a normal female phenotype. They may present in infancy with inguinal hernia or in adolescence with failure of normal pubertal development. The gonads in these girls are testes and they are usually intra-abdominal. Gonadectomy is essential as there is an increased risk of malignancy. The gonadectomy should be performed during infancy or childhood if the diagnosis is made early, or before 16 years of age if the diagnosis is made because of failure of menarche. Some form of vaginoplasty is always required but this should be delayed until adolescence when the patient wants to become sexually active.

Patients with partial androgen insensitivity present with ambiguous genitalia. They represent a complex and an enormously difficult group of patients to manage. One of the most important considerations is to assign gender of rearing.[38] Traditionally, female assignment was performed when it was thought impossible to surgically reconstruct a sexually functional male. This entailed gonadectomy, feminising genitoplasty and vaginoplasty, usually performed in infancy. Long-term gynaecological care is required for all these patients. Recently, this practice of female assignment has been questioned and considerable debate is in progress to decide on the best approach.[39]

True hermaphroditism

This is an extremely rare condition and exists when both ovarian and testicular tissue is present. The forms of presentation can vary greatly. Many of these patients are reared as males but feminise at puberty due to their ovarian function. Management is extremely complex but most patients decide to stay male. If patients have been reared as females every effort should be made to conserve the ovarian tissue.

References

1. Blundon, K. E., Lane, J. W. Diagnostic difficulties in ureteral ectopia. *J Urol* 1960;**84**:463–9
2. Jost, A. Hormonal factors in sex differentiation of the mammalian fetus. *Philos Trans R Soc Lond B Biol Sci* 1970;**259**:119–30
3. Koopman, P., Gubbay, J., Vivian, N., Goodfellow, P., Lovell-Badge, R. Male development of chromosomally female mice transgenic for Sry. *Nature* 1991;**351**:117–21
4. Hughes, I.A., Malone, P. Ambiguous genitalia and intersex. In: Atwell, J.D., editor. *Paediatric Surgery*. London: Arnold; 1998. p. 290–306

5 Arey, L.B. The urinary tract. In: Arey, L.B., editor. *Developmental Anatomy. Textbook and Laboratory Manual of Embryology*, 7th ed. (revised). Philadelphia: W.B. Saunders; 1974. p. 295–314

6 Ives, E., Coffey, R., Carter, C.O. A family study of bladder exstrophy. *J Med Genet* 1980;**17**:139–41

7 Johnston, T.B. Extroversion of the bladder, complicated by the presence of intestinal openings on the surface of the extroverted area. *J Anat* 1913;**48**:89–106

8 Hughes, I.A. Intersex. In: Freeman, N.V., Burge, D.M., Griffiths, D.M., Malone, P.S.J., editors. *Surgery of the Newborn*. Edinburgh: Churchill Livingstone; 1994. p. 781–92

9 Hurwitz, R.S. Easy method of upper pole heminephroureterectomy in duplex systems in children. *Urol Clin North Am* 1990;**17**:115–19

10 International Clearing House for Birth Defects Monitoring Systems. Epidemiology of bladder exstrophy and epispadias. *Teratology* 1987;**36**:221–7

11 Hendren, W.H. Congenital female epispadias with incontinence. *J Urol* 1981;**125**:558–64

12 Mitrofanoff, P. Cystostomie continente trans-appendiculaire dans le traitement des vessies neurologique. *Chirugie Pediatrique* 1980;**21**:297–30

13 Hill, D.E., Chantigan, P.M., Kramer, S.A. Pregnancy after augmentation cystoplasty. *Surgery, Gynaecology and Obstetrics* 1990;**170**:485–7

14 Hall, R., Fleming, S., Gysler, M., McLorie, G. The genital tract in female children with imperforate anus. *Am J Obstet Gynecol* 1985;**151**:169–71

15 Rintala, R.J. Anorectal malformations: an overview. In: Stringer, M.B., Oldham, K.T., Mouriquand, P.D.E., Howard, E.R., editors. *Longterm Outcomes*. Edinburgh: W.B. Saunders; 1998. p. 356–75

16 Rintala, R.J., Mildh, L., Lindahl, H. Fecal continence and quality of life in adult patients with an operated low anorectal malformation. *J Pediatr Surg* 1992;**27**:902–5

17 Malone, P.S., Ransley, P.G., Kiely, E.M. Preliminary report: the antegrade continence enema. *Lancet* 1990;**336**:1217–18

18 Curry, J.I., Osborne, A., Malone, P.S.J. The MACE procedure: experience in the United Kingdom. *J Pediatr Surg* 1999;**34**:338–40

19 Stein, R., Fisch, M., Bauer, H., Friedberg, V., Hohenfellner, R. Operative reconstruction of the external and internal genitalia in female patients with bladder exstrophy or incontinent epispadias. *J Urol* 1995;**154**:1002–7

20 Woodhouse, C.R.J. The gynaecology of exstrophy. *Br J Urol* 1999;**83** Suppl:34–8

21 Bonnet, J. *Philos Trans R Soc Lond B Biol Sci* 1724;**33**:142

22 Stein, R., Stockle, M., Fisch, M., Nakai, H., Muller, S.C., Hohenfellner, R. The fate of the adult exstrophy patient. *J Urol* 1994;**152**:1413–16

23 Krisiloff, M., Puchner, P.J., Tretter, W., Macfarlane, M.T., Lattimer, J.K. Pregnancy in women with bladder exstrophy. *J Urol* 1978;**119**:478–9

24 Burbige, K.A., Hensle, T.W., Chambers, W.J., Leb, R., Jeter, K.F. Pregnancy and sexual function in women with bladder exstrophy. *Urology* 1986;**28**:12–14

25 Matthews, R.I., Perlman, E., Marsh, D.W., Gearhart, J.P. Gonadal morphology in cloacal exstrophy; implications in gender assignment. *BJU International* 1999;**84**:99–100

26 Levitt, M.A., Stein, D.M., Pena, A. Gynaecological concerns in the treatment of teenagers with cloaca. *J Pediatr Surg* 1998;**33**:188–93

27 Arena, F., Romeo, C., Cruccetti, A., Antonuccio, P., Basile, M., Romeo, G. The neonatal management and surgical correction of urinary hydrometrocolpos caused by a persistent urogenital sinus. *BJU International* 1999;**84**:1063–8

28 Hensle, T.W., Chang, D.T. Vaginal reconstruction reconstructive urology. *Urol Clin North Am* 1999;**26**:39–47
29 Hitchcock, R.J.I., Malone, P.S.J. Colovaginoplasty in infants and children. *Br J Urol* 1994;**73**:196–9
30 Hendren, H.W., Atala, A. Use of bowel for vaginal reconstruction. *J Urol* 1994;**152**:752–5
31 Hensle, T.W., Reiley, E. Vaginal replacement in children and young adults. *J Urol* 1998;**159**:1035–8
32 Speiser, P.W. Prenatal treatment of congenital adrenal hyperplasia. *J Urol* 1999;**162**:534–6
33 Lajic, S., Wedell, A., Bui, T-H., Ritzen, E.M., Holst, M. Long-term somatic follow-up of prenatally treated children with congenital adrenal hyperplasia. *J Clin Endocrinol Metab* 1998;**83**:3872–80
34 Bailez, M.M., Gearhart, J.P., Migeon, C., Rock, J. Vaginal reconstruction after initial construction of the external genitalia in girls with salt-wasting adrenal hyperplasia. *J Urol* 1992;**148**:680–2
35 Alizia, N.K., Thomas, D.F.M., Lilford, R.J., Batchelor, A.G.G., Johnson, N. Feminizing genitoplasty for congenital adrenal hyperplasia: what happens at puberty? *J Urol* 1999;**161**:1588–91
36 Schober, J.M. Long-term outcomes and changing attitudes to intersexuality. *Br J Urol* 1999;**83** Suppl:39–50
37 Kuhnle, U., Bullinger, M., Schwarz, H.P. The quality of life in female patients with congenital adrenal hyperplasia: a comprehensive study of the impact of genital malformation and chronic disease on female patients' life. *Eur J Pediatr* 1995;**154**:708–16
38 Glassberg, K.I. Gender assignment and the pediatric urologist. *J Urol* 1999;**161**:1308–10
39 Kipnis, K., Diamond, M. Pediatric ethics and the surgical assignment of sex. *J Clin Ethics* 1998;**9**:398–410

15

Gynaecological malignancy in childhood and adolescence

Khalil Razvi and John H. Shepherd

INTRODUCTION

Malignant disease of the genital tract is rare in prepubertal and adolescent girls. The spectrum of disease also varies markedly from that in the adult. The management of these rare tumours has witnessed a dramatic change over the last few decades and there has been a significant improvement in survival over the last 20 years (Table 1).[1,2] This is largely attributed to the development of multimodality treatment strategies and the centralisation of care in tertiary cancer centres. Thus, expertise is developed as research into the pathogenesis and treatment of these rare conditions is undertaken. Another important factor is the development of national and international multidisciplinary co-operative studies, such as the UK Children's Cancer Study Group (UKCCSG), the Children's Oncology Group in the United States and the international Intergroup Rhabdomyosarcoma Study Group (IRSG). The UKCCSG is the main body responsible for research into the pathogenesis of childhood tumours and is also responsible for the co-ordination of national and international trials in the UK.

Among the more common malignant genital tract tumours of childhood are the genital rhabdomyosarcoma, clear-cell adenocarcinoma of the vagina and cervix, carcinoma of the cervix and ovarian tumours (of which the germ-cell and sex-cord stromal tumours are the most common). Other cancers are even rarer in childhood; these include the endodermal sinus tumour of the vagina, carcinoma of the vulva and carcinoma of the uterine body.

GENITAL RHABDOMYOSARCOMA

Known previously as sarcoma botryoides on account of its grape-like appearance, genital rhabdomyosarcoma is the most common genital-tract neoplasm in children.[3] It is a malignant tumour of mesenchymal origin and mainly arises in the vagina and, less commonly, in the cervix and uterus. Vaginal primaries are more common than cervical[3,4] and are most commonly seen in children less than two years of age,[5] while cervical and uterine lesions peak in the second decade of life.[6] In Western countries, the incidence of rhabdomyosarcoma is lower in the Asian and Afro-Caribbean populations than in the white populations.[7]

Table 1 *Trends in survival rates for children diagnosed with gynaecological malignancy in Britain (adapted from Stiller et al.[1] and Stiller[2])*

Diagnostic group	Two-year survival (%)		Five-year survival (%)	
	1980–82	1989–91	1980–82	1986–88
Rhabdomyosarcoma	59	74	49	56
Ovarian germ cell	83	100	83	85

Pathophysiology

The IRSG has classified rhabdomyosarcomas into three major groupings: embryonal (of which the botryoid type is a variant), alveolar and undifferentiated tumours. Approximately 80% of genital rhabdomyosarcomas are of the embryonal histological subtype.[8] The gross appearance varies from the typical grape-like appearance of the botryoid type to a small simple polyp, a dark haemorrhagic mass or a fleshy bulbous swelling. Histological examination reveals a myxomatous stroma with fusiform cells and cross-striated muscle fibres. Rhabdomyoblasts, which are large cells with a vacuolated eosinophilic cytoplasm, are characteristically seen. Local spread is usually rapid with blood and lymphatic spread occurring later.

Most cases of rhabdomyosarcoma are sporadic and 3.6% are associated with congenital anomalies.[9] There are also well-known associations between rhabdomyosarcomas and familial syndromes including neurofibromatosis, the Li-Fraumeni syndrome and the Beckwith-Wiedemann syndrome. The Li-Fraumeni syndrome has been shown to be associated with germ-line mutations and inactivation of the *p53* tumour-suppressor gene on chromosome 17p3,[10] while the Beckwith-Wiedemann syndrome is associated with abnormalities on chromosome 11p15, where the gene for insulin-like growth factor II (IGF-II) is located.[11] IGF-II has been shown to stimulate rhabdomyosarcoma tumour-cell growth.[12] Associations with maternal use of marijuana and cocaine, exposure to radiation, fetal alcohol syndrome and maternal history of stillbirths have also been described.[13]

Clinical features and investigations

The main clinical feature is that of vaginal bleeding, which may be either minimal or a sudden bright red loss. This is sometimes associated with the passage of a clot or piece of tissue. Although bleeding is a serious symptom in a young girl, it is not always due to malignancy and the presence of a foreign body and precocious puberty need to be excluded. Nevertheless, an examination under anaesthesia is always advisable to exclude malignancy. At examination under anaesthesia, a vaginoscopy, cystoscopy, rectal examination and biopsy are undertaken to confirm diagnosis and delineate the extent of local spread of the disease. Imaging using a chest X-ray, ultrasound, intravenous urography, computed tomography (CT) or magnetic resonance imaging (MRI) and a bone scan are also part of the investigation.

Staging and survival

The clinical grouping system (surgicopathological of staging) developed by the IRSG in 1972 recognises four categories of disease, regardless of site, based on the amount of tumour remaining after initial surgery and the degree of spread at diagnosis (Table 2). Although it is still widely used, there are flaws, including the fact that the differences in surgical treatments between institutions make comparisons difficult and that it excludes other important prognostic variables, such as tumour site and size. Another staging system that has been adopted is the modified pretreatment tumour-nodes-metastasis system that takes these factors into account. This system allows the various tumours to be subdivided into three main risk groups, of which genital rhabdomyosarcomas are considered good prognostic tumours and, hence, low risk. Embryonal tumours are considered intermediate risk while alveolar and undifferentiated tumours, which occur mainly in nongenital sites, are in the high-risk group. Using the tumour-nodes-metastasis staging, all genital tract rhabdomyosarcomas, with or without locoregional extension or nodal disease, are in stage I while those with distant metastases are stage IV. This system has been shown to be highly predictive of outcome in different studies.[14,15]

Table 2 *Rhabdomyosarcoma: clinical grouping system and five-year survival (adapted from Grosfeld[13])*

Group	Characteristics	Five-year survival (%)[a]
I	Localised disease, confined to site of origin or infiltrating beyond site of origin, that is completely resected with no regional lymph node involvement	93
IIa	Grossly resected tumour with microscopic residual disease but without regional lymph node involvement	81
IIb	Complete resection of regional disease with no residual tumour but with involved regional lymph nodes	
IIc	Regional disease with involved lymph nodes grossly resected with evidence of microscopic residual disease or histological involvement of the most distal regional lymph node	
III	Incompletely resected tumour (at least 50% debulked) or biopsy only leaving gross residual disease	73
IV	Distant metastases at time of diagnosis regardless of surgical approach	30

[a]Crist et al.[19]

Treatment

There have been great advances in the treatment of genital rhabdomyosarcomas in the last three decades. Whereas exenterative or other radical surgery was the norm before 1970, it has now been supplanted by chemotherapy and, to a lesser extent, radiotherapy as part of a multimodality treatment regime. During this period, the IRSG completed four sequential prospective trials and the results showed a consecutive decrease in the need for surgical resection in localised vaginal rhabdomyosarcomas. The need for surgical resection was 100% in the IRS-I study and decreased progressively to 70%, 30% and 13% for IRS-II, IRS-III and IRS-IV, respectively.[16]

Complete surgical resection is undertaken only if it is not mutilating or cosmetically damaging and the surgical management of choice is local excision of the tumour. If this is not feasible, a biopsy is undertaken with a view to treating with chemotherapy. In IRS-III, patients with genital rhabdomyosarcomas underwent a biopsy followed by aggressive chemotherapy. Preservation of the bladder, vagina and uterus, without evidence of local recurrence after localised excision, was achieved in 71% of cases.[17] The uterine salvage rate in vaginal rhabdomyosarcoma was 83% while the bladder was preserved in almost all patients.[18] Overall five-year survival for all stages was 70%.[13] More extensive surgery, such as a hysterectomy, vaginectomy or even exenteration, is reserved for the treatment failures. In such instances, 52% of patients will go into complete remission, although survival benefits have yet to be proven.[19]

When response to chemotherapy is not complete and residual recurrent disease is present, a decision has to be taken between surgical resection by hysterocolpectomy or radiotherapy to the pelvis and intracavity brachytherapy. Both have consequences and inevitable morbidity. As fertility will be compromised anyway, the long-term adverse effects of radiotherapy in a growing and developing child can be avoided by surgery, which is, therefore, preferable.

Pelvic reconstructive surgery after radical extirpation of genital rhabdomyosarcoma is possible with good results. Vaginoplasty, using large or small bowel, split-skin grafts and myocutaneous flaps, is usually performed in adolescence prior to starting sexual activity. When bowel is used, the sigmoid colon is usually preferred over other bowel segments and is claimed to give the best long-term result.[20] When the bladder needs to be sacrificed, the options for urinary diversion are many. Many patients will initially have some form of nonrefluxing urinary diversion, usually using a bowel conduit to the abdominal wall. Most would subsequently undergo a functional reconstruction, such as with a continent catheterisable urinary reservoir using bowel, as they approach adulthood.[21]

Chemotherapy is now well established as the mainstay of treatment and vincristine, actinomycin D and cyclophosphamide (VAC) is the gold standard with which other regimens are compared. Recent agents with known activity against this tumour include carboplatin, epirubicin, ifosfamide and etoposide. On the basis of recent data, chemotherapy is now individualised based on risk factors, clinical group and site of disease, which allows stratification of patients into the risk groups mentioned earlier. Patients with low-risk disease and complete tumour excision (which includes most genital rhabdomyosarcomas) are offered vincristine and actinomycin D, with no difference in survival compared with VAC.[19] Those with poor prognosis and metastatic disease are offered a more intensive multi-agent chemotherapy combination in an attempt to improve the dismal survival figures.[22,23] This risk-based management approach aims to improve the survival benefit while minimising long-term morbidity and, hence, improving quality of life.

Radiotherapy, via brachytherapy, also plays a small but important role and can be useful for patients requiring local disease control after surgery and chemotherapy. Ovarian transposition with oophoropexy can be useful to relocate the ovaries away from the radiation field.[5] However, because of its depressive effect on the developing bone, it is sometimes administered through an implant to minimise scatter.[24,25] It also has long-term risks of vaginal, colorectal, urethral and ureteral stenosis.[26] As gynaecological rhabdomyosarcoma is generally low risk, future trials will attempt to reduce the amount of chemotherapy and avoid radiation unless local control is unsuccessful.

CLEAR-CELL ADENOCARCINOMA OF THE VAGINA AND CERVIX

The initial report of an unusual cluster of the rare clear-cell adenocarcinoma of the vagina in a young cohort by Herbst et al.[27] led to the subsequent link with maternal exposure to diethylstilboestrol (DES).[28] This was the first example of prenatal drug exposure-induced carcinogenesis in humans described in the scientific literature. Subsequent studies demonstrated a number of DES-associated non-malignant and anatomical changes of the lower female genital tract, including vaginal adenosis (a precursor lesion to clear-cell adenocarcinoma), transverse vaginal septum, cockscomb cervix and squamous metaplasia/dysplasia.[29,30] It is a disease with a peak incidence in the late teens and early twenties and about 60% have a positive history of DES or other nonsteroidal oestrogen exposure.[31]

Pathophysiology

Although the association with DES is well established, the cellular basis for these changes is still not well understood. Registry data of clear-cell adenocarcinoma cases in the USA, of which there are now more than 700 recorded, has shown that the lifetime risk of clear-cell adenocarcinoma with DES exposure is small at about 1:1000 and that the risk is dose-dependent.[32] This would suggest that other factors might also play a role in carcinogenesis. Factors such as a maternal history of miscarriage and a history of premature birth were identified as risk factors,[33,34] but these may be due to the possibility that such women may have been more likely to have been treated with DES for their poor obstetric histories. DES daughters are also more likely to suffer an adverse pregnancy outcome such as ectopic pregnancy and premature birth.[35] DES-associated clear-cell adenocarcinoma was also noted to be less aggressive and had a better prognosis compared with clear-cell adenocarcinoma independent of DES exposure (Table 3).[36] This mirrors the findings of endometrial cancer associated with unopposed oestrogen replacement therapy[37] and of breast

Table 3 Survival as a function of diethylstilboestrol (DES) exposure and extent of disease in vaginal clear-cell adenocarcinoma (adapted from Waggoner et al.[36])

Stage	DES positive (%)	DES negative (%)	P
All stages			
Five-year	84	69	0.007
Ten-year	78	60	0.008
Stages I and II			
Five-year	89	76	0.025
Ten-year	83	68	0.030
Stages III and IV			
Five-year	41	19	NS
Ten-year	33	0	NS

cancer developing in relation to hormone replacement therapy and oral contraception.[38,39] These data imply that cancers associated with exogenous exposure to oestrogens are less aggressive than their counterparts that occur without this exposure.

The pathology of this lesion reveals a wide variation in size, with the vast majority confined to the vagina and about one-third affecting the cervix. It is histologically similar to adult clear-cell carcinomas, with the characteristic clear cell whereby the cytoplasm appears clear due to a loss of glycogen content. There are three main histological types of clear-cell adenocarcinoma: tubocystic, papillary and solid. The initial spread is local, although lymph node metastases at early stages are not uncommon.

Clinical features and investigations

The cardinal symptom is abnormal vaginal bleeding. Some patients have dyspareunia and others have been discovered on screening after DES exposure was documented. Although most of the vaginal lesions are exophytic on the anterior or posterior vaginal wall, some are submucosal and are only suspected because of nodularity on palpation of the vagina. Diagnosis from exfoliative cytology, although possible, is not reliable.[40] Better detection rates were reported from the Central Netherlands Registry, where 85% of cervical cases and all the vaginal cases had a prior abnormal smear within two years of diagnosis.[41] Although DES is no longer prescribed in pregnancy and most exposed individuals are now in adulthood, it is important that close surveillance and follow-up be maintained. This is because it is still not known if DES-exposed individuals are susceptible to developing clear-cell adenocarcinoma later in life, as in the majority of non-DES-exposed clear-cell adenocarcinoma, who tend to be afflicted in the postmenopausal years.[31]

Unless symptoms warrant it, surveillance of DES-exposed girls is routinely started by the age of 14 years or at the onset of menarche, as it is unusual to develop this tumour earlier. This can initially be done under a light anaesthetic. It is imperative that the whole vagina and cervix are viewed carefully with the aid of the colposcope. Suspicious areas, including bright red areas or areas with an irregular contour, should be biopsied and cytology is also routinely taken from the endocervix, cervix and vagina. A bimanual and rectal examination should be done so that subepithelial nodularity and other structural abnormalities associated with DES exposure are not missed. In the absence of abnormality, this would be repeated annually unless clinically indicated.

Once diagnosis has been made, staging and metastatic investigations proceed as routinely for other cancers of the vagina or cervix. This would usually involve an examination under anaesthesia with biopsy, if this has not already been carried out, cystourethroscopy, proctosigmoidoscopy and uterine curettage, if indicated. Radiological investigations would include an intravenous urography, chest X-ray and CT or MRI scans of the pelvis and abdomen. Staging is the same as the FIGO staging and overall five-year survival is 89% for Stage I/II and 41% for Stage III/IV disease (Table 3).

Treatment

Treatment is by radical surgery in Stages I and II clear-cell adenocarcinoma of the vagina and cervix. Radical hysterectomy (with conservation of the ovaries) with upper (partial) or total vaginectomy and vaginal reconstruction is usually required. Frozen section of the vaginal margins may be used intra-operatively. Pelvic lymphadenectomy is also routinely performed.

Senekjian et al. advocated less radical treatment for patients desirous of fertility and have locally excisable vaginal disease.[42] Suitable tumours are those measuring less than 2 cm in size with a depth of invasion of less than 3 mm, with favourable histology and arising suitably distant from the cervix. A staging laparotomy and pelvic lymphadenectomy is nevertheless performed to confirm the absence of locally advanced disease (one-sixth of Stage I cases have lymph-node metastases) and a wide local excision of the tumour with follow-up brachytherapy is then performed. Alternatively, a laparoscopic approach could be considered. Successful pregnancies have been reported subsequently. Larger tumours are treated with radical radiotherapy and exenterative surgery is usually reserved for central recurrences after radiotherapy.[31]

Advanced vaginal and cervical clear-cell cancer is managed by radiotherapy as in the non-clear-cell counterpart. Unfortunately, there is no known effective chemotherapy for the treatment of this condition. Long-term follow-up of survivors is the norm as late recurrences are not unusual.[31]

CARCINOMA OF THE CERVIX

Carcinoma of the cervix is a rare tumour in the absence of DES exposure. The pathology is usually an adenocarcinoma. The main symptom, as in other malignant tumours of the vagina and cervix, is vaginal bleeding. As in the adult, any suspicious lesion noted on the cervix should be biopsied and subjected to histological review. Once diagnosed, treatment is usually surgical, as brachytherapy is technically challenging in this age group. The long-term adverse effects of radiotherapy also make this less appealing. A radical hysterectomy with partial vaginectomy and lymph node dissection is the procedure of choice in these circumstances. However, the ovaries need not necessarily be removed. It is reasonable in this age group to leave them behind if they appear to be normal. External beam radiotherapy will, however, be recommended if surgical margins are positive for tumour or if lymph node involvement has been documented. The role of more conservative surgery, such as radical trachelectomy, in the management of early-stage cancer to achieve locoregional control while maintaining fertility is one area of promise for the future.[43]

Of probably more important significance in adolescents is the increasing incidence of cervical intraepithelial neoplasia (CIN). This is partly due to the earlier onset of sexual activity as well as the increased incidence of sexually transmitted diseases in this age group and is independent of social class and race. A study of 10 296 paediatric and adolescent Papanicolaou smears in an almost exclusively white, rural and suburban population in New England, USA, revealed that 3.77% were reported to be indicative of CIN and 9.75% had atypical squamous cells of unknown significance (ASCUS).[44] Another smaller study from an inner-city, predominantly Hispanic and African American cohort attending a sexually transmitted diseases clinic, showed 8.4% to have smears indicative of CIN and 12.2% smears indicative of ASCUS.[45] It has also been suggested that ASCUS smears in the adolescent age group, in the absence of lower genital-tract infection, should be referred immediately for colposcopy, as the incidence of CIN is not insignificant.[46] These rates are similar to the adult age group and underscore the importance of implementing early screening in the sexually active adolescent population.

OVARIAN TUMOURS

Ovarian tumours are uncommon and present with management challenges, as early diagnosis is seldom made and many are only picked up at the time of laparotomy, usually as an emergency for acute abdominal pain. The majority of ovarian tumours in this group are benign, although the rates of malignancy vary widely from 9% to 35%.[47-49] Many tumours secrete highly specific and sensitive tumour markers, examples of which are listed in Table 4. Sex-cord stromal tumours may secrete oestrogen, testosterone and inhibin (a peptide produced by granulosa cells) while germ-cell tumours secrete α-fetoprotein, β-human chorionic gonadotrophin and lactic dehydrogenase.

Pathophysiology

The pattern of malignancy differs significantly from the adult, with a predominance of germ-cell and sex-cord stromal tumours. In a review of 648 cases,[49] the most common tumour was dysgerminoma followed by teratoma, endodermal sinus tumour and granulosa-cell tumour. In the same study, the pattern of disease in adolescence mirrored that seen in the adult population, with 38% of girls 13-17 years of age having an epithelial tumour.

The association between dysgenetic gonads in patients having a Y chromosome and malignancy of the gonads has been well recognised, with a life-time risk of developing a malignancy of 30% being reported.[50] The tumour, predominantly dysgerminoma or seminoma, arises from a pre-existing gonadoblastoma and the risks increase significantly after puberty. Hence, prophylactic gonadectomy after puberty is recommended and any young patient with a germ-cell tumour should be karyotyped. Mutations in the androgen receptor gene on the X chromosome in 46XY female gonadal dysgenesis with germ-cell tumours have also been recently described.[51] Furthermore, 6.4% of cases of germ-cell tumours have associated congenital anomalies, predominantly of the musculoskeletal system and spine.[9] This is significantly higher than the incidence among population-based controls and suggests that genetic defects may be a common causal mechanism.

Clinical features and investigations

The clinical presentation in over half the children is usually abdominal pain, for which a laparotomy is undertaken to establish diagnosis. Other findings include abdominal distension, a palpable mass, ascites, acute urinary retention and menstrual disorders in the adolescent.

Table 4 *Tumour markers of ovarian malignancy in children*

Histology	α-fetoprotein	Human chorionic gonadotrophin	Lactic dehydrogenase	Oestradiol
Dysgerminoma	−	±	+	−
Immature teratoma	±	−	±	−
Endodermal sinus tumour	+	−	±	−
Embryonal carcinoma	±	+	±	−
Mixed germ-cell tumours	±	+	+	−
Granulosa-cell tumour	−	−	−	+

Hormonally active tumours such as the granulosa-cell tumour may present with signs of isosexual precocious puberty and even virilisation, although other more common reasons should be excluded, including constitutional causes and intracranial tumours. Differential diagnoses for these tumours include Wilms tumour, an enlarged spleen, a mesenteric cyst, a distended bladder and, in the newborn period, a hydrocolpos.[5]

A gynaecological assessment and ultrasonography should be included as part of the investigation of any girl with abdominal complaints, so that ovarian tumours are not missed. In the case of more advanced disease, this should also include CT or MRI of the chest, abdomen and pelvis and a bone scan. It has been shown that inappropriate surgery for benign neoplasms and functional cysts has been performed because of inadequate investigation preoperatively and that many of the operations were performed as emergencies by non-gynaecologists.[47] Tumour marker levels should also be estimated and, if raised, are useful for monitoring response to treatment. The staging for ovarian tumours is the same as the FIGO staging in the adult, although this has been criticised as being not useful in children with germ-cell tumours, where a system based on risk factors that correlated with outcome has been suggested.[52]

Treatment

Surgical treatment is the rule in the first instance and should be conservative, as salvage rates with adjuvant chemotherapy are good for most of these tumours. Moreover, one cannot totally rely on operative findings or frozen section and it is prudent to reserve more radical surgery for when the final histology and extent of disease is known. The surgical treatment usually undertaken is a staging laparotomy, unilateral salpingo-oophorectomy with debulking surgery, preserving the uterus and the contralateral ovary and tube. If debulking is not possible or hazardous, a biopsy is taken and chemotherapy administered, which will shrink most tumours significantly, thus allowing secondary surgical debulking, if necessary, at a later stage. The contralateral ovary should be biopsied if it appears abnormal or in cases of dysgerminoma (10–15% bilateralism). Preservation of the less affected ovary in bilateral adnexal disease is also feasible with the employment of postoperative chemotherapy and secondary surgical debulking. Fertility-sparing surgery has been shown not to affect the recurrence rate or survival in patients with germ-cell tumours,[53,54] although data on sex-cord stromal tumours are scanty. The availability of sensitive and specific tumour markers, the effectiveness of chemotherapy and better imaging, means that second-look laparotomy is rarely considered necessary with these tumours.

The advent of multi-agent chemotherapy has revolutionised the management of malignant germ-cell tumours. All cases of non-dysgerminomatous germ-cell tumour require postoperative chemotherapy, with the exception of Stage Ia, grade 1 immature teratoma, although a recent study suggested that completely resected tumours of any grade do just as well with surgery alone.[55] The VAC regimen was the first combination used effectively, although higher doses were required to treat advanced disease.[56,57] This was superseded by the platinum-based PVB regimen (cisplatin, vincristine and bleomycin) which gave high cure rates but was also toxic.[58] The effectiveness of etoposide in treating germ-cell tumour in the male[59] led to the development of the PEB regimen (cisplatin, etoposide and bleomycin) which was less toxic but just as effective as the PVB regimen.[60] This remains the gold-standard chemotherapy for paediatric malignant germ-cell tumour. Unfortunately, most of these data are extrapolated from adult studies and comparative paediatric data are lacking. Current efforts are now aimed at tailoring effective but less toxic chemotherapy regimens based on risk scoring and this includes substituting carboplatin for cisplatin and omitting bleomycin from certain tumours with good prognosis. Salvage chemotherapy using ifosfamide, doxorubicin, actinomycin and methotrexate has been used with varying success.

Most patients with pure dysgerminomas present with Stage I disease and surgery alone is effective. Despite it being an extremely radiosensitive tumour, chemotherapy using the PVB or PEB regimens is the treatment of choice for more advanced-stage dysgerminomas, as survival is excellent and the long-term effects of radiotherapy on children are avoided. Recent data from the UKCCSG showed that the overall four-year survival for ovarian germ-cell tumour was 90%.[61] Radiotherapy has little role in the management of germ-cell tumours in children. It may be unavoidable in the presence of residual tumour after surgery and second-line chemotherapy for relapsed disease.[52]

Data on adjuvant treatment of sex-cord stromal tumours are lacking due to the rarity and indolent nature of many of these tumours. Late recurrences are not unusual and, hence, long-term follow-up is needed to establish the efficacy of any treatment modality. Conservative surgery alone is sufficient for patients who present with Stage I disease. The role of chemotherapy in this condition is difficult to define. Adverse prognostic factors such as large tumour size, bilateral disease, nuclear atypia and mitotic rate in granulosa cell tumours and those with poor differentiation, retiform pattern or contain muscle or cartilage in Sertoli-Leydig tumours, have been used to select patients who might benefit from chemotherapy. Platinum-based regimens similar to those for germ-cell tumour are used, although survival benefits remain to be proven.[62-64]

ENDODERMAL SINUS TUMOUR OF THE VAGINA

Endodermal sinus tumour of the vagina is an extremely rare but highly malignant tumour in infants. The clinical appearance is similar to sarcoma botryoides, although histologically it resembles a clear-cell adenocarcinoma, however rare the latter is in infants. The tumour secretes α-fetoprotein, which is a useful tumour marker. It is generally agreed that primary conservative surgery and chemotherapy using the VAC or PEB regimens is the treatment of choice.[65-67] Surgical excision is performed with the aim of removing all local disease. This entails at least a partial vaginectomy. Overall prognosis for this tumour has been poor, although recent data showed a 70% two-year survival rate for all cases of endodermal sinus tumour in children, especially in the pelvis.[66] Recurrent or residual disease requires more extensive surgical extirpation as for sarcoma botryoides.

LONG-TERM EFFECTS OF TREATMENT OF GYNAECOLOGICAL TUMOURS IN CHILDREN AND ADOLESCENTS

Success in the treatment of these cancers has meant that the long-term sequelae of these treatments cannot be overlooked. Survivors are susceptible to suffering slower physical growth as a result of chronic disease, poor nutrition and hypermetabolic states.[68] Radiotherapy causes hypoplasia of the musculoskeletal system as well as asymmetrical fat distribution. Pubertal delay, amenorrhoea, infertility and premature menopause can have long-lasting physical and psychological effects, which need to be carefully addressed, although advances in reproductive technologies have given much hope to these survivors.

Vaginal stenosis from maldevelopment can lead to difficulty with initiating coitus. If ovarian function has been present, this then may result in a haematometra and haematocolpos occurring after a normal menarche. Surgical correction by initial drainage and then reconstruction may be necessary, although difficult, due to the poor development of perineal and pelvic tissues following brachytherapy. Careful surveillance of ovarian function in susceptible individuals should be implemented. There is also a small but appreciable risk of secondary malignancies, especially leukaemia. Long-term renal effects of cisplatin-based chemotherapy have been shown to be mild with no long-term sequelae.[69] Nevertheless, it is important that oncologists and other healthcare professionals entrusted with the care of these young patients are mindful of the long-term risks engendered by their treatments so that these can be minimised. Continued counselling of patients and their parents may be necessary as they mature, even though the treatment has been successful.

Acknowledgement

The authors would like to thank Judith Kingston (consultant in paediatric oncology at St Bartholomew's Hospital, London) for her advice in the preparation of this manuscript.

References

1. Stiller, C.A., Bunch, K.J. Trends in survival for childhood cancer in Britain diagnosed 1971–85. *Br J Cancer* 1990;**62**:806–15
2. Stiller, C.A. Population based survival rates for childhood cancer in Britain, 1980–91. *BMJ* 1994;**309**:1612–16
3. Copeland, L.J., Gershenson, D.M., Saul, P.B., Sneige, N., Stringer, A., Edwards, C.L. Sarcoma botryoides of the female genital tract. *Obstet Gynecol* 1985;**66**:262–6
4. Zeisler, H., Mayerhofer, K., Joura, E.A., Bancher-Todesca, D., Kainz, C., Breitenecker, G. *et al.* Embryonal rhabdomyosarcoma of the uterine cervix: case report and review of the literature. *Gynecol Oncol* 1998;**69**:78–83
5. Dewhurst, J., Shepherd, J.H. Genital tract malignancy in the pre-pubertal child. In: Coppelson, M., editor. *Gynecologic Oncology*, 2nd ed. Edinburgh: Churchill Livingstone; 1992. p. 1047–57
6. Brand, E., Berek, J.S., Nieberg, R.K., Hacker, N.F. Rhabdomyosarcoma of the uterine cervix. *Cancer* 1987;**60**:1552–60
7. Wexler, L., Helman, L. Rhabdomyosarcoma and the undifferentiated sarcomas. In: Pizzo, P., Poplack, D., editors. *Principles and Practice of Pediatric Oncology*, 3rd ed. Philadelphia: Lippincott-Raven; 1997. p. 799–829
8. Weiner, E.S. Rhabdomyosarcoma. In: O'Neill, J.A., Rowe, M.I., Grosfield, J.L. *et al.*, editors. *Pediatric Surgery*, 5th ed. St. Louis: Mosby; 1998. p. 431–45
9. Narod, S.A., Hawkins, M.M., Robertson, C.M., Stiller, C.A. Congenital anomalies and childhood cancer in Great Britain. *Am J Hum Genet* 1997;**60**:474–85
10. Malkin, D., Li, F.P., Strong, L.C., Fraumeni, J.F. Jr, Nelson, C.E., Kim, D.H. *et al.* Germline p53 mutations in a familial syndrome of breast cancer, sarcomas, and other neoplasms. *Science* 1990;**250**:1233–8
11. Li, M., Squire, J.A., Weksberg, R. Molecular genetics of Beckwith-Wiedemann syndrome. *Curr Opin Pediatr* 1997;**9**:623–9
12. El Badry, O.M., Minniti, C., Kohn, E.C., Houghton, P.J., Daughaday, W.H., Helman, L.J. Insulin-like growth factor II acts as an autocrine growth and motility factor in human rhabdomyosarcoma tumors. *Cell Growth Differ* 1990;**1**:325–31
13. Grosfeld, J.L. Risk-based management: current concepts of treating malignant solid tumors of childhood. *J Am Coll Surg* 1999;**189**:407–25
14. Pedrick, T.J., Donaldson, S.S., Cox, R.S. Rhabdomyosarcoma: the Stanford experience using a TNM staging system. *J Clin Oncol* 1986;**4**:370–8

15   Lawrence, W. Jr, Gehan, E.A., Hays, D.M., Beltangady, M., Maurer, H.M. Prognostic significance of staging factors of the UICC staging system in childhood rhabdomyosarcoma: a report from the Intergroup Rhabdomyosarcoma Study (IRS-II). *J Clin Oncol* 1987;**5**:46–54
16   Andrassy, R.J., Wiener, E.S., Raney, R.B., Hays, D.M., Arndt, C.A., Lobe, T.E. et al. Progress in the surgical management of vaginal rhabdomyosarcoma: a 25-year review from the Intergroup Rhabdomyosarcoma Study Group. *J Pediatr Surg* 1999;**34**:731–4
17   Andrassy, R.J., Hays, D.M., Raney, R.B., Weiner, E.S., Lawrence, W., Lobe, T.E. et al. Conservative surgical management of vaginal and vulvar pediatric rhabdomyosarcoma: a report from the Intergroup Rhabdomyosarcoma Study III. *J Pediatr Surg* 1995;**30**:1034–7
18   Corpron, C.A., Andrassy, R.J., Hays, D.M., Raney, R.B., Weiner, E.S., Lawrence, W. et al. Conservative management of uterine pediatric rhabdomyosarcoma: a report from the Intergroup Rhabdomyosarcoma Study III and IV pilot. *J Pediatr Surg* 1995;**30**:942–4
19   Crist, W., Gehan, E.A., Ragab, A.H., Dickman, P.S., Donaldson, S.S., Fryer, C. et al. The Third Intergroup Rhabdomyosarcoma Study. *J Clin Oncol* 1995;**13**:610–30
20   Hensle, T.W., Reiley, E.A. Vaginal replacement in children and young adults. *J Urol* 1998;**159**:1035–8
21   Duel, B.P., Hendren, W.H., Bauer, S.B., Mandell, J., Colodny, A., Peters, C.A. et al. Reconstructive options in genitourinary rhabdomyosarcoma. *J Urol* 1996;**156**:1798–804
22   Ruymann, F., Crist, W., Wiener, E. Comparison of two doublet chemotherapy regimens and conventional radiotherapy in metastatic rhabdomyosarcoma: improved overall survival using ifosfamide/etoposide compared to vincristine/mephalan in IRSG-IV. *Proceedings of the American Society of Clinical Oncology* 1997;**16**:521a
23   Frascella, E., Pritchard-Jones, K., Modak, S., Mancini, A.F., Carli, M., Pinkerton, C.R. Response of previously untreated metastatic rhabdomyosarcoma to combination chemotherapy with carboplatin, epirubicin and vincristine. *Eur J Cancer* 1996;**32A**:821–5
24   Healey, E.A., Shamberger, R.C., Grier, H.E., Loeffler, J.S., Tarbell, N.J. A 10-year experience of pediatric brachytherapy. *Int J Radiat Oncol Biol Phys* 1995;**32**:451–5
25   Gerbaulet, A.P., Esche, B.A., Haie, C.M., Castaigne, D., Flamant, F., Chassagne, D. Conservative treatment for lower gynecological tract malignancies in children and adolescents: the Institut Gustave-Roussy experience. *Int J Radiat Oncol Biol Phys* 1989;**17**:655–8
26   Flamant, F., Gerbaulet, A., Nihoul-Fekete, C., Valteau-Couanet, D., Chassagne, D., Lemerle, J. Long-term sequelae of conservative treatment by surgery, brachytherapy, and chemotherapy for vulval and vaginal rhabdomyosarcoma in children. *J Clin Oncol* 1990;**8**:1847–53
27   Herbst, A.L., Scully, R.E. Adenocarcinoma of the vagina in adolescence: a report of 7 cases including 6 clear cell carcinomas (so called mesonephromas). *Cancer* 1970;**25**:745–57
28   Herbst, A.L., Ulfelder, H., Poskanzer, D.C. Adenocarcinoma of the vagina: association of maternal stilbestrol therapy with tumor appearance in young women. *N Engl J Med* 1971;**284**:878–81
29   Herbst, A.L., Kurman, R.J., Scully, R.E. Vaginal and cervical abnormalities after exposure to stilbestrol *in utero*. *Obstet Gynecol* 1972;**40**:287–98
30   Herbst, A.L., Poskanzer, D.C., Robboy, S.J., Friedlander, L., Scully, R.E. Prenatal exposure to stilbestrol: a prospective comparison of exposed female offspring with unexposed controls. *N Engl J Med* 1975;**292**:334–9
31   Herbst, A.L. Behaviour of estrogen-associated female genital tract cancer and its relation to neoplasia following intrauterine exposure to diethylstilbestrol (DES). *Gynecol Oncol* 2000;**76**:147–56
32   Herbst, A.L. Diethylstilbestrol and adenocarcinoma of the vagina. *Am J Obstet Gynecol* 1999;**181**:1576–8

33   Herbst, A.L., Cole, P., Norusis, M.J., Welch, W.R., Scully, R.E. Epidemiologic aspects and factors related to survival in 384 cases of clear cell adenocarcinoma of the vaginal and cervix. *Am J Obstet Gynecol* 1979;**135**:876–86

34   Melnick, S., Cole, P., Anderson, D., Herbst, A.L. Rates and risks of diethylstilbestrol related to clear cell adenocarcinoma of the vagina and cervix. *N Engl J Med* 1987;**316**:514–16

35   Herbst, A.L., Hubby, M.M., Blough, R.R., Azizi, F. A comparison of pregnancy experience in DES-exposed and DES-unexposed daughters. *J Reprod Med* 1980;**24**:62–9

36   Waggoner, S.E., Mittendork, R.L., Biney, N., Anderson, D., Herbst, A.L. Influence of *in utero* diethylstilbestrol exposure on the prognosis and biologic behaviour of vaginal clear cell adenocarcinoma. *Gynecol Oncol* 1994;**55**:238–44

37   Collins, J., Donner, A., Allen, L.H., Adams, O. Oestrogen use and survival in endometrial cancer. *Lancet* 1980;**2**:961–4

38   Collaborative Group on Hormonal Factors in Breast Cancer. Breast cancer and hormonal contraceptives: collaborative reanalysis of individual data on 53 297 women with breast cancer and 100 239 women without breast cancer from 54 epidemiologic studies. *Lancet* 1996;**347**:1713–27

39   Collaborative Group on Hormonal Factors in Breast Cancer. Breast cancer and hormone replacement therapy: collaborative reanalysis of data from 51 epidemiologic studies of 52 705 women with breast cancer and 108 411 women without breast cancer. *Lancet* 1997;**350**:1047–59

40   Robboy, S.J., Kaufman, R.H., Prat, J., Welch, W.R., Gaffey, T., Scully, R.E. *et al.* Pathologic findings in young women enrolled in the national co-operative DiEthylStilbestrol adenosis (DESAD) project. *Obstet Gynecol* 1979;**53**:309–17

41   Hanselaar, A.G.J.M., Boss, E.A., Massuger, L.F.A.G., Bernheim, J.L. Cytologic examination to detect clear cell adenocarcinoma of the vagina or cervix. *Gynecol Oncol* 1999;**75**:338–44

42   Senekjian, E.K., Frey, R.E., Anderson, D., Herbst, A.L. Local therapy in stage I clear cell adenocarcinoma of the vagina. *Cancer* 1987;**60**:1319–24

43   Shepherd, J.H., Crawford, R.A., Oram, D.H. Radical trachelectomy: a way to preserve fertility in the treatment of early cervical cancer. *Br J Obstet Gynaecol* 1998;**105**:912–16

44   Mount, S.L., Papillo, J.L. A study of 10,296 pediatric and adolescent Papanicolaou smear diagnosis in northern New England. *Pediatrics* 1999;**103**:539–45

45   Edelman, M., Fox, A.S., Alderman, E.M., Neal, W., Shapiro, A., Silver, E.J. *et al.* Cervical Papanicolaou smear abnormalities in inner city Bronx adolescents: prevalence, progression, and immune modifiers. *Cancer* 1999;**87**:184–9

46   Kelly, L., Bleistein, A., Stevens-Simon, C. Should gynecologic maturity change the management of cervical atypia during adolescence? *J Pediatr Adolesc Gynecol* 1999;**12**:203–7

47   Piippo, S., Mustaniemi, L., Lenko, H., Aine, R., Maenpaa, J. Surgery for ovarian masses during childhood and adolescence: a report of 79 cases. *J Pediatr Adolesc Gynecol* 1999;**12**:223–7

48   Hassan, E., Creatsas, G., Deligeorolgou, E., Michalas, S. Ovarian tumors during childhood and adolescence: a clinicopathological study. *Eur J Gynaecol Oncol* 1999;**20**:124–6

49   Breen, J.L., Maxson, W.S. Ovarian tumors in children and adolescents. *Clin Obstet Gynecol* 1977;**20**:607–23

50   Dewhurst, C.J., Ferreira, H.P., Gillett, P.G. Gonadal malignancy in XY females. *J Obstet Gynaecol Br Cwlth* 1971;**78**:1077–83

51   Chen, C.P., Chern, S.R., Wang, T.Y., Wang, W., Wang, K.L., Jeng. C.J. Androgen receptor gene mutations in 46,XY females with germ cell tumours. *Hum Reprod* 1999;**14**:664–70

52   Pinkerton, C.R. Malignant germ cell tumours in childhood. *Eur J Cancer* 1997;**33**:895–902

53   Peccatori, F., Bonazzi, C., Chiari, S., Landoni, F., Colombo, N., Mangioni, C. Surgical management of malignant ovarian germ-cell tumors: 10 years' experience of 129 patients. *Obstet Gynecol* 1995;**86**:367–72

54   Zalel, Y., Piura, B., Elchalal, U., Czernobilsky, B., Antebi, S., Dgani, R. Diagnosis and management of malignant germ cell tumors in young females. *Int J Gynaecol Obstet* 1996;**55**:1–10

55   Cushing, B., Giller, R., Ablin, A., Cohen, L., Cullen, J., Hawkins, E. et al. Surgical resection alone is effective treatment for ovarian immature teratoma in children and adolescents: a report of the pediatric oncology group and children's cancer group. *Am J Obstet Gynecol* 1999;**181**:353–8

56   Smith, J.P., Rutledge, F. Advances in chemotherapy for gynecologic cancer. *Cancer* 1975;**36**:669–74

57   Flamant, F., Schwartz, L., Delons, E., Caillaud, J.M., Hartmann, O., Lemerle, J. Nonseminomatous malignant germ cell tumors in children. Multidrug therapy in stages III and IV. *Cancer* 1984;**54**:1687–91

58   Bokemeyer, C., Berger, C.C., Kuczyk, M.A., Schmoll, H.J. Evaluation of long-term toxicity after chemotherapy for testicular cancer. *J Clin Oncol* 1996;**14**:2923–32

59   Newlands, E.S., Bagshawe, K.D. Epipodophyllin derivative (VP-16–213) in malignant teratomas and choriocarcinomas. *Lancet* 1977;**2**:87

60   Williams, S.D., Birch, R., Einhorn, L.H., Irwin, L., Greco, F.A., Loehrer, P.J. Treatment of disseminated germ-cell tumors with cisplatin, bleomycin, and either vinblastine or etoposide. *N Engl J Med* 1987;**316**:1435–40

61   J. Kingston, Personal communication

62   Muntz, H.G., Goff, B.A., Fuller, A.F. Recurrent ovarian granulosa cell tumor: role of combination chemotherapy with report of a long term response to a cyclophosphamide, doxorubicin and cisplatin regimen. *Eur J Gynaecol Oncol* 1990;**11**:263–8

63   Pectasides, D., Alevizakos, N., Athanassiou, A.E. Cisplatin-containing regimen in advanced or recurrent granulosa cell tumours of the ovary. *Ann Oncol* 1992;**3**:316–18

64   Gershenson, D.M. Management of early ovarian cancer: germ cell and sex cord-stromal tumors. *Gynecol Oncol* 1994;**55**:S62–72

65   Goerzen, J.L., Grant, R.M., Arthur, K., Stuart, G.C.E. Primary endodermal sinus tumor of the vagina in childhood: case report and review of the results of treatment in the literature. *Pediatr Adolesc Gynecol* 1986;**4**:47

66   Davidoff, A.M., Hebra, A., Bunin, N., Shochat, S.J., Schnaufer, L. Endodermal sinus tumor in children. *J Pediatr Surg* 1996;**31**:1075–8

67   Hwang, E.H., Han, S.J., Lee, M.K., Lyu, C.J., Kim, B.S. Clinical experience with conservative surgery for vaginal endodermal sinus tumor. *J Pediatr Surg* 1996;**31**:219–22

68   Schwartz, C.L. Long-term survivors of childhood cancer: the late effects of therapy. *The Oncologist* 1999;**4**:45–54

69   von der Weid, N.X., Erni, B.M., Mamie, C., Wagner, H.P., Bianchetti, M.G. Cisplatin therapy in childhood: renal follow-up 3 years or more after treatment: Swiss Pediatric Oncology Group. *Nephrol Dial Transplant* 1999;**14**:1441–4

16

Anal incontinence – the role of the obstetrician and gynaecologist

Abdul H. Sultan and A. Muti Abulafi

INTRODUCTION

Faecal incontinence is defined as the loss of normal control of bowel action leading to the involuntary passage of flatus and faeces. Incontinence can range from a minor leakage of faeculant fluid, occasional leakage of stool during passage of flatus, to a complete loss of bowel control. It has an estimated prevalence of 4.2/1000 rising to more than 10/1000 in those over 65 years of age.[1] The condition is more common in women than men of young and middle age, although in the elderly it affects both sexes equally.

Patients with incontinence are embarrassed and ashamed to talk about the problem with their doctor and, when they do, they give vague and incomplete information. In the setting of a gynaecology clinic, the condition is commonly encountered in association with other disorders of the pelvic floor such as prolapse and urinary incontinence. It is, therefore, important for the gynaecologist to ask direct questions regarding bowel, bladder and sexual dysfunction. This chapter aims to familiarise the obstetrician and gynaecologist with the anatomy and physiology of the posterior compartment, with pelvic floor disorders and describes the contribution of childbirth trauma to anal incontinence.

ANATOMY AND PHYSIOLOGY

The anal sphincter and pelvic floor

The anal canal is 3–4 cm in length. It is surrounded by two muscles: the internal sphincter, a smooth muscle that represents the expanded distal portion of the circular smooth muscle of the rectum and is innervated by the autonomic nerves. The external sphincter, a striated muscle, is situated around the internal sphincter and extends superiorly to blend with the puborectalis, an important constituent of the levator ani. It is divided descriptively into three parts: subcutaneous, superficial and deep. The innervation of the external sphincter is from the pudendal nerves (S2, S3 and S4) and that of the puborectalis from S3 and S4.

The internal sphincter is almost always contracted and contributes up to 70% of the resting tone. Relaxation occurs in response to certain stimuli such as rectal distension (rectosphincteric reflex) and then only for a short time. The external sphincter, puborectalis and levator ani are constantly active, even during sleep. This activity in the external sphincter contributes further to the resting tone of the anal canal. The activity in these muscles is increased by voluntary squeezing but usually for short periods (up to 60 seconds) and is lowered during defecation (initial straining effort).

The anorectal angle is created and maintained by the constant active contraction of the levator ani and its most central portion, the puborectalis, which passes around the rectum in U-shaped

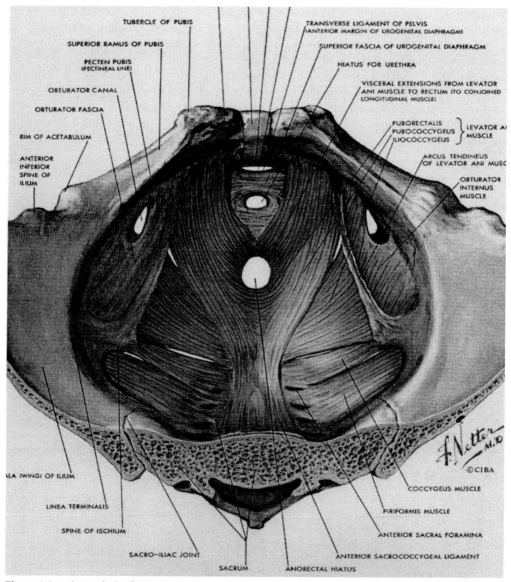

Figure 1 *Lateral view of pelvic floor and anal sphincter complex demonstrating the 'U' shaped puborectalis muscle creating the anorectal angle (reproduced from Mann and Glass,[47] with permission*

fashion, pulling it forward (Figure 1). This allows the anterior wall of the rectum to cover the top of the anal canal as a flap valve. Any increase in the intra-abdominal pressure causes the flap valve to close more tightly preventing rectal contents from entering the anal canal.

Continence and defecation

Normal continence and defecation are achieved by an interplay between a host of sensory and motor inputs. The rectum maintains low intraluminal pressure (rectal compliance) and accommodates slowly the faecal contents, which are propagated slowly down the colon by colonic peristalsis. Once a certain volume is reached, usually 200 ml, a sensation of rectal fullness occurs mediated by sensory stretch receptors in the puborectalis and levator ani. The rectosphincteric inhibitory reflex is activated, causing relaxation of the internal anal sphincter. The faecal bolus descends towards the anal canal with its rich sensory receptors but is prevented from progressing further by the voluntary contraction of the external sphincter. At this point, sensory sampling permits the person to distinguish between flatus, liquid or solid. When socially acceptable, the external sphincter and puborectalis are relaxed together with straining and the anorectal angle is straightened, allowing the rectal contents to be expelled. If the timing is inconvenient the external sphincter and puborectalis remain contracted, returning the luminal contents to the rectum.

Causes of faecal incontinence

Incontinence is usually the result of disturbed sphincter and pelvic floor function (true incontinence). However, it should be remembered that it can still occur in patients with normal sphincter mechanism but with high intraluminal pressure and rapid colonic transit (urge incontinence). It should also be noted that patients with defective sphincter mechanism and low intracolonic and intrarectal pressures and slow rectal transit might not be incontinent. Moreover,

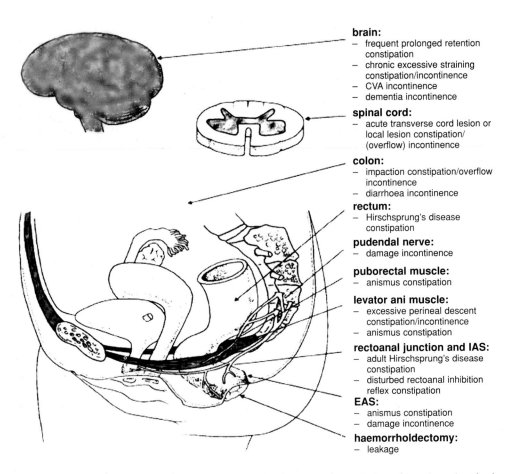

Figure 2 *Schematic representation to demonstrate the sites at which disorders can provoke constipation and incontinence (reproduced from Smout and Akkermans,[48] with permission)*

Table 1 Causes of faecal incontinence

Type of incontinence	Cause	Diagnosis
Normal sphincter		
Urge incontinence		Irritable bowel syndrome
False incontinence		Inflammatory bowel disease
		Short bowel
		Severe diarrhoea
		Cancer
		Faecal impaction with paradoxical diarrhoea
Abnormal sphincter		
True (passive) incontinence	Neurogenic	Cardiovascular accident
		Dementia
		Multiple sclerosis
		Diabetes
		Cauda equina lesions
	Myogenic	Cancer of anus or lower rectum
		Trauma
		– obstetric
		– accidental
		– iatrogenic
		Rectovaginal fistula
		Rectal prolapse
	Idiopathic (thought to be neurogenic)	Descending perineum syndrome

incontinence should be distinguished from minor faecal soiling where the sphincter mechanism and bowel function are normal. In these situations, soiling is the result of local pathology such as mucosal prolapse and prolapsing haemorrhoids. Thus, the causes of faecal incontinence can be classified into colonic (with normal sphincter) and sphincteric (abnormal mechanism) causes (Table 1; Figure 2). This serves to highlight the need for a full assessment of the whole colon, not just the sphincter mechanism, in patients with incontinence.

Colonic causes (normal sphincter mechanism)

Conditions associated with high intraluminal colonic pressure with rapid transit may present with incontinence. Examples include patients with irritable bowel syndrome and inflammatory bowel disorders, rectal cancer or short bowel following extensive resections. Patients with painful anal conditions such as fissures and thrombosed haemorrhoids, or after anal surgery, may develop faecal impaction, which causes activation of the rectosphincteric inhibitory reflex. As a result the anal canal gapes causing faeculant fluid to escape. Therefore, patients with apparent diarrhoea should be given a rectal examination to exclude faecal impaction.

Sphincteric causes (abnormal sphincter mechanism)

The anal sphincter function is impaired when the muscle itself is damaged or disrupted or its nerve supply is defective. Therefore, causes that lead to abnormal sphincter mechanism can be grouped under three main headings: neurogenic, myogenic and idiopathic (probably neurogenic) causes.

Neurogenic

Multiple sclerosis, dementia, stroke and diabetic neuropathy should be considered in patients with incontinence. Lower motor neuron lesions secondary to tumours and lesions of the cauda equina, as well as tabes dorsalis, may also lead to incontinence due to failure of external sphincter and puborectalis function.

Myogenic

Malignant tumours of the anus or the lower rectum, especially those involving the anus, can cause sphincter dysfunction, due to direct involvement of the sphincter muscle by the tumour.

Trauma to the anal sphincter can be classified into three types: obstetric, iatrogenic (surgical) and accidental. Obstetric trauma to the anal sphincter can occur during difficult second-stage labour, forceps delivery and third-degree perineal tears, which usually results in anterior sphincter disruption. Two prospective studies in women undergoing vaginal delivery showed that up to one in three women might sustain occult anal sphincter trauma during their first vaginal delivery.[2,3] One-third of these women had new bowel symptoms after delivery. In another prospective study of 50 patients with symptomatic rectoceles due to obstetric trauma presenting to the authors' unit, 46% were found to have significant sphincter disruption.[4] Obstetric trauma may also cause damage to the pudendal nerve and is a cause of idiopathic incontinence in some patients (see below). Direct accidental injury to the perineum may disrupt the sphincter muscle and damage its blood and nerve supply. Bony fractures may disrupt the pelvic floor and anorectal angle and thereby lead to incontinence. Finally, damage to the sphincter may occur during anal surgery. The internal sphincter is particularly vulnerable during operations for fissures, such as lateral sphincterotomy and manual dilatation, and operations for haemorrhoids. In fistula surgery, most of the internal sphincter and a part of the external sphincter is divided. In these situations, if a pre-existing defect or weakness exists in either the internal or external sphincters, patients are at a high risk of incontinence.

A fistula is an abnormal communication between two epithelial surfaces. Any fistula between the bowel and the perianal skin or vagina will result in faecal leakage and incontinence. Many disease conditions such as inflammatory bowel disease, diverticular disease, cancer and radiotherapy can be responsible. Obstetric trauma is by far the most common cause of rectovaginal fistula.[5] The treatment depends on whether the fistula is to the skin or vagina. However, in general, the treatment is directed at the cause and taking into account the size and location of the fistula.

In patients with rectal prolapse, the full thickness of the rectal wall protrudes through the anus, stretching the sphincter keeping it open and preventing its action. Rectal prolapse is more common in women, especially above the age of 50 years. Interestingly, the majority of these patients are nulliparous and it is therefore unlikely that pregnancy and obstetric trauma have a role in the aetiology.[6] The exact cause is unknown, although it has been observed that, in a large number of patients, there is a history of chronic constipation and straining. It is thought that the prolapse starts as an internal intussusception (Figure 3) of the anterior rectal wall, presumably due to rectal denervation or possibly an inherent weakness in the pelvic floor structures. This activates the rectosphincteric inhibitory reflex causing sphincter relaxation and anal gaping. Further chronic straining will eventually result in complete protrusion of the rectum through the anal canal.

There is no evidence to support a clear association between rectal prolapse and complete uterine prolapse. Reports in the literature are limited to case reports and small series.[7,8] The largest series is by Kupfer and Goligher[9] where only 8 of 83 patients with rectal prolapse had a significant uterine prolapse requiring surgery. However, in our experience, we believe that there is a higher association between lesser degrees of genital and rectal prolapse.[10] It is therefore important to search for these abnormalities by careful history and thorough examination of the vagina and rectum and appropriate investigations.

Table 2 *Causes of constipation*

Origin	Type	Cause
Organic		Cancer
		Diverticular disease
		Fissure *in ano*
Functional	Colonic (slow transit) Constipation – disordered colonic motor activity	Idiopathic
		Drugs
		Endocrine causes
		Psychiatric
		Environmental
	Anorectal constipation	Diminished sensation
		Outlet obstruction
		– rectal intussusception and prolapse
		– rectocele
		– enterocele
		– anismus

Idiopathic (descending perineum syndrome)

This condition was first described by Sir Alan Parks in 1966.[11] Patients usually present with a long history of constipation (Table 2) and marked descent of the perineum on straining. These patients have a prolapse of the anterior rectal wall mucosa, which is interpreted by the patient as luminal content, leading to chronic and habitual straining. As a result of the descent of the pelvic floor, the pudendal nerves supplying the levator ani are put under strain leading to traction neuropathy and eventually faecal incontinence, so-called idiopathic (neurogenic) incontinence.

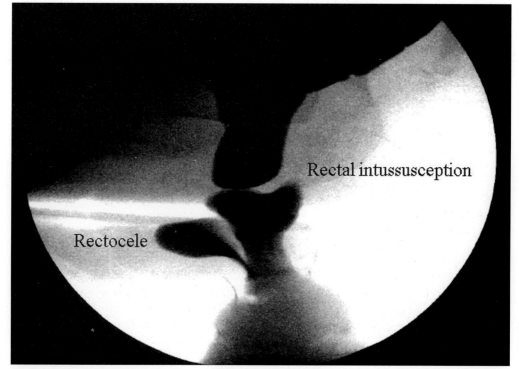

Figure 3 *Defecating proctogram demonstrating a rectocele and a rectal intussusception*

CLINICAL FEATURES

History

Patients with incontinence are ashamed of the problem and embarrassed to talk about it. It is therefore recommended that all patients presenting to a gynaecology clinic, especially those with pelvic floor disorders, be asked this question directly (Table 3). It is even better if the patient fills in a questionnaire prior to the consultation, which includes questions on bowel symptoms and function with special reference to constipation and straining. These questionnaires can be adapted to suit local needs. In the authors' experience, patients are more at ease this way as they will have already thought about their problem and prepared themselves psychologically to face their doctor. Finally, an accurate obstetric and past history should be taken, inquiring about bowel conditions such as colitis, previous bowel or anal operations, diabetes and neurological conditions. At the end of the interview, the gynaecologist should be able to determine if the patient has faecal incontinence or constipation and whether the incontinence is of the urge or true (passive) type or a combination of both.

Examination

If a history of incontinence or constipation is established, patients should have a full general and anorectal examination, including neurological assessment, in addition to the planned gynaecological examination. The main steps of a rectal examination are described below.

Inspection

With the patient lying in the left lateral position, the perineum is inspected for scars of previous anal surgery, episiotomies or perineal tears. The presence of a fresh, deep and painful wound in the anal margins indicates the presence of a chronic fissure *in ano*. It is usually situated at the 6 o'clock or 12 o'clock position. If the wound is situated in any other position, this should alert the clinician

Table 3 *Bowel function questionnaire*

- How often do you open your bowels per week?
- Is your stool hard or soft?
- Is your passage of stool painful?
- Do you strain excessively to open your bowels?
- Do you feel that you emptied yourself completely?
- Is there any mucus or blood in the stool?
- Are you able to control your stool?
- Can you tell the difference between stool and wind?
- Do you lose wind when you do not mean to?
- Do you have any leakage of loose stool?
- How often do you have loose stool per week or day?
- Do you wear pads?
- Do you feel stool coming and you are unable to stop it? (usually urge incontinence)
- Do you feel it after it is too late? (usually true/passive incontinence)

to the possibility of an early cancer. The anus is then inspected for signs of gaping, whether at rest or on parting the buttocks. Patients are then asked to tighten the sphincter 'prevent yourself from passing wind' when often there is little activity in the anal sphincter and instead the buttocks (gluteal muscles) are drawn in to compensate for this. Any lumps or swellings protruding from the anus should be noted at this stage (Table 4). These lumps may not be visible except when patients are asked to strain. On straining, the extent of perineal descent is noted. The vagina is then inspected for signs of rectocele and cystocele.

Palpation

The index finger is introduced gently into the anus and the presence of faecal impaction in the rectum and quality of the anal sphincter are assessed. Both the resting anal tone (internal sphincter) and squeeze pressure (external sphincter) are determined. The anal sphincter is then palpated for sphincter defects with the index finger in the anus and the thumb on the perianal skin. At this stage the patient is asked to strain to elicit paradoxical contraction of the anal sphincter suggestive of anismus. If present, the rectocele is examined with index finger by palpating the anterior rectal wall at rest and on straining. A Sim's speculum is then inserted into the vagina to inspect the anterior and posterior vaginal walls.

Sigmoidoscopy and proctoscopy

While the authors appreciate that these two instruments are not among those normally available in a gynaecology clinic, they are nevertheless mentioned to highlight the importance of examining the rectal and anal mucosa. Conditions such as rectal cancer, rectal inflammation (proctitis), mucosal prolapse and haemorrhoids are easily detected.

Investigations

By the time the history is taken and patient is examined, the following will be apparent:

(1) Type of incontinence: urge, passive or combination of both;

(2) Cause of incontinence: myogenic, neurogenic or a combination of both;

(3) The presence or absence of associated constipation and probable cause.

Table 4 *Causes of lumps protruding from anus*

Site	Cause
Anal canal	Haemorrhoids (prolapsing with or without thrombosis)
	Anal polyps
	Condyloma acuminata
	Cancer
Rectum	Mucosal prolapse
	Full-thickness rectal prolapse
	Polyps
	– adenomas
	– juvenile polyps
Colon	Prolapsing adenomatous polyps

The next step is to refer the patient for investigations. The aim is to obtain an objective evidence of the clinical findings and obtain a base line from which future progress can be monitored. Investigations are usually arranged by the colorectal specialist or, alternatively, they can be arranged by the gynaecologist so that the results are available by the time the patient attends the colorectal clinic.

Anal manometry

This technique studies the activity of the anus and rectum. It measures the anal pressure profile, including the resting and maximum squeeze pressures. Rectal compliance and rectosphincteric anal reflex are also measured.

Pudendal nerve terminal motor latency

Conduction of the terminal part of the nerve is measured and a prolonged latency indicates neurogenic incontinence.

Anorectal sensation

The sensitivity of the rectal and anal mucosa can be determined by electrical stimulation using special electrodes.

Endo-anal ultrasound scan

This technique allows the accurate characterisation of the various constituents of the anal sphincter and detection of structural defects (Figure 4).

Colonic transit studies

Patients are given a special marker-filled capsule to swallow and five days later the positions of the markers within the colon are determined on a plain abdominal X-ray.

Proctogram

This is a contrast X-ray examination whereby the process of defecation is followed as it occurs naturally (Figure 3).

Colonoscopy

This is an important examination, which should be undertaken to ensure that the large bowel is structurally normal and devoid of any organic pathology.

Management

The treatment of incontinence depends on the type of incontinence. Urge incontinence (normal sphincter) occurs as a result of high intracolonic pressure and rapid transit down the colon. Causes such as inflammatory bowel disease and rectal cancer should be treated, as this on its own may cure the problem. In addition, measures aimed at reducing the pressure and transit within the colon may

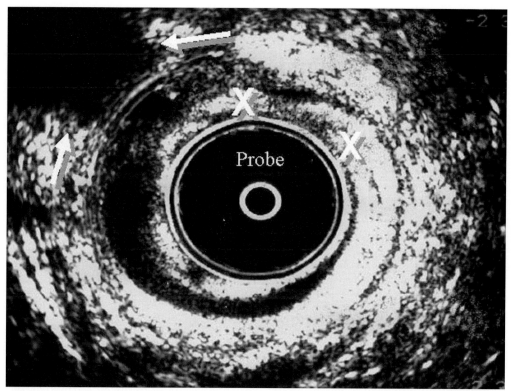

Figure 4 *This patient presented with faecal incontinence dating back to her last delivery when she had a fourth-degree tear repaired; anal endosonography reveals a persistent external sphincter defect (between arrows) and an internal sphincter defect (between crosses)*

be employed. These include slow transit agents such as codeine phosphate or loperamide coupled with antispasmodics. Measures aimed at enhancing the sphincter and pelvic floor function using biofeedback exercises have been tried for some time. The results so far have been mixed but in a study in 1999,[12] biofeedback was reported to be effective in the short term in treating a majority of patients with faecal incontinence, especially of the urge type. It has also been found to be helpful in patients with passive leakage and even those with structural anal sphincter damage. However, a review of eligible trials in the literature concluded that the therapeutic effect of biofeedback is not certain, calling for larger well-designed trials to enable safe conclusions.[13] False incontinence due to faecal impaction is treated by emptying the rectum by suppositories or enemas and, should these fail, then manually under anaesthetic. Naturally, the painful anal condition that caused faecal impaction should also be treated. Faecal soiling due to haemorrhoids or mucosal prolapse is easily controlled by treating the cause.

Management of passive incontinence (abnormal sphincter) depends on whether the abnormality is in the muscle itself or its nerve supply. Naturally, if there is an identifiable cause, such as rectal prolapse, this should be treated first, as doing this may be curative. For example, incontinence associated with rectal prolapse improves in over 90% of patients after abdominal rectopexy[14,15] with evidence of a rise in resting anal sphincter pressures.[16] However, a major problem after rectopexy is constipation and there is some evidence[17,18] that this is reduced by simultaneous sigmoid resection (resection rectopexy).

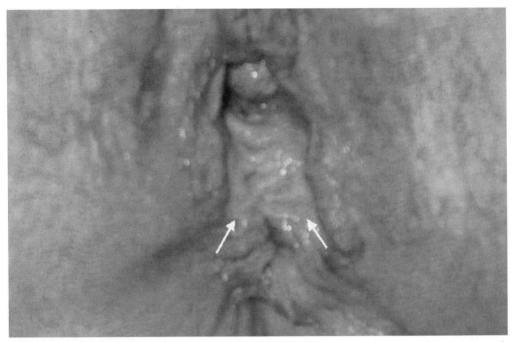

Figure 5 *This photograph demonstrates a severe obstetric anal sphincter injury (between arrows) that was missed; note the absence of the perineum between the vagina and anus, giving rise to a cloacal defect*

Patients with incontinence due to muscle disruption secondary to obstetric trauma usually present to the colorectal surgeon many years after the injury occurred (Figure 5). In these situations, the area of disruption (usually anterior) will have formed scar tissue, which is easily demonstrated on endo-anal ultrasound scan. These patients will benefit from anterior sphincter repair, a procedure aimed at reconstituting the muscle ring, providing the nerve supply is intact. The functional results after the operation are good reaching 80-90%. However, a study from St Mark's Hospital, Harrow, Middlesex, showed deterioration of function with passage of time.[19] In view of this, it is the authors' view that the best chance of achieving good and long-lasting results is to undertake an adequate primary sphincter overlap repair at the time of the injury.

Patients with neurogenic incontinence usually have an intact sphincter muscle but a defective nerve supply. As discussed above, measures aimed at reducing the colonic transit using loperamide or codeine phosphate may be all that is needed. Loperamide is preferable to codeine phosphate as it is also thought to increase anal pressure. Topical phenylephrine ointment is another such drug but this is currently under investigation. Alternative measures include the use of glycerine suppositories or enemas regularly each morning to keep the rectum empty and the patient dry for the rest of the day.

As a last resort prior to consideration of a colostomy, these patients may undergo surgery in the form of post-anal repair. The aim of the operation is to restore the anorectal angle to normal by moving the anorectal junction upwards and forwards. This will also result in elongation and tightening of the anal canal with improvement in the resting tones and squeeze pressures. In a study from St Marks Hospital, 28 of 34 women available for follow-up reported improvement in symptoms.[20] An Australian study[21] reported that, although only 58% improved after surgery, this was an acceptable result since these patients have few alternatives other than complicated procedures or a stoma.

More recently, new treatment modalities[22] such as the electrostimulated gracilloplasty, artificial anal sphincter, sacral nerve stimulation and glutaraldehyde collagen injections into the anal mucosa have become available. However, these treatments still require detailed long-term evaluation and must therefore be only undertaken as a part of controlled trials.

CHILDBIRTH AND THE ANAL SPHINCTER

Acute obstetric anal sphincter rupture

Anal sphincter disruption during vaginal delivery is recognised as a major aetiological factor in the development of faecal incontinence. However, despite conventional primary sphincter repair of acute obstetric injury, anal incontinence is reported by 20-59% of women.[23-25] Consequently, Kamm[26] states that 'Inadequacy of primary third-degree tear repair is the norm at present and cannot be considered negligent practice'. The reason for this poor outcome could be attributed either to operator inexperience or to poor technique.

Sultan et al.[27] interviewed 75 doctors who had practised at least six months in obstetrics and noted that few of them understood the anatomy of the perineum and anal sphincter. Furthermore, only 6% felt that they were adequately trained when they performed their first primary sphincter repair. A much larger study involving all UK consultant obstetricians revealed that less than one-third felt that they had good training in anal sphincter repair.[10] Inadequate training could be attributed to the infrequent occurrence of sphincter disruption. In the UK (where mediolateral episiotomy is practiced) the incidence of recognised sphincter disruption is in the region of 1% as compared with 11% in the USA, where midline episiotomy is favoured.[23]

The conventional primary anal sphincter repair technique employed by obstetricians is by end-to-end approximation of the torn sphincter ends with interrupted or 'figure-of-eight' sutures. Colorectal surgeons performing secondary anal sphincter repair for faecal incontinence favour the overlap technique of repair as long-term follow-up indicates restoration of continence in 76% of patients.[28,29] In view of the unfavourable results reported with the end-to end technique (Figure 4), Sultan et al.[30] attempted the overlap repair technique as a primary procedure in 27 women and also described separate repair of the internal sphincter. It was found[30] that, with this technique, anal incontinence was reduced from 41% to 8% and persistent external sphincter defects were reduced from 85% to 15% when compared with end-to-end repair from another study.[31] However, as this was not a controlled randomised study, the good results may be attributed to operator expertise. A randomised multicentre trial using the technique described is now under way. Nevertheless, this study demonstrates, firstly, that the overlap technique is feasible as a primary procedure in the acute situation and, secondly, it challenges Kamm's statement[26] by demonstrating that, irrespective of the reason for poor outcome, it is possible to achieve more favourable results.

Occult anal sphincter trauma

Until the advent of anal ultrasound, the development of anal incontinence was attributed largely to pelvic neuropathy. However, prospective studies before and after childbirth have shown that up to one-third of women sustain anal sphincter damage that is not recognised at delivery.[2,3] Although only one-third of these women with defects are symptomatic in the short term, it remains to be established whether these women are at higher risk of incontinence in later life. More importantly this finding has raised the question – are these defects really occult or are they in fact missed because the doctor or midwife is not trained appropriately to identify sphincter disruption? It has been shown that only 16% of doctors and 39% of midwives feel that they were trained adequately

Table 5 *Classification of perineal tears*

Degree	Extent of tear
I	Tear involving the vaginal epithelium only
II	Tear of the perineal muscles but not involving the anal sphincter
III	Any involvement of the anal sphincter
a	Less than 50% of external sphincter thickness torn
b	More than 50% of external sphincter thickness torn
c	Internal sphincter torn
IV	Torn anal epithelium

Note: a torn rectal mucosa in isolation is a rare event and should be described as such without inclusion in the above classification

to identify anal sphincter tears.[27] On the other hand, it is possible that the sphincter tear had been recognised but classified as a second-degree tear. A questionnaire sent to all UK consultants[10] and trainees[27] confirmed that up to 40% are still classifying partial and even complete disruption of the sphincter as second degree. The reason for this confusion is partly due to previous teachings[32] and, therefore, for the sake of clarification and consistency, Sultan[33] proposed a comprehensive classification (Table 5).

Instrumental delivery

There is no doubt that, compared with a normal delivery, instrumental delivery is associated with a greater risk of perineal trauma. Although only 4% of women delivered by forceps sustain a third- or fourth-degree tear, up to 50% of those who do tear have an instrumental delivery.[31] MacArthur et al.[34] identified instrumental delivery as the only independent risk factor in the development of faecal incontinence. They reported that 33% of women with new faecal incontinence had an instrumental delivery compared with 14% who never experienced faecal incontinence. It is believed that vacuum extraction is associated with fewer third- and fourth-degree tears than forceps and this view is supported by two large randomised studies. The first study was conducted in the UK,[35] where mediolateral episiotomy is practised and it reported severe vaginal lacerations in 17% of forceps deliveries compared with 11% of vacuum deliveries. The second was a study from Canada,[36] where midline episiotomy is practised, which reported third- to fourth-degree tears in 29% of forceps deliveries compared with 12% of vacuum deliveries. There was no significant difference in neonatal morbidity in the short term with the use of either instrument, although there were more facial lacerations in the forceps group and more retinal haemorrhages and cephalhaematomas in the vacuum group. However, the number that needed phototherapy was similar in both groups.

Occult trauma to the anal sphincter has also been identified more frequently in forceps delivery, occurring in up to 80%.[2] A small randomised study ($n = 44$) confirmed this by identifying occult anal-sphincter defects in 79% of forceps compared with 40% of vacuum deliveries.[37] A five-year follow-up of infants who participated in one centre of a previous multicentre randomised study of forceps and vacuum delivery has confirmed that there was no difference in terms of neurological development and visual acuity with use of either instrument.[38] This provides some consolation to mothers and clinicians alike, who may be concerned about the long-term neurological sequelae of a cephalhaematoma following a vacuum delivery. The vacuum extractor can be less traumatic than forceps to the perineum because no additional space is occupied within the pelvis, vacuum cups detach if undue pressure is applied and an episiotomy is required less often than with forceps.[37] On the basis of this evidence we support the recommendation of the Royal College of Obstetricians and Gynaecologists[39] that the vacuum extractor should be the instrument of choice.

Episiotomy

Episiotomy is the most commonly performed operation in obstetrics (after cutting of the umbilical cord) and yet there is a lack of evidence to support its routine use.[40] On the contrary, there is evidence to suggest that it is associated with an increased risk of trauma to the posterior compartment, including anal sphincter rupture. Interestingly, prevention of anal sphincter rupture is the reason commonly cited in support of performing an episiotomy. There are now considerable observational data to indicate that a reduction in episiotomy rate is not associated with an increase in anal sphincter rupture.[40] However, there are two specific situations when most clinicians and midwives would perform an episiotomy. Firstly, to expedite delivery, for example fetal distress and shoulder dystocia; secondly, to minimise the risk of multiple radial tears which could occur at the time of crowning in the presence of a thick inelastic perineum. Most clinicians would invariably perform an episiotomy during a forceps delivery, although there are some who would question the need for it. Other common indications include malpresentations, such as breech, compound presentations and malpositions, for example persistent occipitoposterior position. It is, therefore, clear that the decision to perform an episiotomy is to a large extent operator dependent. Henrikssen et al.[41,42] performed a study in which they noted that, when midwives who previously had a high episiotomy rate reduced their rate, the prevalence of anal sphincter rupture also reduced. However, this beneficial effect was abolished when midwives with a low rate of episiotomy attempted to reduce it even further. Based on this evidence, it was suggested that the ideal episiotomy rate should lie between 20% and 30% and no more. We believe that, in the light of current evidence, it will soon become a routine requirement to document consent and reasons for performing an episiotomy.

CONCLUSIONS

The role of the gynaecologist and referral to a colorectal specialist

Any history of incontinence to faeces or constipation should trigger a referral to a colorectal specialist with an interest in pelvic-floor disorders. Whether a gynaecologist should examine the anorectum and arrange investigations will depend on the individual concerned. However, we feel that, in an ideal world, gynaecologists should note the following points:

(1) Direct questions should be asked regarding bowel function and, in particular, incontinence, especially of women presenting with uterovaginal prolapse and urinary incontinence.

(2) Constipation should be investigated and treated before any prolapse or incontinence surgery, as this would have an adverse effect on the outcome of surgery. It has been shown that 17% of women presenting with stress incontinence and 83% of women presenting with the sole symptom of uterovaginal prolapse give a history (when asked directly) of excessive straining at stool, with 13% and 61%, respectively, giving a history of constipation.[43]

(3) Women who admit to difficulty in bowel evacuation, especially those resorting to digitation or perineal splinting (supporting the perineum with the finger to facilitate evacuation) should have careful evaluation and consider performing a defaecating proctogram.

(4) Inspection of the perineum and anal sphincter should be part of every gynaecological examination. When bowel symptoms are present, a rectal examination is essential. It is important to refer patients who have a change in bowel habits for colonoscopy, as 18% of women with colorectal cancer will present with faecal incontinence and 34% will admit to the passage of mucus per rectum.[44]

(5) As faecal incontinence may occur *de novo* following a posterior repair, careful assessment of the anal sphincter should be performed prior to surgery.[45]

The role of the obstetrician

As obstetric trauma is regarded as a major aetiological factor in the development of faecal incontinence, the obstetrician must play a crucial role in its prevention.

(1) The single most important factor is improved and focused training. Sultan *et al.*[27] have shown that less than 20% of doctors and 48% of midwives felt that their standard of training was adequate at the time of performing their first unsupervised repair. The anatomy of anal sphincter and perineal muscles was poorly understood. Interestingly, in a survey of UK consultant obstetricians, two-thirds felt that their training in anal sphincter repair was also inadequate.[10] Confusion and variation in the classification of perineal tears is also a source of morbidity following inappropriate management. This could explain the high incidence of 'occult' anal sphincter defects identified by anal ultrasound.

(2) Although instrumental vaginal delivery is a known high-risk factor, there is evidence to suggest that the vacuum extractor is associated with fewer sphincter injuries and should therefore be the instrument of choice.

(3) A high episiotomy rate is associated with an increased risk of anal sphincter trauma and, therefore, its use should be restricted to specific indications and the episiotomy rate should not exceed 30%.

(4) Techniques of vaginal delivery should be modified to those that are associated with the lowest risk of perineal trauma.

(5) To avoid confusion, perineal tears should be reclassified (as above) so that internal sphincter injury as well as the thickness of external sphincter injury is documented and the structures repaired individually.

(6) The technique of primary anal sphincter repair needs further evaluation by a randomised study. However, as 50% of obstetricians are already using the overlap technique,[10] proper training is essential. The consultant must be informed of every anal sphincter rupture and it should be the responsibility of the consultant to decide who is best trained to perform the repair.

(7) A protocol of repair and postoperative management and follow-up must be available in every delivery suite.

(8) An obstetrician with a special interest or a colorectal surgeon should evaluate a woman who has symptoms of impaired anal continence following sphincter repair.

(9) Incontinence surgery is best deferred until the woman's family is complete.

(10) Any woman who has previously had successful continence surgery should be delivered by caesarean section.[46]

The role of a joint pelvic-floor clinic

It is clear that a good proportion of patients presenting to a gynaecology clinic, especially those with minor degrees of genital prolapse and a history of obstetric trauma, will have either symptoms of faecal incontinence or conditions within the rectum that will eventually lead to incontinence. It is important that these conditions are detected early and, if appropriate, treated at the same time as the gynaecological surgery to prevent worsening of the bowel problem and the need for a further anaesthetic to rectify the problem. The concept of the joint pelvic-floor clinic builds on these objectives and helps to boost the confidence of patients. It also serves to focus among trainees the need for a multidisciplinary approach in pelvic-floor disorders and their appropriate management. Ideally, the clinic should be staffed by a gynaecologist, a colorectal specialist and a nurse with an interest in pelvic-floor disorders. Since this is a highly specialised clinic and the patient population is a highly select one, this need not take place more than once a month. In the authors' unit at the Mayday Hospital, the pelvic-floor clinic was established in 1999 and in one year over 80 patients have been seen and 23 joint pelvic operations performed. The most common joint procedure is for vault prolapse associated with urinary incontinence, constipation, rectal intussusception and a rectocele. For such a patient mesh sacrocolpoperineopexy, colposuspension and resection rectopexy would be performed, together with prophylactic bilateral oophorectomy in menopausal women.

References

1. Thomas, T.M., Egan, M., Walgrove, A., Meade, T.W. The prevalence of faecal and double incontinence. *Community Medicine* 1984;**6**:216–20
2. Sultan, A.H., Kamm, M.A., Hudson, C.N., Thomas, J.M., Bartram, C.I. Anal sphincter disruption during vaginal delivery. *N Engl J Med* 1993;**329**;1905–11
3. Donnelly, V., Fynes, M., Campbell, D., Johnson, H., O'Connell, R., O'Herlihy, C. Obstetric events leading to anal sphincter damage. *Obstet Gynecol* 1998;**92**:955–61
4. Tutton, M.G., Sultan, A.H., Swift, I., Abulafi, A.M. Anal sphincter defects in women with rectocoele demonstrated on endoanal ultrasound. Abstract presented at Association of Coloproctology of GB and Ireland. *Colorectal Disease* 2000;**2**(Suppl):54
5. Senatore, P.J. Etiology and classification of rectovaginal fistulas. Seminars in Colon and Rectal Surgery 1999;**10**:3–7
6. Goligher, J.C. Prolapse of the rectum. In: Goligher, J.C., editor. *Surgery of the Anus, Rectum and Colon*, 5th ed. London: Baillière Tindall; 1984. p. 246–84
7. Azpuru, C.E. Total rectal prolapse and total genital prolapse: a series of 17 cases. *Dis Colon Rectum* 1974;**17**:528–31
8. Dekel, A., Rabinerson, D., Ben Rafael, Z., Kaplan, B., Mislovaty, B., Bayer, Y. Concurrent genital and rectal prolapse: two pathologies – one joint operations. *Br J Obstet Gynaecol* 2000;**107**:125–9
9. Kupfer, C.A., Goligher, J.C. One hundred consecutive cases of complete prolapse of the rectum treated by operation. *Br J Surg* 1970;**57**:482–7
10. Abulafi, A.M., Sultan, A.H. Unpublished data
11. Parks, A.G., Porter, N.H., Hardcastle, J. The syndrome of the descending perineum. *Proceedings of the Royal Society of Medicine* 1966;**59**:477–82
12. Norton, C., Kamm, M.A. Outcome of biofeedback for faecal incontinence. *Br J Surg* 1999;**86**:1159–63

13 Norton, C., Hosker, G., Brazzelli, M. Biofeedback and/or sphincter exercises for the treatment of faecal incontinence in adults (Cochrane Review). *The Cochrane Library*, Issue 2. Oxford: Update Software; 2000

14 Madoff, R.D., Watts, J.D., Rothenberger, D.A., Goldberg, S.M. Rectal prolapse: treatment. In: Henry, M.M., Swash, M., editors. *Coloproctology and the Pelvic Floor*, 2nd ed. Oxford: Butterworth Heinemann; 1992. p. 321–46

15 Yoshoika, K., Hyland, G., Keighley, M.R.B. (1989) Anorectal function after abdominal rectopexy: parameters of predictive value in identifying return to continence. *Br J Surg* 1989;**76**:64–8

16 Broden, G., Dolk, A., Holmstrom, B. Recovery of internal anal sphincter following rectopexy: a possible explanation for continence improvement. *Int J Colorectal Dis* 1988;**3**:23–8

17 Deen, K.I., Grant, E., Billingham, C., Keighley, M.R. Abdominal resection rectopexy with pelvic floor repair versus perineal rectosigmoidectomy and pelvic floor repair for full-thickness rectal prolapse. *Br J Surg* 1994;**81**:302–4

18 Xynos, E., Chrysos, E., Tsiaoussis, J., Epanomeritakis, E., Vassilakis, J.S. Resection rectopexy for rectal prolapse. *Surg Endosc* 1999;**13**:862–4

19 Malouf, A.J., Norton, C.S., Engel, A.F., Nicholls, R.J., Kamm, M.A. Long-term results of overlapping anterior anal-sphincter repair for obstetric trauma. *Lancet* 2000;**355**:260–5

20 Setti Carraro, P., Kamm, M.A., Nicholls, R.J. Long-term results of postanal repair for neurogenic faecal incontinence. *Br J Surg* 1994;**81**:140–4

21 Rieger, N.A., Sarre, R.G., Saccone, G.T., Hunter, A., Toouli, J. Postanal repair for faecal incontinence: long term follow-up. *Aust N Z J Surg* 1997;**67**:566–70

22 Vaisey, C.J., Kamm, M.A., Nicholls, R.J. Recent advances in the surgical treatment of faecal incontinence. *Br J Surg* 1998;**85**:596–603

23 Sultan, A.H. Anal incontinence after childbirth. *Curr Opin Obstet Gynecol* 1997;**9**:320–4

24 Gjessing, H., Backe, B., Sahlin, Y. Third degree obstetric tears; outcome after primary repair. *Acta Obstet Gynecol Scand* 1998;**77**:736–40

25 Goffeng, A.R., Andersch, B., Berndtsson, I., Hulten, L., Oresland, T. Objective methods cannot predict anal incontinence after primary repair of extensive anal tears. *Acta Obstet Gynecol Scand* 1988;**77**:439–43

26 Kamm, M.A. Obstetric damage and faecal incontinence. *Lancet* 1994;**344**:730–3

27 Sultan, A.H., Kamm, M.A., Hudson, C.N. Obstetric perineal tears: an audit of training. *J Obstet Gynaecol* 1995;**15**:19–23

28 Jorge, J.M.N., Wexner, S.D. Etiology and management of fecal incontinence. *Dis Colon Rectum* 1993;**36**:77–97

29 Londono-Schimmer, E.E., Garcia-Duperly, R., Nicholls, R.J., Ritchie, J.K., Hawley, P.R., Thompson, J.P.S. Overlapping anal sphincter repair for faecal incontinence due to sphincter trauma: five-year follow-up functional results. *Int J Colorectal Dis* 1994;**9**:110–13

30 Sultan, A.H., Monga, A.K., Kumar, D., Stanton, S.L. Primary repair of obstetric anal sphincter rupture using the overlap technique. *Br J Obstet Gynaecol* 1999;**106**:318–23

31 Sultan, A.H., Kamm, M.A., Hudson, C.N., Bartram, C.I. Third degree obstetric anal sphincter tears: risk factors and outcome of primary repair. *BMJ* 1994;**308**:887–91

32 Sultan, A.H., Kamm, M.A., Bartram, C.I., Hudson, C.N. Perineal damage at delivery. *Contemp Rev Obstet Gynaecol* 1994;**6**:18–24

33 Sultan, A.H. Obstetrical perineal injury and anal incontinence. *Clinical Risk* 1999;**5**:193–6

34 MacArthur, C., Bic, K.D., Keighley, M.R.B. Faecal incontinence after childbirth. *Br J Obstet Gynaecol* 1997;**104**:46–50

35 Johanson, R.B., Rice, C., Doyle, M., Arthur, J., Anyanwu, L., Ibrahim, J. et al. A randomised prospective study comparing the new vacuum extractor policy with forceps delivery. *Br J Obstet Gynaecol* 1993;**100**:524–30

36 Bofill, J.A., Rust, O.A., Schorr, S.J., Brown, R.C., Martin, R.W., Martin, J.N. Jr et al. A randomized prospective trial of obstetric forceps versus the M-cup vacuum extractor. *Am J Obstet Gynecol* 1996;**175**:1325–30

37 Sultan, A.H., Johanson, R.B., Carter, J.E. Occult anal sphincter trauma following randomized forceps and vacuum delivery. *Int J Gynecol Obstet* 1998;**61**:113–19

38 Johanson, R.B., Heycock, E., Carter, J., Sultan, A.H., Walklate, K., Jones, P.W. Maternal and child health after assisted vaginal delivery: five year follow-up of a randomised controlled study comparing forceps and ventouse. *Br J Obstet Gynaecol* 1999;**106**:544–9

39 Royal College of Obstetricians and Gynaecologists Clinical Audit Unit. *Effective Procedures in Maternity Care Suitable for Audit*. London: RCOG; 1997

40 Woolley, R.J. Benefits and risks of episiotomy: a review of the English language literature since 1980. *Obstet Gynecol Surv* 1995;**50**:806–35

41 Henriksen, T.B., Bek, K.M., Hedegaard, M., Secher, N.J. Episiotomy and perineal lesions in spontaneous vaginal deliveries. *Br J Obstet Gynaecol* 1992;**99**:950–4

42 Henriksen, T.B., Bek, K.M., Hedegaard, M., Secher, N.J. Methods and consequences of changes in use of episiotomy. *BMJ* 1994;**309**:1255–8

43 Spence-Jones, C., Kamm, M.A., Henry, M.M., Hudson, C.N. Bowel dysfunction: a pathogenic factor in uterovaginal prolapse and urinary stress incontinence. *Br J Obstet Gynaecol* 1994;**101**:147–52

44 Curless, R., French, J., Williams, G.V., James, O.F. Comparison of gastrointestinal symptoms in colorectal carcinoma patients and community controls with respect to age. *Gut* 1994;**35**:1267–70

45 Kahn, M.A., Stanton, S.L. Posterior colporrhaphy: its effects on bowel and sexual function. *Br J Obstet Gynaecol* 1997;**104**:82–6

46 Sultan, A.H., Stanton, S.L. Preserving the pelvic floor and perineum during childbirth – elective caesarean section? *Br J Obstet Gynaecol* 1996;**103**:731–4

47 Mann, C.V., Glass, R.E., editors. Essential anatomy of anal incontinence. In: *Surgical Treatment of Anal Incontinence*, 2nd ed. London: Springer; 1997. p. 5, fig. 1.4

48 Smout, A.J.P., Akkermans, L.M.A., editors. Rectum, anus and pelvic floor. In: *Normal and Disturbed Motility of the Gastrointestinal Tract*. Petersfield, UK: Wrightson Biomedical; 1994. p. 175

17

Minimal access urogynaecology

Andrew J. S. Tapp

INTRODUCTION

Numerous surgical procedures have been described for the treatment of stress urinary incontinence. The primacy of one surgical technique over another depends upon the perceived cure rate for that operation, the reported morbidity and mortality, the likely impact of the treatment on the patient's life and perhaps some aspects of the health economics of the procedure. The outcomes that may be important to us as medical practitioners may not be weighed similarly by our patients. With cure rates of 80% reported in 1914[1] it is surprising that, despite a multitude of publications, we are still striving for the optimum operation. For the last 30 years, the surgical battle has been largely between the anterior repair and the Burch colposuspension. The former procedure is perceived as having a comparatively low cure rate but reduced morbidity. The trade-off was therefore made and the Burch colposuspension has become the operation of choice in many departments. The Burch colposuspension, however, involves a considerable entry wound and retropubic dissection to produce suitable exposure for a limited surgical procedure. Not surprisingly, with the advent of minimal access surgery in almost all surgical fields, the problem of exposure has been addressed. This has resulted in attempts to mimic the Burch colposuspension procedure using a laparoscopic approach and an explosion of other techniques, some of which have been of dubious value. In the end, with the recognised frequency of genuine stress incontinence and an ageing population, the operation striven for should be minimal access with low morbidity and mortality. It should:

(1) Have little impact on the patient's life save resolving the primary complaint;

(2) Be easy to reproduce;

(3) Be successful in the hands of the general gynaecologist;

(4) Be enduring;

(5) Form part of an integrated resolution of genital prolapse.

Burch[2] described his operative procedure for urinary stress incontinence in 1961. Subsequently, it has been modified in some way by all those who use it to treat genuine stress incontinence. The reported subjective and objective results of the Burch colposuspension vary with the reporting centre, the type of assessment and the duration of follow-up. In his meta-analysis,[3] Jarvis reported subjective and objective cure rates of 89.6% and 84.3%, respectively, at follow-up past 12 months. Results of surgery do decline in a time-dependent manner and may plateau at 69% after 10-12 years,[4] although the subjective cure rate may fall further to 54% at 18 years.[5] The Burch colposuspension also has a significant place in the treatment of recurrent stress incontinence, with subjective and objective cure rates of 88% and 69%, respectively,[6] although such rates may fall to 0% if there have been three previous anti-incontinence procedures.[6] Complications and the adverse short-term and long-term impact of this therapy on a patient's life is perhaps the downfall of the colposuspension. Massive haemorrhage at the time of surgery may occur in 3.6% of patients[7] and 6% may have injury to the urinary tract.[8] In the immediate post-operative period, bacteriuria may be seen in 46% of patients if a urethral catheter is used (21% for suprapubic catheterisation).[9] Wound infection (0.5%),[10] venous thrombosis (1%)[7] and voiding difficulty (25%)[11] are also seen. In the long term, 14.7% of patients suffer from detrusor instability,[4] 22% have symptomatic voiding difficulty and 14% develop urogenital prolapse.[3] Despite the morbidity of the Burch colposuspension, its greater cure rate for urinary incontinence when compared with the anterior repair[12] has resulted in the Burch colposuspension being taken up by most departments as the operation of choice for genuine stress incontinence.

The laparoscopic colposuspension entered the scene ten years ago. Since then, there have been numerous publications describing different techniques, short-term and long-term results, perceived benefits and comparisons with the open technique of Burch colposuspension. Despite this, Lawton and Smith[13] and Lose[14] concluded that the results of a large randomised controlled trial of the two procedures are still needed in order to correctly assess outcomes. Unfortunately, there are not just two procedures. The Burch colposuspension has had numerous modifications since Burch's first publication[2] and there is certainly no uniformity with the laparoscopic Burch colposuspension. In this operation, as in the open Burch colposuspension, access to the cavity of Retzius is required. This can be achieved with a transperitoneal approach[15-17] or an extraperitoneal approach,[18] using for the latter either direct insufflation or balloon dissection.[19-21] With the transperitoneal approach, the upper border of the bladder can be demarcated by instilling 300 ml of saline, as occasional fundal bladder entry is seen. The transperitoneal approach allows the pelvic organs to be inspected, if this is desired, and concomitant laparoscopic surgery can be undertaken. The extraperitoneal approach provides less room for the surgeon to operate but, with experience, this is not a problem. Closure of the peritoneum after a transperitoneal approach is not necessary.[15]

The most popular technique for attaching the paravaginal tissue to the ipsilateral iliopectineal ligament is with sutures (PDS, Ethibond® or Gortex®). One can argue over technique, but some authors find it easier to place the suture from upwards down through Coopers ligament before coming on to the vagina using a suture holder from the contralateral side,[22] while others place the suture through the vagina first. Single suture placement on either side jeopardises the cure rate (58%), whereas two-suture placement on either side gives a cure rate comparable with the open Burch (83%).[23] Rather than tying it into place the suture may be stapled.[24] Mesh held in place with staples is another popular approach to the suspension.[18,25] Five-year results with mesh suspension are satisfactory (88%). Another proposed alternative to create elevation of the bladder neck and its fixture to the pubic bone is fibrin glue.[26] Peri-operative complications are uncommon and blood loss is certainly less than with the open Burch colposuspension.[27] However a 5–7%[19] rate of inferior epigastric artery injury has been reported and entry into the bladder is seen in between 1.6%[20,28] and 2.5%[19] of patients, although in some series neither of these complications is encountered.[16] Although operating times of under 30 minutes in 89% of cases of laparoscopic colposuspension have been reported[20] most would agree that the total time for a laparoscopic colposuspension is greater than for an open colposuspension.[29] The operation of laparoscopic colposuspension, however it is performed, is moderately technically demanding and it can take up to 30 cases before the operating time is stabilised.

The postoperative period following a laparoscopic Burch colposuspension is certainly different from that of an open Burch colposuspension. The mean hospital stay for the former need only be 0.9 days,[19] with 95% of patients ready to be discharged on the day of the operation,[24] although in other studies 60% of patients need to stay overnight,[18] with a mean inpatient stay of 2.2 days.[18] Ninety-five percent of patients are discharged without a catheter[28] and patients are back to normal activity after 7[19] to 14[28] days and have returned to work after 17 days.[19] Cure rates vary depending on the study but rates of 89.8% at six months[19] and 90.6% at two years[16] have been reported. Whether one uses sutures or mesh seems to be unimportant with regard to the outcome.[30] Although comparable results in retrospective studies between open and laparoscopic Burch colposuspension have been reported[29] this is not consistently seen.[27] Indeed, in Burton's[31] prospective randomised comparison of laparoscopic Burch colposuspension with open Burch colposuspension, the latter was significantly more likely to resolve urinary stress incontinence. Complications are less common following the laparoscopic Burch colposuspension[27] but 20% of women may develop detrusor instability after this operation.[21]

It is doubtful whether the laparoscopic colposuspension will ever find acceptance among the general body of gynaecologists as one of the operations they would offer to their patients with genuine stress incontinence. The advantage of the minimal access approach is evident but the technique is demanding and it has not been shown to be superior to the open Burch colposuspension with regard to the primary aim of the surgical procedure. If, however, laparoscopic surgery is undertaken by an endoscopic surgeon for another reason, in a patient with concomitant urodynamically proven genuine stress incontinence, then the laparoscopic Burch colposuspension may be the most appropriate bladder-neck procedure to perform and, in this circumstance, the procedure is likely to remain in use.

Transvaginal bladder-neck needle suspension techniques were introduced by Pereyra.[32] His own technique was subsequently modified into what we now understand as the Pereyra procedure.[33] This procedure was joined by the Stamey[34] and the Raz[35] procedures. Although these procedures gained considerable popularity in the 1980s and early 1990s, this popularity has waned. Surgical results, however, are still published in the modern literature and require continuing consideration of these operations as viable techniques. Jongen and Brouwer[36] report a comparison of the modified Pereyra using a permanent suture with the Burch colposuspension. In their 97 patients, satisfaction rates for the Pereyra and colposuspension were 86% and 81%, respectively. Grofit et al.,[37] after a mean of 90 months follow-up, reported that the overall success rate following a Stamey procedure was 65.5%, although in patients with pure stress incontinence this rose to 93%. Gilja et al.[38] found the Raz procedure to produce similar results to the Burch colposuspension at three years (80.4% and 89.3%, respectively) and felt, based on pure success rates, that there was no reason to prefer a particular operation. This conclusion tends to go against the general flow of publication, where the objective success rates of the Pereyra procedure may be as low as 50% at six months[39] although Jarvis[3] found it to be successful in 70% at over 12 months follow-up. Objective success with the Stamey procedure may be even poorer, with rates of 40%[40] to 80%[41] reported. Masson and Govier[42] seem to concur with this general feeling, reporting that, four years after a Pereyra procedure, only 14% of patients had no leakage, 42% had mild leakage and 44% moderate or severe leakage. Four years after the Pereyra procedure, 53% of their population were still wearing pads. Although bladder perforation at the time of needle suspension is of little significance if identified, transgression of the suspending sutures or buffers, in the case of the Stamey procedure, into the bladder is a genuine problem and one that has put off many surgeons from continuing with these techniques. Although the transvaginal bladder-neck needle suspension techniques are easy to perform, are quick and have limited immediate morbidity, the perceived cure rates seem to have resulted in a partial retreat. Not surprisingly, further development of these needle suspensions has taken place, particularly with the placement of the needle though the ipsilateral iliopectineal ligament, thereby relying on this structure to supply support rather than the rectus sheath[43] and indeed such a procedure can be performed under laparoscopic control.[44]

Bone anchor fixation for the support of the bladder neck has been explored in a number of ways. The bone anchor may be used to anchor a Z-shaped suture that is placed in the ipsilateral vaginal skin just lateral to the urethra; a bone anchor may be used to anchor a suburethral sling or a bone anchor may be driven directly through the vagina lateral to the urethra into the pubic bone behind. In the case of the first variant of these anchoring techniques, a bone anchor is applied to the pubic tubercle through two small transverse suprapubic incisions on either side of the midline, using a hand drill and a guide. A modified needle is passed through the retropubic space into the vaginal wall 1 cm lateral to the bladder neck. The suture is then passed through a total of three points in the vaginal skin to make a Z shape and subsequently withdrawn through the suprapubic wound. The vaginal suture is then tied on to the bone anchor.[45,46] Such a technique may be associated with a subjective cure rate of 94% at 12 months,[46] although at 18 months this may be only 68%.[45] Bone anchor placement can result in chronic pain[47] and, indeed, pubic osteomyelitis and pubic bone granuloma formation[48] have required removal of the bone anchors. Instead of using the normal vaginal skin supported on either side of the urethra as a sling, Mersilene®,[49] Gortex®[50] or polypropylene[51] can be placed under the urethra and then these synthetic slings can be fixed with bone anchors. Such techniques in selected patients, some with recurrent incontinence, may produce subjective cure rates of 100%, 88.9% and 91.4%, respectively.

Perhaps the most interesting advance in minimal access urogynaecology over the last three years has been the use of tension-free vaginal tape. This technique can be conducted under local or low spinal anaesthetic. It may also be combined with other vaginal surgical procedures for genital prolapse. Placement of the Prolene tape is via two small suprapubic incisions and one longitudinal

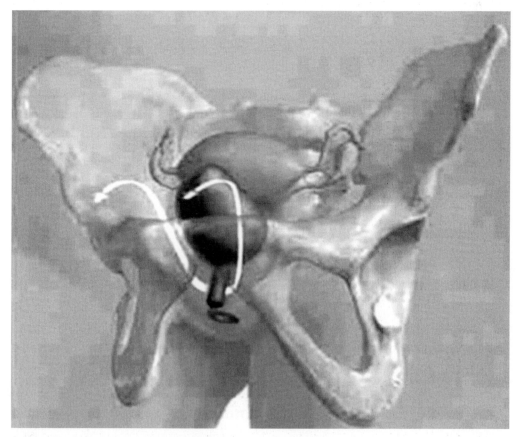

Figure 1 *Tension-free vaginal tape placement at the mid-urethra; it is inserted by one vertical suburethral incision and two transverse abdominal incisions; the tape is placed with no tension*

vaginal incision at the point of the mid-urethra (Figure 1). The Prolene tape is mounted on two 5-mm needles that are passed from the vaginal incision to the anterior abdominal-wall incisions on either side. Inadvertent bladder perforation is identified during the procedure by cystoscopy. The Prolene 'sling' is placed under the mid-urethra without tension and its efficacy can be checked during the surgical procedure by asking the patient to cough with a full bladder. At one year[52] and three years[53,54] objective cure rates of 91% and 86–90%, respectively, are seen and a further 6–11% of patients are significantly improved. Despite fears of tape erosion into the urethra or transgression into the bladder this has not been reported. The mean operating time is between 28[52] and 29 minutes.[53] Intra-operative complications include inadvertent bladder perforation, seen in up to 4.3% of cases,[55] and blood loss of greater than 200 ml requiring indwelling catheterisation and vaginal tamponade in up to 16%.[55] A small incidence of uncomplicated haematoma may be seen post-operatively (1.5%).[52] Ninety percent of patients are able to void spontaneously without a significant residual within 24 hours and are also able to leave the hospital at this time.[52] A further 10% require a temporary indwelling catheter.[53] Prolonged catheterisation (more than ten days) is rare (less than 1%).[52]

Such a surgical technique, with a high cure rate and limited morbidity with a rapid return to full activity, fulfils the requirements of a desirable minimal access surgical intervention for urinary stress incontinence. However, this technique must be approached with caution, awaiting confirmatory results from other centres, long-term studies and comparisons with current surgical techniques. Despite the lack of data, 70 000 procedures have been conducted worldwide and at least 4000 will be conducted in the UK in the year 2000; 170 consultants in the UK are now using this technique.

CONCLUSIONS

Surgical developments in the field of urogynaecology abound, with well over 150 techniques for the treatment of urinary stress incontinence described in the literature. Minimal access surgery enables the introduction of techniques that limit morbidity, cost and convalescence. Unfortunately, despite the numerous operative techniques that have entered the field, the lack of long-term data and supporting comparative studies has resulted in many falling by the wayside. What is needed is a highly successful procedure with low adverse impact on the patient that can be widely used and can be combined with other procedures for genital prolapse.

References

1. Kelley, H.A., Dumm, W. Urinary incontinence in women without manifest injury to the bladder. *Surg Gynecol Obstet* 1914;**18**:444–50
2. Burch, J.C. Urethrovesical fixation to Coopers ligament for correction of stress incontinence, cystocele and prolapse. *Am J Obstet Gynecol* 1961;**81**:281–90
3. Jarvis, G.J. Surgery for stress incontinence. *Br J Obstet Gynaecol* 1994;**101**:371–4
4. Alcalay, M., Monga, A., Stanton, S. Burch colposuspension: a 10–20 year follow-up. *Br J Obstet Gynaecol* 1995;**102**:740–5
5. Laursen, H., Farlie, R., Rasmussen, K.L., Aagard, J. Colposuspension Burch – an 18 year follow-up study. *Neurourol Urodyn* 1984;**3**:201–7
6. Amye-Obu, F.A., Drutz, H.P. Surgical management of recurrent stress urinary incontinence: a 12-year experience. *Am J Obstet Gynecol* 1999;**181**:1296–307

7   Demirci, F., Yucel, N., Ozden, S., Delikara, N., Yalti, S., Demirci, E. A retrospective review of perioperative complication in 360 patients who had Burch colposuspension. *Aust N Z J Obstet Gynaecol* 1999;**39**:472–5

8   Pow-Sang, J.M., Lockart, J.L., Suarez, A., Lansman, H., Politano, V. Female urinary incontinence: perioperative selection, surgical complications and results. *J Urol* 1986;**136**:831–3

9   Anderson, J.T., Heisterberg, S., Hebjorn, S. Suprapubic versus transurethral bladder drainage after surgery for stress urinary incontinence. *Obstet Gynecol* 1987;**69**:546

10 Stanton, S.L., Cardozo, L.D. Results of the colposuspension operation for incontinence and prolapse. *Br J Obstet Gynaecol* 1979;**86**:693–7

11 Lose, G., Jorgensen, L., Mortensen, S.O., Molsted-Pedersen, L., Kristensen, J.K. Voiding difficulties after colposuspension. *Obstet Gynecol* 1987;**69**:33–7

12 Kammerer-Doak, D.N., Dorin, M.H., Rogers, R.G., Cousin, M.O. A randomized trial of Burch retropubic urethropexy and anterior colporrhaphy for stress urinary incontinence. *Obstet Gynecol* 1999;**93**:75–8

13 Lawton, V., Smith, A.R. Laparoscopic colposuspension. *Semin Laparosc Surg* 1999;**6**:90–9

14 Lose, G. Laparoscopic Burch colposuspension. *Acta Obstet Gynecol Scand* 1998;**168**:29–33

15 Lam, A.L., Jenkins, G.J., Hyslop, R.S. Laparoscopic Burch colposuspension for stress incontinence preliminary results. *Med J Aust* 1995;**162**:18–21

16 Papasakelariou, C., Papasakelariou, B. Laparoscopic bladder neck suspension. *J Am Assoc Gynecol Laparosc* 1997;**4**:185–9

17 Teichman, J.M. Laparoscopic Burch colposuspension. *Tech Urol* 1995;**1**:19–27

18 von Theobald, P., Guillaumin, D., Levy, G. Laparoscopic preperitoneal colposuspension for stress urinary incontinence. *Surg Endosc* 1995;**9**:1189–92

19 Yang, S.-C., Park, D.-S., Lee, J.-M., Graham R.W. Laparoscopic extraperitoneal bladder neck suspension (LEBNS) for stress urinary incontinence. *J Korean Med Sci* 1995;**10**:426–30

20 Hannah, S.L., Chin, A. Laparoscopic retropubic urethropexy. *J Am Assoc Gynecol Laparosc* 1996;**4**:47–52

21 Tay, K.P., Lim, P.H.C., Ravintharam, T. Laparoscopic bladder neck suspension for urinary stress incontinence in women: our first 20 patients. *Int J Urol* 1996;**3**:278–81

22 Wattiez, A., Boughizane, S., Alexandre, F., Canis, M., Mage, G., Pouly, J.-L. et al. Laparoscopic procedures for stress incontinence and prolapse. *Curr Opin Obstet Gynecol* 1995;**7**:317–21

23 Persson, J., Wolner-Hanssen, P. Laparoscopic Burch colposuspension for stress urinary incontinence: a randomised comparison of one or two sutures on each side of the urethra. *Obstet Gynecol* 2000;**95**:151–5

24 Henley, C. The Henley staple-suture technique for laparoscopic Burch colposuspension. *J Am Assoc Gynecol Laparosc* 1995;**2**:441–4

25 Ou, C.S., Rowbotham, R. Five-year follow-up of laparoscopic bladder neck suspension using synthetic mesh and surgical staples. *J Laparoendosc Adv Surg Tech A* 1999;**9**:249–52

26 Kiilholma, P., Haarala, M., Polvi, H., Makinen, J., Chancellor, M. Sutureless endoscopic colposuspension with Fibrin sealant. *Tech Urol* 1995;**1**:81–3

27 Su, T.-H., Wang, K.G., Hsu, C.-Y., Wei, H.-J., Hong, B.-K. Prospective comparison of laparoscopic and traditional colposuspension in the treatment of genuine stress incontinence. *Acta Obstet Gynecol Scand* 1997;**76**:576–82

28 Iosif, C.S. Laparoscopic surgery for stress urinary incontinence. *Urol Int* 1996;**57**:180–4

29 Miannay, E., Losson, M., Lanvin, D., Querleu, D., Crepin, G. Comparison of open retropubic and laparoscopic colposuspension for treatment of stress urinary incontinence. *Eur J Obstet Gynecol Reprod Biol* 1998;**79**:159–66

30. Ross, J. Two techniques of laparoscopic Burch repair for stress incontinence. A prospective randomised study. *J Am Assoc Gynecol Laparosc* 1996;**3**:351–7
31. Burton, G. A three-year prospect randomised urodynamic study comparing open and laparoscopic colposuspension. *Neurourol Urodyn* 1997;**16**:353–4
32. Pereyra, J.C. A simplified surgical procedure for the correction of stress incontinence in women. *Western Journal of Surgery* 1959;**67**:223–6
33. Pereyra, A.J., Lebheriz, T.B. The revised Pereyra procedure. In: Buchsbaum, H., Schmidt, J.D., editors. *Gynaecologic and Obstetric Urology*. Philadelphia, PA: W.B. Saunders; 1978. p. 208–22
34. Stamey, T.A. Endoscopic suspension of vesical neck for urinary incontinence. *Surg Gynecol Obstet* 1973;**136**:547–54
35. Raz, S. Modified bladder neck suspension for female stress incontinence. *Urology* 1981;**17**:82–4
36. Jongen, V.H., Brouwer, W.K. Comparison of the modified Pereyra procedure using permanent suture material and Burch urethropexy. *Eur J Obstet Gynecol Reprod Biol* 1999;**84**:7–11
37. Grofit, O.N., Landau, E.H., Shapiro, A., Pode, D. The Stamey procedure for stress incontinence long-term results. *Eur Urol* 1998;**34**:339–43
38. Gilja, I., Puskar, D., Mazuran, B., Radej, M. Comparative analysis of bladder neck suspension using Raz, Burch and transvaginal Burch procedures: a three-year randomised prospective study. *Eur Urol* 1998;**33**:298–302
39. Weil, A., Reyes, H., Bischoff, P., Rottenburg, R.D., Krauer, F. Modifications of urethral rest and stress profiles after 3 different types of surgery for urinary stress incontinence. *Br J Obstet Gynaecol* 1984;**91**:46–55
40. Mundy, A.R. A trial comparing the Stamey bladder neck suspension procedure with colposuspension for stress incontinence. *Br J Urol* 1983;**55**:687–700
41. Hilton, P. A clinical and urodynamic study comparing the Stamey bladder neck suspension and suburethral sling procedures in the treatment of genuine stress incontinence. *Br J Obstet Gynaecol* 1989;**96**:213–20
42. Masson, D.B., Govier, F.E. Modified Pereyra bladder neck suspension in patients with intrinsic sphincter deficiency and bladder neck hypermobility: patient satisfaction with a mean follow-up of 4 years. *Urology* 2000;**55**:217–21
43. Darai, E., Perdu, M., Benifla, J-L., Madelenot, P. Percutaneous needle colposuspension to Coopers ligament for the treatment of stress incontinence in women: a report of 82 cases. *Eur J Obstet Gynecol Reprod Biol* 1997;**74**:53–5
44. Pelosi, M., Pelosi, M. Laparoscopic assisted transpectineal needle suspension of the bladder neck. *J Am Assoc Gynecol Laparosc* 1998;**5**:39–46
45. Schultheiss, D., Hofner, M., Oelke, M., Grunewald, V., Jonas, U. Does bone anchor fixation improve the outcome of pericutaneous bladder neck suspension in female stress urinary incontinence. *Br J Urol* 1998;**82**:192–5
46. Dmochowski, R., Appell, R. Percutaneous bladder neck suspension: technique and results. *Tech Urol* 1996;**2**:147–53
47. Bernier, P., Zimmern, P. Bone anchor removal after bladder neck suspension. *Br J Urol* 1998;**82**:302–3
48. Fitzgerald, M.P., Gitelis, S., Brubaker, L. Pubic osteomyelitis and granuloma after bone anchor placement. *Int Urogynecol J Pelvic Floor Dysfunct* 1999;**10**:346–8
49. Kovac, S.R., Cruikshank, S.H. Pubic bone suburethral stitch ligation for recurrent urinary incontinence. *Obstet Gynecol* 1997;**98**:624–7

50 Chloe, J.M., Staskin, D.R. Gortex patch sling: seven years later. *Urology* 1999;**54**:641–6
51 Hom, D., Desautel, M., Lumerman, J., Feraren, R., Badlani, G. Pubo vaginal sling using polypropylene mesh and Vesica bone anchors. *Urology* 1998;**51**:708–13
52 Ulmsten, U., Falconer, C., Johnson, P., Jumaa, M., Lanner, L., Nilsson, C.G. *et al.* A multicentre study of tension free vaginal tape (TVT) for the surgical treatment of stress urinary incontinence. *Int Urogynecol J Pelvic Floor Dysfunc* 1998;**9**:210–13
53 Ulmsten, U., Johnson, P., Rezapour, M. A three-year follow-up of tension free tape for surgical treatment of female stress urinary incontinence. *Br J Obstet Gynaecol* 1999;**106**:345–50
54 Olsson, I., Kroon, U. A three-year postoperative evaluation of tension free vaginal tape. *Gynecol Obstet Invest* 1999;**48**:267–9
55 Wong, A.C., Lo, T.S. Tension free vaginal tape: a minimally invasive solution to stress urinary incontinence in women. *J Reprod Med* 1998;**43**:429–34

18

HRT forever

William Thompson and Karen A. McKinney

INTRODUCTION

Hormone replacement therapy (HRT) is one of the few medical interventions that has the potential of improving morbidity and mortality in postmenopausal women. Furthermore, there is increasing evidence that HRT can be important in improving quality of life and, in particular, psychological wellbeing.[1] Although the major causes of mortality in older women are cancer, cardiovascular disease and cerebrovascular accident, chronic conditions that are non-fatal exact a toll of morbidity and altered lifestyle. With increasing life expectancy of the female population, the problems of postmenopausal women are now a major public health concern. Women can now expect to live one-third of their life after the menopause.

For some women, menopause is the beginning of an era of ageing with its connotations of diminishing abilities and competence. However, to others it is the beginning of a new and promising period of life, free from worries about contraception, pregnancy and menstruation. In this context, women in many cultures view the menopause as a natural process and taking medication should therefore be avoided. Health professionals, on the other hand, are much more likely to perceive the menopause as a 'medical problem' or a deficiency disease requiring treatment. However, the wider use of HRT is not accepted by all. A survey in 1994[2] reported that only 64% of gynaecologists and 56% of GPs thought that all women should be offered HRT. With regard to the use of HRT in the elderly, Handa *et al.*[3] reported an incidence of 6.1% in US women aged over 65 years. Women in the highest income groups were over four times more likely to use oestrogen than women in lower income groups. HRT use was negatively associated with age, decreasing by some 12% with each year of life. A further study in the USA, by Cauley *et al.*,[4] reported a 13.7% current use of oral HRT in women over 65 years of age.

One of the major limitations in the evaluation of long-term HRT is the identification of a control group. Women taking HRT often have healthier lifestyles and are more likely to seek medical advice than those women who decide against treatment.[5] In spite of this, the epidemiological evidence supporting the beneficial effects of HRT is overwhelming in its uniformity and consistency.

Against the background of increasing public awareness and expectations of HRT, tertiary referral menopause clinics are treating increasing numbers of patients with complicated medical histories. In our experience, these patients often have concerns which include protection against many of the diseases of ageing, especially osteoporosis and cardiac disease.[6] These findings suggest that menopausal women in both the UK and USA are well-informed about the potential protective benefits of HRT and now expect an improvement in the quality of their lives well beyond the relief of menopausal symptoms.

THE BENEFITS OF LONG-TERM HRT

Protection against cardiovascular disease

Coronary heart disease causes at least one-third of all deaths in postmenopausal women in northern and eastern Europe and North America, as well as being a major cause of morbidity.[7] The incidence of cardiovascular disease rises in both sexes with age. However, the menopause has a substantial and additional effect upon women.[8] Rates of coronary heart disease are relatively low in premenopausal women but rise sharply after the menopause. Oestrogen deficiency leads to potentially adverse changes in certain metabolic parameters such as lipids, insulin secretion and metabolism, body fat distribution and arterial blood flow. Most epidemiological evidence supports a protective role for oestrogen against the risk of cardiovascular morbidity and mortality.[9-11] A meta-analysis in 1998 also found a 35% reduced coronary risk in women who had ever used oestrogen.[12] The major limitation of these observational studies is selection bias. Women who use oestrogen tend to be more health conscious, leading healthier lifestyles, and are of higher socio-economic status than non-users.[13] There is also a danger of physician selection of relatively healthy women for oestrogen therapy.[14]

The Women's Health Initiative is a study of more than 27 000 healthy postmenopausal women who were randomly allocated to placebo or oestrogen alone or in combination with progestin.[15] In contrast with the evidence for HRT cardioprotection, preliminary findings released by this study[15] show that women taking HRT suffer slightly more cardiovascular events in the first two years than women taking placebo. As less than 1% of the women enrolled had a cardiovascular event, this trend may well disappear over the course of the study. Based on the ten-year duration of follow-up, final results will not be available until 2008.

The European Women's International Study of Long Duration Oestrogen after Menopause (WISDOM),[16] which has a similar design and sample size, is also currently under way. Both these trials are large enough to assess multiple benefits and risks of hormone therapy including the primary prevention of cardiovascular disease.

The evidence on the role of oestrogen in the secondary prevention of cardiovascular disease has been questioned. The Heart and Estrogen/Progestin Replacement Study (HERS) was a randomised placebo-controlled trial of conjugated oestrogen and medroxyprogesterone acetate in postmenopausal women with coronary heart disease.[17] The HERS results provided no evidence that hormone therapy was useful for secondary prevention in women with coronary heart disease. There were difficulties in interpreting the excess risk of recurrent coronary events in the first year of the trial followed by a reduced risk in the last two years of the trial. The limitation of this study was the short duration of follow-up.

As coronary heart disease is the leading cause of death in women, beneficial effects of oestrogen on the cardiovascular system should drive the decision for hormone therapy. However, the magnitude of cardioprotection afforded by oestrogen and whether protection differs between different hormone regimens remains uncertain. The results from large randomised controlled trials currently in progress will address some of these issues.

Prevention of stroke

Despite a decline in mortality from stroke over the past few decades it remains the third leading cause of death in women in developed countries. A 50-year-old white woman has a 20% lifetime probability of developing stroke and an 8% probability of dying from it.[18] The association of HRT and stroke is not as consistent as that of oestrogen and coronary heart disease. Psaty *et al.*[19] summarised the literature on this subject and concluded that there was little, if any, association.

A significant reduction in stroke mortality was associated with oestrogen use in two cohort studies of elderly women. The National Health and Nutrition Examination Survey[20] enrolled 1910 menopausal women and followed them for an average of 12 years. Oestrogen users had a 31% reduction in stroke incidence and a 63% reduction in stroke mortality.[20] In the Leisure World Cohort in southern California,[21] long-term and current use of oestrogen had a strong protective effect with an overall 46% reduction in the risk of death from stroke and a 79% reduction in recent users. However, other studies have failed to demonstrate a protective effect of HRT on the risk of stroke. A large Danish study[22] found no indication that postmenopausal oestrogen influenced the risk of stroke. There was also a failure to observe protection against stroke in the Nurse's Health Study[23] in striking contrast to the Leisure World Cohort.

In the Cardiovascular Health Study in Australia,[24] current use of oestrogen and oestrogen plus a progestogen was associated with reduced carotid intimal–medial thickness. In a three-year lovastatin trial, investigators found that in the placebo group intimal–medial thickness tended to regress in HRT users but to progress in non-users.[25]

Studies using transcranial Doppler ultrasonography have found oestrogen-related differences in bloodflow velocity, pulsatility index and vasomotor reactivity. Vasomotor reactivity is lower in postmenopausal women compared with premenopausal women[26] and flow resistance of the internal carotid and middle cerebral arteries is increased.[27] Furthermore, the time since menopause correlates with the pulsatility index in the circulation.[28] It has been shown that oestrogen replacement therapy increases the blood velocity and decreases resistance in the cerebral microcirculation.[29] Even with this confusing mix of results, the epidemiological evidence supports a beneficial impact of postmenopausal HRT on stroke mortality, possibly by decreasing the severity of the stroke.

Prevention of osteoporosis

The current lifetime risk of an osteoporotic fracture for a 50-year-old woman is estimated to be 40%.[18] As the proportion of elderly women in society increases, so does the frequency of osteoporotic fractures, which in turn places an additional burden on health resources. Many studies have shown that oestrogen therapy arrests early postmenopausal bone loss[30] and this manifests itself in a lower fracture rate.[31] HRT offers protection from accelerated postmenopausal bone loss and an estimated reduction to 0.28 in the relative risk of death from femoral neck fracture, as well as an ability to improve the quality of life. Prevention of osteoporosis is one of the most important reasons for long-term, or indeed, forever HRT, since its beneficial effect lessens with time without therapy.

Tooth loss

Oral alveolar bone loss, which can lead to tooth loss, is strongly correlated with the development of osteoporosis. Even in women without established osteoporosis there is a correlation between spinal bone density and number of teeth.[32]

There was a significant reduction in tooth loss among oestrogen users in the Leisure World Cohort[33] and this beneficial effect was greater with increasing duration of oestrogen use. The Nurses' Health Study[34] also found a 25% reduction in risk of tooth loss in current oestrogen users.

Beneficial effects on cancer

In older women who take HRT it is important to consider the potential effects of such treatment on the development of cancer. Postmenopausal HRT can be administered to all patients with cervical, ovarian or vulval malignancies as none of these cancers appear to be adversely affected.

Women who have undergone a hysterectomy and who have had Stage I adenocarcinoma of the endometrium may use oestrogen therapy without fear of recurrence, but the combination of oestrogen and progestin is recommended in view of the protective action of the progestin. There are no data about the risk in women with more advanced disease. However, if the tumour is oestrogen-receptor positive, a period of approximately five years without recurrence should improve the safety of hormone therapy. A similar approach should be used in patients previously treated for endometrioid tumours of the ovary.

Melanomas can be oestrogen- or progesterone-receptor positive; therefore it has been suggested that there may be a possible association between the use of hormone therapy and development of melanoma. Epidemiological evidence has confirmed that HRT appears to have no adverse effects on the incidence, prevalence or course of melanoma and its use is not contraindicated in women with a history of melanoma or who are at risk of the disease.[35,36]

Mortality rates for colorectal cancer have declined over the last decade in women more than men.[37] This may be due to women having healthier dietary and lifestyle patterns as well as a potential protective effect of HRT.[38] Two recent meta-analyses demonstrated a 20% reduction in the risk of colon cancer among current users.[39,40] These epidemiological data support the hypothesis that HRT confers protection against colorectal cancer. The exact biological mechanism of this effect remains uncertain. Bile acids are direct colon carcinogens and HRT may alter bile-acid synthesis and secretion leading to reduced concentrations in the colon.[41] Oestrogens inhibit the growth of colon cancer cells *in vitro*[42] and the oestrogen receptor itself may play a role in tumour suppression.[43] HRT also lowers the risk of colorectal adenomatous polyps, which are precursor lesions of colon cancer.[44] It appears that HRT use has a favourable effect on colorectal cancer but additional research is required to confirm the chemopreventative potential of HRT.

Dementia

Dementia is a major health problem in elderly patients, with prevalence rising exponentially with increasing age. As female longevity continues to increase, the number of women with dementia and in need of care will increase dramatically over the next few decades. Alzheimer's disease is the most common form, with vascular dementia and dementia with Lewy bodies also prevalent. Oestrogen increases choline acetyltransferase, the enzyme needed to synthesise acetylcholine.[45] This suggests that oestrogen enhances the cholinergic function known to be deficient in Alzheimer's disease, the classical symptom of which is memory deficit.[46]

The Leisure World Cohort[47] indicated that Alzheimer's disease occurred less frequently in oestrogen users and the effect was greater with increasing dose and duration of use. Furthermore, the age of onset of Alzheimer's disease was later in women who had taken oestrogen. Recent reports suggest a protective effect against Alzheimer's disease possibly because HRT increases cerebral blood flow and neuronal stimulation.[47] This is now supported by a meta-analysis demonstrating a 29% decrease in dementia in HRT users.[48] Furthermore, the administration of oestrogen to patients with Alzheimer's disease has modified the clinical course of the disease by improving cognitive performance.[49] This potential benefit of oestrogen therapy, especially in older women, would be a strong argument for long-term treatment.

Cognitive function

Over the past decade, the mechanism by which oestrogen affects the structure and function of neurones in the brain involved in memory has been elucidated. The ageing process itself may partially account for cognitive decline, independent of any hormone effect. Overall, studies that have investigated an association between oestrogen and memory suggest a positive impact on short- and long-term verbal memory in women but minimal effect on visual-spatial memory.[50] A further study found that the addition of oestrogen therapy to women treated with a gonadotrophin-releasing hormone agonist reversed cognitive deficits significantly more than placebo.[51]

The evidence suggests that oestrogen may protect specific cognitive functions that are compromised by ageing of the brain and diseases that alter such functions. These effects may be even more important in elderly women in whom some degree of neuronal death has occurred as a result of the natural ageing process. In such cases, exogenous oestrogen may optimise residual functioning.

Quality-of-life issues

Oestrogen seems to have many potential effects on the eye. Sex-steroid receptor mRNA is present in numerous ocular tissues indicating that these sites probably represent target organs for androgen, oestrogen and progestin action.[52]

Postmenopausal women often present with symptoms of keratoconjunctivitis sicca and symptoms improve after short-term HRT.[53] Recent evidence suggests a relationship between the onset of menopause and the development of glaucoma, with HRT reducing the intra-ocular pressure.[54] Epidemiological studies have also suggested a role for oestrogen in protecting against cataract.[55] Postmenopausal women on HRT and younger women taking oral contraceptives display a decreased prevalence and severity of cataract.[56] Oestrogen appears to reduce the risk of macular degeneration, which is the most common cause of visual handicap in the western world.[57] The mechanism involved is unknown but oestrogen may protect against atherosclerosis and microcirculation failure in the retina.[9]

Rheumatic diseases, especially osteoarthritis and musculoskeletal pain, are extremely common in the elderly and are a major cause of immobility. The chronic pain associated with joint disease can often lead to depression and a further deterioration in quality of life. There are no definitive data on the effect of HRT on rheumatic diseases, especially rheumatoid arthritis.[58] There appears to be no benefit in osteoarthritis but some alleviation of symptoms has been observed in carpal tunnel syndrome and fibromyalgia.

Genital atrophy

The oestrogen-dependent nature of the urogenital tissues means that genitourinary atrophy can lead to a variety of symptoms that affect both ease and quality of life. The incidence of detrusor instability increases with age as a result of mucosal thinning in the bladder and urethra.[59] Older women are more prone to intrinsic sphincter deficiency, asymptomatic bacteriuria and detrusor hyperactivity with impaired contractility.[60] Recurrent urinary tract infections are effectively prevented by postmenopausal HRT.[61] Oral oestrogen restores the vaginal flora and, therefore, older patients require fewer antibiotics. There is conflicting evidence on whether HRT improves genuine stress incontinence. However, the majority of cases of urinary incontinence in elderly women are a mixed problem with a significant component of detrusor instability that can definitely be improved by oestrogen therapy.

Sexual function

Studies have suggested that interest in sexual activity waned in women as they aged. However, the most reliable predictor of continued sexual satisfaction is the enjoyment of sex in earlier years.[62] HRT can help with sexual problems caused by atrophic changes, loss of libido and difficulty reaching orgasm. Androgen therapy may help some women, with improvement in psychological well-being and an increase in sexually motivated behaviour.[63] However, for older women, the lack of a partner is often the main problem.[64]

ADVERSE EFFECTS OF LONG-TERM HRT

The two main reasons for poor compliance with HRT are fear of cancer and vaginal bleeding and both these factors are extremely important in the older woman requiring long-term therapy. Breast cancer is the most common cancer in women. However, the leading cause of death in women is cardiac disease, which accounts for 34% of deaths compared with 3–4% of deaths resulting from breast cancer.[65] There have been many epidemiological studies of the relationship between HRT and breast cancer. However, a consistent pattern of risk has not been demonstrated. The latest reports from the Nurses' Health Study represent 16 years of follow-up (1976–92).[66,67] This analysis revealed that women who had used oestrogen in the past were not at increased risk of breast cancer but there was an increased risk in current users. However, this finding of an increased relative risk in current users was not definitive and not free from confounding variables. In contrast, a case-control study in Washington State, USA, focused on long-term use and could detect no adverse impact of HRT on the risk of breast cancer.[68] In an attempt to resolve these conflicting reports, researchers formed a collaborative group and re-analysed 90% of the world-wide evidence on oestrogen and breast cancer.[69] Among current and recent users of HRT there is a small increased relative risk of breast cancer of approximately 2.3% for each year of use (Table 1). This report suggests that there will be an extra 12 cases of breast cancer by the age of 70 years for every 1000 women who start HRT at the age of 50 years and continue for 15 years. The mortality rates of women who were taking oestrogen at the time of breast-cancer diagnosis have documented improved survival rates.[69] This probably reflects earlier diagnosis in users, as the greater survival rate in current users is associated with a lower frequency of late-stage disease. There is also evidence to suggest that oestrogen users develop better-differentiated tumours and that detection bias is not the only explanation for better survival.

The data on breast cancer and oestrogen therapy remain inconclusive and lacking in consistency. However, this lack of a definitive answer is actually reassuring as this indicates that there is unlikely to be a major effect of oestrogen therapy on breast-cancer risk. This issue is being addressed in several new studies, including the Women's Heath Initiative study in the USA (to be completed in 2008)[15] and the European WISDOM trial (to be completed in 2011).[16] These large randomised trials will eliminate the effect of bias and should clarify this issue.

In those with an intact uterus, unopposed oestrogens should be avoided, as there is a 20% incidence of endometrial hyperplasia after one year of use.[70] The addition of cyclically administered

Table 1 *Excess risk of breast cancer and duration of use of HRT in a woman starting treatment at age 50 years (after Collaborative Group on Hormonal Factors in Breast Cancer[69])*

HRT use (years)	Cumulative incidence over next 20 years	Excess risk/1000
Never	45	Nil
5	47	2
10	51	6
15	57	12

progestogen for a minimum of ten days each cycle would appear to prevent the development of endometrial cancer.[71] However, there have been conflicting reports of a three-fold increased risk of endometrial cancer with five years of cyclical therapy.[72,73] Reluctance to accept menstrual bleeding is an important cause of poor continuance in older women with an intact uterus.[74] There is evidence that absence of withdrawal bleeding may improve long-term compliance.[75] The continuous-combined oestrogen and progestin method of treatment avoids bleeding in 80% of patients after six months of treatment.[76] There is another advantage of the continuous-combined regimen, namely the reduction in the incidence of endometrial cancer.[72]

The importance of other non-life threatening adverse effects affecting compliance should not be dismissed, especially in older women. There are now many oestrogen preparations and routes of administration – for example, patches and gels – that avoid the first-pass effect through the liver and therefore reduce the dosage required and, thus, the adverse effects. Many women have intolerance to progestogens. Intrauterine devices containing a progestogen offer an alternative to oral progestogens and initial studies appear to confirm that they maintain an atrophic endometrium. Further studies are needed to confirm that such a treatment regimen would be acceptable to older women.

Women are concerned about the potential weight gain that may occur with hormonal therapy. This aspect was studied in a double-blind prospective fashion by the PEPI Trial,[77] in which patients were followed on placebo and various HRT regimens. All groups in the study gained weight but the placebo group gained the most weight. In spite of this evidence it is still difficult to convince women that weight gain is an effect of ageing and lowered basal metabolic rate and not an adverse effect associated with HRT.

Three studies have suggested that postmenopausal HRT was associated with a two- to three-fold risk of venous thromboembolism.[78-80] These studies tried to control for risk factors for venous thromboembolism except a family history of the condition. In view of recent knowledge regarding the Leiden mutation and its impact on venous thromboembolism with oral contraceptives, this is an important consideration and would inject bias into the case group. The incidence of idiopathic venous thromboembolism in this age group is approximately 1/10 000 women per year. If these studies are correct this would increase the incidence to about 3/10 000 per year. Recent data of an increased risk of deep venous thrombosis in both the HERS secondary prevention study[17] and data obtained on the effect of raloxifene support previous observational studies.[81] Even if we accept that this is a real risk, it remains confined to short-term current users and would not diminish the emphasis on long-term use for preventative health benefits.

FUTURE PROSPECTS FOR HRT

Selective oestrogen receptor modulators (SERMS) are characterised by their binding affinity to α and β oestrogen receptors. These compounds, which include tamoxifen and its analogues such as raloxifene and droloxifene, have mixed oestrogen agonist and antagonist effects depending on the target issue. The goal of developing these drugs is to derive the potential benefits of postmenopausal oestrogen replacement without oestrogenic adverse effects (such as vaginal bleeding and mastalgia) and avoiding the potential risks.

Two SERMS are currently approved for clinical use: tamoxifen (for adjuvant therapy and treatment of breast cancer and prevention of breast cancer in high-risk women) and raloxifene (for the prevention of osteoporosis). Raloxifene prevents postmenopausal osteoporosis with only a few adverse effects including increase risk of VTE (similar to oestrogen), hot flushes and leg cramps.[82] The effect of raloxifene on cardiovascular risk factors has been partially evaluated. It has a favourable effect on the lipid profile decreasing low-density lipoprotein (LDL) cholesterol and lipoprotein(a) with minimal effects on total high-density lipoprotein cholesterol.[83] The overall long-term effect of raloxifene on the cardiovascular system awaits the results of the RUTH (Raloxifene Use for the Heart trial) which is currently underway.[84] Raloxifene does not increase the risk of endometrial hyperplasia or cancer.[83]

Another SERM currently in development is droloxifene for the treatment of metastatic breast cancer and osteoporosis in postmenopausal women. Unfortunately, its uterotropic effects limit its usefulness in women who have not had a hysterectomy.[85] Other SERMS are also currently under evaluation for efficacy and safety. These drugs may prove to be the next generation of postmenopausal hormone therapy specifically targeted for the older patient.

Another promising development is the development of phyto-oestrogens, which have a weak affinity for oestradiol receptors. The low incidence of breast cancer and cardiovascular disease in Asian Pacific populations compared with Western societies has been attributed to a higher dietary intake of soy proteins.[86,87] However, soy phyto-oestrogens have several deficiencies compared with oestrogen. They do not appear to prevent the development of osteoporosis associated with oestrogen deficiency.[88] There are cardiovascular benefits [89,90] but the reduction of LDL cholesterol and triglycerides seems dependent on the soy protein and not the phyto-oestrogen extract.[91]

Another limiting factor is that the dietary quantity of soy protein required to achieve phyto-oestrogen levels that would relieve vasomotor symptoms remains unacceptably high. Soy phyto-oestrogen may have a role as an adjunct to HRT retaining the beneficial effects of oestrogen on vasomotor symptoms, cardiovascular system, bones and brain. The extent to which the combination may attenuate adverse effects of oestrogen on the breast and endometrium requires further evaluation.

The benefits of long-term HRT outweigh the risks in the majority of women. The development of new formulations further enhance the risk/benefit profile of treatment. HRT forever is not an unrealistic prospect within the foreseeable future.

References

1 Purdie, D.W., Empson, J.A.C., Crichton, C.C., MacDonald, L. Hormone replacement sleep quality and psychological well-being. *Br J Obstet Gynaecol* 1996;**102**:735–9
2 Norman, S.G., Studd, J.W.W. A survey of views on hormone replacement therapy. *Br J Obstet Gynaecol* 1994;**101**:879–87
3 Handa, V.L., Landerman, R., Hanlon, J.T., Harris, T., Cohen, H.J. Do older women use oestrogen replacement. *J Am Geriatr Soc* 1996;**44**:1–6
4 Cauley, L.A., Cummings, S.R., Black D.M., Mascioli, S.R., Seely, D.G. Prevalence and determinants of estrogen replacement therapy in elderly women. *Am J Obstet Gynecol* 1990;**163**:1438–44
5 Barratt-Connor, E. Postmenopausal estrogen and prevention bias. *Ann Intern Med* 1991;**115**:455–6
6 McKinney, K.A., Severino, M., McFall, P., Thompson, W. The treatment-seeking women at menopause: a comparison between two university menopause clinics. *Menopause* 1998;**5**:174–7
7 Wenger, N.K. Coronary heart disease – an older woman's major health risk. *BMJ* 1997;**315**:1085–90
8 Gordon, T., Kannel, W.B., Hjortland, M.C., McNamara, P.M. Menopause and coronary heart disease. The Framingham Study. *Ann Intern Med* 1978;**89**:157–61

9   Stampfer, M.J., Colditz, G.A., Willet, W.C., Manson, J.E., Rosner, B., Speizer, F.E. et al. Postmenopausal estrogen therapy and cardiovascular disease. *N Engl J Med* 1991;**325**:756–62
10 Hunt, K., Vessey, M., McPherson, K. Mortality in a cohort of long-term users of hormone replacement therapy: an updating analysis. *Br J Obstet Gynaecol* 1990;**97**:1080–6
11 Stampfer, M.J., Colditz, G.A. Oestrogen therapy and coronary heart disease: a quantitative assessment of the epidemiological evidence. *Prev Med* 1991;**20**:27–63
12 Barrett-Connor, E., Grady, D. Hormone replacement therapy, heart disease and other considerations. *Annu Rev Public Health* 1998;**19**:55–72
13 Wenger, N.K. Postmenopausal hormone therapy. Is it useful for coronary prevention? *Cardiol Clin* 1998;**16**:17–25
14 Vandenbrouke, J.P. Postmenopausal oestrogen and cardioprotection. *Lancet* 1991;**337**:833–4
15 McGowan, J.A., Pottern, L. Commenting on The Women's Health Initiative. *Maturitas* 2000;**34**:109–12
16 Vickers, M.R., Meade, T.W., Wilkes, H.C. Hormone replacement therapy and cardiovascular disease. The case for a randomised controlled trial. *CIBA Found Symp* 1995;**1991**:150–60
17 Hulley, S., Grady, D., Bush, T., Furberg, C., Herrington, D., Riggs, B. et al. Randomised trial of estrogen plus progestin for secondary prevention of coronary heart disease in postmenopausal women. Heart and Estrogen/Progestin Replacement Therapy Study (HERS) Research Group. *JAMA* 1998;**280**:605–13
18 Grady, D., Rubin, S.M., Pettiti, D.B., Fox, C.S., Black, D., Ettinger, B. et al. Hormone therapy to prevent disease and prolong life in postmenopausal women. *An Intern Med* 1992;**117**:1016–41
19 Psaty, B.M., Heckbert, S.R., Atkins, D., Siscovik, D.S., Koepsell, T.D., Wahl, P.W. A review of the association of estrogens and progestins with cardiovascular disease in postmenopausal women. *Arch Intern Med* 1993;**153**:1421–7
20 Finucane, F.F., Madams, J.H., Bush, T.L., Wolf, P.H., Kleinman, J.C. Decreased risk of stroke among postmenopausal hormone users. *Arch Intern Med* 1993;**153**:73–9
21 Henderson, B.E., Paganini-Hill, A., Ross, R.K. Decreased mortality in users of estrogen replacement therapy. *Arch Intern Med* 1991;**151**:75–8
22 Boysen, G., Nyboe, J., Appleyard, M., Sorensen, P.S., Boas, J., Somnier, F. et al. Stroke incidence and risk factors in Copenhagen, Denmark. *Stroke* 1988;**19**:1345–53
23 Grodstein, F., Stampfer, M.J., Manson, J.E., Colditz, G.A., Willett, W.C., Rosner, B. et al. Postmenopausal estrogen and progestin use and the risk of cardiovascular disease. *N Engl J Med* 1996;**335**:453–61
24 Jonas, H.A., Kronmal, R.A., Psaty, B.M. Current estrogen-progestin and estrogen replacement therapy in elderly women: association with carotid atherosclerosis. *Am J Epidemiol* 1996;**6**:314–23
25 Espeland, M.A., Applegate, W., Furberg, C.D., Lefkowitz, D., Rice, L., Hunninghake, O. Estrogen replacement therapy and progression of intimal-medial thickness in the carotid arteries of postmenopausal women. *Am J Epidemiol* 1995;**142**:1011–19
26 Matteis, M., Troisi, E., Monaldo, B.C. Caltagirone, C., Silvestrini, M. Age and sex differences in cerebral hemodynamics. A transcranial Doppler study. *Stroke* 1998;**29**:963–7
27 Penotti, M., Nencioni, T., Gabrielli, L., Farini, M., Castiglioni, E., Polvani, F. Blood flow variations in internal carotid and middle cerebral arteries induced by postmenopausal hormonal replacement therapy. *Am J Obstet Gynecol* 1993;**169**:1226–32
28 Ganger, K.F., Byas, S., Whitehead, M., Crook, D., Meire, H., Campbell, S. Pulsatility index in internal carotid artery in relation to transdermal oestradiol and time since menopause. *Lancet* 1991;**338**:839–42
29 Belfort, M.A., Saade, G.R., Snabes, M., Dunn, R., Moise, K.J. Jr, Cruz, A. et al. Hormonal status affects the reactivity of the cerebral vasculature. *Am J Obstet Gynecol* 1995;**172**:1273–8

30   Lindsay, R., Hart, D.M., Forrest, C., Baird, C. Prevention of spinal osteoporosis in oophorectomised women. *Lancet* 1980;**ii**:1151–4
31   Hutchinson, T.A., Polansky, S.M., Feinstein, A.R. Postmenopausal oestrogens protect against fractures of hip and distal radius. *Lancet* 1979;**ii**:705–9
32   Krall, E.A., Dawson-Hughes, B., Papas, A., Garcia, R.I. Tooth loss and skeletal bone density in healthy postmenopausal women. *Osteoporosis Int* 1994;**4**:104–9
33   Paganini-Hill, A. The benefits of estrogen replacement therapy on oral health. The Leisure World Cohort. *Arch Intern Med* 1995;**155**:2325–9
34   Grodstein, F., Colditz, G.A., Stampfer, M.J. Postmenopausal hormone use and tooth loss: a prospective study. *JADA* 1996;**127**:372–7
35   Hartmann, B.W., Huber, J.C. The mythology of hormone replacement therapy. *Br J Obstet Gynaecol* 1997;**104**:163–8
36   Smith, M.A., Fine, J.A., Barnhill, R.L., Berwick, M. Hormonal and reproductive influences and risk of melanoma in women. *Int J Epidemiol* 1998;**27**:751–7
37   La Vecchia, C., Negri, E., Levi, F., Decarli, A., Boyle, P. Cancer mortality in Europe: effects of age, cohort of birth and period of death. *Eur J Cancer* 1998;**34**:118–41
38   McMichael, A.J., Potter, J.D. Reproduction, endogenous and exogenous sex hormones and colon cancer: a review and hypothesis. *J Natl Cancer Inst* 1980;**65**:1201–7
39   Herbert-Croteau, N. A meta-analysis of hormone replacement therapy and colon cancer in women. *Cancer Epidemiol Biomarkers Prev* 1998;**7**:653–9
40   Grodstein, F., Newcomb, P.A., Stampfer, M.J. Postmenopausal hormone therapy and the risk of colorectal cancer: a review and meta-analysis. *Am J Med* 1999;**106**:574–82
41   McMichael, A.J., Potter, J.D. Host factors in carcinogenesis: certain bile acid metabolic profiles that selectively increase the risk of proximal colon cancer. *J Natl Cancer Inst* 1985;**75**:185–91
42   Lointier, P., Wildrick, D.M., Boman, B.M. The effects of steroid hormones on a human colon cancer cell *in vitro*. *Anticancer Res* 1992;**12**:1327–30
43   Issa, J.P., Ottaviano, Y.L., Celano, P., Hamilton, S.R., Davidson, N.E., Baylin, S.B. Methylation of the oestrogen receptor CpG islands links ageing and neoplasia in the human colon. *Nat Genet* 1994;**7**:536–40
44   Chen, M.J., Longnecker, M.P., Morgenstern, H. Recent use of HRT and the prevalence of colorectal adenomas. *Cancer Epidemiol Biomarkers Prev* 1998;**7**:227–30
45   Luine, V.N. Estradiol increases choline acetyltransferase activity in specific basal forebrain nuclei and projection areas of female rats. *Exp Neurol* 1985;**80**:484–90
46   Bartus, R.T., Dean, R.L., Beer, B., Lippa, A.S. The cholinergic hypothesis of memory dysfunction. *Science* 1982;**217**:208–417
47   Paganini-Hill, A., Henderson, V.W. Estrogen replacement therapy and the risk of Alzheimer's disease. *Arch Intern Med* 1996;**156**:2213–17
48   Yaffe, K., Sawaya, G., Lieberburg, I., Grady, D. Estrogen therapy in postmenopausal women. Effects on cognitive function and dementia. *JAMA* 1998;**279**:688–95
49   Henderson, V., Paganini-Hill, A., Emanuel, C.K., Dunn, M.E., Buckwalter, J.G. Estrogen replacement therapy in older women: comparisons between Alzheimer's disease cases and non-demented control subjects. *Arch Neurol* 1994;**51**:896–900
50   Barrett-Connor, E., Kritz-Silverstain, D. Estrogen replacement therapy and cognitive function in older women. *JAMA* 1993;**260**:2637–41
51   Sherwin, B.B., Tulandi, T. 'Add-back' estrogen reverses cognitive defects induced by a gonadotrophin releasing hormone agonist in women with leiomyomata uteri. *J Clin Endocrinol Metab* 1996;**81**:2545–9

52 Wickham, L.A., Rocha, E.M., Gao, J., Krenzer, K.L., da Silviera, L.A., Toda, I. et al. Identification and hormonal control of sex steroid receptors in the eye. *Adv Exp Med Biol* 1998;**438**:95–100

53 Vavilis, D., Agorastos, T., Vakiani, M., Jafetas, J., Panidis, D., Donstantinidis, T. The effect of transdermal estradiol on the conjunctiva in postmenopausal women. *Eur J Obstet Gynecol Reprod Biol* 1997;**72**:93–6

54 Sator, M.O., Akramian, J., Joura, E.A., Nessman, A., Wedrich, A., Gruber, D. et al. Reduction of intraocular pressure in a glaucoma patient undergoing hormone replacement therapy. *Maturitas* 1998;**29**:93–5

55 Klein, B.E.K. Lens opacities in women in Beaver Dam, Wisconsin: is there evidence of an effect of sex hormones? *Trans Am Ophthalmol Soc* 1993;**91**:517–44

56 Klein, B.E.K., Klein, R., Ritter, L.L. Is there evidence of an estrogen effect of age-related lens opacities? *Arch Ophthalmol* 1994;**112**:85–91

57 The Eye Disease Case-Control Study Group. Risk factors for idiopathic macular holes. *Arch Ophthalmol* 1996;**114**:545–54

58 Vandenbrouke, J.P., Witteman, J.C.M., Valkenburg, H.A., Boersma, J.W., Cats, A., Festen, J.J. et al. Non-contraceptive hormones and rheumatoid arthritis in perimenopausal and postmenopausal women. *JAMA* 1986;**255**:1299–301

59 Agency for Health Care Policy and Research. *Clinical Practice Guidelines. Urinary Incontinence in Adults.* Rockville, MD; 1992 (Publication no. 902–0038)

60 Ouslander, J.G. Ageing and the lower genital tract. *Am J Med Sci* 1997;**314**:214

61 Raz, R., Stamm, W.E. A controlled trial of intravaginal estriol in postmenopausal women with recurrent urinary tract infection. *N Engl J Med* 1993;**329**:753–5

62 Goldstein, M.K., Teng, N.N.H. Gynaecological factors in sexual dysfunction of the older women. *Clin Geriatr Med* 1991;**7**:41–61

63 Sherwin, B.B., Gelfand, M.M. The role of androgen in the maintenance of sexual functioning in oophorectomised women. *Psychosom Med* 1987;**49**:397–409

64 Diokno, A.C., Brown, M.B., Herzog, A.R. Sexual function in the elderly. *Arch Intern Med* 1990;**150**:197–200

65 Cummings, S.R., Black, D.M., Rubin, S.M. Lifetime risks of hip, Colles or vertebral fracture and coronary heart disease among white postmenopausal women. *Arch Intern Med* 1989;**149**:2445–8

66 Colditz, G.A., Stampfer, M.J., Willett, W.C. Type of postmenopausal use and risk of breast cancer: 12-year follow-up from the Nurses Health Study. *Cancer Causes Control* 1992;**3**:433–9

67 Colditz, G.A., Hankinson, S.E., Hunter, D.J., Willett, W.C., Manson, J.E., Stampfer, M.J. et al. The use of estrogens and progestins and the risk of breast cancer in postmenopausal women. *N Engl J Med* 1995;**332**:1589–93

68 Stanford, J.L., Weiss, N.S., Voigt, L.F., Daling, J.R., Habel, L.A., Rossing, M.A. Combined estrogen and progestin hormone replacement therapy in relation to risk of breast cancer in middle-aged women. *JAMA* 1995;**274**:137–42

69 Collaborative Group on Hormonal Factors in Breast Cancer. Breast cancer and hormone replacement therapy: collaborative re-analysis of data from 51 epidemiological studies of 52,705 women with breast cancer and 108,411 women without breast cancer. *Lancet* 1997;**350**:1047–59

70 Woodruff, J.D., Pickar, J.H. Incidence of endometrial hyperplasia in postmenopausal women taking conjugated estrogens (Premarin) with medroxyprogesterone acetate or conjugated estrogens alone. The Menopause Study Group. *Am J Obstet Gynecol* 1994;**170**:1213–23

71 Pike, M.C., Peters, R.K., Cozen, W., Probst-Hensch, N.M., Felix, J.C., Wan, P.C. et al. Estrogen-progestin replacement therapy and endometrial cancer. *J Natl Cancer Inst* 1997;**89**:1110–16

72 Weiderpass, E., Adami, H.O., Baron, J.A., Magnusson,, C., Bergstrom, R., Lindgren, A. et al. Risk of endometrial cancer following estrogen replacement with and without progestins. *J Natl Cancer Inst* 1999;**91**:1131–7

73 Beresford, S.A., Weiss, N.S., Voigt, L.F., McKnight, B. Risk of endometrial cancer in relation to use of oestrogen combined with cyclic progestogen therapy in postmenopausal women. *Lancet* 1997;**349**:458–61

74 Williams, S.R., Frenchek, B., Speroff, T., Speroff, L. A study of combined continuous ethinyl estradiol and norethindrone acetate for postmenopausal hormone replacement. *Am J Obstet Gynecol* 1990;**162**:438–46

75 Ettinger, B., De-Kun, I., Klein, R. Continuation of postmenopausal hormone replacement therapy: comparisons of cyclic versus continuous combined schedules. *Menopause* 1996;**3**:185–9

76 Archer, D.F., Pickar, J.H., Bottiglioni, F. Bleeding patterns in postmenopausal women taking continuous combined or sequential regimens of conjugated estrogens with medroxyprogesterone acetate. The Menopause Study Group. *Obstet Gynecol* 1994;**83**:686–92

77 Writing Group for the PEPI Trial. Effects on oestrogen or oestrogen/progestin on heart disease risk factor in postmenopausal women. *JAMA* 1995;**273**:199–208

78 Daly, E., Vessey, M.P., Hawkins, M.M., Carson, J.L., Gough, P., Marsh, S. Risk of venous thromboembolism in users of hormone replacement therapy. *Lancet* 1996;**348**:977–80

79 Jick, H., Derby, L.E., Myers, M.W., Vasilakis, C., Newton, K.M. Risk of hospital admission for idiopathic venous thromboembolism among users of postmenopausal oestrogens. *Lancet* 1996;**348**:981–3

80 Grodstein, F., Stampfer, M.J., Goldhaber, S.Z. Prospective study of exogenous hormones and risk of pulmonary embolism in women. *Lancet* 1996;**348**:983–7

81 Cummings, S.R., Eckert, S., Kreuger, K.A., Grady, D., Powles, T.J., Cauley, J.A. et al. The effect of raloxifene on risk of breast cancer in postmenopausal women. Results from the MORE randomised trial. *JAMA* 1999;**281**:2189–97

82 Walsh, B., Kuiler, L., Wild, R., Paul, S., Farmer, M., Lawrence, J. et al. Effects of raloxifene on serum lipids and coagulation factors in healthy post-menopausal women. *JAMA* 1998;**179**:1444–51

83 Kovidhunkit, W., Shoback, D.M. Clinical effects of raloxifene hydrochloride in women. *Ann Intern Med* 1999;**130**:431–9

84 Barrett-Connor, E., Wenger, N.K., Grady, D., Mosca, L., Collins, P., Kornitzer, M. et al. Coronary heart disease in women, randomised clinical trials HERS and RUTH. *Maturitas* 1998;**31**:1–7

85 Gradishar, W.J., Jordan, V.C. Clinical potential of new anti-estrogens. *J Clin Oncol* 1997;**15**:840–52

86 Knight, D.C., Eden, J.A. A review of the clinical effects of phyto-estrogens. *Obstet Gynecol* 1996;**87**:897–904

87 Wu, A.H., Ziegler, R.G., Nomura, A., West, D.W., Kolonel, L.N., Horn-Ross, P.L. et al. Soy intake and breast cancer in Asians and Asian Americans. *Am J Clin Nutr* 1998;**68**:1437–43S

88 Scambia, G., Mango, D., Signorile, P.G., Angeli, R.A., Palena, C., Gallo, D. et al. Clinical effects of a standardised soy extract in postmenopausal women: a pilot study. *Menopause* 2000;**7**:105–11

89 Washburn, S., Burke, G.L., Morgan, T., Anthony, M.S. Effect of soy protein supplementation

on serum lipids, blood pressure and menopausal symptoms in perimenopausal women. *Menopause* 1999;**6**:7–13

90 Anderson, J.W., Johnstone, B.M., Cook-Newell, M.E. Meta-analysis of the effects of soy protein intake on serum lipids. *N Engl J Med* 1995;**333**:276–82

91 Nestel, P.J., Yamashita, T., Sasahara, T., Pomeroy, S., Dart, A., Komesaroff, P. *et al.* Soy isoflavones improve systemic arterial compliance but not plasma lipids in menopausal and perimenopausal women. *Arterioscler Thromb Vasc Biol* 1997;**17**:3392–8

19

Bilateral uterine artery embolisation for fibroids

Woodruff J. Walker

INTRODUCTION

Arterial embolisation is not a new technique and has been carried out for at least four decades. It has been mainly used in the control of haemorrhage[1] and for palliation and control of symptoms in malignancies. More recently, it has been used for the control of obstetric and gynaecological bleeding, particularly for postpartum (where it may be life saving)[2] and post-caesarean haemorrhage and following gynaecological surgery.[3] In 1995, embolisation was reported as being employed for the management of uterine myoma, the first case being carried out at L'Hôpital Lariboisière under Professor Ravina.[4] The technique was initially used to occlude the vascular supply to the fibroids in order to reduce haemorrhagic complications following surgery but it was found that in many cases the fibroids shrunk and surgery was unnecessary.

At the Royal Surrey County Hospital in Guildford, an observational trial of fibroid embolisation is in progress that commenced in 1996 and has so far treated over 300 patients.

PROTOCOL AND TECHNIQUE

There are some minor variations in technique between centres. The protocol at the Royal Surrey County Hospital is described in this chapter.

Prior to the procedure, the patient is interviewed by the consultant radiologist (WJW) carrying out the procedure. The technique and trial results are explained to the patient and, in particular, complications that may occur are fully discussed. It is important not to give the patient a false expectation and to prevent any confusion with regard to outcome. It must be explained that fibroid embolisation kills and shrinks the fibroids but does not eliminate them, except in the small group of patients who pass their fibroids. If the patient requires preservation of fertility it is explained that fibroid embolisation has not been fully assessed in this area and, although patients who were previously infertile have become pregnant after the procedure, the efficacy of the technique in this respect is as yet not fully established. It is particularly important that patients with large complex fibroid masses in whom neither myomectomy nor fibroid embolisation is likely to be effective in terms of fertility should not be given a false expectation.

On the day of the procedure, a diclofenac suppository 100 mg is administered per rectum one hour prior to the procedure. During the procedure intravenous sedation is administered in the form of a titrated mixture of fentanyl and midazolam. Antibiotics are given intravenously: gentamicin 120 mg, ampicillin 500 mg and metronidazole 500 mg.

A 4F Pigtail catheter is then passed into the lower aorta via the right femoral artery using a right groin approach and a flush pelvic arteriogram carried out, which provides a 'road map' of the pelvic arteries. The Pigtail catheter is then exchanged for a 4F Cobra 2 catheter, which is passed over the aortic bifurcation and into the left common iliac artery under fluoroscopic imaging. A microcatheter is then introduced through the 4F catheter into the uterine artery and passed approximately one-third to halfway along its length. Particles of polyvinyl alcohol (PVA) are then injected into the uterine artery until flow in the vessel ceases. The main uterine artery is then occluded with Gelfoam' pledgets or coils. Should spasm in the uterine artery develop, aliquots of 300 μg of glyceryl trinitrate are injected into the uterine artery.

The procedure itself generates little pain but the patient may experience severe pain during the 12–24 hours following the procedure. This may be adequately controlled with a patient-controlled analgesia pump set to deliver aliquots of 2.5 mg of morphine intravenously. This is backed up with diclofenac suppositories and maximum strength co-codamol tablets. The patient is kept in hospital for two nights and discharged the following morning. No prophylactic antibiotics are administered after the procedure.

There are small differences in technique in other centres. In some centres, microcatheters are not used and, where spasm develops and flow is restricted in the uterine arteries, particles are simply forced into the vessel. Some centres administer epidural anaesthesia and others give prophylactic antibiotics following the procedure.

Unlike in most series, at the Royal Surrey it is the radiologist who looks after the patient during her stay in hospital. In most centres the patient is then discharged under the care of the gynaecologist with the radiologist playing little part in follow-up. At the Royal Surrey the opposite is the case. All patients are followed up at regular intervals by the radiologist in addition to the gynaecologist or general practitioner. The radiologist (WJW) places himself on 24-hour call for all his patients at all times. This is particularly important where the radiologist is being referred patients by different gynaecologists around the country, as the gynaecologists looking after those patients may have little experience of fibroid embolisation. The radiologist, however, will have an accumulated experience of many cases and is therefore in a good position to advise the patient over the telephone in the event of the development of problems. At the Royal Surrey, should any complications develop, the facilities are available to deal with those complications, even where patients are not local, or we will liaise with the local gynaecologist, depending on the circumstances of the individual case. It is important that every patient who is embolised has a named individual that they can contact in the event of any worries or concerns or the development of symptoms.

All Royal Surrey patients enter an observational trial that has obtained ethical approval and this is important as the procedure has a SERNIP C rating (safety and efficacy of the procedure not proven and should be the subject of an observational trial). The patients are followed up at regular intervals, six weeks, three months, six months and then six-monthly. They have ultrasound scans at each visit, blood tests for hormone levels, iron stores and a full blood count and at 0 and 6 months magnetic resonance imaging (MRI) is performed. At each visit patients are required to fill out a detailed questionnaire.

RESULTS OF FIBROID EMBOLISATION

Results of this procedure have been reported elsewhere.[5-8] An average reduction in fibroid volume of 40% was achieved at six weeks, 54% at three months, 63% at six months and 73% at one year. This demonstrated that shrinkage continues in the period from six months to one year. The response rate to our questionnaires was 94% and this indicated an average improvement in the symptoms of 78%, periods improving in 80%, pressure symptoms in 84% and abdominal discomfort in 71%; 94% of patients indicated that they were satisfied with the procedure and 97.5% said they would recommend it to a friend.

Complications

There were two infective complications leading to hysterectomy and these have been reported elsewhere.[5-8] One of these was a tubo-ovarian abscess for which hysterectomy was carried out at three weeks. The second was a chronic fibroid infection for which a hysterectomy was carried out approximately three months after the embolisation. The case of the woman who developed a tubo-ovarian abscess is interesting, in that there was no infection in the fibroid itself and when the pathological specimen was examined it was found that there were particles of PVA in the ovarian vessels. This patient had been embolised with 150–200 micron particles as well as 355–500 micron particles and this may have been the reason for the appearance of these particles in the ovarian arteries. A number of other patients have experienced intermittent discharges, one of whom required a hysteroscopic resection of fibroid debris to resolve the symptoms. A 33-year-old Afro-Caribbean patient had a chronic actinomycotic infection of her endometrial cavity 18 months after the procedure. She had a huge fibroid mass the size of a 30-week pregnancy and had a number of episodes of infection in the follow-up period. A patient with fibroids and adenomyosis haemorrhaged at six weeks and required a blood transfusion. She was treated conservatively.

Ovarian failure

Of 153 patients under 45 years of age in the study, three patients (2%) stopped having periods. However, one of these had only one ovary, which was itself affected by an endometrioma. A second patient was one of the few embolised with 150–250 micron particles (in most cases embolisation is carried out with 355–500 micron particles) and it is possible that the small size of particles caused passage into the ovarian arteries. The third patient had no predisposing factors for her ovarian failure.

Failures

Of 300 patients so far embolised, four elected to have hysterectomies because of an inadequate response to embolisation. In two patients neither uterine artery could be embolised because of unusual anatomy and in a further two patients only one uterine artery could be catheterised and the patients refused a second attempt as their symptoms resolved. Two patients with adenomyosis and fibroids did not respond to embolisation.

Passage of fibroids

Seven patients passed intact fibroids and the largest of these was 12 cm in diameter.[9]

Pregnancies

Four patients have become pregnant. One of these patients had a 6×5×5 cm fibroid after embolisation. A second patient had an 18-week sized uterus before embolisation, with no normal tissue evident on MRI. After the embolisation, having passed much fibroid tissue, she was left with a virtually normal uterus. The third patient passed a 12-cm submucous fibroid after the embolisation. The fourth patient had an embolisation of a submucous fibroid followed by hysteroscopic resection. All these patients have continuing pregnancies except the third, who elected to have an abortion as the pregnancy was unintentional.

DISCUSSION

Since fibroid embolisation was first commenced in France over 6000 cases have been performed in the USA, France and the UK and medium term results have been reported.[5-8,10-13] These series all demonstrate a success rate of over 85% for fibroid embolisation and a low complication rate. There are some minor variations in technique between groups some using standard angiographic catheters and others microcatheters. At the Royal Surrey the use of microcatheters is preferred in order to maintain bloodflow around the catheter, so that the maximum number of particles can be delivered into the uterine artery. If a standard catheter is used, this often results in flow restriction or spasm around the catheter and particles need to be forced into the uterine artery. Some interventionalists complete the process of occlusion of the uterine artery with coils, as at the Royal Surrey, and others use absorbable gelatin sponge (Gelfoam™). Recently, the author has commenced using a combination of coils and Gelfoam™ to complete the occlusion of the uterine arteries. There is some variation in the degree of shrinkage in different series. Our group[10] and the Ravina group[11] report higher shrinkages compared with that of the USA group.[13] This may be because our group and the French group use smaller particles (150–200 microns and 355–500 microns as opposed to the 500–700 microns used by the USA group). The smaller particles may be expected to cause a distal block in the uterine arteries and, therefore, cause a more profound infarction. However, this may be associated with an increased complication rate and both patients who suffered infections leading to hysterectomy in our series were embolised with 150–200 micron particles in addition to 355–500 micron particles. We have now ceased using 150–200 micron particles. It should also be noted that the patient with a tubo-ovarian abscess in our series was found to have particles in the ovarian arteries at pathology.

It is the view of the author that MRI is particularly useful for assessment of patients undergoing fibroid embolisation. The fibroids can be more accurately mapped using MRI and the endometrium and junctional zone are more consistently visualised in cases of complex fibroid masses than with ultrasound. All but Stage I carcinoma[14,15] of the endometrium can be excluded, the ovaries accurately assessed and non-gynaecological pathology can be picked up. MRI is particularly important for the exclusion of adenomyosis. In our series, embolisation failed in two patients with adenomyosis. We believe this is due to the diffuse nature of the hypervascularity in adenomyosis as contrasted with the peripheral hypervascularity and relative central hypovascularity of fibroids. The latter renders fibroids easy to infarct, which is not the case with adenomyosis. Finally, because MRI is more reproducible it is more accurate in the assessment of fibroid shrinkage than ultrasound.

Ovarian failure is a recognised complication of embolisation.[11] We were surprised at how infrequently it occurred, with an incidence of only 2%. But if possible predisposing factors are excluded, such as the use of small particles (150–200 microns) and prior ovarian compromise, then only one patient developed to ovarian failure, giving an incidence of less than 1%. It is also important to realise that premature menopause occurs in over 3.3% of women under the age of 45 years.[16] In addition, none of our three patients with ovarian failure expressed any dissatisfaction at the result.

Since infection is the main complication of fibroid embolisation and this has already caused one death,[17] the question of prophylactic antibiotics arises. In both patients who had infections leading to hysterectomy prophylactic antibiotics were administered for five days following the procedure (ampicillin and metronidazole together with gentamicin, at the time of the procedure). We now only administer prophylactic antibiotics at the time of the procedure and not subsequently. This is the practice of most groups.

The safety of fibroid embolisation has been called into question.[17] In the world experience there are two known deaths from fibroid embolisation. One case has been published[17] and a second occurred in Milan where a 65-year-old patient with two small fibroids underwent fibroid embolisation and died suddenly, 24 hours after the procedure, from a pulmonary embolus. She had been catheterised and immobilised following the embolisation. This case was reported in the 1999 survey on the safety of fibroid embolisation conducted by the Society of Cardiovascular and Interventional Radiology. The survey received data on 4500 patients who had undergone fibroid embolisation in the USA. Approximately 1500 cases of fibroid embolisation have so far been carried out in Europe. This gives a total figure for fibroid embolisation in Europe and the USA of 6000, of which two patients have died. The mortality rate for hysterectomy for benign disease excluding complications of pregnancy is 1:1600.[18]

Embolisation of a uterine sarcoma is of concern. However, it should be realised that the incidence of uterine sarcoma is rare, less than 0.2%.[19] Unfortunately, it is not possible to distinguish uterine sarcoma either clinically (as it has been shown that rapid growth of the fibroid is not an indication of malignancy[20]) or by any imaging techniques. Uterine sarcomas are silent until they metastasise and, with long waiting lists in the UK, are likely to be missed surgically as well as radiologically. It needs to be borne in mind that the mortality of 1:1600 for hysterectomy for benign disease excluding pregnancy is greater than the incidence of uterine sarcoma.

The efficacy of fibroid embolisation with regard to fertility is unknown. In the Royal Surrey series, there were four pregnancies. Pregnancies have also been reported in other series.[10,11] However, the published evidence is scanty, whereas the literature on pregnancy following myomectomy is extensive, although it lacks a correlation with MRI assessment of the type of fibroids. There would appear to be some clear indications for embolisation in patients who desire to retain fertility. The first is where the only treatment on offer is a hysterectomy and the second where the patient has undergone previous myomectomies.

Much has already been established concerning the efficacy and safety of fibroid embolisation but much is still unknown. The optimal technique has yet to be established. Is it necessary, for example, to occlude the uterine arteries as well as the branches of the uterine artery? What is the most appropriate embolic substance? Are prophylactic antibiotics useful or not? What types of fibroid are most appropriately treated? Are there any imaging modalities which can predict likely outcome? Currently, fibroid embolisation has a SERNIP C rating, which means that this is still at the trial stage. However, the large number of women who have benefited from the procedure, exemplified by the high satisfaction rate on short- and medium-term follow-up, would indicate that this technique may well have a place in the gynaecologist's therapeutic armamentarium.

References

1. Walker, W.J., Goldin, A.R., Shaff, M.I. et al. Per catheter control of haemorrhage from the superior and inferior mesenteric arteries. *Clin Radiol* 1980;**31**:71–80
2. Walker, W.J. Successful internal iliac artery embolisation with glue in a case of massive obstetric haemorrhage. *Clin Radiol* 1996;**51**:442–4
3. Wells, I. Internal iliac artery embolisation bleeding in the management of pelvic bleeding. *Clin Radiol* 1996;**51**:825–7
4. Ravina, J.H., Herbreteau, D., Ciraru-Vigneron, N., Bouret, J.M., Houdart, E., Aymard, A. et al. Arterial embolisation to treat uterine myomata. *Lancet* 1995;**346**:671–2
5. Walker, W.J. Bilateral uterine artery embolization for fibroids. In: Sheth, S., Sutton, C., editors. *Menorrhagia*. Oxford: Isis Medical Media; 1999. p. 185–94

6   Goodwin, S.C., Walker, W.J. Uterine artery embolization for the treatment of uterine fibroids. *Curr Opin Obstet Gynaecol* 1998;**10**:315–20
7   Walker, W. Arterial embolization in obstetrics and gynaecology with particular reference to uterine fibroids. *Advances in Gynaecology and Obstetrics* 1999;**16**:2–8
8   Walker, W., Green, A., Sutton, C. Bilateral uterine artery embolisation for myomata – results, complications and failures. *Journal of Minimally Invasive Therapy* 1999;**8**:449–54
9   Jones, K., Walker, W.J., Sutton, C. Sequestration and extrusion of intramural fibroids following arterial embolization: a case series. *Gynaecological Endoscopy* 2000;**9**:309–14
10 Worthington-Kirsch, R.L., Popky, G.L., Hutchins, F.L. Uterine arterial embolization for the management of leiomyomas: quality-of-life assessment and clinical response. *Radiology* 1998;**208**:625–9
11 Ravina, J.H., Bouret, J.M., Ciraru-Vigneron, N., Aymard, A., Houdart, E., Ledfref, O. et al. Particulate arterial embolization: a new treatment for uterine leiomyomata-related hemorrhage. *Presse Méd* 1998;**27**:299
12 Ravina, J.H., Bouret, J.M., Ciraru-Vigneron, N., Repiquet, D., Herbreteau, D., Aymard, A. et al. Recourse to particular arterial embolisation in the treatment of some leiomyoma. *Bull Acad Natl Med* 1997;**181**:223–43
13 Goodwin, S.C., Vedantham, S., McLucas, B., Forno, A.E., Perrella, R. Preliminary experience with uterine artery embolisation for uterine fibroids. *J Vasc Interv Radiol* 1997;**8**:517–26
14 Hricak, H., Rubinstein, L.V., Gherman, G.M., Karstaedt, N. MR imaging evaluation of endometrial carcinoma: results of an NCI Co-operative Study. *Radiology* 1991;**179**:829–32
15 Scoutt, L.M., McCarthy, S., Flynn, S.D., Lange, R.C., Long, F., Smith, R.C. et al. Clinical stage I endometrial carcinoma: pitfalls in preoperative assessment with MR imaging. *Radiology* 1995;**194**:567–72
16 Cassou, B., Derriennic, F., Monfort, C., Dell'Accio, P., Touranchet, A. Risk factors of early menopause in two generations of gainfully employed French women. *Maturitas* 1997;**26**:165–74
17 Vashisht, A., Studd, J., Carey, A., Burn, P. Fatal septicaemia after fibroid embolisation. *Lancet* 1999;**354**:307–8
18 Wingo, P.A., Huezo, C.M., Rubin, G.L., Ory, H.W., Peterson, H.B. The mortality risk associated with hysterectomy. *Am J Obstet Gynecol* 1986;**152**:803–8
19 Davies, A., Magos, A.L. Indications and alternatives to hysterectomy. *Baillière's Clin Obstet Gynaecol* 1997;**11**:61–75
20 Parker, W.H., Fu, Y.S., Berek, J.S. Uterine sarcoma in patients operated on for presumed leiomyoma and rapidly growing leiomyoma. *Obstet Gynecol* 1994;**83**:414–18

Further reading

Royal College of Obstetricians and Gynaecologists, Royal College of Radiologists. *Clinical Recommendations on the Use of Uterine Artery Embolisation in the Management of Fibroids. Report of a Joint Working Party*. London: RCOG Press; 2001.

20

Vault prolapse

Patrick Hogston

INTRODUCTION AND DEFINITION

Vaginal vault prolapse refers to prolapse of the apex of the vagina and can, therefore, occur before or after hysterectomy. Most gynaecologists tend to use the term in association with post-hysterectomy patients and this is the terminology used in this chapter. Vault prolapse is commonly associated with enterocele and other support defects. In some cases all support has failed, resulting in total vaginal eversion (Figure 1). Enterocele is a hernia of peritoneum through a defect in normal endopelvic fascia resulting in peritoneum (usually containing small bowel) being in direct contact with vaginal epithelium. Therefore, post-hysterectomy enterocele can occur in the absence of vault prolapse if the uterosacral ligaments are intact and the fascial defect is between the rectovaginal and pubocervical fascia.

The surgical treatment of vaginal vault prolapse poses specific difficulties for the gynaecological surgeon. It is perhaps fortunate that many patients do not require surgical correction. However, as patients with vault prolapse often have other types of vaginal prolapse or urinary incontinence, decisions on management present their own difficulties. Surgical treatment is thus complex, carries a greater risk and is more prone to failure than other types of pelvic reconstructive surgery.

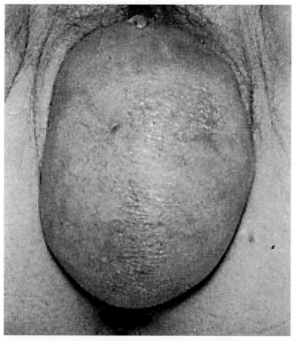

Figure 1 *Total vaginal eversion after previous hysterectomy*

EPIDEMIOLOGY AND AETIOLOGY

The epidemiology of vaginal prolapse, particularly after hysterectomy, is poorly documented for many reasons. The incidence of vault prolapse is typically quoted to be between 0.3% and 43%[1] and up to 30% of operations for prolapse or incontinence are repeat operations.[2] The question, therefore, remains open as to whether these figures could be improved by attention to surgical technique.

Such a variation highlights the difficulty in performing population studies and reflects bias in referral patterns. Many patients are asymptomatic and hence will never be seen. Baden and Walker reported on 864 patients undergoing various reparative procedures for prolapse and incontinence.[3] Only 22% of patients with uterine or vault prolapse were symptomatic, although the more severe the prolapse the more likely it was to be symptomatic.

Marchionni et al.[4] reviewed 2670 hysterectomies performed at one institution between 1983 and 1987. Five hundred patients were randomly selected and asked to participate in the study; 448 (90%) agreed and were examined 9–13 years after hysterectomy (308 abdominal, 20 vaginal without prolapse, 120 vaginal with repair for prolapse). Five of the 2670 (0.2%) had presented with symptomatic vault prolapse. Of the 448 asymptomatic patients, 20 had a degree of vault prolapse. Six patients with vault prolapse had previously undergone abdominal hysterectomy for benign disease (total 308). No patient had vault prolapse after vaginal hysterectomy alone (20 cases). Fourteen patients with vault prolapse had undergone vaginal hysterectomy for prolapse and a further five had vaginal but not vault prolapse, an overall incidence of post-hysterectomy prolapse of 15.8% (19:120).

The factors leading to the first operation for prolapse may still exist and there is evidence of pelvic neuropathy in women with prolapse and incontinence. However, in some women, neuropathy is made worse by vaginal repair and this may contribute to surgical failure.[5] In addition, the widespread use of colposuspension for stress incontinence predisposes to vaginal vault prolapse and enterocele in up to 17% of cases.[6] With an increase in life expectancy, the number of women requiring treatment for recurrent prolapse is likely to continue to increase for the foreseeable future.

ASSESSMENT AND DOCUMENTATION

The diagnosis is usually obvious, although the supine position may underestimate the degree of prolapse, as may examination first thing in the morning or if a pessary has been in use. Examination in the standing position may be helpful.

There is no universally accepted system for describing the position of the pelvic organs and experienced gynaecologists do not always agree in their assessment of the same patient. Vaginal vault prolapse is usually associated with other vaginal support defects. In the USA, gynaecologists commonly use Baden's 'half-way' system which refers to each part of the vaginal prolapse with reference to the hymen.[3] In order to standardise terminology, the International Continence Society has recently introduced the Pelvic Organ Prolapse Quantitation (POP-Q) system, which allows accurate description of physical findings as well as meaningful comparisons between published data.[7] Once the gynaecologist has been instructed thoroughly in its use, it is an accurate and reproducible method of documentation.[8]

INVESTIGATIONS

Although unusual, upper tract conditions, such as hydronephrosis and even renal failure, have been described with complete prolapse and, hence, renal assessment by biochemistry and ultrasound will need to be considered in such patients.

Postmicturition residual urine measurement by catheterisation or ultrasound will identify patients in chronic retention who may also have voiding difficulty after any surgery. Additional investigations, such as cystometry, will be required if incontinence is present but occult stress incontinence is increasingly recognised as a potential problem. Veronikis[9] reported 83% of patients with massive pelvic organ prolapse to have occult stress incontinence using urethrocystometry and urethral pressure profiles after prolapse reduction, whereas Versi[10] reported that occult stress incontinence occurs in 28% of patients using video-urodynamics. Occult detrusor instability can also occur. The availability of these investigations will determine their use but, if surgery is contemplated in women with severe prolapse, some assessment for occult stress incontinence is essential.

Investigations such as dynamic fluoroscopy or ultrasound can demonstrate the presence or absence of enterocele, which can save tedious dissection in the operating theatre.

TREATMENT

Conservative measures such as pelvic floor exercises, electrical stimulation or weighted cones may still be useful, although after previous failed surgery these are less likely to succeed. Vaginal pessaries are useful in the frail or infirm but no treatment may be an option for this group also.

For most women requiring treatment surgery will usually provide the best option. Particular care is required for patients with medical problems but age *per se* is not a major risk factor under 80 years. A study of 66 478 patients over 65 years of age undergoing surgery for stress incontinence showed a mortality of 3.3 per 1000.[11] Only 2.6% of patients were over 85 years of age and the mortality for this group was 1.6%. However, the population over 80 years is growing and will place increasing demands on medical and surgical services. The rate and quality of healing depends on oestrogen[12] and the use of hormone replacement therapy before surgery in postmenopausal women is recommended.

PREVENTION OF VAULT PROLAPSE AT PRIMARY HYSTERECTOMY

Fifty percent of patients with vaginal vault prolapse present within two years[1] of hysterectomy and hence it seems reasonable to conclude that surgical technique is likely to be relevant in this group. The uterosacral-cardinal ligament complex is required to support the vaginal vault after hysterectomy and maintenance of vaginal length is important. There is continued debate as to whether vaginal prolapse is due to stretching or tearing of these fascial supports. Similarly, in uterine prolapse the uterosacral ligaments may be detached from the cervix or torn near their sacral attachment. If one accepts the above argument then the surgical challenge is finding these defects during surgery. This will radically change the way prolapse surgery is performed. Length of the vagina is important so that the vagina is compressed against the pelvic floor and not telescoped upon itself by increases in intra-abdominal pressure.

Concern is often expressed as to the position of the ureter when trying to support the vaginal vault. The position of the ureter at vaginal hysterectomy for prolapse has been studied by DeLancey,[13] who has shown increasing separation between the cervix and ureter with increasing uterine prolapse descent. This means that patients with the largest prolapse can safely undergo the necessary shortening, sometimes up to 15 cm. Whether this shortening is in fact finding the detached caudal end of the ligament previously torn as the cause of the prolapse may be academic but it is important to use strong tissue. Many techniques of vault support are described in the literature, most using the pedicle sutures themselves to resuspend the vault. McCall[14] described his technique of culdoplasty in 1957, later modified by Nicholls.[15] Separate sutures placed through the full thickness of the vaginal skin, peritoneum and uterosacral ligaments obliterate the cul-de-sac and suspend the vault by the uterosacral ligaments. This also results in lengthening of the vagina. McCall originally used silk but since sutures need removal in 20% of cases delayed absorbable material such as polyglactin or polyglycolic acid may be preferable. Scientific evaluation of this method suggests an 85% success rate at nine years.[16] Information from the Mayo Clinic[16] on a series of 693 patients with post-hysterectomy vault prolapse identified only 47 (6.8%) patients with a previous vault repair after vaginal hysterectomy by this technique.

There is no published evidence that sacrospinous fixation at the time of primary vaginal hysterectomy and repair offers any advantage and this only increases the complication rate.[17]

SURGICAL APPROACHES TO POST-HYSTERECTOMY VAULT PROLAPSE

Pelvic floor repair for post-hysterectomy prolapse can be technically challenging and may involve repair of all vaginal supports. Anaesthetic considerations are paramount and regional anaesthesia may be appropriate to reduce opiate use, if nothing else. Adequate time must be allowed for pelvic reconstructive surgery and the aim is to restore structure and function, particularly for sexually active women.

Postoperative care is also important, particularly for the elderly, and strategies to avoid postoperative confusion and hypothermia need to be considered.

Vaginal approaches

Culdoplasty and uterosacral ligament suspension

Post-hysterectomy vault prolapse is typically associated with enterocele formation. However, enterocele can occur *de novo* from a break in the pericervical fascial ring. This defect can thus be repaired after ligating the enterocele sac and ensuring the apposition of rectovaginal and pubocervical fascia. However, in the majority of cases the vagina must also be suspended. This is also the case in surgical treatment of procidentia (third-degree uterine prolapse). Suspension can be performed by either high uterosacral ligament or sacrospinous ligament fixation as both result in effective vault support with preservation of vaginal length.[18]

McCall's original technique was to be used at the time of primary vaginal hysterectomy. This, therefore, needs some modification in the case of previous hysterectomy, not least because the uterosacral ligaments can be difficult to define. This is due to retraction closer to the sacrum although it is claimed[19] that they can always be found. Shull and Bachofen[19] describe a technique of high uterosacral ligament suspension to ensure that the remnants of the uterosacral ligaments are identified posterior and medial to the ischial spine as close to the sacrum as possible. It is then necessary to reattach the ligaments to the pubocervical and rectovaginal fascia to re-establish complete fascial integrity. However, there is concern over the position of the ureter and ureteric occlusion has been reported in up to 10% of cases.[20] This may be because of kinking due to the high purse-string suture often used to close the peritoneum. It is routine practice in many centres in the USA to perform cystoscopy with intravenous indigo carmine to ensure ureteral patency.[19] An alternative is to use ureteral stents to delineate the position of the ureter. There is scepticism from many surgeons as to whether this technique is really feasible for total vault eversion.

The Mayo Clinic reported the use of McCall's culdoplasty in 693 patients with post-hysterectomy prolapse.[16] Complications such as infection and bladder or rectal damage were low at 3% and there were no long-term sequelae. A postal survey of 660 patients operated on between 1976 and 1987 produced an 80% response. Only 36 (5.2%) patients had a definite second operation; 493 (71%) patients had no further operation after a mean of 8.8 years. Data on 164 (23.7%) were incomplete. Similar results were given for high uterosacral suspension, with only a 5% failure in 220 patients at one year.[21] There were only two instances of ureteral obstruction identified and dealt with at the time of surgery.

It has been further suggested that laparoscopy could be used to identify and tag the uterosacral ligaments.[22] The enterocele was then opened vaginally and excised. The sutures were then retrieved and used to support the vaginal vault and the pericervical ring reconstructed. These authors used 2–0 braided polyester but did have some problems with suture erosions. The addition of laparoscopy to otherwise vaginal surgery needs to be fully evaluated, as there will be the added risk of laparoscopy.

Sacrospinous fixation

In patients with total vaginal eversion, it may be difficult to find sufficient uterosacral ligament strength and Nichols[15] popularised sacrospinous ligament fixation for this indication. After opening the posterior vaginal wall and incising the right rectal pillar the sacrospinous ligament is identified. Two permanent sutures are placed through the ligament at least two fingerbreadths medial to the ischial spine. The sutures are attached to the vaginal skin and held until the vagina is two-thirds closed. When the sutures are tied, the vaginal apex is firmly attached to the surface of the sacrospinous ligament without a suture bridge. Unilateral fixation is usually sufficient but bilateral fixation can be considered in severe cases. Anatomically, there are concerns that the vagina is not supported on the left side in cases of right fixation and that the procedure produces an iatrogenic para-rectal fascial defect. However, there is good evidence that it is a successful procedure.

Over 1200 cases are reported in the literature but follow-up times are often not specified or are less than one year.[23] The overall success rate in published series is between 77% and 92% but early reports used absorbable sutures which are not recommended. The number of procedures performed in the UK is estimated at between 2000 and 3500 per year[24] but the success rate and complications have been reported in the literature for less than 100 patients.[25] The advantages of the vaginal route include a high success rate, fewer complications, less pain and a shorter hospital stay. There is also the opportunity to repair other defects. Specific complications include buttock pain in 3% of patients due to damage to a small nerve running through the sacrospinous ligament. This settles spontaneously by six weeks. However, gluteal pain and lumbar plexus neuropathy require immediate removal of sutures that have been incorrectly placed. Cystocele is frequently reported as a long-term problem after sacrospinous fixation but most studies have not compared results of similar patients undergoing pelvic floor repair with and without sacrospinous fixation.[26] It is possible that factors other than the sacrospinous fixation determine subsequent cystocele. *De novo* stress incontinence is rare.

Although infrequent, serious complications have been reported and, with the more widespread use of the technique, many are likely to go unreported. Life-threatening haemorrhage from laceration of the hypogastric venous plexus or inferior gluteal artery, resulting in death, has occurred.[27] Anatomic variations mean that the inferior gluteal artery may arise from the posterior division of the internal iliac artery and, hence, ligation of the hypogastric artery may increase pulse pressure and make matters worse rather than help (Figure 2). Vascular clips, packing or embolisation are suggested in these difficult situations and involvement of other colleagues is vital.

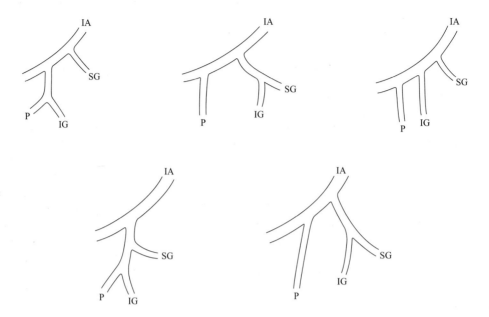

Figure 2 *Branching patterns of internal iliac artery; IA, internal iliac; SG, superior gluteal; IG, inferior gluteal; P, pudendal*

Other vaginal operations

Other vaginal operations include iliococcygeal fixation of the vagina. Partial vaginectomy, which is itself a treatment, seems to have been performed concomitantly but this will also result in a short vagina.[23] Obliterative procedures such as colpocleisis still have a place and can be performed under local anaesthetic.

Abdominal approach

Several authors have described the use of sacrocolpopexy interposing mesh between the vagina and sacrum.[1] The disadvantage of laparotomy is clear, particularly in the elderly, with more complications and a longer recovery time. Positioning the mesh retroperitoneally involves careful dissection to avoid the ureter, middle sacral vessels, common iliac vein and mesocolon. Non-absorbable sutures are used to attach the mesh to vagina and sacrum with careful assessment of length to avoid over correction. Synthetic mesh is used and success rates in excess of 90% at five years are reported.[1] A concomitant colposuspension can be performed if stress incontinence is present, although it is often necessary to repair vaginally any rectocele and deficient perineum. Serious operative complications occur in low numbers in the literature but are under reported by occasional operators. Severe haemorrhage causing death can occur from presacral veins and the surgeon needs to be aware of the options available, including thumbtacks and magnetic applicators. Postoperative intestinal obstruction can occur if the mesh is not buried and graft extrusion and vaginal rupture can occur due to poor vascularity of the cuff itself.

The abdominal procedures have been performed via laparoscopy as opposed to laparotomy.[28] Operating time is longer but the risks of surgery seem similar in experienced hands. Initial success seems acceptable but longer-term results are awaited.

TREATMENT OF OCCULT AND GENUINE STRESS INCONTINENCE

The management of cystocele and incontinence is dealt with in Chapter 16. However, it is important to raise the issue here, as many patients with vault prolapse will have clinical or occult genuine stress incontinence (GSI). Although vaginal techniques such as pubo-urethral ligament plication to elevate the urethra and urethrovesical junction and Kelly's plication of the bladder neck to eliminate funnelling are described, reliable data are not available.[15]

Colombo et al.,[29] from Milan, have addressed this issue in a randomised controlled trial of cystopexy alone versus cystopexy and pubo-urethral ligament plication in 102 continent patients undergoing surgery for prolapse. Four patients in each group (8%) had postoperative stress incontinence at one year. Colombo et al.[30] further investigated women undergoing surgery for prolapse who had either stress incontinence or potential stress incontinence (defined as 'positive stress test with repositioning') by randomising 109 patients to either concomitant pubo-urethral ligament plication or Pereyra suspension. With a minimum five-year follow-up, Pereyra suspension provided significantly better results for potential incontinence (100% versus 76% objective). However, for incontinent patients the cure rate was only 57% and not significantly different in either arm. Complications were higher for the Pereyra group, particularly the need for further anti-incontinence surgery. Veronikis,[31] however, reported a 56% incidence of low-pressure urethra as a cause of occult GSI and proposed a sling urethropexy using Mersilene mesh or fascia lata with a 100% success at one year.

The surgeon is often left with the dilemma of a combined vaginal and abdominal operation with increased operating time and morbidity. The optimum therapy for patients with urogenital prolapse and occult GSI thus remains to be determined, although with clinical stress incontinence a colposuspension is still the standard operation. As the morbidity of abdominal surgery is primarily the sacrocolpopexy there is the option of correcting the prolapse vaginally and then performing a coloposuspension.[19]

SUTURE MATERIAL

The ideal suture for vaginal surgery does not exist. If prolapse is regarded in the same way as a hernia, that is a distinct break in connective tissue support, the surgeon would use non-absorbable sutures of great strength. This is largely impractical in the vagina because of the substantial risk of suture erosion, dyspareunia and fistula formation. However, nothing less than delayed absorbable suture is logical, as connective tissue will only have 25% of its strength at three weeks, the time at which rapidly absorbable sutures will have disappeared.[32] Such material should, therefore, be used for culdoplasty and rectocele repair. In the anterior compartment, polytetrafluoroethylene (PTFE) has many attractive features, being a permanent monofilament suture that handles well and is incorporated into adjacent structures during healing. Some practise with knot tying is required as they tend to slip. The use of permanent polyester and polypropylene for posterior compartment repair has been described. However, suture erosion is a problem and follow-up data are required over a long period of time.[22]

SELECTION OF OPERATION

Table 1 shows a comparison of different methods of vaginal vault repair. Experienced operators report high success rates with most procedures, with vaginal operations having less morbidity. However, it is difficult to know what are the success rates in general gynaecological practice, particularly with occasional operators. Vault prolapse is a complicated problem and expertise is best concentrated. Therefore, it is likely that not all gynaecologists will deal with this problem. In younger women with concomitant urinary stress incontinence, the abdominal approach is likely to be more appropriate, since colposuspension would be the operation of choice to treat the stress incontinence.

In the absence of incontinence or cystocele, reported success rates are similar for vaginal and abdominal approaches and, thus, the major difference is in the occurrence of complications. Laparoscopic treatment is not recommended outside specialised centres due to expense, time and the need for a long learning curve for a relatively uncommon condition.

For elderly patients it seems clear that vaginal surgery carries less risk, lower morbidity, shorter hospital stay and faster return to normal activities. A comparative study from Canada reported a large personal series of 130 vaginal sacrospinous fixations and 80 abdominal sacrocolpopexies over six years.[33] It is not clear why one operation was chosen over the other, although 59 of the abdominal group (74%) also had a colposuspension. The failure rate over a mean of three years was 2% in both groups, perhaps highlighting good case selection for the procedures.

The only randomised study of vaginal versus abdominal surgery for recurrent prolapse was reported by Benson.[34] Of 101 patients randomised, 88 completed the study and half the patients had complete pelvic organ prolapse. Abdominal sacrocolpopexy showed a higher success rate and the need for fewer subsequent operations. However, the number of procedures performed on each patient was more than three and, hence, interpretation is difficult.

CONCLUSIONS

Vaginal vault prolapse is a difficult condition to manage and not one for the occasional operator. From published series, both vaginal and abdominal approaches appear equally effective (Figure 3) and individual patient assessment by a surgeon regularly performing such procedures would appear to be the key to success rather than the procedure *per se*.

Table 1 *Comparison of different methods of vaginal vault repair*

Method of repair	Advantages	Disadvantages
McCull culdoplasty	Low risk Good published results	Difficulty identifying uterosacral ligaments in advanced cases
High uterosacral suspension and fascial defect repair	Anatomically based	Difficulty identifying defects Minimal published data Risk of ureteric occlusion
Sacrospinous fixation	Easily learnt Good published results	Relies on small area of support Unilateral fixation leaves other side unsupported Risk of serious complications
Open sacrocolpopexy	Good published results Can combine with colposuspension	High risk of morbidity May need vaginal repair of other defects
Laparoscopic sacrocolpopexy	Lower morbidity in experienced hands Can combine with colposuspension	Long learning curve Expensive Success data awaited

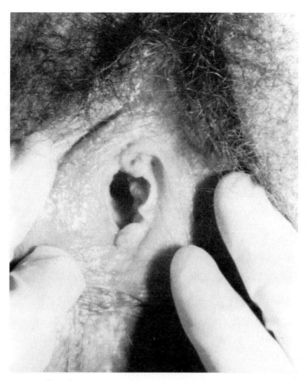

Figure 3 *Successful reconstruction of post-hysterectomy prolapse*

References

1. Toozs-Hobson, P., Boos K., Cardozo L. Management of vaginal vault prolapse. *Br J Obstet Gynaecol* 1998;**105**:13–17
2. Olsen, A.L., Smith, V.J., Bergstrom, J.O., Colling, J.C., Clark, A.L. Epidemiology of surgically managed pelvic organ prolapse and urinary incontinence. *Obstet Gynecol* 1997;**89**:501–6
3. Baden, W.F., Walker, T. *Surgical Repair of Vaginal Defects*. Philadelphia: Lippincott; 1992
4. Marchionni, M.D., Bracco, G.L., Checcucci, V., Crarbaneanu, A., Coccia, E.M., Megacci, F. et al. True incidence of vaginal vault prolapse. *J Reprod Med* 1999;**44**:679–84
5. Welgoss, J.A., Vogt, V.Y., McClellan, E.J., Benson J.T. Relationship between surgically induced neuropathy and outcome of pelvic organ prolapse surgery. *Int Urogynecol J Pelvic Floor Dysfunct* 1999;**1**:111–14
6. Wiskind, A.K., Creighton, S.M., Stanton, S.L. Incidence of genital prolapse after the Burch colposuspension. *Am J Obstet Gynaecol* 1992;**167**:399–405
7. Bump, R.C., Mattiason, A., Bo, K., Brubaker, L.P., DeLancey, J.O., Klarskov, P. et al. The standardisation of terminology of female pelvic organ prolapse and pelvic floor dysfunction. *Am J Obstet Gynecol* 1996;**175**:10–17
8. Steele, A., Mallipeddi, P., Welgoss, J., Soled, S., Kohli, N., Karram, M. Teaching the Pelvic Organ Prolapse Quantitation system. *Am J Obstet Gynecol* 1998;**179**:458–64
9. Veronikis, D.K., Nichols, D.H., Wakamatsu, M.M. The incidence of low-pressure urethra as a

function of prolapse-reducing technique in patients with massive pelvic organ prolapse (maximum descent at all vaginal sites). *Am J Obstet Gynecol* 1997;**177**:1305–14

10   Versi, E., Griffiths, D.J., Giovanini, D. Video-urodynamic diagnosis of occult genuine stress incontinence (GSI) in patients with anterior vaginal wall relaxation. *J Soc Gynecol Investig* 1998;**5**:327–30

11   Muller, K. Operating on the elderly woman. *Curr Opin Obstet Gynecol* 1997;**3**:300–5

12   Ashcroft, G.S., Dodsworth, J., van Boxtel, E., Tarnuzzer, R.W., Horan, M.A., Schultz, G.S. et al. Estrogen accelerates cutaneous wound healing associated with an increase in TGF-B1 levels. *Nat Med* 1997;**3**:1209–15

13   DeLancey, J.O., Strohbehn, K., Aronson, M.P. Comparison of ureteral and cervical descents during vaginal hysterectomy for vaginal prolapse. *Am J Obstet Gynecol* 1998;**179**:1405–10

14   McCall, M. Posterior culdoplasty. *Obstet Gynecol* 1957;**10**:595–602

15   Nichols, D.H., Randall, C.L. *Vaginal Surgery*, 4th ed. Baltimore: Williams and Wilkins; 1996

16   Webb, M.J., Aronson, M.P., Ferguson, L.K, Lee, R.A. Post hysterectomy vaginal vault prolapse: primary repair in 693 patients. *Obstet Gynecol* 1998;**92**:281–5

17   Colombo, M., Milani, R. Sacrospinous ligament fixation and modified McCall culdoplasty during vaginal hysterectomy for advanced vaginal prolapse. *Am J Obstet Gynecol* 1998;**179**:13–20

18   Elkins, T.E., Hopper, J.B., Goodfellow, K., Gasser, R., Nolan, T.E., Schexnayder, M.C. Initial report of anatomic and clinical comparison of the sacrospinous ligaments fixation to the high McCall culdoplasty for vaginal cuff fixation at hysterectomy for uterine prolapse. *Journal of Pelvic Surgery* 1995;**1**:12–17

19   Shull, B.L., Bachofen, C. Enterocele and rectocoele. In: Walters, M.D., Karram, M.M., editors. *Urogynaecology and Reconstructive Pelvic Surgery*, 2nd ed. St Louis: Mosby; 1999. p. 221–234

20   Barber, M., Visco, A., Weidner, A., Amundsen, C.L., Bump, R.C. Bilateral uterosacral ligament vaginal vault suspension with site-specific endopelvic fascia defect repair for treatment of pelvic organ prolapse. *Am J Obstet Gynecol* 2000;**183**:1402–11

21   Shull, B.L., Bachofen, C., Coates, K.W., Kuehl, T.J. A transvaginal approach to the repair of apical and other associated sites of pelvic organ prolapse with uterosacral ligaments. *Am J Obstet Gynecol* 2000;**183**:1365–74

22   Miklos, J.R., Kohli, N., Lucente, V., Saye, W.B. Site-specific fascial defects in the diagnosis and surgical management of enterocele. *Am J Obstet Gynecol* 1998;**179**:1418–23

23   Sze, E.H., Karram, M.M. Transvaginal repair of vault prolapse: a review. *Obstet Gynecol* 1997;**89**:466–75

24   Carey, M.O., Slack, M.C. Transvaginal sacrospinous colpopexy for vault and marked uterovaginal prolapse. *Br J Obstet Gynaecol* 1994;**101**:536–40

25   J. Hawkins, Corey Brothers Ltd, Brittacy Hill, London. Personal communication

26   Holley, R.L., Varner, R.E., Gleason, B.P., Apffel, L.A., Scott, S. Recurrent pelvic support defects after sacrospinous ligament fixation for vaginal vault prolapse. *J Am Coll Surg* 1995;**180**:444–8

27   Barksdale, P.A., Elkins, T.E., Sanders, C.K., Jaramillo, F.E., Gasser, R.F. An anatomic approach to pelvic hemorrhage during sacrospinous ligament fixation of the vaginal vault. *Obstet Gynecol* 1998;**91**:715–18

28   Mahendran, D., Prashar, S., Smith, A.R., Murphy D. Laparoscopic sacrocolpopexy in the management of vaginal vault prolapse. *Gynecol Endosc* 1996;**5**:217–22

29   Colombo, M., Maggioni, A., Zanetta, G., Vignaci, M., Milani, R. Prevention of postoperative stress urinary incontinence after surgery for genitourinary prolapse. *Obstet Gynecol* 1996;**87**:266–71

30 Colombo, M., Maggioni, A., Scalambrino, S., Vitobello, D., Milani, R. Surgery for genitourinary prolapse and stress incontinence: a randomised trial of posterior pubourethral ligament plication and Pereyra suspension. *Am J Obstet Gynecol* 1997;**176**:337–43

31 Veronikis, D.K., Nichols, D.H., Wakamatsu, M.M. The incidence of low-pressure urethra as a function of prolapse-reducing technique in patients with massive pelvic organ prolapse (maximum descent at all vaginal sites). *Am J Obstet Gynecol* 1997;**177**:1305–14

32 Sanz, L.E. Sutures in gynaecologic surgery. *Contemporary Ob/Gyn* 1998;**43**:57–72

33 Hardiman, P.J., Drutz, H.P. Sacrospinous vault suspension and abdominal colposacropexy: success rates and complications. *Am J Obstet Gynecol* 1996;**175**:612–16

34 Benson, J.T., Lucente, V., McClellan, E. Vaginal versus abdominal reconstructive surgery for the treatment of pelvic support defects: a prospective randomised study with long-term outcome evaluation. *Am J Obstet Gynecol* 1996;**175**:1418–22

21

Rectovaginal endometriosis

Jeremy T. Wright, David B. Redwine and Norman Ratcliffe

INTRODUCTION

Rectovaginal endometriosis with obliteration of the cul-de-sac is regarded as one of the most challenging conditions in gynaecology. In women with this condition, invasive endometriotic disease of the cul-de-sac involves the uterosacral ligaments, the posterior cervix, frequently the rectovaginal septum and the anterior bowel wall. Such advanced rectovaginal disease is a cause of much pelvic pain and discomfort including dysmenorrhoea, low abdominal pain, dyspareunia and dyschezia.[1] Treatment options include hormone regulation or anti-inflammatory drugs and analgesics to control symptoms or surgery, either thermal ablative surgery or excision. The success rate of these individual treatments is poorly documented and variable.

This chapter explores the history, incidence and aetiology of rectovaginal endometriosis, together with the relevant clinical history, examination and treatment.

HISTORY

Endometriosis is perceived as a relatively modern problem but it is well described in the pathological literature of the 17th century.[2] Perhaps the first known description is by the German physician Daniel Shroen in 1690.[3] He describes 'pelvic sores and inflammations that have the tendency to form adhesions that link viscera together'. He was remarkably perceptive in this description of non-ovarian endometriosis. He went on to suggest that it was a relatively common disease and he stated categorically 'this is a female disorder characteristic of those who are sexually maturing'.

There then followed a number of other European studies in the 18th century[4-7] whose authors, although lacking microscopes and histology, still saw the clinical pathology of endometriosis in detail. Louise Brotherson, a Scottish doctor, wrote in 1776: 'In its worst stages, this disease affects the well-being of the female patient totally and adversely, her whole spirit is broken, yet she lives in fear of still more symptoms such as further pain, the loss of consciousness and convulsions'.[8]

CLINICAL LITERATURE

The often spectacular surgical presentations of endometriosis have made the disease a favourite of descriptive morphologists. Cullen[9-12] wrote extensively on rectovaginal endometriosis, describing adenomyomas of the rectovaginal septum and of the rectal wall; his descriptions stand up well to those of later authors. Classic descriptions of adenomyomas of the rectovaginal septum appear in the literature in 1929.[13] Other case reports occur in the literature from 1921,[14,15] with advice, in 1949,[16] that pregnancy will cure the disease. An early case series in the literature from 1940[17] studied a group of 31 patients, six of whom were treated by castration with surgery or radium, achieving good symptomatic relief and decreasing the size of the lesions. Among 25 treated by conservative surgery, 92% had reduction of symptoms but only 19% had reduction of nodule size.

Despite advice as long ago as 1951[18] that hysterectomy and bilateral salpingo-oophorectomy should be accompanied by excision of bowel implants this procedure is only rarely carried out today.

Although histological diagnosis is regarded as important in all other branches of surgery, it is rare for the diagnosis to be confirmed histologically, except on extirpated portions of bowel. Uterosacral ligament disease is rarely confirmed by biopsy.

The first proposal that rectovaginal adenomyomas were separate entities from peritoneal endometriosis was in 1950,[19] which was to be echoed by Donnez et al. in 1998.[20] In 1950, Holmes[21] presented a case series of 145 patients with endometriosis, of whom 23 were noted to have nodules on rectal examination. He felt that excision was too dangerous and that the treatment should be bilateral oophorectomy. This series prolonged the debate between the protagonists of excision of the disease[18] and those who felt that this was too dangerous.[21] Henriksen, as early as 1955,[22] made the point that medical treatment was not particularly effective in his hands.

The clinical literature on the subject consists largely of case reports from all over the world, all of which highlight the apparent rarity of the condition and the need for segmental bowel resection. Many of the reports are in surgical[23] rather than gynaecological journals, typically consisting of between one and six cases.

The vast majority of patients in these reports were treated surgically at laparotomy by segmental resection of the bowel, although treatment of coexisting pelvic disease was usually recommended.[24] Superficial excision of seromuscular disease appeared in the surgical literature in 1973.[25]

THE PATHOLOGY OF RECTOVAGINAL ENDOMETRIOSIS

Definition and incidence

Endometriosis is defined as the presence of tissue which resembles endometrium, but which is located outside the uterus. Endometriosis tissue is not identical to eutopic endometrium, having multiple enzymatic,[26] histologic,[27] chromosomal[28] and immunohistochemical[29] differences from native endometrium.

Pelvic endometriosis affects 5–10% of menstruating women.[30] The incidence of bowel involvement in such women varies greatly between published series with reported incidences of 3–34%. In many cases, bowel involvement is serosal and nonsymptomatic but, with deeper involvement, symptomatic disease may result and require treatment to control symptoms or to exclude malignancy.

The sites of bowel involvement are, in descending order of frequency, rectosigmoid, ileum, appendix and caecum. In cases of rectosigmoid involvement the disease is usually located anteriorly on the antimesenteric aspect of the bowel, such distribution being relevant to techniques of surgical ablation.[1]

Women who have ovarian endometriosis are more likely to have bowel involvement than those without ovarian disease and, in women who have confirmed endometriosis of the bowel, approximately 97.2% have coexisting pelvic disease.[31]

Histology of endometriosis

Histological definition depends on the recognition of both stromal and glandular components of endometrium in microscopic sections (Figure 1). Confusion may arise if lesser histological criteria are accepted for diagnosis. Frequently, there is evidence of bleeding from adjacent capillaries that

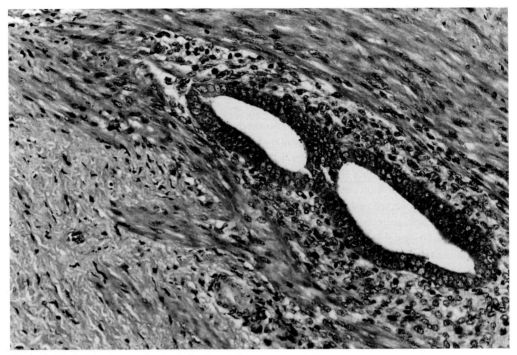

Figure 1 *Histological appearance of rectovaginal endometriosis*

may be recent or old and is often characterised by blood-derived pigment within macrophages. However, many subtle lesions lack any haemorrhage at all.[32] Although commonly associated with endometriotic foci, the presence of haemorrhage, haemosiderin or cells resembling endometrial stroma without associated glandular tissue do not in themselves establish the diagnosis histologically. Biologically active lesions are frequently associated with fibrosis that may be dense and adhesive. In bowel lesions there may be striking hypertrophy of smooth muscle reminiscent of the changes seen in adenomyosis of the uterus. The varying histology may represent a wider spectrum of oestrogen-dependent non-endometriotic causes of pelvic pain originating in the peritoneum.

Morphological changes attributable to cyclical hormonal stimulation have been described in 44–80% of resected samples[27] but often the epithelial changes seen in eutopic endometrium in the luteal phase of the cycle are impaired or absent in synchronously removed endometriotic foci.[33-35]

PATHOGENESIS

For more than a century the pathogenesis of endometriosis has generated tremendous debate of both clinical and academic interest, as a better understanding of the origin of endometriosis is likely to lead to more rational and effective therapy.

Traditionally pelvic endometriosis has been recognised in three forms:

(1) Peritoneal endometriosis;

(2) Ovarian endometriosis;

(3) Rectovaginal endometriosis.

Peritoneal lesions have for long been thought to be due to either retrograde menstruation and peritoneal implantation, or the so-called metastatic theory historically associated with Sampson[36] and, more recently, Nisolle et al.[32] The latter authors have compared eutopic endometrium with peritoneal and rectovaginal endometriotic tissue using a variety of parameters. These include mitotic activity, stromal vascularisation, epithelial to stromal ratios, quantitative immunohistochemical characteristics, including hormone receptor status, as well as differing therapeutic responses to gonadotrophin-releasing hormone agonists and lynestrenol. By comparing such parameters, Nisolle et al.[32] concluded that rectovaginal disease appears to be different from peritoneal disease and that the observed variation in oestrogen receptor and progesterone receptor content suggests that the regulatory mechanisms of rectovaginal endometriosis differ from those of eutopic endometrium.

In addition, Nisolle et al.[32] also hypothesised that rectovaginal endometriosis is not due to deep-infiltrating implanted endometriosis but most likely derives from embryologically determined rests of Müllerian tissue within the rectovaginal septum.

The Müllerian origin of rectovaginal endometriosis is supported by Redwine,[37,39] who also extends the concept of Mülleriosis to include peritoneal and other sites of endometriosis in both men and women. He questions most of the evidence supporting the retrograde menstruation/implantation hypothesis as it is mostly circumstantial. A problem with Sampson's hypothesis is that convincing histological demonstration or robust photomicrographic evidence of recent attachment of shed endometrial fragments to peritoneum in early peritoneal lesions is lacking, despite the extensive literature on the subject. If retrograde menstruation were to result in attachment of shed endometrial fragments to peritoneum, evidence would be available. The lack of such robust evidence must question Sampson's theory of origin. Cullen's work also shows clear evidence that rectovaginal adenomas are separate entities and make retrograde menstruation unlikely as a cause.

The gratifying and protracted clinical response to excision of endometriosis tissue obtained by several specialist centres[20,24,39,40] would seem surprising if the disease were being reimplanted on a monthly basis and argues strongly for derivation of the disease from developmentally abnormal or metaplastic Müllerian tissue.

DIFFERENTIAL DIAGNOSIS OF RECTOVAGINAL ENDOMETRIOSIS

The major clinical differential diagnoses to be considered are primary malignancies of the colon and rectum, inflammatory bowel disease, diverticulitis, pelvic inflammatory disease and pelvic abscess. However, in women of reproductive age endometriosis is far more common than any of the above conditions and it should be considered first in women with pelvic pain, dysmenorrhoea or dyspareunia.

Clinical features

A 1995 review[39] of the symptomatology of rectovaginal endometriosis presented a group of patients in whom severe backache, lower abdominal pain, dyschezia and constipation predominated. Diarrhoea can become a problem when laxatives are used frequently, although some patients complain of diarrhoea with the menstrual flow. Associated features are severe dyspareunia and, sometimes, heavy, painful periods.[39] Patients may also rarely present with rectal or sigmoid stricturing.[40] If a detailed history is taken, it is common to find that symptoms started from menarche and either have been ignored or treated as primary dysmenorrhoea, usually with oral contraceptives. Concomitant pelvic endometriosis and ovarian cysts are also frequently reported. Despite these severe symptoms, there is rarely any systemic upset and general examination is usually normal apart from mild lower abdominal tenderness. Patients frequently resist pelvic examination because they know that it will be painful and this may well be interpreted as having a psychological cause, sometimes leading to years of ill-advised psychosexual counselling. They also suffer rectal pain with the passage of stool and flatus and sometimes even sitting down. As part of the initial assessment, it is useful to ask the patient to rate their symptoms on a simple ranked ordinal scale that will allow later comparison. The interrelationship of the severity of different symptoms can then be explored, as can the effectiveness of any intervention.

Pelvic examination

Pelvic examination should be gentle and thorough. Speculum examination should particularly concentrate on examination of the posterior vaginal fornix. This is best achieved by tipping a bivalve speculum posterior to the cervix and opening it up so as to expose the vaginal epithelium posterior to the cervix, which may of itself cause some discomfort in patients with rectovaginal disease. Rectovaginal disease can frequently be seen invading the vaginal epithelium (Figure 2) and can be identified by the disruption of normal rugae in the overlying vagina, epithelial piling, distortion and small bluish cysts. It is invariably retained within the boundaries of the uterosacral ligaments.

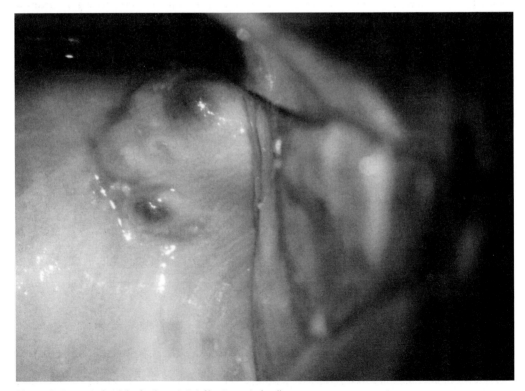

Figure 2 *Rectovaginal nodule of endometriosis infiltrating vaginal wall*

Bimanual vaginal examination should then assess the size, position and mobility of the uterus. An assessment should then be made for adnexal tenderness and the presence of any ovarian enlargement. The remainder of the examination is performed only with the internal hand while the examiner regards the facial and body expressions of the patient. Patients with the disease will usually grimace, if not cry out and push up on the table, away from the examiner's hand. The uterosacral ligaments should be gently palpated and stroked for any tender nodularity, which is more common on the left than the right. Palpation of the pouch of Douglas will often reveal a tender, fixed nodule of endometriosis that may involve the rectovaginal septum. This can frequently be confirmed on rectal examination or by concomitant rectal and vaginal palpation. Rectal examination should be part of the routine assessment of rectovaginal disease.

Investigation

Investigations are usually unrewarding. Levels of serum CA125 may be marginally raised, particularly in the presence of ovarian endometriomas and there may be a slight rise in erythrocyte sedimentation rate. Colonoscopy and sigmoidoscopy is described in much of the surgical literature but mostly with negative results for endometriosis, although this may rule out primary bowel problems. Passage of the instrument or contrast past a rectosigmoid stricture may be difficult but the mucosa is largely intact and the reports commonly describe extrinsic compression. Trans-anal ultrasound examination has been employed to delineate the lesions but this requires specially modified rectal probes and, frequently, distension of the rectum with a liquid medium, therefore making it unsuitable for everyday use.[41] Although localised, ultrasonographic techniques have proved useful in defining the extent of proven or suspected endometriosis of the rectovaginal septum.[42] It is important to remember that there are no radiological or diagnostic imaging findings specific for endometriosis and unequivocal diagnosis requires microscopic examination.

Most vaginal ultrasound probes are not suitable for demonstrating the pouch of Douglas, so most nodular lesions are missed on ultrasound examination. However, with experience they can be demonstrated. Modern magnetic resonance imaging techniques can also demonstrate endometriotic lesions. However, all these tests largely confirm what can be found on digital examination; no test is in itself diagnostic, nor do any of them eliminate the patient's pain or the need for surgical evaluation of that pain. Ureteric compression or infiltration is more common than it was thought to be and pre-operative assessment of renal function by ultrasound or intravenous pyelography is wise.

Laparoscopy

Laparoscopy is a major diagnostic tool, although it is frequently inadequate and carried out by unsupervised doctors in training. The following problems may arise:

(1) The patient will not be put in sufficiently steep Trendelenberg position to allow proper inspection of the pouch of Douglas.

(2) There will be inadequate visualisation because of either poor equipment or poor patient position. Unless the patient is appropriately placed on the operating table, vaginal and uterine manipulation is impeded.

(3) Appropriate laparoscopic inspection involves inspection of the whole of the pelvic peritoneum including both ovarian fossae and the anterior and posterior cul-de-sacs. This requires manipulating these structures and moving bowel and fluid out of the posterior cul-de-sac.

(4) Many diagnostic laparoscopies are carried out using a suprapubically placed Veress needle as the second port for manipulation, which is entirely inadequate to allow for proper visualisation. Ideally, a laterally placed 5-mm port should be employed to allow access for a suction irrigation probe.

(5) Laterally placed ports run the risk of inferior epigastric injury but, as these vessels are constant in position, they can always be avoided. The inferior epigastrics are always situated in a triangle between the obliterated umbilical vessels and the insertion of the round ligament and they can usually be identified visually by observing them laparoscopically through the anterior parietal peritoneum. The laterally placed port can be inserted when the abdomen is fully inflated and the point directed medially. This can either be under direct vision or by supporting the abdominal wall from the peritoneal side with the laparoscope just medial to the point of insertion of the 5-mm trocar and directing the trocar so that it passes directly under the laparoscope and into the pneumoperitoneum. Control of the tension on the abdominal wall will ensure that there is no rapid or explosive insertion of the trocar leading to possible damage of underlying viscera.

(6) Having adequately inspected the pelvis using either the sucker irrigator or a pair of forceps, the pelvis, particularly the pouch of Douglas and uterosacral ligaments, should be inspected for areas of nodularity while they are on the stretch by pushing the uterus out of the pelvis with the intrauterine manipulator. Nodular endometriosis is classically hard and the probe will appear to click over it. Ideally, these areas should be treated by excision biopsy but, regrettably, this is rarely undertaken. In these circumstances, biopsies of at least one of the endometriotic lesions should be undertaken to confirm the diagnosis histologically, with plans for later referral for specialist surgical care.

Rectovaginal disease is often not associated with florid flame haemorrhages or active vascular change; on the contrary, frequently an apparently small vascular lesion on the uterosacral ligament may be the tip of a large rectovaginal nodule. Associated fibromuscular metaplasia and fibrosis usually gives a yellowish or whitish appearance, occasionally with overlying haemorrhagic discoloration. Frank rectovaginal endometriosis will be diagnosed by observing dense adhesive fibrotic disease with obliteration of the pelvic cul-de-sac. Involvement of the rectum can be identified visually as 'the rounded rectum' (Figure 3), indicating a round bulge in the rectal wall at the point of attachment to the posterior cervix as the uterus is held in extreme anteversion and elevation by an intrauterine manipulator. Rectal involvement is uncommon if the surface of the rectum is flat at its point of adherence to the posterior cervix.

TREATMENT

The treatment of this disease has been a matter of some controversy. The pathology is that of dense fibrosis with relatively small areas of poorly hormone-responsive endometriosis. Although oestrogen and progesterone receptors can be demonstrated in this tissue, hormonal manipulation will do little to suppress the disease.[43] Even if there is some suppression during the time that hormones are administered, the disease and the symptoms will return once hormone manipulation is stopped, since no medicine eradicates endometriosis. The majority of case reports in the literature have dealt with disease in the bowel but have not tackled the surrounding pelvic fibrosis with its associated invasive endometriosis. This type of disease requires excision. The surgical series with the best postoperative results are those in which pelvic as well as intestinal endometriosis is tackled radically.

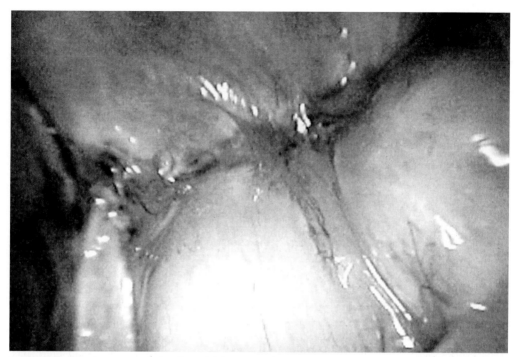

Figure 3 *Laparoscopic appearance of a bowel 'rounded' by rectovaginal nodule of endometriosis*

Surgical treatment of rectovaginal disease requires meticulous preparation of the patient, both emotionally and physically. Detailed and adequate counselling is important and should be backed up by appropriate written material. Also, women should receive osmotic and physical bowel preparation with 'on table' lavage if there is any faecal residue.

In a series of 130 women[24] who had undergone aggressive surgical management by laparotomy of advanced colorectal endometriosis, including low anterior resection, sigmoid resection, disk excision of the rectal wall, or right hemicolectomy, 90% of the patients reported good relief of their pelvic symptomatology and there was a crude pregnancy rate of 44%. There was no significant morbidity.

In a further study[44] of 163 cases of bowel endometriosis there was also good symptomatic relief. Colonic surgery was carried out by general surgeons, and gynaecologists carried out multiple excision biopsies of small endometriotic implants.

In all the literature, the morbidity is extremely low when a deliberate decision is taken to excise the areas of endometriosis in the rectovaginal septum or bowel but rises when there is an attempt to dissect the adhesive disease binding the rectum to the posterior cervix. This probably results from small, unrecognised tears developing which are held open by the surrounding fibrosis, allowing for faecal soiling. One of the great difficulties of assessing the extent of the disease is, of course, its adhesive nature.

The laparoscopic management of rectovaginal endometriosis has mostly been pioneered in the USA and in Europe. The approaches of the various schools are different. The biggest modern published series is by Donnez *et al.*[20] Their technique is based on the principle that the disease is adenomyosis of the rectovaginal septum and that endometriotic involvement of the rectal muscularis or mucosa does not occur. They demonstrated plaque disease on double-contrast barium enema and this is described as 'perivisceritis'. The technique they describe is to stay within the uterosacral ligaments and dissect the cervix free from the rectum. Once the rectum is free, the vaginal adenomyoma is removed transvaginally and the defect sutured. Any residual endometriosis is ablated using a CO_2 laser that is also the primary tool of dissection. Good symptomatic relief is claimed for this method but there has been no objective follow-up. Complications included the bowel lumen being entered on three occasions, although there was no significant morbidity from this. There remains controversy about their opinions that the bowel wall is almost never involved. The vast majority of the other literature on this subject describes endometriotic lesions involving the muscularis propria, although penetration to the mucosa is rare.

A similar technique has been employed by Wood et al.[45] in a small series using gasless laparoscopy and an abdominal elevator. Theoretically, this allows a simultaneous laparoscopic and vaginal approach to ease the dissection and no morbidity was reported.

Nezhat et al.[46] have reported laparoscopic dissection and partial proctectomy using a stapling technique, as have Reich et al.,[47] who reported on a series of 100 women. Both these groups advised the use of a CO_2 laser but, in subsequent reports, Reich has used cold-scissor dissection with bipolar diathermy. Scissor dissection has the advantage of allowing constant palpation of the tissue, allowing soft, normal tissue to be distinguished from firmer, fibrotic, diseased tissue.

Many surgical techniques for the management of rectovaginal endometriosis share two flaws. The first is only treating the adhesions, not the disease. When encountering obliteration of the cul-de-sac an attempt is made only to dissect the rectum from the uterus, cervix and uterosacral ligaments, by incision through the disease. Hence, nothing is done to the disease remaining on either side of the incision. When this part of the dissection is completed, the surgeon is left with a broad, raw area extending from the posterior cervix, down across the cul-de-sac and on to the anterior bowel wall. All invasive disease is still present and the raw surfaces remaining make identification of residual disease or unrecognised bowel injury problematic. Secondly, there remains concern over the ability of thermal ablation techniques alone to eradicate invasive disease completely and safely.

The approach adopted by two clinical authors[48] is a radical *en bloc* dissection using unipolar electrodiathermy delivered through 3-mm scissors at high settings (90 W cutting, 50 W coagulation). These high settings allow a high power density with rapid cutting of tissue by vaporisation and little lateral thermal spread.

When there is involvement of the vaginal mucosa it is helpful first to delineate this using a vaginal approach prior to the laparoscopy. Using a pencil electrode and coagulation current, the nodule is outlined by incision of the vaginal mucosa, which is then extended into the softer tissue of the rectovaginal septum posteriorly, followed by blunt finger dissection laterally. Usually, little bleeding is encountered. This will considerably ease the final stages of the laparoscopic dissection.

The laparoscopic dissection begins with incisions lateral and parallel to the uterosacral ligaments in normal peritoneum followed by blunt undermining of the uterosacral ligament. An important technical point is the need to keep the tissue to be cut under strong tension applied through the graspers and this is also facilitated by keeping the uterus in extreme anteversion, patient positioning being all-important. This prevents tissue 'pillowing' around the electrode and reduces the risk of inadvertent tissue damage. The electrosurgical current should be delivered in short, sharp bursts so that the tissue is divided with the minimum of lateral thermal spread. A transverse incision is created across the cervix or fundus above the line of adherence of the bowel. An intrafascial dissection with electrosurgery is then carried down toward the rectovaginal septum. The uterosacral ligaments are transected at the cervical insertions in this process. No attempt is made to dissect in the plane of adherence of the bowel. The lateral fatty attachments of the bowel to the pelvic side-walls are severed. Only when the rectum is mobilised completely and free along its length is the endometriotic area excised. If it involves the vaginal mucosa, the vagina is opened at this point and because of the mobility of the rectum, it is often possible to dissect disease off the rectum and undertake a repair transvaginally. The hypertrophied muscular layers of the bowel wall frequently allow the surgeon to bluntly peel the affected layers off underlying mucosa (mucosal skinning, as described by Redwine[48]). If the vagina is opened before the laparoscopic dissection is complete, adequate pneumoperitoneum can be maintained by placing a wet laparotomy pack in the vagina.

In 70% of cases, the rectal mucosa is not penetrated during resection, in which case a laparoscopic repair can be undertaken by just closing the seromuscular layer. If dense submucosal fibrosis causes the mucosa to be penetrated during the dissection, the disk of diseased tissue can be removed transrectally and a two-layer repair undertaken. The repair can be checked for leaks by underwater trans-anal air pressure examination. This approach, together with meticulous attention to haemostasis and peritoneal toilet, is associated with a low morbidity.

In the authors' American and English series,[49] excision of rectovaginal disease using this technique is associated with good symptom relief, low morbidity and a short one- or two-day hospital stay.

Garry et al.[50] have recently reported improvement in the quality of life using physical wellbeing scores in a group of 57 patients over a four-month period, the first major UK paper on the subject.

The management of rectovaginal endometriosis for gynaecologists with little intestinal surgical experience will frequently require close co-operation between coloproctologists and gynaecologists with a special interest in the disease. There are few gynaecologists in the UK who would consider undertaking rectal surgery and equally there are few coloproctologists who understand the pathology of endometriotic disease involving the bowel. This is a disease of the seromuscularis of the bowel that rarely involves the mucosa. In particular, it usually only involves the antimesenteric border of the bowel and, therefore, limited disk resection of the bowel is frequently all that is required.

MANAGEMENT STRATEGIES

With increased planning and interest it is possible for patients to be offered the appropriate laparoscopic surgery by trained and interested individuals. Such surgery requires meticulous planning and patient preparation with time spent with the patient to allow them to understand its benefits and shortcomings. However, with the severe symptoms that these patients suffer, together with their lack of response to hormone manipulation, the majority of patients with rectovaginal disease will require extensive surgery, which we suggest is best performed laparoscopically. This should ideally be performed by surgeons with a particular interest in the disease and there is now a strong argument for the specialty of 'benign gynaecology' to undertake this sort of surgery in specialist subregional centres. There is increasing evidence that the majority of gynaecological surgery can now be performed laparoscopically, safely and with decreased morbidity to the patient. This is certainly true of endometriosis in general and rectovaginal disease in particular. Much of this is nodular and fibrotic requiring excision. It has been demonstrated internationally in many centres that the laparoscopic approach is both safe and efficacious and, with appropriate training, can be used for women with this condition.

References

1 Redwine, D.B. Treatment of endometriosis of the cul-de-sac. In: Nezhat, C., editor. *Endometriosis: Advanced Management and Surgical Techniques*. Berlin: Springer Verlag; 1995. p. 105–15
2 Knapp, V.J. How old is endometriosis? Late 17th and 18th century European descriptions of the disease. *Fertil Steril* 1999;**72**:10–14
3 Shroen, D. *Disputatio Inauguralis Medica de Ulceribus Uteri*. Jena: Krebs; 1690. p. 6–17
4 Tailford, R. *Dissertatio Medica Inauguralis de Ulcere Uteri*. Louvain: Theodorum; 1765. p. 7–14
5 Duff, A. *Dissertatio Inauguralis Medica de Metritide*. Louvain: Haak; 1769. p. 6–31
6 Ludgers, A. *Dissertatio Medico-practica Inauguralis de Hysteritide*. Louvain: Wiskoff; 1776. p. 3–32
7 Gebhard, J. *Dissertatio Medica de Inflammatione Uteri*. Marburg: Rayroff; 1786. p. 30–2
8 Brotherson, L. *Dissertatio Medica Inauguralis de Utero Inflammatione Ejusdem*. Edinburgh: Balfour and Smellie; 1776. p. 16–22
9 Cullen, T.S. Adenomyoma of the recto-vaginal septum. *JAMA* 1914;**62**:835–9
10 Cullen, T.S. Adenomyoma of the recto-vaginal septum. *JAMA* 1916;**67**:401–6
11 Cullen, T.S. Adenomyoma of the recto-vaginal septum. *Johns Hopkins Hospital Bulletin* 1917;**321**:343–8
12 Cullen, T.S. The distribution of adenomyomas containing uterine mucosa. *Arch Surg* 1920;**1**:215–83
13 Read, C.D., Roques, F. Results of the operative treatment of endometriomata. *BMJ* 1929;**i**:1159–60
14 Payne, F.L. The clinical aspects of pelvic endometriosis. *Am J Obstet Gynecol* 1940;**39**:373–82
15 Sampson, J.A. Perforating haemorrhagic (chocolate) cysts of the ovary. *Arch Surg* 1921;**3**:245–323
16 Cullen, T.S. The distribution of adenomyomas containing uterine mucosa. *Arch Surg* 1920;**1**:215–83
17 Beecham, C.T. Surgical treatment of endometriosis. *JAMA* 1949;**139**:971–2
18 Huffman, J.W. External endometriosis. *Am J Obstet Gynecol* 1951;**62**:1243–52
19 Fallon, J., Brosnan, J.T., Manning, J.J., Moran, W.G., Meyers, J., Fletcher, M.E. Endometriosis: a report of 400 cases. *Rhode Island Medical Journal* 1950;**33**:15–23
20 Donnez, J., Nisolle, M., Gillerot, S., Smets, M., Bassil, S., Csanas-Rou, F. Rectovaginal septum adenomyotic nodules: a series of 500 cases. *Br J Obstet Gynaecol* 1998;**104**:1014–18
21 Holmes, W.R. Endometriosis. *Am J Obstet Gynecol* 1942;**43**:255–66
22 Henriksen, E. Endometriosis. *Am J Surg* 1955;**90**:331–6
23 Graham, B., Mazier, W.P. Diagnosis and management of endometriosis of the colon and rectum. *Dis Colon Rectum* 1988;**31**:952–6
24 Randolph Bailey, H., Ott, M.T., Hartendorp, P. Aggressive surgical management for advanced colorectal endometriosis. *Dis Colon Rectum* 1994;**37**:747–53
25 Ponka, J.L., Brush, B.E., Hodgkinson, C.P. Colorectal endometriosis. *Dis Colon Rectum* 1973;**16**:490–9
26 Leyendecker, G., Kunz, G., Noe, M., Herbertz, M., Mall, G. Endometriosis: a dysfunction and disease of the archimetra. *Hum Reprod Update* 1998;**4**:752–62
27 Metger, D.A., Olive, D.L., Haney, A.F. Limited hormonal responsiveness of ectopic endometrium: histologic correlation with intrauterine endometrium. *Hum Pathol* 1988;**19**:1417–24

28 Kitawaki, J., Noguchi, T., Amatsu, T., Maeda, K., Tsukamoto, K., Yamamoto, T. *et al.* Expression of aromatase cytochrome P450 protein and messenger ribonucleic acid in human endometriotic and adenomyotic tissues but not in normal endometrium. *Biol Reprod* 1997;**57**:514–19

29 Jones, R., Bulmer, J., Searle, R. Immunohistochemical characterisation of proliferation, oestrogen receptor and progesterone receptor expression in endometriosis; comparison of eutopic and ectopic endometrium with normal cycling endometrium. *Hum Reprod* 1995;**10**:3272–9

30 Higgs, H., Noronha, F., Ramos Dias, J.L. Intestinal endometriosis. *Acta Med Port* 1995;**8**:635–8

31 Redwine, D.B. Ovarian endometriosis: a marker for more extensive pelvic and intestinal disease. *Fertil Steril* 1999;**72**:310–15

32 Nisolle, M., Paindaveine, B., Bourdon, A., Berliere, M., Casnas-Roux, F., Donnez, J. Histologic study of peritoneal endometriosis in infertile women. *Fertil Steril* 1990;**53**:984–8

33 Bergqvist, A., Ferno, M. Oestrogen and progesterone receptors in endometriotic tissue and endometrium: comparison according to localisation and recurrence. *Fertil Steril* 1993;**60**:63–8

34 Janne, O., Kauppila, A., Kokko, E., Lantto, T., Ronnberg, L., Vikho, R. Oestrogen and progestin receptors in endometriosis lesions: comparison with endometrial tissue. *Am J Obstet Gynecol* 1981;**141**:562–6

35 Tamaya, T., Motoyama, T., Ohono, Y., Ide, N., Tsurusaki, T., Okada, H. Steroid receptor levels and histology of endometriosis and adenomyosis. *Fertil Steril* 1979;**10**:3272–9

36 Sampson, J.A. Peritoneal endometriosis due to menstrual dissemination of endometrial tissue into the peritoneal cavity. *Am J Obstet Gynecol* 1927;**14**:422–69

37 Redwine, D.B. Mülleriosis: the single best fit model of the origin of endometriosis. *J Reprod Med* 1988;**33**:915–19

38 Lauchlan, S.C. The secondary Müllerian system revisited. *Int J Gynecol Pathol* 1994;**13**:73–9

39 Redwine, D.B., Sharp, D.R. Laparoscopic surgery for intestinal and urinary endometriosis. *Advanced Laparoscopic Surgery. Baillière's Clin Obstet Gynaecol* 1995;**9**:775–94

40 Borsellino, G., Buonaguidi, A., Veneziano, S., Borsellino, V., Mariscalco, G., Minnici, G. Endometriosis of the large intestine: a report of two clinical cases. *Minerva Ginecol* 1993;**45**:443–7

41 Schroder, J., Lohnert, M., Doniec, J., Dohrmann, P. Endoluminal ultrasound diagnosis and operative management of rectal endometriosis. *Dis Colon Rectum* 1997;**40**:614–17

42 Athey, P.A., Diment, D.D. The spectrum of sonographic findings in endometriomas. *J Ultrasound Med* 1989;**8**:487–91

43 Managing endometriosis. *Drug Ther Bull* 1999;**37**:25–32

44 Weed, J., Ray, J. Endometriosis of the bowel. *J Obstet Gynaecol* 1987;**69**:727–30

45 Wood, C., Maher, P., Hill, D. Laparoscopic removal of endometriosis in the Pouch of Douglas. *Aust N Z J Obstet Gynaecol* 1993;**33**:295–9

46 Nezhat, C., Nezhat, F., Pennington, E., Nezhat, C.H., Ambroze, W. Laparoscopic disk excision and primary repair of the anterior rectal wall for the treatment of full-thickness bowel endometriosis. *Surg Endosc* 1994;**8**:682–5

47 Reich, H., McGlynn, F., Salvat, J. Laparoscopic treatment of cul-de-sac obliteration secondary to retrocervical deep fibrotic endometriosis. *J Reprod Med* 1991;**36**:516–22

48 Redwine, D.B. Laparoscopic en bloc resection for treatment of the obliterated cul-de-sac in endometriosis. *Reprod Med* 1992;**37**:695–8

49 Wright, J.T., Shafik, A. Quality of life following radical excision of recto-vaginal endometriosis associated with complete obliteration of the posterior cul de sac. *Gynaecol Endosc* 2001;**10**:in press
50 Garry, R., Clayton, R., Hawe, J. The effect on endometriosis and its radical laparoscopic excision on quality of life indicators. *J Obstet Gynaecol* 2000;**107**:44–54

22

Surrogate pregnancy

David D. Boyle

INTRODUCTION

The literal meaning of the word surrogate is 'substitute' and, where applied to reproduction, implies that a substitute is being used to carry a pregnancy. The practice is also known as surrogacy or surrogate motherhood, although the latter has controversial connotations about the differentiation between the carrying and delivery of a fetus and the motherhood that follows.

Surrogacy is not new; the first record is in the Holy Bible and refers to the use of Sarah's handmaiden Hagar as a surrogate (*Genesis* Chapter 16, verses 1–16). Sarah advised her husband, Abraham, to 'go into' Hagar and, as a result, Ishmael was born. This was what is now known as partial surrogacy and it is assumed that couples have used it as a remedy for their childlessness since time began. It is only since the advent of assisted reproductive technology and *in vitro* fertilisation (IVF) that full surrogacy has become possible. The first reported successful pregnancy from full surrogacy was in the USA in 1985[1] and the first in the UK followed treatment at Bourn Hall in 1989.[2] Surrogacy carries with it many controversial legal, ethical and social issues which have brought it into the public domain and created interest and concern, which have been heightened by some well-publicised events. The first of these was the birth of a baby to British housewife Kim Cotton, following a commercial surrogacy arrangement through an American agency.[3] There have been 'tug of love' cases where the host has refused to part with the baby after its birth. In 1999, the commercial arrangement in the USA between a British homosexual couple and an American host encapsulated many of the public's concerns. The surrogate acted for financial gain. The product, a baby girl, is now being reared in what many would regard as an unsuitable environment, is of uncertain paternity and the natural mother is now expressing regret that she is not being involved in the raising of her daughter. Has the child's welfare been well served in this arrangement?

ETHICAL ISSUES

The ethical problems associated with surrogacy are centred round a woman allowing herself to be used to nurture a fetus, which, when born, she will not keep, whether or not it is genetically hers. On the one hand, this is considered as a devaluation of human dignity and, when exchange of money for financial gain is involved, a form of prostitution where the uterus rather than the vagina is rented. On the other hand, it is seen as an altruistic act which equates reproductive labour with manual labour and anticipates that the surrogate mother can regard her role as one of a facilitator, enabling her to divorce herself from an emotional attachment to the product of her labour, as a craftsman can hand over his product without remorse.

Commercialisation of the process is felt to worsen the dehumanising process by turning the product, or child, into a commodity. As such, the surrogate is offering herself at a price, to produce a child, which she sees as a source of income. This process is regarded as 'baby farming' or likened to a 'baby factory'. The view is held that financial gain is not a proper motive with which to enter a surrogacy arrangement. However, for the have-nots, i.e. the infertile, there may be no other way to obtain a child and, whether payment is involved or not, for them it is a means to an end and if adoption is precluded it is the only solution to their problem.

Surrogacy is now a real option for only a limited number of couples. It is offered and taken up in only a small number of countries. It is illegal in most Australian states and most European countries, and in many countries it is not practised for ethical or religious reasons. In many countries, including the UK and some American states, it takes place because of lack of legislation to prohibit it rather than legislation to permit it.

Most Christian churches take the view that surrogacy is contrary to the unity of marriage and to the dignity of procreation. Judaism permits surrogacy, as do Hinduism and Buddhism. According to the Quran 'Our mothers are those who provide the womb and give birth' and Islam dictates that pregnancy should follow legitimate marriage, thus forbidding surrogacy.

TERMINOLOGY

The woman who carries the pregnancy is the surrogate but she is also referred to as the host or gestational mother and she and her partner as the host couple. The woman who will become the social mother of the child is referred to as the commissioning mother and she and her partner as the commissioning couple.

Partial surrogacy

This is also known as traditional surrogacy, genetic surrogacy or straight surrogacy and involves the fertilisation of the surrogate's egg by the sperm of the male partner of the commissioning couple (the commissioning father). This may be by natural insemination or, probably more commonly nowadays, by artificial insemination. Should the commissioning father be infertile or not want to pass on a genetic disorder (for example, Huntington's chorea) donor sperm may be used and the commissioning couple will then have no genetic input to the child.

Full surrogacy

This is also known as gestational surrogacy, IVF surrogacy, host surrogacy or gestational carrier pregnancy and has only been possible since the introduction of IVF. In this situation, the surrogate has no genetic input to the pregnancy. Most commonly, the gametes are from the commissioning couple and involve egg retrieval from the commissioning mother who has ovarian tissue but no uterus or a non-functioning uterus, IVF using sperm from the commissioning father and, finally, transfer of embryo(s) into the uterus of the surrogate mother. However, there may be circumstances where the gametes of the commissioning couple are not used and are substituted by donor sperm, donor oocytes or even donated embryos. If neither of the commissioning parents has genetic input to the pregnancy then a Parental Order cannot be obtained (see below).

THE MEDICAL PROFESSION

It is only since advances in medical science have allowed full surrogacy that the medical profession has shown a major interest in all the aspects of surrogacy. This is because there was, and still is, no necessity for a medical person to be involved with a partial surrogacy arrangement. The views taken by the British Medical Association (BMA) have highlighted the wavering of opinion about this controversial treatment. In March 1984, and following a number of reports of doctors' involvement with surrogacy arrangements and the possible coercion of individuals to act against their own best interests, the BMA Council issued a statement which concluded that 'it considers that it is unethical for a doctor to become involved in techniques and procedures leading to surrogate motherhood'. The Surrogacy Arrangements Act,[4] which was passed in 1985 and is discussed below, caused the BMA to carry a motion at its Annual Representatives Meeting in 1985[5] which stated 'That this meeting agrees with the principle of surrogate births in selected cases with careful controls'. The BMA's Board of Science was commissioned to produce a report and in due course *Surrogate Motherhood* was published in1987.[6] This report concluded that the interests of childless couples were outweighed by legitimate social considerations opposing surrogacy. Protection of the interests of the child was the main concern and, following discussion at the Annual Representatives Meeting in 1987,[7] the meeting rejected the principle of surrogacy and advised that 'doctors should not participate in any surrogacy arrangements until the appropriate ethical safeguards and controls were agreed'. A working party, under the chairmanship of Sir Malcolm MacNaughton, led to the publication in August 1990 of a report which gave doctors guidelines within which to act.[8] It stated that 'it would not be possible or desirable to prevent the involvement of doctors in surrogacy, especially as the Government does not intend to make the practice illegal'.

Subsequently, the BMA published a report which stated that 'Surrogacy is an acceptable option of last resort in cases where it is impossible or highly undesirable for medical reasons for the intended mother to carry a child herself'.[9] No further advice has been forthcoming from the BMA, which now seems to accept that as long as the practice is not illegal then it is better that doctors are involved where needed. However, it remains with the strongly held view that not only should surrogacy be seen as a last resort but also the welfare of the child should be properly protected.

THE LAW IN THE UK

In 1985, the Warnock Committee recommended that it should be rendered criminal to create or operate agencies which recruited women for surrogate pregnancies or made surrogate arrangements, whether for profit or not.[10] It also recommended that it be rendered criminal for professionals (i.e. doctors) to knowingly assist in the establishment of a surrogate pregnancy and that all surrogate arrangements be illegal contracts and therefore unenforceable in Court. This was not a unanimous opinion and in an 'Expression of Dissent'[10] two members stated that 'there are ... rare occasions when surrogacy could be beneficial to couples as a last resort ... In the best interests of all concerned, however, and particularly in the best interests of the child that may ensue, we think that stringent care and control is necessary'. The sort of control that was envisaged by them was the licensing of agencies, referral through a consultant gynaecologist and the provision of counselling. These are issues being considered in the current review of surrogacy referred to below.

Government considered that surrogacy should not be encouraged, but did not legislate against the involvement of professionals in surrogacy arrangements and set out that, where it did take place, firstly, there should be no financial inducement to encourage it and third parties should not make a profit and, secondly, that the surrogate mother should not be bound to give up her child. Subsequently, the Surrogacy Arrangements Act[4] was passed making it a criminal offence to make surrogacy arrangements on a commercial basis, while permitting the payment of expenses to the surrogate by the commissioning couple. It also made it a criminal offence to carry or distribute any advertising related to recruitment for surrogacy.

The Human Fertilisation and Embryology Act 1990[11] includes three sections related to surrogacy. In section 27, it makes it clear 'that the woman who carries the baby is the legal mother'. In section 30 it sets out the conditions which must be met to allow the court to make a Parental Order for the child to be treated in law as the child of the commissioning couple. These conditions include that:

(1) The child is genetically related to at least one of the commissioning couple;

(2) The surrogate mother has consented to the making of the Order;

(3) The commissioning couple are married to each other;

(4) The commissioning couple are both 18 years of age or over;

(5) No money, other than expenses, has been paid to the surrogate.

If all the conditions are met, an application for a Parental Order may be made and must be supported by a detailed written report from an independent specialist social worker. The alternative is for the commissioning couple to apply to adopt the child under the terms of the Adoption Act 1976. Finally, Section 36 of the Human Fertilisation and Embryology Act makes it clear that the woman who carries the baby is the legal mother and this remains so until the granting of a Parental Order or completion of the adoption process.

Naturally, the social services have a central role to play. In order to protect the welfare of the child they are required to make enquiries when they are aware that a child has been, or is going to be, born subsequent to a surrogacy arrangement. If they consider that the child is being or may be harmed they can seek a Care Order under the provision of the Children Act 1989.

It is clear that the issues raised in the last 20 years have provided much debate and genuine concern about surrogacy and how it should be regulated and adequately legislated for. Opinion has changed from the extreme of the Warnock Committee's recommendation to make it illegal to its current apparent acceptance. Consequently, a consultation process is being undertaken by Brazier *et al.* to consider the questions of payments to surrogate mothers and the regulation of surrogate arrangements and also to advise whether changes are needed to the existing legislation.[12]

INDICATIONS FOR SURROGACY

It is estimated that at least one in ten couples wanting children experience some difficulty and a small number of these will see surrogacy as a possible solution.

In a survey of licensed clinics in the UK, Balen and Hayden[13] found that the main reasons for requiring surrogacy were:

(1) Congenital absence of the uterus;

(2) Surgical removal of the uterus with conservation of the ovaries after either uterine or cervical cancer or obstetric haemorrhage;

(3) Medical conditions preventing pregnancy (for example severe heart disease);

(4) Recurrent implantation failure at IVF (8–10 attempts).

There are other indications which do not fall easily into one of these groups. For example, the patient who has a uterus which cannot function because of Asherman syndrome or the patient with recurrent early pregnancy loss, whether or not associated with an identifiable problem such as antiphospholipid syndrome.

It would be generally regarded as unacceptable to pursue surrogacy on nonmedical grounds.

The woman who saw it as a means of avoiding pregnancy and delivery for personal, social or career reasons would not be seen by the majority to have an acceptable indication for treatment.

A commissioning couple will almost certainly have had contact with the medical profession before realising their plight and may have been given advice about how to proceed. In a survey of all licensed clinics that perform surrogacy in the UK, it was found that only 29 clinics perform IVF surrogacy and that there are approximately 60–70 cases treated each year.[13] Because full surrogacy involves IVF it must take place in a licensed centre and so these figures should be reliable. The Human Fertilisation and Embryology Authority (HFEA) does not record IVF surrogacy separately from IVF and, therefore, exact figures are not known. In effect, surrogacy in the UK is working on two levels. Full surrogacy is subject to the regulations of the HFEA, while partial surrogacy is unregulated. Some licensed centres do assist with partial surrogacy but there is no requirement for a couple to seek treatment through a clinic and, as a result, there is no accurate record of numbers seeking or receiving treatment. Even though the majority of couples proceed through an agency, the best known and largest of which is Childlessness Overcome Through Surrogacy (COTS), the children that result should be known to the social services through the adoption or Parental Order procedures. However, there is no record of the number of babies born.

Commissioning couples can either recruit their own host, who would usually be known to them as a friend or relative, or seek an introduction through an agency. There are no regulations with regard to the host but most clinics have their own guidelines and an agency will give detailed instructions to both commissioning couple and host.

Where IVF is involved, the HFEA guidelines must be adhered to and these are set out in the most recent code of practice.[14] The commissioning couple are to be treated as donors and, therefore, the female should usually be 38 years of age or under and the male should usually be 55 years of age or under. Each should have their hepatitis B, hepatitis C and human immunodeficiency virus status checked as should the host and her partner. Blood groups of all parties may also be requested and, in some cases, cystic fibrosis screening is carried out.

COUNSELLING

Before proceeding to treatment, thorough counselling of all parties is advisable. The HFEA lays great emphasis on the welfare of the child and each licensed clinic has its own method of fulfilling this responsibility not only to the child but also to the adults in the arrangement and their other children and extended families. In many instances, a local ethics committee will scrutinise each arrangement. The agencies strongly recommend that those taking part in partial surrogacy obtain or employ a specialist counsellor.

There are many issues to discuss and they should all be fully explored before treatment is contemplated. These involve detailed consideration of all the outcomes. If pregnancy does not occur will the host feel guilty or the commissioning couple feel angry? If miscarriage occurs whose fault is it – the embryo or the uterus? If, in the eyes of the commissioning couple, the host does not take proper care of herself, for example smokes or drinks excessive alcohol, what will their reaction be? If the baby is abnormal or stillborn how will all parties react and what will the reaction of other children be to a baby with no pregnancy or a pregnancy with no baby? Finally, and most in the public eye, what will happen if the host (legal mother) decides to keep the baby? All these and other potential problems must be explored with the help of an experienced specialist counsellor who will also give advice on either the application for a Parental Order or the details of the adoption process.

Other professionals should be involved. Both parties should seek independent legal advice. This should take into account the orders referred to above, which will transfer the legal status of the child and will ensure that there is nothing likely to prevent the commissioning couple from becoming the legal parents, for example previous involvement with social services or the payment of unreasonable expenses. Expenses should be agreed in principle in advance and detailed records kept. Legal advice may involve a contract or agreement between the parties, even though it is currently unenforceable in law, and also the making of wills to ensure adequate provision for the child should something untoward happen to the commissioning couple before the child is handed over.

Finally, advice should be given about the insurance that the commissioning couple should purchase in order to protect the host and her family against serious illness or even death as a result of the pregnancy.

TREATMENT

The medical treatment required to achieve a surrogate pregnancy is part of routine practice in any licensed assisted reproduction unit.

With full IVF, the requirement to quarantine sperm means that either already quarantined frozen sperm is used or, if fresh sperm is used, the embryos obtained are quarantined before transfer into the host uterus.[14] If fresh embryo transfer is planned then ovulation induction in the commissioning mother must be co-ordinated with endometrial preparation in the host mother. This is standard practice in the much more common process of ovum donation.

For partial surrogacy, where the host will be inseminated, she requires to avoid unprotected intercourse with her partner, learn to identify the fertile time of her cycle and how to perform the insemination. Infertility clinics may help with this process and agencies give detailed instructions as well as recommending the parties to seek medical help.

OUTCOMES OF TREATMENT

There is incomplete information about the outcomes of surrogacy arrangements. There is no published information about partial surrogacy as it is not regulated and there is no obligation to register such treatment or any pregnancy or birth that results. In the ten years 1988–98, COTS is aware of 254 births as a result of arrangements under their supervision.[15] Four of their arrangements have been unsuccessful in that the host kept the child. They were all in the early days when their guidelines about preparation and counselling were either not fully developed or not followed. There are two reports about the results of full surrogacy in the UK. Meniru and Craft reported on their experience with full surrogacy following hysterectomy.[16] There was an overall pregnancy rate of 27.3% per cycle of treatment. The age of the commissioning mother was the most influential factor, the pregnancy rate being 50% (four pregnancies in eight cycles) in those of 37 years of age or less and falling to 15.4% (two pregnancies in 13 cycles) in those over 37 years of age. Of the six pregnancies, two miscarried and both of these were with older women. These numbers are small but they demonstrate results similar to those obtained with standard IVF.

Brinsden reported on 37 couples who received treatment at Bourn Hall Clinic by full surrogacy between 1990 and 1997 and the results demonstrate the success of this treatment (Table 1).[2] Twenty-four clinical pregnancies resulted from 75 commenced host cycles (32% pregnancies per cycle) and from 66 embryo transfers (36.4% pregnancies per embryo transfer). Again, these compare well with standard IVF. There were no serious clinical, ethical or legal problems in this series because Bourn Hall has a rigorous information-giving, patient selection and counselling process for patients. Difficulties have arisen through failure of treatment, unreasonable expectations and the occurrence of miscarriage, so emphasis is laid on the need for support counselling, which may be required for many years after treatment.

Table 1 *Results of treatment by IVF surrogacy at Bourn Hall Clinic 1990–97*

Genetic mother cycles	
Number of mothers starting treatment	37
Mean age at start of treatment (years)	32 (range 22–40)
Total stimulation cycles	61 (mean 1.6; range 1–5)
Mean number of oocytes recovered	10 (range 2–4)
Mean number of embryos frozen/cycle	5.4 (range 0–13)
Host surrogate cycles	
Number of hosts starting treatment	41
Number of started cycles	75
Number of cycles to embryo transfer	66 (88%)
Mean number of transfer cycles/host	1.6
Mean number of embryos transferred	2.2
Final outcome	
Clinical pregnancies per genetic couple	24/37 (64.8%)
Clinical pregnancies per host surrogate	24/41 (58.5%)
Delivered or continuing pregnancies per genetic couple	16/37 (43.2%)
Delivered or continuing pregnancies per host surrogate	16/41 (39.0%)

The experience of surrogacy in the USA is much more extensive than in the UK, but again there is little report of outcome. Three such reports confirm that the physical outcome of treatment is in keeping with standard IVF and they are reassuring about the obstetric and the perinatal outcomes.[17-19]

CONCLUSIONS

Partial surrogacy has existed for many years and by the nature of its conduct little debate surrounded it. However, in the past 20 years and because of full surrogacy, society has become interested and both development of the law and regulation of the process have become necessary. Clearly, this means of dealing with infertility is here to stay. Practically, it is easy to accomplish but should be preceded by careful thought, preparation and guidance by skilled professional counsellors. The vast majority of those currently involved with the provision of this service wish to see it regulated – but by whom and to what degree? The present review by Brazier *et al.*[14] should provide a way forward and the general willingness to see that action follows their recommendations should ensure results.

A surrogacy arrangement involves many more than two people. It affects the surrogate and her family, the commissioning couple and their families, not to mention the resultant child and its future family. Too little is known about the outcome of surrogate pregnancy in terms of its long-term effect on all those involved. Van den Akker studied the function and responsibilities of organisations dealing with surrogacy in the UK and found no systematic in-depth study on the procedures and impact of surrogacy on the vital parties.[20] The consensus of opinion among the organisations involved was that regulation of the process would be beneficial to all concerned and it should be accompanied by both long-term follow-up of the psychosocial and physical health of participants and more research to determine best practice.

References

1   Utian, W.H., Sheean, L., Godfarb, J.M., Kiwi, R. Successful pregnancy after *in vitro* fertilisation – embryo transfer from an infertile woman to a surrogate. *N Engl J Med* 1985;**313**:1351–2

2. Brinsden, P.R. *A Textbook of* In Vitro *Fertilization and Assisted Reproduction*. Carnforth: Parthenon; 1999
3. Cotton, K., Winn, D. *Baby Cotton for Love and Money*. London: Dorling Kindersley; 1985
4. Surrogacy Arrangements Act. London: HMSO; 1985
5. British Medical Association. *Annual Representative Meeting Report*. London; 1985
6. British Medical Association. *Surrogate Motherhood. Report of Board of Science and Education*. London; 1987
7. British Medical Association. *Annual Representatives Meeting Report*. London; 1987
8. British Medical Association. *Surrogacy: Ethical Considerations. Report of the Working Party on Human Infertility Services*. London; 1990
9. Morgan, D. *Changing Conceptions of Motherhood: the Practice of Surrogacy in Britain*. London: BMA; 1996
10. Department of Health and Social Security. *Report of the Committee of Inquiry into Human Fertilisation and Embryology*. London: HMSO; 1984
11. Human Fertility and Embryology Act. London: HMSO; 1990
12. Brazier, M., Golombok, S., Campbell, A. *Surrogacy. Review for the UK Health Minister of Current Arrangements for Payments and Regulation*. London: DoH; 1997
13. Balen, A.H., Hayden, C.A. British Fertility Society survey of all licensed clinics that perform surrogacy in the UK. *Human Fertility* 1998;**1**:6–9
14. HFEA. *Code of Practice for Clinics Licensed by the Human Fertilisation and Embryology Authority*. London; 1998
15. Surrogate Babies. BBC television programme; 2000
16. Meniru, G.I., Craft, I.L. Experience with gestational surrogacy as a treatment for sterility resulting from hysterectomy. *Hum Reprod* 1997;**12**:51–4
17. Schnitzer, J.J., Marrs, R.P. Gestational surrogacy seminars. *Reproductive Endocrinology* 1995;**13**:204–9
18. Parkinson, J., Tran, C., Tan, T., Nelson, J., Batzofin, J., Serafini, P. Perinatal outcome after *in vitro* fertilization – surrogacy. *Hum Reprod* 1998;**14**:671–6
19. Corson, S.L., Kelly, M., Braverman, A.M., English, M.S.N. Gestational carrier pregnancy. *Fertil Steril* 1998;**69**:670–4
20. van den Akker, O.B.A. Functions and responsibilities of organizations dealing with surrogate motherhood in the UK. *Human Fertility* 1998;**1**:10–13

23

What do we do with the pregnant athlete?

Michael M. Dooley

Girl power! Nature or nurture, training or programming. It is a brave man who even tries to address the complicated relation between sex and sport.[1]

HISTORY OF WOMEN AND SPORT

Women have taken part in sport since ancient times and particularly in the competitions of the Herean Games of 1000 BC that were staged specifically for women. The Herean Games, the origins of which stem from an ancient fertility rite, were held at Olympia and were dedicated to the Goddess Hera who was the sister-wife of Zeus. Ancient Greeks did not worry about sex discrimination, as women were traditionally prohibited from participating in the Ancient Olympic Games. They could not even enter the playing areas or the stadium as spectators.

In the Roman era, women engaged in horse riding and swimming and, in the 10th and 12th centuries, Asian women were pictured taking part in sport. During the Middle Ages and the Renaissance, women and men put leisure activities aside.

The development of the Modern Olympics was a turning point for modern women and sport. Baron Pierre DeCoubertin took the initiative to revive the Olympic Games for all male athletes of the countries of the world, regardless of national rivalries, jealousies and differences of all kinds and with all considerations of politics, race, religion, wealth and social status eliminated. As the last Ancient Olympic Games had taken place in Athens in AD 393, with DeCoubertin's enthusiasm, a conference at Sorbonne, Paris, in 1894 put forward the vision that the Games of the First Olympiad of the modern cycle would take place in Athens in 1896.

DeCoubertin was adamantly opposed to competitive sports for women. His games were intended to emulate the male ideals of Ancient Greece and the ethos of sport in Victorian public schools. With time, women were gradually introduced into the Games.

At the Olympic Games in 1900, women competed in golf and tennis. At those Games, Charlotte Cooper of Great Britain became the first Modern Olympic champion by winning a gold medal for tennis. In 1912, swimming was included in the programme but track and field events were not introduced until the Amsterdam games of 1928. These events consisted of 100-metre, 400-metre relay and 800-metre races, high jump and discus throwing. American female physical educators strongly opposed female elite competitions. In 1928, many women collapsed after the 800-metre race and it was not re-introduced into the programme until 1960. In 1984 women ran the marathon and in 1988 they also ran the 10 000 metres.

Opinions about women and sport have changed but not without resistance. In 1928, a woman from the University of Illinois stated, 'Women can never hope successfully to compete in the men's world of athletics, and when they do they not only endanger their health but at the end become awkward, ugly and in every way unattractive'.[2]

Since the 1970s, there has been a rising awareness of the contribution of sport to the wellbeing of women. At the centennial Olympic Congress, held in Paris in 1994, a major theme was women in sport. On the basis of the Congress' final report, the International Olympic Committee (IOC) took the following stance. The IOC:

(1) Encourages women to participate in sport and to become integrated within sports organisations;

(2) Invites the National Federations, the International Federations, the National Organising Committees and other national organisations to ensure that women serve in the various executive bodies in order to allow them to make a significant contribution to the evolution of the sport and the Olympic movement;

(3) Decides that the National Organising Committees will establish as a goal to be achieved by 31 December 2000 that at least 10% of all positions in their decision-making structures be reserved for women and that by the year 2005 this percentage is to be increased to 20%;

(4) Recommends that International Federations take measures to train coaches and administrators;

(5) Encourages the National Organising Committees to undertake programmes to promote women in sport and in its technical and administrative structures;

(6) Wishes that regular consultation about questions relating to the progress of women athletes in the various countries be organised.

It is of interest to compare the world records for women and men. In swimming, the highest speeds attained by women are on average 90.4% of those reached by men. In track events, women's performances are at the same ratio; with top speeds at the 89.3% level. In speed skating, women reach 91% of men's world record speeds. In cycling the figure is 83.8%. The large difference between women and men in world records in track and field events is evident in the high jump, with the women's cross bar at 85.3% of the men's 2.45 metres, and the long jump, in which the best woman jumped 84% of Mike Powell's 8.95 metres.[3]

What is interesting is the development of results for women and men over the years. It does appear that women's records have gradually crept closer to the men's levels. Speculation that women will eventually catch up with men's world records in the marathon sooner than in any other event has gained worldwide interest from the mass media.[4] Whipp and Ward[4] extrapolated from world record progression, expressed as mean running velocity versus historical time for women and men, respectively, and concluded that women may overtake men in the marathon by the year 2000 and in the 200-metre sprint by the year 2005.

HISTORY OF PREGNANCY AND SPORT

'... the Hebrew women are not as the Egyptian women, for they are lively and are delivered ere the midwife come unto them.' (*Exodus* Chapter 1, verse 19)

Throughout history, recommendations for exercise have been based on common-sense principles based on the relationship between maternal physical activity and birth outcomes. In Biblical times, as can be seen in the above quote, it was recognised that Hebrew slave women had easier labours than did their Egyptian masters. One may speculate that Hebrew slave women, while being physically prepared for the demands of childbirth, delivered growth-restricted babies; it may also be due to the high incidence of premature labours. It may be that the sedentary lifestyle of Egyptian women predisposed them to the delivery of large babies and associated dystocia.

An excellent review of pregnancy and exercise has already been published and a summary is included in this chapter.[2] Aristotle, in the third century AD, also attributed difficult childbirth to a sedentary maternal lifestyle.[5] Two thousand years later, in 1788, James Lucas, Surgeon at the Leeds General Infirmary in the UK, strongly advocated maternal exercise in a paper presented to the Medical Society of London. Lucas suggested that maternal exercise could decrease the size of the infant and allow easier passage through the maternal pelvis.[6]

Alexander Hamilton in 1781,[6] in his *Treatise of Midwifery*, stated in his chapter 'Rules and cautions of conduct of pregnant women' that pregnant women should exercise only in moderation, avoiding 'agitation of the body from violent or improper exercise such as jolting in a carriage, riding on horseback, dancing and whatever disturbs the body or mind'.

Jennings, in 1808,[7] stated 'It is a common opinion that breeding women ought to live indolently and feast luxuriously as they are able, lest by exercise they should injure, or by abstinence debilitate the unborn child ... Those ladies who are accustomed to idleness and who of course cannot take considerable degree of exercise without consequent soreness or even fever, ought by no means to indulge in riding on horseback, running or romping, in any stage of pregnancy ...'.[7]

Stapoole, in 1892,[8] wrote 'When you neglect, risk or injure your own health during pregnancy, you do a direct injustice to, and commit a real crime against your unborn baby'.

Moving to the 20th century, a theme developed for moderation in exercise and the need for outdoor air. A handbook for mothers published in 1913[9] provided the following advice: 'the prospective mother ... should stop the moment she begins to feel tired ... Women who have laborious household duties to perform do not require as much exercise as those who lead a sedentary life; but they do require just as much fresh air ... All kinds of violent exertion should be avoided – a rule which at once excludes sweeping, scrubbing ... The use of a sewing machine is emphatically forbidden'.

Between 1933 and 1947, Dick Read developed specific progressive breathing patterns and physical exercise for improving health, muscle tone and sense of wellbeing as well as decreasing the pain of childbirth.[10] The goal of Dick Read's programme was to create a birth experience unhampered by mechanical, pharmacological and mental factors. In more modern times, during the period of sweeping social change in the 1960s, prenatal exercise established itself as a permanent component of childbirth preparation and many of the earlier radical ideas involving physical and psychological control of childbirth became *de rigeur* in prenatal programmes.

In a 1977 book entitled *Exercises for Increased Awareness in Education and Counselling in Childbirth*, Kitzinger[11] wrote that exercise should aim at developing poise and a sense of wellbeing. On discussing pelvic-floor exercises she wrote, 'There is, therefore, room for exercises, always and flowing, which increases in women a happy consciousness of this part of their body as both good, clean and right, and is under their control'.

An article in the *Wall Street Journal*[12] appearing on 17 August 1984 discussed the enormous changes in expectations and procedures of childbirth during the last generation. It stated that 'Today's middle class mother-to-be is often older and more ambitious than her mother was ... She approaches childbirth as she does any activity: she studies and prepares and trains as though labour was a bar examination or sales campaign. She is so programmed to be in control, however, that if something goes wrong and childbirth doesn't meet her high expectations, she faces a profound sense of guilt and failure. That's the downside risk of new motherhood. The variables a mother-to-be can control include diet and exercise. So the conscientious career woman ... plunges into prenatal exercise classes that strengthen her back, abdomen and pelvic muscles. She also keeps going as long as she can'.[12]

In view of the current trends towards a more physically active society, the medical community has an obligation to investigate, design and promote activities that will be safe and maintain the wellbeing of both mother and fetus. With more and more women doing strenuous exercise and becoming elite athletes before childbirth, it is the role of doctors to make sure that they are given appropriate advice.

WHY ARE WOMEN (AND MEN) EXERCISING MORE?

There are multifactorial reasons why exercise is increasing in both men and women. There is a general increase in the awareness of the health benefits of exercise. School education systems are allowing more exercise and, indeed, legislation changes and media interest have improved this. The modern image of young women is changing from the 'Monroe' era of sitting on a bar stool smoking a cigarette to the sporty woman of the 21st century wearing a leotard. Women are becoming more aware of the benefits to the cardiovascular system and general physical endurance and work capacity of doing exercise. They are equally aware that it reduces adiposity, improves physical appearance and allows them to be more flexible. Not only has medical endorsement supported this but cultural changes and being far more socially acceptable has greatly encouraged women to do more exercise.

The White Paper, *Saving Lives: Our Healthier Nation*,[13] states that the Government will build on many existing initiatives including 'wide-ranging and affordable sports and leisure opportunities at local neighbourhood level'. With a dramatic increase in the number of women taking part in sport there is an urgent need to develop our understanding of the beneficial and negative effects of exercise for the female. This knowledge is needed across all the different stages of the woman's life.

Until recently, most obstetricians advised pregnant women to avoid exercise throughout gestation. There was no consideration for their present state of fitness, their present exercise habits or their medical or obstetric conditions. In the author's opinion, this advice is no longer acceptable. Indeed, many women find it necessary to be physically active for financial, social or personal reasons and many others choose an active lifestyle because they enjoy it and believe it to be beneficial in many ways.

PHYSIOLOGICAL CHANGES IN PREGNANCY AND EXERCISE

Pregnancy is distinguished by a multitude of physiological and endocrine adjustments directed towards the creation of an optimal environment for the fetus. There is no system in the body that is not affected by the normal physiological changes of pregnancy. Exercise is a process in which chemical energy is transformed into movement or muscular tension in isometric exercise and inevitably into heat. Understanding and comparing physiological changes of pregnancy and exercise is needed to help the pregnant mother clinically.

Cardiovascular alteration in pregnancy

In pregnancy, there is a large increase in blood volume, averaging 45–50% by term in 20–100% of women, depending on size and parity.[14] There is also an increase in cardiac output, reaching a maximum increment of more than 50% above nonpregnant levels by late pregnancy.

Cardiac output is a product of stroke volume and heart rate, both of which increase during pregnancy. Stroke volume rises by eight weeks of gestation and continues to increase to its maximum level during the second trimester. Left ventricular mass increases and there is a decrease in systemic vascular resistance and diastolic blood pressure. The increased cardiac output that occurs throughout pregnancy is accompanied by large increases in blood volume to the uterus, placenta, kidneys and skin.[14]

Cardiovascular changes during exercise

Acute exercise leads to an increase in cardiac output proportional to the intensity of the exercise. Major increment in cardiac output supplies the exercise in skeletal muscle and a small increment supplies the heart. The cardiac output response during exercise is greater during pregnancy than in the nonpregnant state.[14] The pregnancy-induced rise in cardiac output at low exercise intensities is related to increase in both heart rate and stroke volume. At high exercise intensity, however, increases in stroke volume account for more of the gain in cardiac output than do increases in heart rate.[14]

Haemodynamic alterations in pregnancy and exercise

Red blood cell mass increases throughout pregnancy. Plasma volume increases early in pregnancy at a faster rate than the rise in red blood cell mass. There is, therefore, a dilutionary anaemia that worsens until the second trimester and then remains at a plateau. Plasma volume expansion correlates with increased birth weight and favourable outcome. Failure of plasma volume expansion during pregnancy has been associated with low birth weight and fetal growth restriction.[14]

When one compares social exercise with exercise in training it is known that chronic endurance training also leads to an increased blood volume, partly due to an increase in intravascular plasma protein content.[15] Red blood cell volume also expands with chronic training but this increases less than that occurring in plasma volume. As a result, chronic exercise can cause a dilutionary anaemia.[15]

The combined effects of pregnancy and endurance training produce haemodynamic changes that are greater than those seen with either pregnancy or training alone. Thus, during the second and third trimesters, pregnant exercisers demonstrate a greater blood volume, plasma volume and red blood cell volume compared with sedentary pregnant women.[14]

Pulmonary alterations in pregnancy and exercise

During pregnancy, tidal volume increases, total lung capacity decreases, functional residual capacity decreases, residual volume decreases, respiratory reserve volume decreases, alveolar ventilation increases and inspiration capacity decreases. In addition, respiratory rate increases slightly, tidal volume increases appreciatively and oxygen consumption increases moderately. Respiratory minute volume increases causing a decrease in alveolar CO_2.[16]

Exercise ventilation during pregnancy increases more than option uptake, possibly because of the direct effect of progesterone and an increase in sensitivity to carbon dioxide.[16]

Thermoregulation in pregnancy

Maternal temperature is normally about 0.5°C higher than follicular-phase temperatures as a result of the thermogenic effect of progesterone.[17] Fetal temperature is normally about 0.5°C higher than maternal temperature due to the higher fetal placental metabolic rate that results from growth and development. This fetal-maternal temperature gradient ensures the fetal heat is always transferred to the mother and represents the only mechanism by which the fetus can dissipate heat.[17]

The fetal-maternal temperature gradient of 0.5°C observed at rest is initially reduced during exercise and is eventually reversed in prolonged maternal exercise as the maternal temperature rises. This reversal of the fetal-maternal temperature gradient leads to a transfer of heat from mother to fetus. Animal studies have demonstrated that the fetal temperature quickly exceeds the maternal temperature as a result of maternal heat dissipation. The fetal temperature may remain elevated for more than one hour and probably for several hours. Thus, the fetal temperature can remain significantly elevated long after the maternal temperature returns to normal.[17]

Alteration in weight in pregnancy and exercise

During pregnancy, maternal weight gain includes the fetus, placenta, amniotic fluid in the uterus, breasts, intravascular fluid and adipose tissue. Endurance exercise training promotes less weight gain than occurs in sedentary women and with cessation of training there is promotion of weight gain. Pregnant women who exercise see similar effects. Those who continue to exercise throughout pregnancy gain less weight than sedentary pregnant individuals.[18]

Musculoskeletal alteration in pregnancy and exercise

Several investigations have demonstrated progressive development of maternal peripheral joint laxity throughout pregnancy. The causes and consequences of these joint changes remain to be shown. Ireland[19] stated that during pregnancy the female body undergoes many hormonal and anatomic changes that affect the musculoskeletal system. These changes may cause various musculoskeletal complaints, predisposing to injury, or alter the course of pre-existing conditions. These changes need to be taken into account when counselling women who wish to exercise during their pregnancy. Any treatment of musculoskeletal conditions during pregnancy must include the potential effects on the mother and fetus.[20]

BENEFITS AND SAFETY CONSIDERATIONS OF EXERCISE IN PREGNANCY

Scientific research has demonstrated that exercise and training are beneficial in general and it has thus been assumed that it is safe in pregnancy.

There are several potential concerns about exercise in pregnancy, such as the increase in fetal temperature mentioned above.[21] Physical activity can increase maternal core temperature, which in turn can cause the fetal temperature to rise. Repeated episodes of maternal hyperthermia in animals have been associated with adverse effects such as an increased incidence of fetal malformation when exposed early in pregnancy, decreased potential learning ability and decreased birthweight when exposure occurs in the last half of pregnancy.[21-23]

To try to prevent adverse fetal effects in the human it has been recommended that the core temperature should not exceed 38°C when exercising.[24-26]

When giving advice on exercise and pregnancy, it is important to specify both the intensity and duration because it is this combination that determines the temperature response. O'Neill[27] looked specifically at cycling and confirmed that there was no contraindication to cycling for 30 minutes at a maternal heart rate of around 140 beats per minute or exercising for 15 minutes at a rate of around 155 beats per minute.[27]

When assessing safety, there is a need to take into consideration the different groups of women who exercise. The prepregnancy sedentary group needs different advice from the prepregnancy elite professional athlete group.

A recent study examined the effects of exercise on physical and psychological variables in sedentary primigravidae.[28] The data from this study suggest that a vigorous exercise programme can lead to significant improvements in aerobic fitness at similar lactate concentrations compared with a control group and can be well tolerated by low-risk, sedentary primigravidae without any deleterious effects occurring to the woman or her unborn child.

PREGNANCY OUTCOME WITH EXERCISE

Perinatal morbidity and mortality statistics can assess pregnancy outcome by birthweight and neonatal growth and development. Although studies have demonstrated higher litter mortality in rats trained during pregnancy regardless of prepregnancy training, no similar effects have been demonstrated in humans.[29] Differences have been observed among animal species and their response to exercise during pregnancy and it remains unclear whether conclusions about humans can be drawn from any of the animal species that have been studied. To date, specific studies have demonstrated no adverse effects from exercise in the periconceptual period and throughout pregnancy, upon the instance of failure to conceive, spontaneous abortion, congenital abnormalities, abnormal presentation, premature rupture of membranes or premature labour.[14]

The relationship of maternal exercise to labour, delivery and the health of the newborn was assessed by Rice.[30] Thirty women were interviewed and divided into active and sedentary groups. Neonates of active women showed slightly higher one-minute Apgar scores and no difference in fetal weight or five-minute Apgar scores. Active women indicated lower perceived exertion during labour, longer delivery times and no differences in gestational length, maternal weight gain and time during the first stage of labour.[30]

PSYCHOLOGICAL EFFECTS OF EXERCISE

Mood changes have been reported to occur in many women following pregnancy. It is well documented that exercise is associated with reductions in anxiety and depression. Results indicate that anxiety and depression decreased significantly ($P < 0.05$) following exercise and quiet rest. Furthermore, exercise was associated with significant decreases ($P < 0.05$) in total mood disturbance as well as significant increases ($P < 0.05$) in vigour in physically active postpartum women.[31]

PREVENTION OF DISEASE IN PREGNANCY AND EXERCISE

Apart from overall health benefits there are specific diseases that can benefit from exercise. The physiological and psychological benefits of physical exercise are not only available to healthy women, but have also proven to be valuable for the prevention and treatment of illnesses such as gestational diabetes.[32] The activation of large groups of muscles allows for improved glucose utilisation by simultaneously increasing insulin sensitivity.[32]

GENERAL SAFETY CONSIDERATIONS OF EXERCISE AND PREGNANCY

It is important that the following safety considerations are followed:[3]

(1) Avoiding prolonged or strenuous exertion during the first trimester;

(2) Avoiding isometric exercises or straining while holding the breath;

(3) Maintaining adequate nutrition and hydration; drinking fluids before and after exercise. Dehydration can be generally assessed by the colour of the urine;

(4) Avoiding exercising in warm, humid environments;

(5) Avoiding exercising while lying on the back after the fourth month of pregnancy;

(6) Avoiding activities that involve physical contact or danger of falling; wearing adequate protective clothing;

(7) Periodic rest periods may help to minimise possible hypoxic or temperature stresses to the fetus;

(8) Knowing reasons when to stop exercise and consulting an obstetrician immediately if they occur;

(9) Informing any medical officer who needs to know, so that if an injury does occur appropriate care can be provided;

(10) Not concealing the pregnancy.

Advice on when to discontinue exercise

There are many reasons to discontinue exercise and consult an obstetrician and these include:[3]

(1) Bloody discharge from the vagina;

(2) Persistent contractions;

(3) Absence of fetal movement or alteration of fetal movement;

(4) Persistent headaches and/or visual disturbances, unexplained dizziness or fainting;

(5) Elevation of pulse rate or blood pressure persisting after exercise;

(6) Insufficient weight gain;

(7) Excessive fatigue, palpitations or chest pain;

(8) Unexplained abdominal pain;

(9) Sudden swelling of the ankles, face or hands;

(10) Premature rupture of membranes;

(11) Swelling, pain and redness in the calf of one leg;

(12) Evidence of intrauterine growth restriction;

(13) Abnormal Doppler blood flow;

If the woman has any doubts about the continuation of exercise then she should stop; negative thoughts will lead to negative events.

Absolute contraindications to exercise

There are many absolute contraindications to exercise during pregnancy and these include:[3]

(1) Clinically significant valvular or ischaemic heart disease;

(2) Diabetes mellitus with peripheral vascular disease (medical opinion should be obtained);

(3) Uncontrolled hypertension;

(4) Cervical weakness;

(5) A history of three or more miscarriages, especially in the second trimester;

(6) Vaginal bleeding or placenta praevia;

(7) Premature rupture of the membranes;

(8) Pre-eclampsia;

(9) Intrauterine growth restriction/abnormal Doppler blood flow;

(10) Low percentage of body fat, eating disorders; concern must be addressed to the individual, who may already be at risk of osteoporosis;

(11) Multiple pregnancy.

Relative contraindications to exercise in pregnancy

(1) History in previous pregnancy of premature labour, intrauterine growth restriction;

(2) Anaemia or iron deficiency;

(3) Significant pulmonary disease;

(4) Mild valvular or ischaemic heart disease;

(5) Low physical fitness prior to the pregnancy;

(6) Prescription of drugs which can alter cardiac output or blood flow distribution;

(7) Obesity, when excessive exercise may cause additional strain; now is not the time to reduce weight and take on new sports activities.

Risks may exceed benefits of exercise. A consultation needs to occur with the obstetrician and consideration should be given for the type and duration of the exercise as well as the experience of the athlete.[3]

ADVICE FOR EXERCISE AND PREGNANCY FOR SPECIFIC SPORTS

It is safe to state that on the basis of the current state of scientific research in this area, physical exercise is to be recommended during pregnancy as long as women are aware of the potential danger, in some sports more than others, and of possible contraindications.

It is often the type of activity, not the length of time in which the pregnant woman participates, that is a problem. Activities that require sudden forceful contact should be avoided, for example boxing, football, soccer and hockey. In these sports abdominal trauma and abruption may occur. Other sports that may be associated with an increase of injury include downhill skiing, ice-skating, gymnastics, horseback riding and mountain climbing. Water skiing should be avoided as it can forcefully push water into the genitals causing miscarriage.[33] Scuba diving can lead to the formation of nitrogen bubbles and should be avoided, although experimental data are not conclusive.[34,35]

Activities not known to increase pregnancy risk include jogging, swimming, cycling, golf, racket sports, cross-country skiing, low-impact skiing and walking.[36]

Jogging

Many women have found jogging to be an excellent from of exercise and want to continue for as long as possible into the pregnancy. This activity is not one that should be initiated after pregnancy has begun. In published studies of exercise throughout pregnancy, women who averaged 1.5–2.5 miles per day had no apparent deleterious effects.[18] Studies have demonstrated a voluntary reduction of mileage during gestation.[37,38]

Important guidelines include:

(1) Not beginning a jogging programme while pregnant; the risk of musculoskeletal injuries is increased;

(2) Reducing mileage to less than two miles per day;

(3) If temperature and humidity are high, not exercising; adverse conditions may cause fetal loss;

(4) Giving special attention to terrain and running surface because of connective tissue changes associated with pregnancy;

(5) Wearing running shoes and proper support.

Aerobics

In the last five to ten years, women have wanted to get the benefit of aerobic workouts associated with jogging but without running alone and have searched for other ways to exercise. Aerobics combine dance with an aerobic workout. Because aerobics are weight-bearing exercises, the same concerns associated with jogging should be considered by a mother during the progress of her pregnancy. Again, close obstetric follow-up may be needed in intense exercise programmes.

Specific exercises that should be avoided include over-extension exercises performed on the back. There is a need to avoid hard surfaces when exercising and to limit repetitive movements to ten. It is important that the woman warms up gradually and cools down properly.

Cycling

Cycling is not without risk. On a stationary bicycle, heat dissipation may become a problem and exercising out of doors in traffic and smog may have unknown negative effects on both mother and fetus. Cycling may cause low-back stress and should be avoided out of doors in high temperatures and high pollution levels.

Swimming

Swimming is a non-weight-bearing aerobic activity. Many consider swimming to be the most adequate aerobic exercise for the pregnant woman. Throughout the pregnancy, the mother may be able to maintain a given distance but take longer to complete it.[38] Respiratory changes may make swimming difficult in late pregnancy. Swimming in water that is either too cold or too hot should be avoided and jacuzzi temperatures of about 38.5°C should be avoided.

Due to thermoregulatory advantages, the beneficial effects of immersion and its joint protective character, 'aquatic exercise' can be highly recommended during pregnancy.

Psychologically speaking, physical exercise offers a variety of benefits such as encouragement of co-operation and competition, which can be experienced as fun and gratifying.

ELITE ATHLETES

As indicated earlier, the number of elite female athletes competing in Olympic and World Championships has shown a dramatic increase, as has the number of women participating in professional sports. With this added interest there has been an increase in professional women's sports, including the formation of several professional women's football teams.

The management of the elite athlete is different from that of the recreational athlete. As a result of personal goals and financial incentives, the elite athlete must continue intense training throughout what has historically been referred to as her childbearing years. Some individuals may delay their family or try to deliver during the 'off season'. Pregnant athletes who intend to continue training at a high level of intensity could lessen the risks by seeking closer medical supervision from an appropriately skilled physician. There is, however, little evidence-based medicine on the course and complication of pregnancy in the professional or elite athlete. Being accustomed to training at a high intensity level before pregnancy, professional and elite athletes may place themselves at increased risk of overuse injuries, not realising they are pregnant and that there are pregnancy-related changes in joints and ligaments (Table 1).

The use of anabolic steroids among elite athletes is well documented.[40] Anabolic steroid use may, therefore, not only have significant adverse effects including clitoral enlargement, facial hair and acne on the female athlete but also could cause significant problems for the fetus.

In the author's experience, athletes need to be encouraged to inform the relevant authorities about their pregnancies so that appropriate attention and care can be provided. Concealing the pregnancy must be actively discouraged.

An air of openness must be encouraged but there is always the question of the selection of athletes for competition. The British Equestrian Federation, for example, has approached this problem by encouraging athletes to inform the honorary medical officer about becoming pregnant and making it clear that this may not affect selection. However, participation in the team rather than as an individual may be restricted.

Osteoporosis in pregnancy is a rare clinical problem of unknown aetiology. If the bone loss results from pregnancy alone, it should improve towards normal after delivery. The elite athlete

Table 1 *Risks of exercise in pregnancy for the elite athlete*

Risks	Advice
Maternal	
Musculoskeletal injuries	As there are changes in joint and ligament laxity there is a need to discuss this with the athlete and consider a change in her training
Cardiovascular complications	It is important to monitor maternal heart rate. The athlete needs to be aware of the danger of palpitations and tachycardia
Vaginal bleeding or premature labour	Stop training
Development of other medical conditions	These include pre-eclampsia and diabetes. Full discussion must take place with the medical team
Drug abuse and fetal problems	Avoid
Fetal	
Fetal distress	Be alert to fetal activity; in the presence of any complication, stop training and resume after medical clearance
Intrauterine growth restriction	Stop training
Fetal malformations	Avoid hyperthermia and dehydration immediately after conception and weeks thereafter
Fetal injuries	Avoid sports in which there is a higher probability of blunt trauma after 16–20 weeks of gestation

Adapted from Hale and Artal[39]

who presents in pregnancy is, however, another problem and, where bone density was low before pregnancy, due to some other secondary cause, significant postpartum improvement may not be expected.[41] Appropriate advice before pregnancy is important to maximise bone density. Dietary advice is required throughout this period. Post-pregnancy advice includes a careful evaluation of the benefits and risks of breastfeeding and a careful, staged return to exercise.

Delivery for the elite athlete

Delivery in the elite athlete is equally controversial. There is some pressure from individuals to have elective caesarean sections in order to have a timed delivery, perhaps earlier than they would have a vaginal delivery. Indeed, in certain sports, such as horse-riding, this may be seen as an advantage because of a fear of damage to the perineum.

Postpartum for the elite athlete

The return to full physical activity to overcome the de-training process that occurred during pregnancy is the primary concern of the athlete after delivery. Most want to start training immediately. There are few sources of data to indicate the optimum time for resuming physical activity and the decision should be an individual one. The relaxation of ligaments and joints does not disappear significantly before the second postpartum week and in most instances not until at least four to six weeks postpartum. As a result, it is has been recommended that the women does not consider returning to an exercise training routine until after a two-week check up, after which conditioned training can begin.[42]

Consideration must also be given to diet, especially if the woman is breastfeeding. There is no known contraindication to breastfeeding and exercise but the quality of milk may differ after exercise.[39]

Pregnancy, for the elite athlete as in the general population, should not be a state of confinement. Unrestricted, or even restricted, physical activity involves a certain degree of risk that must be recognised. Acceptance of the various risks then becomes a personal choice.

POSTPARTUM EXERCISE IN GENERAL

Postpartum exercise does depend on the mode of delivery. Gradual but regular exercise at least three times per week should start soon after delivery. Ballistic movements, extreme stretching, heavy weightlifting and weight-resistant machines should be avoided for up to 12 weeks or longer if joint laxity persists. Target heart rates and limits should be established in consultation with a sports physician. It is important that women remember to take fluids liberally.

LEGAL ASPECTS OF EXERCISE AND PREGNANCY

Negligence is usually the legal basis for law suits. To be found negligent a doctor must meet the four elements of negligence: duty, breach, causation and damages. With respect to pregnancy, it is important that appropriate advice is given to the individual. It is not only the physician whose duty to care must be to the woman. There are, equally, other individuals and professional bodies who need to address the situation. Many questions remain unanswered. It is important that individual authorities allow an air of openness but prevention of a pregnant athlete from competing may be an infringement of their legal rights. It is important that the environmental conditions are appropriate. It is necessary also that individual physicians at sports events, and physicians in general, are aware of the complications of exercise and pregnancy.

Exercise itself implies some risk. By participation there is an implication that the player knew and assumed the risk of injury.

A review by the Medical Defence Union[43] stated that the duty of care of medical officers at sporting events includes advice to organisers of the extent of medical resources needed for the event and to ensure that these facilities are available throughout the event. There is no place for 'token doctors' at sporting events.

GUIDELINES TO EXERCISE AND PREGNANCY

In 1985, the American College of Obstetricians and Gynecologists developed a set of guidelines for women who plan to exercise during their pregnancy.[24]

(1) During pregnancy, women can continue to exercise and derive health benefits even from mild-to-moderate exercise routines. Regular exercise (at least three times per week) is preferable to intermittent activity;

(2) Women should avoid exercise in the supine position after the first trimester. Such a position is associated with decreased cardiac output in most pregnant women; because the remaining cardiac output will be preferentially distributed away from splanchnic beds (including the uterus) during vigorous exercise, such regimens are best avoided during pregnancy. Prolonged periods of motionless standing should also be avoided;

(3) Women should be aware of the decreased oxygen available for aerobic exercise during pregnancy. They should be encouraged to modify the intensity of their exercise according to maternal symptoms. Pregnant women should stop exercising when fatigued and not exercise to exhaustion. Weight-bearing exercises may, under some circumstances, be continued at intensities similar to those prior to pregnancy throughout pregnancy. Non-weight-bearing exercises may, under some circumstances, be continued at intensities similar to those prior to pregnancy throughout pregnancy. Non-weight-bearing exercises such as cycling or swimming will minimise the risk of injury and facilitate the continuation of exercise during pregnancy;

(4) Morphologic changes in pregnancy should serve as a relative contraindication to types of exercise in which loss of balance could be detrimental to maternal or fetal well-being, especially in the third trimester. Furthermore, any type of exercise involving the potential for even mild abdominal trauma should be avoided;

(5) Pregnancy requires an additional 300 kcal per day in order to maintain metabolic homeostasis. Thus, women who exercise during pregnancy should be particularly careful to ensure an adequate diet;

(6) Pregnant women who exercise in the first trimester should augment heat dissipation by ensuring adequate hydration, appropriate clothing and optimal environmental surroundings during exercise;

(7) Many of the physiological and morphological changes of pregnancy may persist four to six weeks postpartum. Thus, prepregnancy exercise routines should be resumed gradually based on a woman's physical capability.

CONCLUSION

In the absence of either obstetric or medical complications, pregnant women can continue to exercise and derive related benefits. Women who have achieved cardiovascular fitness prior to pregnancy should be able to safely maintain that level of fitness throughout pregnancy and the postpartum period.

Women may need to modify their exercise patterns depending on physiological and pathological changes during the pregnancy and the type of exercise they are taking.

With adequate attention to detail and following appropriate advice, exercise during pregnancy has no deleterious effect on the fetus.[24]

The lead professional should be involved in making decisions regarding exercise and further expert evidence-based advice must be obtained where appropriate.

References

1. Macauley, D. Editorial. *Br J Sports Med* 1999;**4**:223–4
2. Artal, R., Gardin, S.K. Historical perspectives of physiological adaptations to pregnancy. In: Artal, R., Wiswell, R., Drinkwater, B., editors. *Exercise in Pregnancy*, 2nd ed. Baltimore, MD: Williams & Wilkins; 1991. p. 1–7
3. Mottola, M.F. Exercise and pregnancy – what do I tell my pregnant athlete? In: Harries, M., Williams, C., Stanish, W.D., Micheli, L.J., editors. *Oxford Textbook of Sports Medicine*, 2nd ed. Oxford: Oxford Medical Publications; 1998. p. 779–86
4. Whipp, B.J., Ward, S.A. Will women soon outrun men? *Nature* 1992;**355**;25
5. Vaughn, K. *Exercise Before Childbirth*. London: Faber and Faber; 1951. p. 11–29
6. Kerr, J.M.M., Johnson, R.W., Phillips, M.H. *Historical Review of British Obstetrics and Gynaecology*. London: Livingstone; 1954
7. Jennings, S.K. *Married Lady's Companion or Poor Mans Friend*. New York: Lorenzo Dow; 1808. p. 77–80
8. Stapoole, F. *Advice to Women on the Care of Their Health Before, During and After Confinement*. London: Cassel; 1892
9. Slemmons, J.M. *The Prospective Mother: a Handbook for Women During Pregnancy*. New York: Appleton; 1913. p. 125–35
10. Dick Read, G. An outline of the conduct of physiological labour. *Am J Obstet Gynecol* 1947;**54**:702–6
11. Kitzinger, S. *Exercises for Increasing Body Awareness and Education and Counselling for Childbirth*. London: Baillière Tindall; 1977. p. 165–71
12. Cox, M. Many professional women apply career lessons to job of childbirth. *Wall Street Journal*, Section 2, 17 August 1984
13. Department of Health. *Saving Lives: Our Healthier Nation*. London: The Stationery Office; 1999
14. Warren, M.P., Shangold, M.M. *Sports Gynaecology: Care of the Athletic Female*. Oxford: Blackwell Science; 1996
15. Capeless, E.L., Clapp, J.F. Cardiovascular changes in early phase of pregnancy. *Am J Obstet Gynecol* 1989;**161**:1449–3
16. Artal, R., Wiswell, R., Romen, Y., Dorey, F. Pulmonary responses to exercise in pregnancy. *Am J Obstet Gynecol* 1986;**154**:378–83
17. Clapp, J.F. The changing thermal response to endurance exercise during pregnancy. *Am J*

Obstet Gynecol 1991;**165**:1684–9

18 Carpenter, M.W., Sady, S.P., Sady, M.A., Haydon, B., Coustan, D.R., Thompson, P.D. Effect of maternal weight gain during pregnancy an exercise performance. *J Appl Physiol* 1990;**68**:1173–6

19 Ireland, M.L. The effects of pregnancy on the musculoskeletal system. *Clin Orthop* 2000;**372**:169–79

20 Calguneri, M., Bird, H.A., Wright, V. Changes in joint laxity occurring during pregnancy. *Ann Rheum Dis* 1982;**41**:126–8

21 Bell, R., O'Neill, M. Exercise and pregnancy. *Birth* 1994;**21**:85–95

22 Jonson, K.M., Lyle, J.G., Edwards, M.J., Penny, R.H.C. Effect of prenatal heat stress on brain growth and serial discrimination reversal learning in the guinea pig. *Brain Res Bull* 1976;**1**:133–50

23 Bell, A.W., Wilkening, R.B., Meschia, G. Some aspects of placental function in chronically heat stressed ewes. *J Dev Physiol* 1987;**9**:17–19

24 American College of Obstetricians and Gynecologists. *Women and Exercise.* Washington, DC: ACOG; 1992 (ACOG Technical Bulletin No. 173)

25 Bell, R., Palma, S. Antenatal exercise and birth weight. *Aust N Z J Obstet Gynaecol* 2000;**40**:70–3

26 Bell, R., O'Neill, M. Exercise and pregnancy: a review. *Birth* 1994;**21**:85–95

27 O'Neill, M.M. Maternal rectal temperature and fetal heart responses to upright cycling in late pregnancy. *Br J Sports Med* 1996;**30**:32–5

28 Marquez-Sterling, S., Perry, A.C., Kaplan, T.A., Halberstein, R.A., Signorile, J.F. Physical and psychological changes with vigorous exercise in sedentary primigravidae. *Med Sci Sports Exerc* 2000;**32**:58–62

29 Wilson, N.C., Gisolfi, C.V. Effects of exercising rats during pregnancy. *J Appl Physiol* 1980;**48**:34–40

30 Rice, P.L., Fort, I.L. The relationship of maternal exercise on labour and health of the new born. *J Sports Med Phys Fitness* 1991;**31**:95–9

31 Koltyn, K.F., Schultes, S.S. Psychological effects of an aerobic exercise session and a rest session following pregnancy. *J Sports Med Phys Fitness* 1997;**37**:287–91

32 Carpenter, M.W. The role of exercise in pregnant women with diabetes mellitus. *Clin Obstet Gynecol* 2000;**43**:56–64

33 Kizer, K.W. Medical hazards of the water skiing douche. *Ann Emerg Med* 1980;**9**:268–90

34 Bolton-Klug, M.E., Leher, A.E., Lanphier, E.H., Rankin, J.H. Lack of harmful effects from simulated dives in pregnant sheep. *Am J Obstet Gynecol* 1986;**146**:48–51

35 Bolton, M.E. Scuba diving and fetal well-being: a survey of 208 women. *Undersea Biomedical Research* 1980;**7**:183–9

36 Hauth, J.O., Gilstrap, L.C., Widmer, K. Fetal heart rate reactivity before and after maternal jogging during the third trimester. *Am J Obstet Gynecol* 1982;**142**:545–7

37 Jarrett, J.C., Spellacy, W.N. Jogging during pregnancy an improved outcome? *Obstet Gynecol* 1983;**61**:705–9

38 Katz, J. *Swimming Through Your Pregnancy, the Perfect Exercise for Pregnant Women.* New York: Dolphin Books, Doubleday; 1983

39 Hale, R.W., Artal, R. Pregnancy in the elite and professional athlete – a stepwise clinical approach. In: Artal, R., Wiswell, R., Drinkwater, B., editors. *Exercise in Pregnancy*, 2nd ed. Baltimore, MD: Williams and Wilkins; 1991. p. 231–7

40 Perry, P.H., Anderson, K.H., Yates, W.R. Elicit anabolic steroid use in athletes: a case series analysis. *Am J Sports Med* 1990;**18**:422–8

41 Phillips, A.J., Ostlere, S.J., Smith, R. Pregnancy associated osteoporosis: does the skeleton recover? *Osteoporos Int* 2000;**11**:449–54
42 Hale, R.W., Milne, L. The elite athlete and exercise in pregnancy. *Semin Perinatol* 1996;**20**:277–84
43 Allen, M. Medical officers in sporting events. *Journal of the Medical Defence Union* 2000;**16**:8–9

24

Trial of scar?

Harold Gee

INTRODUCTION

A trial, by definition, will result in success or failure. When we attempt to deliver a woman vaginally following a previous caesarean delivery, two unknowns are on trial: whether vaginal delivery can be achieved and whether the scar will remain intact. The sentence for failure of vaginal delivery (20–40%) is the increased risk of emergency compared with elective caesarean section. Emergency caesarean section carries 1.5 times more risk of maternal mortality than elective caesarean section and, in many respects, the risk can be managed by timely intervention, skilled surgeons and appropriate prophylaxis against infection and thromboembolism. But what of scar rupture and dehiscence? The occurrence is low (0.8 %) but the morbidity and mortality are significant[2] and, inevitably, diagnosis is after the event. Thus, a trial of vaginal delivery may be acceptable but should we ever undertake 'trial of scar'?

This chapter confines itself to attempted vaginal delivery after lower segment caesarean section. Classical caesarean section is held to give a high risk of scar rupture; its rarity means there are few data and its clinical impact is small. American data may contain cases of vertical lower segment incisions that are uncommon in UK practice. Meta-analysis has shown no difference between transverse and vertical lower segment incisions.[3]

The terms 'dehiscence' (a silent, virtually avascular separation of the scar) and 'rupture' (catastrophic, haemorrhagic separation) are used loosely in the literature and the distinction is probably academic, since both interfere with uterine physiology and fetal oxygenation, although clearly one is more dramatic than the other. Both are to be avoided.

OUTCOME OF ATTEMPTED VAGINAL DELIVERY AFTER PREVIOUS CAESAREAN DELIVERY

There are over 120 articles in the literature documenting the outcome of delivery after previous caesarean section in nearly 150 000 cases. Most are retrospective observational studies. These have been performed in a variety of clinical settings and populations. Despite this, the findings are remarkably consistent:

(1) 70% of cases are considered suitable for an attempt at vaginal delivery;

(2) 73% of attempts result in vaginal delivery;

(3) 0.8% experience scar complications (rupture or dehiscence);

(4) Approximately 9/1000 result in perinatal mortality;

(5) Approximately 10/100 000 result in maternal mortality.

Perinatal and maternal mortality rates are hard to interpret because background population rates are unknown and it is impossible to ascertain the accuracy of the data. Meta-analysis increases the power of individual studies for uncommon events but the limitations of this technique must be taken into account.[3,4] A meta-analysis comparing perinatal mortality from vaginal birth after caesarean section with elective repeat caesarean section showed no difference,[3] although there were more neonates with low Apgar scores in the previous caesarean section group. Not surprisingly, this association was stronger in those patients who did not achieve vaginal delivery compared with those who did. Major maternal morbidity such as hysterectomy, major operative injury and uterine rupture were significantly increased (OR 1.8; CI 1.1–3.0).[5]

Thus, two-thirds to three-quarters of those who attempt vaginal delivery will be successful and experience minimal morbidity and mortality. One-quarter to one-third will fail, thereby increasing their morbidity. Furthermore, this morbidity, when it does occur, is more likely to be serious. Three percent of those who are unsuccessful will be at risk from scar complication and its associated risks (*vide infra*).

The data given above are of interest but they do not help to formulate management for the individual. Here, it is of more use to know what are her chances of success or failure. Furthermore, should she fail, will she be unfortunate enough to be in the group, albeit small, who suffer a scar complication. She would also be right and sensible to seek assurances from her attendants about their ability to cope safely with complications; that is, can we manage the risks?

DECISION ANALYSIS

Clinicians would ideally like to have a test that would determine the result of an attempt at vaginal delivery with 100% specificity and sensitivity. Such a test is not available. In a theoretical analysis, it has been shown that sensitivity and specificity must reach 75% before a reasonable trade-off is achieved between a reduction in morbidity and the total rate of caesarean section.[6] Tests with poorer sensitivities and specificities may be of use when lower than average rates of vaginal delivery are achieved in a particular delivery unit. Thus, units practising vaginal delivery for women who have previously delivered by caesarean section should audit their outcomes and devise policies for selection according to their success rates and the sensitivity and specificity of selection criteria (assuming they are available).

PREDICTION OF THE LIKELIHOOD OF VAGINAL DELIVERY

The likelihood of vaginal birth is proportional to the patient's and the supervising clinician's motivation.[7-10]

Caesarean section for malpresentation or when vaginal delivery has previously been achieved carries an 84–85% chance of success, compared with 67% for those who have failed to progress'.[4] The type of aberrant progress in labour, whether during the first or second stages, does not seem to affect this rate of success.[11] In these cases, pelvimetry has been shown to be of no value in improving the prediction of outcome.[12,13] More sophisticated tests, such as fetal pelvic index, require further clinical assessment.[14,15]

Two previous caesarean sections do not alter the vaginal delivery rate nor the scar complication rate, unless the second caesarean section was a failed attempt at vaginal delivery.[3,16-18] There are published series on twin[19-21] and breech[22] deliveries after previous caesarean section. Complications are comparable with the figures given above for singleton cephalic 'trials' and vaginal delivery rates are comparable with those in labour with unscarred uteruses.

The outcome of induced labour after previous caesarean section has also been documented in observational studies, mainly using local prostaglandin E_2.[23-29] Scar complications occurred in 1.1%

(95% CI 0.1–2.1%) which is similar to spontaneous labour after previous caesarean section.[30] However, retrospective analysis of intrapartum stillbirths has identified a worrying number of cases in which scar rupture has occurred in association with repeated doses of vaginal prostaglandins.[31] Clearly, caution should be exercised if induction of labour is to be undertaken. The management of cases should be planned by the consultant in charge and safeguards should be in place regarding maximum dosages of any uterotonic agent and duration of the attempt. There are two small randomised trials, one for oxytocin versus vaginal prostins,[32] the other for mifepristone.[33] Significant complications do not appear to be evident but both studies lack power due their small numbers. There has been one randomised study on misoprostol versus oxytocin for induction of labour,[34] but the study was terminated due to two scar complications in 17 cases.

These criteria apply to conditions prior to labour. Prognostic factors have been identified and weighted to allow the clinician to gauge the likelihood of vaginal delivery from the clinical features at the time of admission in labour.[35] The main favourable factors are:

(1) Age less than 40 years;

(2) Previous vaginal birth;

(3) Vaginal birth since caesarean section;

(4) Indication other than failure to progress;

(5) Good cervical effacement;

(6) Cervical dilatation greater than 4 cm.

These variables have been weighted and combined in a scoring system. The predictive value in practice appears promising. With high scores (8–10 out of 10) almost 100% of women will deliver vaginally, whereas poor scores give only a 40–50% chance. An admission scoring system does not avoid emergency caesarean section but it does facilitate counselling at a relatively early stage in the labour.

PREDICTION OF SCAR INTEGRITY

Women who have failed a previous 'trial of scar' are three times more likely to experience scar complications than those without such a history.[3]

Ultrasound has been used to measure scar thickness at 36–38 weeks of gestation.[36] Measurement has to be within fractions of a millimetre, which is on the limit of resolution. With a cut-off point of 3.5 mm, the test has a good negative predictive value (99.3%) but a less impressive positive predictive value (11.8%) in a series of 642 scans with 25 scar defects.

Endoscopy has been used to examine the scar from within the uterus on admission after rupture of the membranes.[37] This is a small series ($n = 52$). Such a procedure is of interest but more evaluation is required and its predictive value needs to be assessed.

PRACTICE POINTS TO SAFEGUARD SCAR INTEGRITY IN LABOUR

Delivery of a patient with a previous caesarean section should be planned and supervised by a senior clinician with adequate experience of the procedure. All those in attendance should be educated in their role and points of management, particularly cardiotocograph interpretation. Plans should be well documented and local guidelines should specify policies for maternal and fetal intrapartum surveillance and augmentation.

Every case of scar complication should be investigated as part of the audit process.[31] The standard cervimetric limits should be used for judging progress in labour.[38] Women who have only delivered by caesarean section progress like nulliparae while those who have delivered vaginally should be judged by multiparous criteria.

The amount of delay behind an action line that is acceptable is a trade-off between scar complication risk and increased risk from operative intervention. A two-hour delay is likely to give a 0.8% scar complication and a caesarean section rate of 36% (sensitivity 71%; specificity 78%) whereas a three-hour action line gives a 1.6% scar complication and a 27% caesarean rate (sensitivity 43%; specificity 96%).[39]

Progress in the first stage of labour is due to transfer of tension from the myometrium to the cervix. Poor progress may be a sign that this process is inefficient due to yielding of a weak scar. When the scar ruptures, uterine activity may cease totally – a well-recognised sign. Intrauterine pressure monitoring has been advocated[40] but intrauterine pressure also depends upon wall tension. Thus, in a scarred uterus, poor progress in labour may be due to hypotonus or scar weakness.

There is no evidence that intrauterine pressure monitoring helps with this differentiation and it may be misleading.[41] Palpation and timing of repetition frequency may not sound so scientific but may tell us better what we need to know. Augmentation of uterine activity with oxytocin does not appear to be associated with an increased incidence of scar rupture[3] but extreme care should be exercised. Its use should be restricted to those women whose poor progress is specifically due to poor rates of uterine contractions (less than three in ten minutes), all other possibilities having been excluded.

Fetal heart rate abnormality is a sensitive indicator of scar complications but is after the event. No pattern prior to the event is predictive.[41,42] Continuous electronic fetal monitoring is mandatory.

Careful monitoring of the mother's pulse and blood pressure is important and this can easily be done continuously. Blood pressure is late in showing circulatory loss. Epidural analgesia can be used safely.[43]

MANAGING THE RISK

Scar complications can occur at any time during labour, including the second stage.[41]

As noted earlier, meta-analysis of attempted vaginal birth overall does not show increased perinatal or maternal mortality compared with elective caesarean section. The incidence of scar rupture and dehiscence is remarkably constant, even in units with the highest of standards. In most cases, scar complications do not have premonitory features which could be acted upon to reduce the risks. One study has looked at the maternal and perinatal consequences of scar rupture.[2] In this study the scar complication rate was 0.87%, which is in keeping with other studies. There was one maternal death in 99 cases; 19% of women required hysterectomy. The perinatal mortality rate was 6/1000 and 5% of neonates were severely asphyxiated; 39% had Apgar scores of less than seven at five minutes (12% had scores of less than four) and 42% had an umbilical artery pH of less than 7.00. Analysis was made of the time between noting prolonged fetal heart rate deceleration and delivery. Neonatal mortality and morbidity was avoided if this interval was less than 17 minutes. This is a much more stringent limit than the 30 minutes usually quoted for decision-delivery interval for fetal distress. Rehearsal of procedures to cope with the eventuality of scar rupture is recommended for these cases followed by continuing audit of performance. It is questionable whether the risk can be managed without these practices in place and, without them, should attempted vaginal delivery after previous caesarean section ever be advocated and undertaken?

References

1. Lilford, R.J., van Coeverden, H.A., Moore, P.J., Bingham, P. The relative risks of caesarean section (intrapartum and elective) and vaginal delivery: a detailed analysis to exclude the effects of medical disorders and other acute pre-existing physiological disturbances. *Br J Obstet Gynaecol* 1990;**97**:883–92
2. Leung, A.S., Leung, E.K., Paul, R.H. Uterine rupture after previous cesarean delivery: maternal and fetal consequences. *Am J Obstet Gynecol* 1993;**169**:945–50
3. Rosen, M.G., Dickinson, J.C., Westhoff, C.L. Vaginal birth after cesarean: a meta-analysis of morbidity and mortality. *Obstet Gynecol* 1991;**77**:465–70
4. Rosen, M.G., Dickinson, J.C. Vaginal birth after cesarean: a meta-analysis of indicators for success. *Obstet Gynecol* 1990;**76**:865–9
5. McMahon, M.J., Luther, E.R., Bowes, W.A. Jr., Olshan, A.F. Comparison of a trial of labor with an elective second cesarean section. *N Engl J Med* 1996;**335**:689–95
6. Macones, G.A. The utility of clinical tests of eligibility for a trial of labour following caesarean section: a decision analysis. *Br J Obstet Gynaecol* 1999;**106**:642–6
7. Murphy, M.C., Harvey, S.M. Choice of a childbirth method after cesarean. *Womens Health* 1989;**15**:67–85
8. McClain, C.S. The making of a medical tradition: vaginal birth after cesarean. *Soc Sci Med* 1990;**31**:203–10
9. Goldman, G., Pineault, R., Potvin, L., Blais, R., Bilodeau, H. Factors influencing the practice of vaginal birth after cesarean section. *Am J Public Health* 1993;**83**:1104–8
10. Fraser, W., Maunsell, E., Hodnett, E., Moutquin, J.M. Randomized controlled trial of a prenatal vaginal birth after cesarean section education and support program. Childbirth Alternatives Post-Cesarean Study Group. *Am J Obstet Gynecol* 1997;**176**:419–25
11. Jongen, V.H., Halfwerk, M.G., Brouwer, W.K. Vaginal delivery after previous caesarean section for failure of second stage of labour. *Br J Obstet Gynaecol* 1998;**105**:1079–81
12. Krishnamurthy, S., Fairlie, F., Cameron, A.D., Walker, J.J., Mackenzie, J.R. The role of postnatal X-ray pelvimetry after caesarean section in the management of subsequent delivery. *Br J Obstet Gynaecol* 1991;**98**:716–18
13. Thubisi, M., Ebrahim, A., Moodley, J., Shweni, P.M. Vaginal delivery after previous caesarean section: is X-ray pelvimetry necessary? *Br J Obstet Gynaecol* 1993;**100**:421–4
14. Thurnau, G.R., Scates, D.H., Morgan, M.A. The fetal-pelvic index: a method of identifying fetal-pelvic disproportion in women attempting vaginal birth after previous cesarean delivery. *Am J Obstet Gynecol* 1991;**165**:353–8
15. Ferguson, J.E. IInd, Newberry, Y.G., De Angelis, G.A., Finnerty, J.J., Agarwal, S., Turkheimer, E. (1998) The fetal-pelvic index has minimal utility in predicting fetal-pelvic disproportion. *Am J Obstet Gynecol* 1998;**179**:1186–92
16. Phelan, J.P., Ahn, M.O., Diaz, F., Brar, H.S., Rodriguez, M.H. Twice a cesarean, always a cesarean? *Obstet Gynecol* 1989;**73**:161–5
17. Hansell, R.S., McMurray, K.B., Huey, G.R. Vaginal birth after two or more cesarean sections: a five-year experience. *Birth* 1990;**17**:146–50
18. Granovsky-Grisaru, S., Shaya, M., Diamant, Y.Z. The management of labor in women with more than one uterine scar: is a repeat cesarean section really the only 'safe' option? *J Perinat Med* 1994;**22**:13–17
19. Strong, T.H. Jr, Phelan, J.P., Ahn, M.O., Sarno, A.P. Jr. Vaginal birth after cesarean delivery in the twin gestation. *Am J Obstet Gynecol* 1989;**161**:29–32

20. Miller, D.A., Mullin, P., Hou, D., Paul, R.H. Vaginal birth after cesarean section in twin gestation. *Am J Obstet Gynaecol* 1996;**175**:194–8
21. Odeh, M., Tarazova, L., Wolfson, M., Oettinger, M. Evidence that women with a history of cesarean section can deliver twins safely. *Acta Obstet Gynecol Scand* 1997;**76**:663–6
22. Sarno, A.P. Jr, Phelan, J.P., Ahn, M.O., Strong, T.H. Jr. Vaginal birth after cesarean delivery. Trial of labor in women with breech presentation. *J Reprod Med* 1989;**34**:831–3
23. MacKenzie, I.Z. Previous caesarean section and labour induction with PGE_2. In: Egarter, C., Husslein, P., editors. *Prostaglandins for Cervical Ripening and/or Induction of Labour*. Vienna: Facultas Universtatsverlag; 1988. p. 53–7
24. Goldberger, S.B., Rosen, D.J., Michaeli, G., Markov, S., Ben-Nun, I., Fejgin, M.D. The use of PGE_2 for induction of labor in parturients with a previous cesarean section scar. *Acta Obstet Gynecol Scand* 1989;**68**:523–6
25. Norman, M., Ekman, G. Preinductive cervical ripening with prostaglandin E_2 in women with one previous cesarean section. *Acta Obstet Gynecol Scand* 1992;**71**:351–5
26. Blanco, J.D., Collins, M., Willis, D., Prien, S. Prostaglandin E_2 gel induction of patients with a prior low transverse cesarean section. *Am J Perinatol* 1992;**9**:80–3
27. Stone, J.L., Lockwood, C.J., Berkowitz, G., Alvarez, M., Lapinski, R., Valcamonico, A. et al. Use of cervical prostaglandin E_2 gel in patients with previous cesarean section. *Am J Perinatol* 1994;**11**:309–12
28. Williams, M.A., Luthy, D.A., Zingheim, R.W., Hickok, D.E. Preinductive prostaglandin E_2 gel prior to induction of labor in women with a previous cesarean section. *Gynecol Obstet Invest* 1995;**40**:89–93
29. Flamm, B.L., Anton, D., Goings, J.R., Newman, J. Prostaglandin E_2 for cervical ripening: a multicenter study of patients with prior cesarean delivery. *Am J Perinatol* 1997;**14**:157–60
30. Vause, S., Macintosh, M. Use of prostaglandins to induce labour in women with a caesarean section scar. *BMJ* 1999;**31**:1056–8
31. Confidential Enquiry into Stillbirths and Death in Infancy. *Fifth Annual Report*. London: Maternal and Child Health Research Consortium; 1998
32. Taylor, A.V.G., Sellers, S., Ah Moye, M., MacKenzie, I.Z. A prospective random allocation trial to compare vaginal prostaglandin E_2 with intravenous oxytocin for labour induction in women previously delivered by caesarean section. *J Obstet Gynaecol* 1993;**12**:333–6
33. Lelaidier, C., Baton, C., Benifla, J.L., Fernandez, H., Bourget, P., Frydman, R. Mifepristone for labour induction after previous caesarean section. *Br J Obstet Gynaecol* 1994;**101**:501–3
34. Wing, D.A., Lovett, K., Paul, R.H. Disruption of prior uterine incision following misoprostol for labor induction in women with previous cesarean delivery. *Obstet Gynecol* 1998;**91**:828–30
35. Flamm, B.L., Geiger, A.M. Vaginal birth after cesarean delivery: an admission scoring system. *Obstet Gynecol* 1997;**90**:907–10
36. Rozenberg, P., Goffinet, F., Phillippe, H.J., Nisand, I. Ultrasonographic measurement of lower uterine segment to assess risk of defects of scarred uterus. *Lancet* 1996;**347**:281–4
37. Petrikovsky, B.M. Endoscopic assessment of the integrity of the postcesarean uterine wall before a trial of labor. Transcervical Endoscopy Registry. *J Reprod Med* 1994;**39**:464–6
38. Chazotte, C., Madden, R., Cohen, W.R. Labor patterns in women with previous cesareans. *Obstet Gynecol* 1990;**75**:350–5
39. Khan, K.S., Rizvi, A., Rizvi, J.H. Risk of uterine rupture after the partographic 'alert' line is crossed – an additional dimension in the quest towards safe motherhood in labour following caesarean section. *Journal of the Pakistan Medical Association* 1996;**46**:120–2

40 Arulkumaran, S., Gibb, D.M., Ingemarsson, I., Kitchener, H.C., Ratnam, S.S. Uterine activity during spontaneous labour after previous lower-segment caesarean section. *Br J Obstet Gynaecol* 1989;**96**:933–8

41 Beckley, S., Gee, H., Newton, J.R. Scar rupture in labour after previous lower uterine segment caesarean section: the role of uterine activity measurement. *Br J Obstet Gynaecol* 1991;**98**:265–9

42 Menihan, C.A. Uterine rupture in women attempting a vaginal birth following prior cesarean birth. *J Perinatol* 1998;**18**:440–3

43 Sakala, E.P., Kaye, S., Murray, R.D., Munson, L.J. Epidural analgesia: effect on the likelihood of a successful trial of labor after cesarean section. *J Reprod Med* 1990;**35**:886–90

25

Maternal suicide

Carol A. Henshaw

INTRODUCTION

The *Report on Confidential Enquiries into Maternal Deaths 1994–96* (CEMD) was the first report to devote a separate chapter to deaths from psychiatric causes.[1] It concluded that 'psychiatric illness leading to suicide is a significant factor in at least 10% of maternal deaths'. The report highlights inadequacies in recording and assessing risk factors and poor liaison between professional groups. Recommendations are provided that are designed to improve services for women with mental health problems in the hope that these deaths can be prevented, although there are considerable impediments to their implementation.

POSTNATAL MENTAL DISORDER

There is significant psychiatric morbidity consequent upon childbirth. Non-psychotic postnatal depression follows 13% of deliveries.[2] At least two per 1000 new mothers develop a psychotic illness, usually a mood disorder.[3] Approximately two-thirds of these will experience a depressive psychosis and one-third a manic episode. Postnatal morbidity is predominantly depressive in nature, depression being the mental disorder most closely associated with suicide. In addition, women who are suffering a wide range of other mental disorders from chronic schizophrenia or neurosis to substance abuse, learning disability and personality disorder, become pregnant. These disorders may make women vulnerable to suicide or self-harm through psychosis, alcohol or drug consumption, or poor impulse control that may occur in some personality disorders.

Despite this substantial morbidity, the suicide rate for postpartum women is lower than would be expected. A study comparing the observed to expected mortality ratios for suicides in England and Wales over the period 1973–84, found that the standardised mortality ratio (SMR) in postnatal women was 0.17, one sixth of that expected.[4] Those who did commit suicide after childbirth often did so in the first month, coinciding with the peak onset of puerperal psychosis.

Postnatal suicides tend to use more violent methods, a reversal of the usual trend of women using non-violent methods such as overdose. Self-incineration, jumping from bridges or in front of trains occurred more often than would be expected in this study. An excess of violent methods was also reported in a Swedish study examining maternal deaths between 1980 and 1988.[5] Several of the cases reported in the CEMD died by violent means including jumping from tall buildings, hanging and self-incineration. The timing and choice of method strongly suggests that many of these postnatal suicides were psychotic at the time of death.

DELIBERATE SELF-HARM IN POSTNATAL WOMEN

Rates of deliberate self-harm in a consecutive six-month sample of women attending an accident and emergency department were examined.[6] Rates of deliberate self-harm, like suicide rates, were lower in those women who had delivered a child in the previous year compared with those who had not.

It is proposed that the presence of a fetus or infant is protective and may act in an inhibitory way in those who experience suicidal ideation. This hypothesis is supported by the findings of a study in Seattle.[7] A sample of the public was asked what would prevent them from committing suicide if they were distressed. The most common answers were child concerns, religion and fear of pain. The responses were used to compile the Reason for Living Inventory that was then given to a sample of inpatients who had experienced suicidal ideation or had harmed themselves. The only difference between the two groups was that those who had not harmed themselves were more likely to cite child concerns.

SUICIDE IN PREGNANT WOMEN

The rate of non-psychotic depression during pregnancy is similar to that occurring postpartum,[8] although onsets of psychosis are less common.[3] The ratio for suicide during pregnancy in Appleby's study[4] was 0.05 of that for all pregnant women. More recent data from the USA confirm the low rates during pregnancy.[9] This study examined all autopsy reports from female residents of New York City 10-44 years of age who committed suicide between 1990 and 1993, in order to ascertain how many were pregnant.[9] The age- and race-adjusted risk of suicide in pregnant women was found to be one-third that in nonpregnant women. Women who self-harm or commit suicide during pregnancy usually use the customary female method of self-poisoning.

Deliberate self-harm in pregnancy

A review in 1968[10] estimated that between 5% and 12% of women attempting suicide were pregnant. In 1984, 0.07% of calls to a USA metropolitan poison control centre were from or about pregnant women and the attempt reported was usually her first.[11] Half of the overdoses were taken during the first trimester, most commonly using an over-the-counter analgesic, iron or a vitamin. In Budapest, an inpatient toxicology centre serving a population of three million found that 2.8% of the 22 969 women admitted between 1985 and 1993 were pregnant.[12] Eighty-seven percent had ingested drugs and the peak period for overdose was the first postconceptual month, with the second highest rate in the following month. The rates of deliberate self-harm later in pregnancy were significantly lower. Another study, however, found that rates were more evenly distributed over pregnancy and that most deliberate self-harm occurred during the second trimester.[13]

A Swedish study found that issues relating to pregnancy and interpersonal difficulties were cited as the main provoking factors for deliberate self-harm in pregnant women.[14] This was also the case in a series of 15 pregnant women who had self-harmed in Philadelphia. They were compared with 131 nonpregnant women who had also self-harmed. Although the methodology is not fully described, the pregnant women cited prior loss of children (through death, termination or adoption), desire for a termination or the potential loss of a partner as reasons for their act.[15]

A retrospective case-report study of patients referred to a psychiatry-obstetric consultation service in Atlanta, found that 19% had reported some suicidal feelings during pregnancy.[16] This was more likely to occur in women reporting a history of physical abuse, sexual abuse or both. Of 742 women attending University of Virginia obstetric clinics, who were screened for physical abuse, past or present, 10.9% admitted to past abuse and were significantly more likely to have a psychiatric history and 20% of those who had been abused had harmed themselves.[17]

Two of the 559 women who self-poisoned in Budapest died[18] and, in the 213 overdoses occurring during the first month of gestation, over 80% ended in fetal loss. Of the 111 pregnant women who contacted the USA poison control centre in the study described above,[11] 55% had mild or nonexistent symptoms and 45% major or life-threatening problems. Much of the literature in this area consists of single case studies so it is difficult to gain a clear picture of maternal and fetal morbidity relating to deliberate self-harm. The Budapest group also studied live births in 777 women who had had previously self-poisoned months or years before the birth and found significantly lower birthweights in this population when compared with the partners of men who had self-poisoned.[19] However, it is not clear to what extent this might be the result of other factors not controlled for.

ADOLESCENTS

Young women appear to be particularly vulnerable to suicide. Appleby's study[4] found teenage pregnant women to have a risk of suicide five times greater than all pregnant women and offered the explanation that, as there seemed to be an absence of prior psychiatric history in this group, it may be related to the impact of unwanted pregnancy.

Thirty years ago, Gabrielson, in New Haven, followed up women under the age of 18 years who had given birth. Fourteen of the 105 women for whom he had follow-up data attempted suicide, although in the majority this was later than the first year after delivery. The members of this group were more likely to be single, living in a poor area, to be Roman Catholic, have had a complicated pregnancy and a sexually transmitted disease since delivery.[20] A more recent study of 352 pregnant teenagers from lower socio-economic backgrounds in San Francisco, found 18% to have prior suicidal thoughts or actions, particularly if they also had a history of physical or sexual abuse.[21] However, the group was not followed up during or after pregnancy to ascertain actual rates of self-harm over that period.

PREGNANCY LOSS

The SMR for women who had experienced a stillbirth was 1.05, six times higher than that for all postnatal women and similar to that of all women in the general population.[4] All of the women who experienced a stillbirth had no other children and could, therefore, be considered as being without the protective effect of a child. Such women may leave hospital quickly and may be reluctant to remain in contact with health professionals. The low rates of stillbirth may lead to a sense of isolation, with women not knowing anyone with similar experience. There are active voluntary organisations to offer help but they may be more acceptable to, or more easily accessed by, middle-class women, leaving other groups with less support.

Termination of pregnancy

A Finnish study,[22] linking birth, termination and hospital discharge registers with suicide statistics, confirmed the low rates in postnatal women but found that rates were higher in those who had been admitted to hospital for treatment of a miscarriage and higher still in those who had experienced a termination of pregnancy during the year before death. It was not possible to determine whether this was a direct effect of mental health at termination or a more complex interaction of common risk factors. Rates of psychiatric disorder overall are no greater after termination than after childbirth.[23] However, those undergoing termination who had prior psychiatric histories in this study were at greater risk whatever the pregnancy outcome, whereas those without such a history were at increased risk of deliberate self-harm following termination. Again the assumption was that common risk factors were involved.

ETHNIC COMMUNITIES

Suicide rates are high in young Asian women in the UK, with 20% of those who commit suicide killing themselves by burning.[24] An earlier study found an association between deliberate self-harm and pregnancy in young West Indian women[25] in the UK and a descriptive study of Turkish women resident in Berlin found two-thirds of those seeking a termination were experiencing suicidal ideation.[26] There may be particular stressors surrounding unwanted pregnancy in some ethnic communities.

CHRONIC MENTAL ILLNESS

Two of the cases described in the CEMD[1] had histories of chronic mental illness, one a recurrent depressive disorder and the other bipolar disorder (manic depressive illness). The second woman had had her prophylactic medication discontinued prior to conceiving. Bipolar patients are at considerable risk of relapse, especially of mania, on discontinuation of lithium or other maintenance therapy.[27] The risk can be reduced somewhat by a gradual rather than rapid discontinuation. These women are also at substantial risk of recurrence (over 50%) following delivery.[28] Relapse of a psychotic illness may involve considerable risk to the woman, her fetus or infant and others before she can be treated. Treatment may involve admission (perhaps under the Mental Health Act) and may require considerable amounts of medication.

Such patients require careful evaluation of the risks of relapse versus any potential risk to the fetus of continuing with medication. The risk of fetal exposure to lithium is now known to be less than previously believed[29] but each case requires careful individual evaluation by someone aware of all the issues at stake. Certainly, prophylaxis immediately following delivery should be offered. This could involve re-starting lithium or, if the woman wishes to breastfeed, an alternative medication such as an anti-psychotic. Women with prior non-psychotic postpartum depressions or recurrent depressive disorder may benefit from antidepressant prophylaxis.

PROBLEMS IN IDENTIFICATION AND RISK ASSESSMENT

Of the five indirect deaths during pregnancy described in the CEMD,[1] four clearly had current or past psychiatric disorders but lack of information made this impossible to ascertain for the fifth. Lack of information, poor recognition of mental disorder and the risks involved, together with poor liaison between professionals, are cited as being pertinent.

Of the 18 indirect and late indirect deaths occurring after delivery, 11 involved a depressive illness, five of which may have been psychotic, and two had a chronic mental illness. Substance abuse was a factor in five deaths. Again, there are issues concerning the importance of the patient's history and acting on serious warning signs such as plans to commit suicide.

RECOMMENDATIONS

Antenatal booking

The first recommendation relates to the antenatal booking interview. It is suggested that the midwife should take details about current or past maternal psychiatric disorder, substance abuse, social problems and self-harm. Such sensitive and stigmatised topics require careful appraisal and a sufficiently private environment in order to encourage disclosure. In recent years, partners and other relatives have been encouraged to attend antenatal appointments and to participate in the process. Many appointments take place in the woman's own home. Under these circumstances, it may be difficult to ensure the privacy which is required in order to undertake a full assessment of these areas. Women may be fearful that disclosing mental illness, substance abuse or physical abuse will result in their children being taken into care.

Clearly, responsibility does not end at booking. Those caring for pregnant or postpartum women need to be aware of the implications of suicidal ideation and threats and what action to take. Many of the CEMD suicides had made threats prior to killing themselves but this was often not taken seriously or acted upon.

Many midwives have little experience of psychiatry during their preregistration training and few have undergone training since registration. The majority of midwives surveyed in two adjacent health districts[30] indicated that, while they agreed they had a role to play in managing perinatal mental disorder, they lacked the skills and confidence to do so. Few had been given any formal training. The CEMD refers to 'techniques being piloted' but does not elaborate. Clearly, should these interventions prove successful, there are resource implications in ensuring all midwives undertaking booking assessments and antenatal care receive appropriate training.

Liaison

Midwives should also ensure that they are familiar with statutory and voluntary services for the mentally ill and how to access them locally. They may be managed by a different trust on a different site from maternity services. This will become more likely with the move towards specialist mental health trusts and may make liaison work more difficult. Community midwives may find that they can meet with, for example, community psychiatric nurses also working in primary care settings. Women with severe mental disorders will have their care co-ordinated via the Care Programme Approach with regular review meetings involving all the relevant professionals, the patient and carers. This provides a forum whereby the midwife can link up with all concerned.

Midwives undertaking postnatal care need to be aware of the early symptoms of mental illness arising in the puerperium. Such symptoms are often nonspecific, for example sleep disturbance and agitation, but may be the precursor of florid psychotic symptoms.

Most of these measures are to be incorporated into auditable standards for midwifery care in the near future but clearly each service has to develop a training strategy for its staff.

Specialist services

The CEMD proposes the identification of a clinician in each district who should manage a perinatal mental health service on a sessional basis. Current shortages of psychiatrists and other mental health professionals make this unlikely to be achievable in the short term even if sufficient resources can be identified. Perinatal psychiatry is not an identified subspecialty of psychiatry leading to a CCST and training posts do not exist on all higher training rotations. There are, however, a growing number of psychiatrists who have gained relevant experience and a number of societies, including the Marcé Society and the British Society for Psychosomatic Obstetrics and Gynaecology, which seek to educate and research this area as well as pressing for improved services.

Current specialist services are patchy. Mother-and-baby inpatient units exist in some centres and can act as a focus for services linked in to obstetric, primary care and generic mental health services. These could have a training and consultation or liaison role. However, this is not universal and many women who require admission still face the choice between admission without their baby to a general psychiatric setting or transfer to a mother-and-baby unit at some considerable distance. Some trusts feel they have addressed the issue by the provision of a small number of beds attached to a general psychiatric ward. Such units are usually without specialist psychiatric cover, designated and skilled nursing staff or nursery nurses. Infants in this setting may be particularly vulnerable.[31]

Some areas have developed health-visitor screening and counselling intervention for non-psychotic postnatal depression.[32] However, in places this has been implemented without considering links with, or the implications for, secondary mental health services. This approach clearly does not meet the needs of the more severely ill mother nor of those women with disorders other than depression and it may not screen pregnant women.

Psychological autopsy

Obstetricians and paediatricians have led the field for years with multidisciplinary detailed audit of perinatal morbidity and mortality. Psychiatrists have been slow to follow and only in recent years has the National Confidential Enquiry into Suicides been instituted. Many psychiatric services do not hold open local multidisciplinary review of suicides or 'near misses', which could provide a valuable means of learning and re-shaping services. Where such incidents involve pregnant or postpartum women there is a clear case for a joint review with maternity services.

SUMMARY

The greater focus on psychiatric causes of maternal mortality in the CEMD should be welcomed by all who care for pregnant and recently delivered women and their infants. It remains for the recommendations to be taken seriously and resourced adequately. Only then might we see a reduction in these frequently preventable deaths.

References

1. Drife, J., Lewis, G., editors. *Why Mothers Die: Report on Confidential Enquiries into Maternal Deaths in the UK 1994–96*. London: The Stationery Office; 1998
2. O'Hara, M.W., Swain, A.M. Rates and risks of postpartum depression: a meta-analysis. *International Review of Psychiatry* 1996;**8**:37–54
3. Kendell, R.E., Chalmers, J., Platz, C. The epidemiology of puerperal psychosis. *Br J Psychiatry* 1987;**150**:662–73
4. Appleby, L. Suicide during pregnancy and in the first postnatal year. *BMJ* 1991;**302**:137–40
5. Högerg, U., Innala, E., Sandström, A. Maternal mortality in Sweden, 1980–88. *Obstet Gynecol* 1994;**84**:240–4
6. Appleby, L., Turnbull, G. Parasuicide in the first postnatal year. *Psychol Med* 1995;**25**:1087–90
7. Linehan, M.M., Goodstein, J.L., Nielsen, S.L., Chiles, J.A. Reasons for staying alive when you are thinking of killing yourself: the Reason for Living Inventory. *J Consult Clin Psychol* 1983;**51**:276–86
8. Green, J.M., Murray, D. The use of the Edinburgh Postnatal Depression Scale to explore the relationship between antenatal and postnatal dysphoria. In: Cox, J., Holden, J., editors. *Perinatal Psychiatry: Use and Misuse of the Edinburgh Postnatal Depression Scale*. London: Gaskell; 1994. p. 180–98
9. Marzuk, P.M., Tardiff, K., Leon, A.C., Hirsch, C.S., Portera, L., Hartwell, N. *et al.* Lower risk of suicide during pregnancy. *Am J Psychiatry* 1997;**154**:122–3
10. Whitlock, F.A., Edwards, J.E. Pregnancy and attempted suicide. *Compr Psychiatry* 1968;**9**:1–12

11 Rayburn, W., Aronow, R., DeLancey, B., Hogan, M.J. Drug overdose during pregnancy: an overview from a Metropolitan Poison Control Center. *Obstet Gynecol* 1984;**64**:611–14
12 Czeizel, E., Timar, L., Susansky, E. Timing of suicide attempts by self-poisoning during pregnancy and pregnancy outcomes. *Int J Gynaecol Obstet* 1999;**65**:39–45
13 Lester, D. The timing of attempted suicide during pregnancy. *Acta Paediatrica Hungarica* 1987;**28**:259–60
14 Otto, U. Suicidal attempts made by pregnant women under 21 years. *Acta Paedopsychiatrica* 1965;**32**:276–88
15 Lester, D., Beck, A.T. Attempted suicide and pregnancy. *Am J Obstet Gynecol* 1988;**158**:1084–5
16 Farber, E.W., Herbert, S.E., Reviere, S.L. Childhood abuse and suicidality in obstetrics patients in a hospital-based urban prenatal clinic. *Gen Hosp Psychiatry* 1996;**18**:56–60
17 Hillard, P.J.A. Physical abuse in pregnancy. *Obstet Gynecol* 1985;**66**:185–90
18 Czeikel, A.E., Mosonyi, A. Monitoring of early human fetal development in women exposed to large doses of chemicals. *Environ Mol Mutagen* 1997;**30**:240–4
19 Czeikel, A.E, Szabados, A., Sasansky, E. Lower birth weight of offspring born after self-poisoning of parent. *Mutat Res* 1992;**269**:35–9
20 Gabrielson, I.W., Klerman, L.V., Currie, J.B., Tyler, N.C., Jekel, J.F. Suicide attempts in a population pregnant as teenagers. *Am J Public Health* 1970;**60**:2289–301
21 Bayatpour, M., Wells, R.D., Holford, S. Physical and sexual abuse as predictors of substance abuse and suicide among pregnant teenagers. *J Adolesc Health* 1992;**13**:128–32
22 Gissler, M., Hemminki, E., Lönnqvist, J. Suicide after pregnancy in Finland, 1987–94: register linkage study. *BMJ* 1996;**313**:1431–4
23 Gilchrist, A.C., Hannaford, P.C., Frank, P., Kay, C.R. Termination of pregnancy and psychiatric morbidity. *Br J Psychiatry* 1995;**167**:243–8
24 Raleigh, S. Suicide patterns and trends in people of Indian subcontinent and Caribbean origin in England and Wales. *Ethn Health* 1996;**1**:55–63
25 Burke, A.W. Socio-cultural determinants of attempted suicide among West Indians in Birmingham: ethnic origin and immigrant status. *Br J Psychiatry* 1976;**129**:261–6
26 Berzewski, H. Psychological and social disorders of Turkish women during an unaccepted pregnancy in a foreign country. *Int J Soc Psychiatry* 1984;**30**:275–82
27 Suppes, T., Baldessarini, R.J., Faedda, G.L., Tohen, M. Risk of recurrence following discontinuation of lithium treatment in bipolar disorder. *Arch Gen Psychiatry* 1991;**48**:1082–8
28 Cohen, L.S., Sichel, D.A., Robertson, L.M., Heckscher, E., Rosenbaum, J.F. Postpartum prophylaxis for women with bipolar disorder. *Am J Psychiatry* 1995;**152**:1641–5
29 Cohen, L.S., Friedman, J.M., Jefferson, J.M., Johnson, J.W., Weiner, M.L. A reevaluation of risk of *in utero* exposure to lithium. *JAMA* 1994;**271**:146–50
30 Stewart, C., Henshaw, C. Unpublished data
31 Brockington, I. *Motherhood and Mental Health*. Oxford: Oxford University Press; 1996. Services. p. 555–83
32 Holden, J.M., Sagovsky, R., Cox, J.L. Counselling in a general practice setting: a controlled study of health visitor intervention in the treatment of postnatal depression. *BMJ* 1989;**298**:223–6

26

Fetal hydrops

David James

INTRODUCTION, DEFINITION AND AETIOLOGY

Fetal hydrops is a syndrome associated with high perinatal morbidity and mortality at all gestational ages.[1-4] It is defined as the occurrence of fluid in two or more body compartments (ascites, pleural or pericardial effusions) together with oedema. However, many would use the term when any of these features are present. It is conventionally classified into immune and non-immune causes. In developed countries, the ratio of non-immune to immune causes is at least 9:1.[5] There are many causes or associations with fetal hydrops and these are summarised in Table 1.[6]

INCIDENCE

Although the incidence of fetal hydrops is commonly quoted as 1/1000 there is considerable regional variation.[7] Thus, for example α-thalassaemia is the most common cause of hydrops in South-East Asia, accounting for up to 25% of perinatal mortality, whereas it is relatively rare elsewhere.[8,9] Hydrops is also subject to seasonal variation, especially with parvovirus B19 epidemics.[10]

PATHOPHYSIOLOGY

Hydrops occurs when the microvascular fluid exchange regulatory systems in the fetus and placenta are disturbed. These fluid exchange mechanisms in the fetus are gestationally dependent and poorly understood. No simple, single mechanism explains fetal hydrops in the wide range of clinical settings (Table 1). Our understanding of fetal hydrops is based on animal research complemented by limited studies in human fetuses.

The fluid-dominated environment of the fetus and the specific physiological characteristics of the fetal heart and the lymphatic system make it particularly susceptible to hydrops. Recent animal research together with clinical study suggests that raised central venous pressure (CVP) is a critical step in the pathophysiology of hydrops. Indeed, some fetal medicine centres advocate the clinical use of umbilical venous pressure (UVP) in the investigation and management of some cases of fetal hydrops, given the apparent importance of CVP and the lymphatic system in such research.[11,12] It also follows from this work that some of the traditional pathophysiological forces, such as colloid oncotic pressure, are apparently less important than they were formerly thought to be.

OUTLOOK FOR THE FETUS

The main fetal risks from hydrops are:

(1) Death from the underlying pathophysiology, invasive fetal investigations or fetal treatment. The mortality rate ranges between 50% and 90%;

(2) Complications of the various invasive diagnostic and therapeutic procedures, including miscarriage, preterm labour, trauma and maternal red-cell alloimmunisation;

(3) Infant morbidity, both in the short and long term depends on the underlying diagnosis and treatment undertaken.

Table 1 *Abnormalities associated with hydrops (reproduced with permission from Smoleniec et al.[43])*

Immune
Anti-D rhesus antibodies
Antibodies to K in Kell system
Antibodies to Fya in Duffy system

Non-immune

'*Idiopathic*'/*unknown*
Anaemia (other than alloimmunisation)
Homozygous α-thalassaemia
Chronic fetomaternal transfusion
Twin-to-twin transfusion and variants
Erythroleukaemia

Cardiovascular
Severe congenital heart disease (atrial septal defect, ventricular septal defect, hypoplastic left heart, pulmonary valve insufficiency, Ebstein's anomaly, subaortic stenosis, atrioventricular canal defect, tetralogy of Fallot, premature closure of foramen ovale)
Premature closure of ductus (? indomethacin therapy)
Myocarditis (coxsackie, cytomegalovirus, parvovirus B19)
Large atrioventricular malformation
Tachyarrhythmias (supraventricular tachycardia, atrial flutter)
Bradyarrhythmias (heart block)
Wolff–Parkinson–White syndrome
Intracardiac tumours (teratoma, rhabdomyoma)
Cardiomyopathy (e.g. fibroelastosis)
Myocardial 'infarction'
Arterial calcification

Chromosomal
Trisomies
Turner syndrome (45XO)
Triploidy

Pulmonary
Cystic adenomatous malformation
Pulmonary lymphangiectasia
Pulmonary hypoplasia
Diaphragmatic hernia
Chondrodysplasia
Bronchogenic cysts and other tumours
Pulmonary sequestration
Congenital hydro-/chylothorax

Renal
Congenital nephrosis (Finnish type)
Renal vein thrombosis
Urethral obstruction (atresia, posterior valves)
Spontaneous bladder perforation
Cloacal malformation
Prune belly

Table 1 *Abnormalities associated with hydrops (reproduced with permission from Smoleniec et al.[43]) continued.*

Infection (intrauterine)
Parvovirus B19 (either by anaemia, myocarditis or hepatitis)
Syphilis
Cytomegalovirus
Toxoplasmosis
Herpes simplex
Leptospirosis
Chagas disease

Liver
Hepatic calcifications
Hepatic fibrosis
Congenital hepatitis
Cholestasis
Polycystic disease
Biliary atresia
Familial cirrhosis

Genetic metabolic disease (may have effect via the liver)
Gaucher's disease
GM_1 gangliosidosis
Mucopolysaccharidosis (types VIa and VII)
Iron-storage disease
Anomalies (many associated with fetal immobility)
Achondroplasia
Achondrogenesis type 2
Thanatophoric dwarfism
Sacrococcygeal teratoma
Arthrogryphosis
Multiple pterygium syndrome
Neu-Laxova syndrome
Pena-Shokeir type 1 syndrome
Noonan syndrome
Myotonic dystrophy
Neuronal degeneration

Miscellaneous
Cystic hygroma
Meconium peritonitis
Fetal neuroblastosis
Tuberous sclerosis
Small bowel volvulus
Amniotic band syndrome
Torsion of ovarian cyst
Polysplenia syndrome

Placental
Vein thrombosis
Chorioangioma
True cord knots

Maternal
Diabetes mellitus
Pre-eclampsia
Severe anaemia
Hypoalbuminaemia

OUTLOOK FOR THE MOTHER

Maternal risks of fetal hydrops include:

(1) Before labour and delivery: pre-eclampsia ('mirror' syndrome),[13] anaemia, hydramnios and placental abruption from invasive fetal procedures;[14]

(2) During labour and delivery: dystocia (e.g. hydrops from large tumours), caesarean delivery, placental abruption, postpartum haemorrhage (primary and secondary) and retained placenta.

DIAGNOSIS

Hydrops is the excessive, extravascular accumulation of fluid in the interstitial compartment secondary to disruption of the normal intravascular interstitial fluid homeostatic mechanisms. The excessive accumulation of interstitial fluid, particularly in serous cavities (peritoneal, pleural, pericardial), placenta and amniotic fluid, facilitates the sonographic diagnosis of fetal hydrops. Classically, as described above, the sonographic diagnosis of hydrops requires the presence of generalised oedema plus the accumulation of fluid within two or more serous cavities, although clearly many of the pathologies leading to such a diagnosis go through phases where fluid is only recognised sonographically in one site.

MANAGEMENT OVERVIEW

Fetal hydrops presents clinically in one of several ways:

(1) By chance from:
   - ultrasound examination;
   - fetal heart rate recording.

(2) As part of assessment for:
   - 'large-for-dates' (hydramnios);
   - reduced fetal movements;
   - placental abruption;
   - maternal diabetes;
   - maternal pre-eclampsia ('mirror syndrome').

Once fetal hydrops is identified, the mother should be counselled regarding the importance of trying to make a diagnosis based on maternal and fetal investigations (Tables 2 and 3); the prognosis, namely the fetal risks both in the short and long term, which are influenced by the diagnosis and by any invasive procedures undertaken in diagnosis and treatment; and whether treatment is possible. A comprehensive search in the mother and fetus for the 'cause' usually involves antenatal invasive procedures (Tables 2 and 3). The severity, gestational age, ultrasonographically identified anomalies and the parents' wishes influence the decision to perform these procedures. The ultrasound scan may identify an associated cause in more than 50% of cases.[6] A diagnosis may not be possible in 15–26%.[6,14] The most common invasive procedures are fetal blood sampling and amniocentesis. Fetal blood sampling will yield more information more quickly but the associated mortality rates may be higher than when the invasive procedures are performed for nonhydropic indications, especially when the fetus is thrombocytopenic (for example, parvovirus B19 infection) and when it is technically more difficult.[14,15]

Polymerase chain reaction investigation is an important advance in the diagnosis of fetal

Table 2 Maternal investigations for fetal hydrops

Type	Investigations
History	Previous fetal hydrops or diagnosis causing hydrops
	Previous baby with jaundice
	Ethnic origin
Blood	Complete blood count
	Blood group and antibody screen (titre if antibodies present)
	Electrophoresis (depending upon ethnic background)
	Glucose-6-phosphate dehydrogenase and pyruvate kinase carrier status
	α-fetoprotein
	Serological test for:
	– syphilis
	– parvovirus B19
	– toxoplasmosis
	– cytomegalovirus
	– herpes simplex virus
	– coxsackie
	Urate, urea and electrolytes
	Liver function including albumin
	Kleihauer–Betke test
	Test of glucose tolerance
	Lupus anticoagulant and anti-Ro if fetal bradycardia

Table 3 Fetal investigations for fetal hydrops

Type	Investigations
Ultrasound	Sites and severity of hydrops
	Detailed real-time ultrasound for congenital abnormality and abnormality of placenta and cord
	Fetal echocardiography, pulsed and colour Doppler studies and M-mode
	Amniotic fluid volume
	Biophysical assessment (non-stress testing or biophysical profile score)
Invasive (mainly fetal blood)	Haematological tests: full blood count, haemoglobin electrophoreses (depending on ethnic background), group and Coombs
	Infection: serological tests for acute phase specific immunoglobulin M antibodies for infection; culture; electron microscopy for rapid diagnosis of parvovirus B19
	Blood gas analysis and pH estimation to provide an indication of the immediate well-being of the fetus
	Umbilical vessel (venous) pressure
	Karyotype (blood, placenta, ascitic or pleural fluids are suitable sources)
	Liver function tests (albumin)
	White-cell enzymes (Gaucher's, mucopolysaccharidoses)

infection. If not available, a maternal infection screen should be performed before the fetal screen in order to optimise the use of the relatively small fetal sample.

If the heart is displaced from its normal midline position by a unilateral or asymmetrical bilateral pleural effusion, the fetal chest can be punctured and the effusion(s) drained to determine the effect of decompression on lung re-expansion and the restoration of the heart to its normal midline position. The measurements of the intrathoracic pressure and the UVP before and after the drainage may be used prognostically. The measurement of UVP is used by some as a surrogate for fetal CVP. However, it requires an otherwise unnecessary cordocentesis if the diagnosis is apparent, since most laboratory studies can typically be performed on the pleural fluid.

Table 4 *Approximate survival rates (%) for major causes of fetal hydrops (reproduced with permission from Smoleniec et al.[43])*

Cause	Gestation at presentation	
	< 24 weeks	≥ 24 weeks
Anaemia		
Alloimmune	24–74	31–92a
Non-immune	25	22a
Cardiovascular	7	29a
Chromosomal	0	27
Pulmonary	0	46a
Renal	0	20
Infection	50 (2 cases)	11a
Anomalies	0	13
Miscellaneous	0	25
'Idiopathic'	0	2
Lymph	1	

a Potential treatment available (blood transfusion for fetal anaemia, correction of cardiac arrthymia, treatment of twin-to-twin transfusion syndrome, shunt insert for hydro-/chylothorax) (Data from Stangenberg et al.[44] and Hutchinson et al.[45])

The optimal time for counselling about prognosis (Table 4) is when the results of the maternal and fetal investigations are available. After counselling, the patient may elect to undergo a termination of pregnancy if legal at the given gestational age.

TREATMENT

The proportion of cases amenable to antenatal treatment varies in each reported series since they are generally small in number and reflect variation in local referral practices. It is likely that no more than 20–30% of cases are candidates for treatment.[16]

Currently, the only causes of fetal hydrops amenable to therapy are those associated with:

(1) Fetal anaemia;

(2) Fetal arrhythmia;

(3) Hydrothoraces;

(4) Twin-to-twin transfusion syndrome;

(5) Type I cystic adenomatoid malformation;

(6) Tumours.

Anaemia

In South-east Asia, thalassaemia is the main cause of fetal hydrops. The prognosis for homozygous α-thalassaemia is not as good as for other causes of fetal anaemia.[17]

Fetal blood transfusion is the only therapeutic option for the treatment of hydrops secondary to anaemia. The principles, in general, are the same whether the anaemia is secondary to parvovirus B19 infection (see below) or chronic fetomaternal haemorrhage. However, the prognosis for both these conditions may be worse than that for haemolytic disease secondary to red blood cell alloimmunisation.[17]

If fetomaternal haemorrhage is the cause of the hydrops, screening for further episodes of haemorrhage is vital as these may be fatal. However, their occurrence and severity is unpredictable and delivery may be considered once the pregnancy has reached an appropriate gestation.

There are no effective antenatal treatments for glucose-6-phosphate dehydrogenase deficiency and erythroleukaemia. Gene therapy may prove possible in the future and interdisciplinary counselling involving paediatric colleagues and clinical geneticists is advisable.

Cardiovascular anomalies

Cardiac anomalies are the most common anatomical abnormalities associated with fetal hydrops.[6] In general, hydrops associated with a structurally abnormal heart carries a poor prognosis, as the anomaly is usually severe.[18] Those hydropic fetuses with an arrhythmia but a structurally normal heart usually respond to either transplacental or direct fetal therapy. For a more detailed discussion the reader is referred to other texts.[19,20] In general, the prognosis is good.

Pulmonary anomalies

The prognosis for hydrops for these conditions is generally poor and the therapeutic options limited. However, the place of fetal surgery (open and minimally invasive) for thoracic lesions (congenital cystic adenomatoid malformations, pulmonary sequestrations) appears promising; for example, there have been case reports of successful *in utero* drainage of such lesions.[21] There are several different therapeutic strategies (e.g. tracheal occlusion, iatrogenic gastroschisis) aimed at improving the outcome from diaphragmatic hernia; however, they must be regarded as experimental at present.[22] The main exception to the above generalisation about poor prognosis is hydrops associated with hydrothorax causing cardiac displacement. The diagnosis of congenital hydrothorax is a diagnosis of exclusion: excess pleural fluid in the absence of another detectable cause. Hydrothoraces typically present after 24 weeks of gestation when lung development has already entered the canalicular phase. The lymphocyte content of the fluid is not relevant to either prognosis or diagnosis.[23] Although it has been known since the early 1980s that the placement of a thoracoamniotic shunt could reverse the hydrops,[24] the rate of success among reported series has been variable.[23] This suggests more than one mechanism may underlie the hydrops. Draining the thorax permits the heart to return to its normal midline position. An initially elevated UVP associated with an elevated intrathoracic pressure which normalise after the effusions have been drained, suggests that the intrathoracic pressure is associated with the pathophysiology. It may be causing mechanical impairment of cardiac output or it may be related to impaired lymph return to the heart. If the effusion recurs, placement of a thoracoamniotic shunt is more likely to be curative. On the other hand, if the UVP is normal prior to decompression of the chest or remains elevated after the chest has been drained and the heart has returned to its normal midline position, the placement of a thoraco-amniotic shunt is not as likely to be beneficial.

Tumours

Fetal surgery for surgically correctable conditions, in particular fetal thoracic lesions and sacrococcygeal teratoma, is at an early research or developmental stage, with only a few cases having been treated in centres with the necessary expertise.[21]

Chromosomal anomalies

Chromosomal anomalies may be found in about 13% of cases, some of which will be associated with anatomical anomalies.[6] It is important to exclude aneuploidy before offering antenatal therapy, especially in cases of hydrothorax. The main therapeutic option is pregnancy termination. Careful counselling of the family is important.

Infection

Fetal infection may be found in at least 8% of cases.[25] The application of polymerase chain reaction technologies is revealing an increasing number of previously unsuspected fetal infections. The most common infectious causes of hydrops include parvovirus B19, cytomegalovirus, syphilis and toxoplasmosis. Apart from parvovirus, little can currently be done antenatally to treat these conditions once they have produced fetal hydrops.

Parvovirus B19 infection is a relatively newly recognised cause of human fetal hydrops.[26,27] It is estimated that 23–50% of pregnant women are susceptible to parvovirus infection.[28,29] It occurs in three-to-five-year epidemic cycles,[30] when it may be the leading cause of hydrops in a region.[10] The risk of fetal hydrops may be higher in mothers with asymptomatic infection.[10] The fetal hydrops is mainly associated with anaemia but can also be caused by myocarditis[31,32] and hepatitis.[33] The risk of fetal loss is greatest in the first 20 weeks of pregnancy, with most reported cases in the second trimester.[34] However, the true incidence of first-trimester losses due to parvovirus infection is unknown. The interval from maternal infection to fetal death has been variably reported at 1–16 weeks[35] with the majority of cases having a range estimated to be 3–5 weeks.[34]

Management depends on severity. Serial ultrasound scans are used to assess severity.[36] In mild to moderate hydrops that shows improvement on serial scans, no fetal investigation or treatment is necessary.[33] A fetal blood sample may also yield useful information. If the fetus is not severely hydropic, not severely thrombocytopenic, not acidaemic and shows an increased reticulocyte response, this suggests that spontaneous recovery is under way. In severe cases, fetal intrauterine transfusion is indicated.[33,36] Myocarditis secondary to parvovirus has been treated with fetal digitalisation. Infant follow-up is mandatory in view of the risk of congenital red-cell aplasia.[37]

Other causes

Fetal akinesia is another condition associated with fetal hydrops that has been encountered in regional units. It has a large number of causes and carries a poor prognosis. The risk of recurrence is generally low but may be influenced by the cause if it is identified. Recurrent idiopathic non-immune hydrops has been reported[38,39] and postulated to be related to a recessive gene. There are few therapeutic options available for antenatal treatment of other causes of fetal hydrops.

Fetal sites of fluid collection and the amount of fluid (severity) may be helpful in the management of hydrops once the cause is ascertained.[33,36] In general, the absence of amniotic fluid is a poor prognostic sign. Fetal heart dimensions are another means of assessing severity.[11]

The UVP measurement is helpful in the management of fetal hydrops. If the pressure is raised and therapy reduces it, the prognosis is better than if there is no effect. Hydrops characterised by an elevated UVP not remedied by either surgical or medical therapy is usually progressive and the fetus either dies or requires preterm delivery for postnatal therapy.[12] Hydropic fetuses with a normal UVP have not, to date, been amenable to antenatal therapy.[40] Infection, arrhythmia and twin-to-twin transfusion syndrome are the only causes of spontaneously reversible hydrops that have been clearly diocumented.[41] For a detailed discussion of the management of twin-to-twin transfusion syndrome the reader is referred elsewhere.[42]

Fetal hypoproteinaemia and hypoalbuminaemia appear to be secondary effects. There is no evidence to suggest that the practice of giving the fetus albumin is of value.

CONCLUSIONS

Fetal hydrops is a serious condition with a complex pathophysiology. It is associated with a wide range of pathologies carrying a poor prognosis overall. However, survival is not impossible. It is important to try and make a diagnosis not only to provide an explanation for parents but also to identify those cases, approximately one-third, where antenatal therapy is possible.

References

1. Scoll, M.A., Sharland, G.K., Allen, L.D. Is the ultrasound definition of fluid collections in non-immune hydrops fetalis helpful in defining the underlying cause or predicting outcome? *Ultrasound Obstet Gynecol* 1991;**1**:309–12
2. Gough, J.D., Keeling, J.W., Castle, B., Iliff, P.J. The obstetric management of non-immunological hydrops. *Br J Obstet Gynaecol* 1986;**93**:226–34
3. Carlton, D.P., McGillivray, B.C., Schreiber, M.D. Nonimmune hydrops fetalis: a multidisciplinary approach. *Clin Perinatol* 1989;**16**:839–51
4. Holzgreave, W., Holzgreave, B., Curry, C.J.R. Non-immune hydrops fetalis: diagnosis and management. *Semin Perinat* 1985;**9**:52–67
5. Smoleniec, J.S., James, D. Fetal hydrops – is the prognosis always poor? *J Obstet Gynaecol* 1994;**14**:142–5
6. Keeling, J.W. Fetal hydrops. In: Keeling, J.W., editor. *Fetal and Neonatal Pathology*, 2nd ed. London: Springer-Verlag; 1993. p. 253–71
7. Machin, G.A. Hydrops revisited: literature review of 1414 cases published in the 1980s. *Am J Med Genet* 1989;**34**:366–90
8. Thumasathit, B., Nondasuta, A., Silpisornkosol, S., Lousuebsakul, B., Unchalipongse, P., Mangkornkanok, M. Hydrops fetalis associated with Bart's hemoglobin in northern Thailand. *J Pediatr* 1968;**73**:132–8
9. Ireland, J.M., Luo, H.Y., Chui, D.H.K., Chu, B., Yuan, J., Hsea, Y.E. Detection of the (—SEA) double α-globin gene deletion by a simple immunologic assay for embryonic zeta-globin chains. *Am J Hematol* 1993;**44**:22–8
10. Smoleniec, J.S., Pillai, M., Caul, E.O., Usher, J. Subclinical transplacental parvovirus B19 infection: an increased fetal risk? *Lancet* 1994;**343**:1100–1
11. Johnson, P., Sharland, G., Allan, L.D., Tynan, M.J., Maxwell, D.J. Umbilical venous pressure in nonimmune hydrops fetalis: correlation with cardiac size. *Am J Obstet Gynecol* 1992;**167**:1309–13
12. Weiner, C.P. Umbilical pressure measurement in the evaluation of nonimmune hydrops fetalis. *Am J Obstet Gynecol* 1993;**168**:817–23
13. Nicolaides, K., Gainey, H. Pseudotoxemic state associated with severe Rh isoimmunisation. *Am J Obstet Gynecol* 1964;**89**:41–5
14. Weiner, C.P., Wenstrom, K.D., Sipes, S.L., Williamson, R.A. Risk factors for cordocenteses and fetal intravascular transfusion. *Am J Obstet Gynecol* 1993;**165**:1020–5
15. Maxwell, D.J., Johnson, P., Hurley, P., Neales, K., Allan, L., Knott, P. Fetal blood sampling and pregnancy loss in relation to indication. *Br J Obstet Gynaecol* 1991;**98**:892–7
16. Hansmann, M., Gembruch, U., Bald, R. New therapeutic aspects in nonimmune hydrops fetalis based on 402 prenatally diagnosed cases. *Fetal Ther* 1989;**4**:29–36
17. Weiner, C.P., Williamson, R.A., Wenstrom, K.D., Sipes, S.L., Grant, S.S., Widness, J. Management of fetal hemolytic disease by cordocentesis. I. Prediction of fetal anemia. *Am J*

Obstet Gynecol 1991;**165**:546–53
18. Allan, L.D., Crawford, D.C., Sheridan, R., Chapman, M.G. Aetiology of non-immune hydrops: the value of echocardiography. *Br J Obstet Gynaecol* 1986;**93**:223–5
19. Meijboom, E.J., van Engelen, A.D., van de Beek, E.W., Weijtens, O., Lautenschutz, J.M., Benatar, A.A. Fetal arrhythmias. *Curr Opin Cardiol* 1994;**9**:97–102
20. Rizzo, G., Capponi, A., Chaoui, R., Taddei, F., Arduini, D., Romanini, C. Blood flow velocity waveforms from peripheral pulmonary arteries in normally grown and growth-retarded fetuses. *Ultrasound Obstet Gynecol* 1966;**8**:87–92
21. Bullard, K.M., Harrison, M.R. Before the horse is out of the barn: fetal surgery for hydrops. *Semin Perinatol* 1995;**19**:462–73
22. Shaw, K.S., Filiatrault, D., Yazbeck, S., St-Vil, D. Improved survival for congenital diaphragmatic hernia based on prenatal ultrasound diagnosis and referal to a combined obstetric-pediatric surgical centre. *J Pediatr Surg* 1994;**29**:1268–9
23. Rodeck, C.H., Fisk, N.M., Fraser, D.I., Nicolini, U. Long-term *in utero* drainage of fetal hydrothorax. *N Engl J Med* 1988;**319**:1135–8
24. Weiner, C.P., Varner, M.W., Pringle, K.C., Hein, H.A., Williamson, R.A., Nielsen, C. Antenatal diagnosis and treatment of nonimmune hydrops fetalis secondary to pulmonary extralobar sequestration. *Obstet Gynecol* 1986;**68**:275–80
25. Barron, S.D., Pass, R.F. Infectious causes of hydrops fetalis. *Semin Perinatol* 1995;**19**:493–501
26. Brown, T., Anand, A., Ritchie, L.D. Clewley, J., Reid, T. Intrauterine parvovirus infection associated with hydrops fetalis. *Lancet* 1984;**ii**:1033–4
27. Knott, P.D., Welply, G.A., Anderson, M.J. Serologically proved intrauterine infection with parvovirus. *BMJ* 1984;**289**:1660
28. Mortimer, P.P., Cohen, B.J., Buckley, M.M., Cradock-Watson, J.E., Ridehalgh, M.K., Burkhardt, F. et al. Human parvovirus and the fetus. *Lancet* 1985;**ii**:1012
29. Klopper, P.E., Morris, D.J. Screening for viral and protozoal infections in pregnancy: a review. *Br J Obstet Gynaecol* 1990;**97**:974–83
30. Anderson, L.J. Human parvoviruses. *J Infect Dis* 1990;**161**:603–8
31. Porter, H.J., Quantrill, A.M., Flemming, K.A. B19 parvovirus infection of the myocardium. *Lancet* 1988;**i**:535–36
32. Naides, S.J., Weiner, C.P. Antenatal diagnosis and palliative treatment of non-immune hydrops fetalis secondary to parvovirus B19 infection. *Prenat Diagn* 1989;**9**:105–14
33. Smoleniec, J.S., Pillai, M. Fetal hydrops associated with parvovirus B19 infection: management. *Br J Obstet Gynaecol* 1994;**101**:1079–81
34. Public Health Laboratory Service Working Party on Fifth Disease. Prospective study of human parvovirus (B19) infection in pregnancy. *BMJ* 1990;**300**:1166–70
35. Rodis, J.F., Hovick, T.J., Rosengren, S.S., Tattersall, P. Human parvovirus infection in pregnancy. *Obstet Gynecol* 1988;**72**:733–8
36. Fairley, C.K., Smoleniec, J.S., Caul, O.E., Miller, E. Observational study of effect of intrauterine transfusions on outcome of fetal hydrops after parvovirus B19 infection. *Lancet* 1995;**346**:1335–7
37. Brown, K.E., Green, S.W., Antunez de Mayolo, J.A., Bellanti, J.A., Smith, S.D., Smith, T.J. et al. Congenital anaemia after transplacental parvovirus infection. *Lancet* 1994;**343**:895–96
38. Windebank, K.P., Bridges, N.A., Ostman-Smith, I., Stevens, J.E. Hydrops fetalis due to abnormal lymphatics. *Arch Dis Child* 1987;**62**:198–200
39. Onwude, J.L., Thornton, J.G., Mueller, R.H. Recurrent idiopathic non-immunologic hydrops fetalis: a report of two families, with three and two affected siblings. *Br J Obstet Gynaecol* 1992;**99**:854–6

40 Moise, K.J., Carpenter, R.J., Hesketh, D.E. Do abnormal Starling forces cause fetal hydrops in red cell alloimmunisation? *Am J Obstet Gynecol* 1992;**167**:907–12

41 Achiron, R., Rabinowitz, R., Aboulafia, Y., Diamant, Y., Glaser, J. Intrauterine assessment of high-output cardiac failure with spontaneous remission of hydrops fetalis in twin-twin transfusion syndrome: use of two-dimensional echocardiography, Doppler ultrasound and color flow mapping. *J Clin Ultrasound* 1992;**20**:271–7

42 Shalev, E., Zalel, Y., Ben-Ami, M., Weiner, E. First trimester ultrasonic diagnosis of twin reversed arterial perfusion sequence. *Prenat Diagn* 1992;**12**:219–22

43 Smoleniec, J., Weiner, C., James, D. Fetal hydrops. In: James, D.K., Steer, P.J., Weiner, C.P., Gonik, B., editors. *High Risk Pregnancy: Management Options*, 2nd ed. London: W.B. Saunders. p. 327–41

44 Stangenberg, M., Selbing, A., Lingman, G., Westgren, M. Rhesus immunisation: new perspectives in maternal-fetal medicine. *Obstet Gynecol Surv* 1991;**46**:189–95

45 Hutchinson, A.A., Drew, J.H., Yu, V.Y.H., Williams, M.L., Fortune, D.W., Beischer, N.A. Nonimmunologic hydrops fetalis: a review of 61 cases. *Obstet Gynecol* 1982;**59**:347–52

27

The edge of viability

B. Garth McClure and Angela H. Bell

INTRODUCTION

A major recurring problem for obstetricians is what to do for women who present in very early preterm labour, that is from 22 to 26 weeks of gestation. Our predecessors in obstetrics practised against the background knowledge that live-born babies of less than 28 weeks of gestation were extremely unlikely to survive and were termed 'previable'. For example, Crosse,[1] in Birmingham, reported a 100% mortality in babies born at less than 28 weeks of gestation up to the year 1946. Statistics such as these continued to affect obstetricians and paediatricians well into the 1960s. Even as late as 1969, it was felt that babies of less than 1500 g who required assistance because of respiratory failure should not receive it, as the prognosis was so poor. However, this is not now the case because of the many major advances in neonatal intensive care over the past 30 years. Obstetricians now practise their art more in the public gaze than ever before, with decisions being constantly scrutinised by an ever more aware public, which has constantly increasing expectations. These expectations are fortified to some extent by neonatologists, who are seldom loathe to proclaim their successes, and by the national press who repeatedly assail us with tales of 'miracle babies' who have survived at incredibly low gestational ages with apparently little residual harmful effect.

Obstetricians should, however, be aware of the fact that neonatologists are talking about the survival of babies who are born alive and about whom decisions have often been made in the labour ward as to whether to perform intensive care or not. Even with this selection, the outcome of babies born from 23 to 25 weeks of gestation is not rosy, with poor survival rates, moderate or serious disabilities in some, neurobehavioural dysfunction and poor school performance in others. These words are easy to write, but we should reflect that, when we say that a child has a moderate or serious disability, we mean that the child and family will be significantly handicapped physically, emotionally and financially. These problems are not resolved quickly, but will last a lifetime, the long-term survival of children with cerebral palsy, for example, being over 20 years.[2] It is of the utmost importance that obstetricians in practice bear this in mind when counselling and treating mothers in early preterm labour. Further, we should also recognise that, in this era when we are impaled upon the spear of evidence-based medicine, there is remarkably little evidence upon which to base a rational decision.

SURVIVAL

Every maternity hospital should know what the intact survival rate is for babies who have presented in preterm labour within their unit and also in their geographical region. This varies considerably from country to country and from hospital to hospital.

Data from Scotland[3] may reflect the situation in the UK. In a study of 625 646 single births over a ten-year period to 1994, the neonatal death rate fell from 795/1000 live births at 24 weeks of gestation to 9/1000 live births at 36 weeks. The rates at 25 and 26 weeks of gestation were 518/1000 and 396/1000 live births, respectively. Kramar et al.,[4] studied 114 infants born between

23 and 27 weeks of gestation in a tertiary centre in Texas and found survival to six months of 13% at 23 weeks of gestation, rising to 75% at 26 weeks. A Japanese study[5] of 1655 babies of less than 600 g admitted to neonatal intensive care units, found a survival rate of 28% to hospital discharge. Hussain et al.[6] studied 405 infants of between 22 and 27 weeks of gestation who had been actively resuscitated in three tertiary perinatal centres in Connecticut, USA; 69% survived to discharge. Unfavourable outcome, defined as death or major morbidity, was seen in more than 85% of infants of 23 and 24 weeks of gestation, falling to 70% at 25 weeks, 57% at 26 weeks and 39% at 27 weeks.

These studies were primarily concerned with liveborn babies who had been admitted to intensive care units and many cases excluded stillbirths and babies who died in the labour ward. The Trent Region of the UK has produced birthweight and gestational age-specific survival tables for babies known to be alive at the onset of labour.[7] Based on a population of 240 000 live births, stillbirths and late fetal losses of more than 22 weeks of gestation, they show the harsh reality of predicted survival rates ranging from 8% at 23 weeks, 20% at 24 weeks to 40% at 25 weeks. Within these survival tables, survival depended upon birthweight in each gestational age band. At the Royal Maternity Hospital, the Regional Perinatal Centre for Northern Ireland, McGinn[8] studied 72 babies from January 1997 to the end of December 1999. Infant mortality including stillbirths and deaths in labour wards were counted. The survival rates were similar to Trent with 13% survival at less than 24 weeks of gestation, 20% at less than 25 weeks and 34% at less than 26 weeks.

It should be noted that the latter studies are based on survival to discharge and take no account of long-term morbidity. A further study in Trent[9] showed that babies born at less than 26 weeks of gestation had only a 12% chance of surviving normally to two years of age.

COUNSELLING

Counselling of mothers in early preterm labour and their partners is extremely difficult. Perhaps the first thing to be recognised is that young parents approaching these major problems often have absolutely no experience of their situation and may be extremely frightened. On the other hand, there are groups of parents who have unrealistically high expectations for themselves and their babies. Counselling should be given by obstetricians and paediatricians and should be done by the most senior staff available and as well in advance of delivery as possible. Anecdotally, we have often found that the opinions of junior staff are often more optimistic than those of their senior colleagues. It is often of benefit to include a senior nurse in the counselling group, as they often have clear insights into the neonatal management of these babies and of the long-term outcome.

Consideration may also be given to having as part of the counselling team someone who has experience of what 'handicap' really means. In our experience, the explanation of handicap by others may be understated, thus allowing young parents to become unrealistic.

The language used should be clear, concise and devoid of medical jargon. It is important to remember the likelihood that the majority of young parents have little or no medical knowledge. Unit survival rates and regional survival rates should be available to parents at the time of counselling. Unit figures alone should not be used to avoid local bias in management. This information should be supplemented by knowledge and frank discussion of the risks of serious handicap in survivors.

Parents should also be informed that decisions made in advance may need to be revised following assessment of the baby after birth if examination shows it is more mature and vigorous than anticipated. The American Academy of Pediatrics Policy Document[10] states that 'Parents should understand that the decisions about neonatal management made before delivery may be altered depending on the condition of the neonate at birth, the postnatal gestational age assessment and the infants' responses to resuscitative and stabilization measures'.

PLACE OF BIRTH

Common sense dictates that if a baby is to be born very prematurely, and for whom all possible means of treatment are to be given, that baby should be born in hospital where these problems are commonly faced. This statement needs to be tempered with considerations of distance, family support and financial constraints but, broadly speaking, it seems to be sensible that babies should be born where experts are available. It has recently been suggested that one explanation of the difference in survival rates between Australia and the UK[11] is the management of small babies in small hospitals within the UK, in contrast to the situation in Australia, where these babies are cared for in larger units. Appropriate counselling should be given to parents prior to transfer to ensure that transfer does not lead to them having unrealistic hopes for the outcome of their baby.

GESTATIONAL AGE OR SIZE

Assessment of gestational age and size is fraught with difficulty, since the menstrual dates may be uncertain and the prognosis for the baby changes with each extra week or each few hundred grams of birthweight. In a woman with a regular menstrual cycle, clinical assessment of gestational age is appropriate. A policy statement in 1995[10] from the American Academy of Pediatrics Committee on Fetus and Newborn with the American College of Obstetricians and Gynecologists Committee on Obstetric Practice, recommended that clinical assessment to determine gestational age is usually appropriate for women with regular menstrual cycles and that the known last menstrual period was confirmed by early examination. The statement goes on to say that fetal measurements by ultrasound should not be used to alter the estimated gestational age unless there is a discrepancy of two or more weeks. In addition, it states that 'Even in ideal circumstances, the 95% confidence limits for a formula-based estimate of fetal weight are ±15–20%'.

Many obstetricians believe it is possible to assess fetal weight accurately. When both gestational age and weight are clearly established, the prognosis may be clarified, as survival at each gestational age varies with birthweight. For example, the Trent study[7] showed that survival will vary at 25 weeks of gestation from 19% at birthweight of 500 g to 50% if the birth weight is over 1000 g. However, it should be stressed that it is extremely uncommon for estimations of fetal weight to be so precise.

TOCOLYTICS AND STEROIDS

Since perinatal mortality is related to gestational age and birthweight, it seems sensible to delay preterm labour using β-adrenergic agonists. Unfortunately, systematic reviews of tocolytics do not show an impact on perinatal mortality. In a large Canadian study,[12] which compared ritodrine with a placebo, pregnancies were stratified by gestational age at enrolment. In those who enrolled from 20 to 23 weeks of gestation, there was no difference in perinatal mortality. In those from 24 to 27 weeks of gestation 'there was a trend towards a lower infant mortality in the ritodrine group'.

The major breakthrough in the management of preterm labour was the discovery by Liggins and Howie[13] of the effect of prenatal steroids on fetal lung maturation. In spite of the many reservations of obstetricians with regard to possible harm to the mother, prenatal steroids are standard practice in the management of preterm labour.

A systematic review by Crowley[14] concluded that antenatal steroids are associated with a reduction in neonatal mortality, a reduction in the severity of the respiratory distress syndrome and a lower risk of intraventricular haemorrhage. This applied to a wide band of gestational ages but she highlighted that there was little evidence of effect prior to 28 weeks of gestation because of a paucity of data. This question was clarified by Piper,[15] who showed a reduction in neonatal mortality with combined tocolytics and steroids at 24-28 weeks of gestation.

A question mark remains over the effect of prenatal steroids on the fetus. Crowley[14] identified no adverse consequences of a single course of steroids on short- or long-term neurodevelopment. However, animal models studying repeated steroid use have shown a delay in cerebral myelination[16] and a recent study in Australia[17] suggested that babies may be at increased risk of neurological impairment after repeated use of prenatal steroids.

REASONS FOR DELIVERY AND SURVIVAL

Obstetricians undertake early delivery either in the maternal or fetal interest. The authors of this chapter have no experience as obstetricians and, therefore, are not in a position to comment on delivery in the maternal interest.

The outcome for the baby appears not to be affected by the reason for preterm delivery. Wolf et al.[18] studied 535 consecutive liveborn single infants with birthweights between 500 g and 1499 g, and concluded that the principal pregnancy complications did not alter the pre-discharge survival of liveborn infants. The complications studied were premature rupture of the membrane, idiopathic preterm labour, antepartum haemorrhage, pregnancy-induced hypertension and other 'complications'. They did demonstrate an association between predischarge morbidity and pregnancy complication, such as a higher incidence of patent ductus arteriosus after antepartum haemorrhage, although there was no difference in mortality. These babies were, however, somewhat larger and more mature than those under discussion here, having mean gestational ages of more than 26 weeks. Iannucci et al.[19] studied babies of 500–800 g in a regional perinatal centre and studied the outcome in relation to preterm labour with no antecedent rupture of membranes, premature rupture of the membranes, those delivered because of 'non-reassuring maternal or fetal status' and a fourth group which included all patients with multiple gestations. The study population was 111 neonates and Iannucci et al.[19] concluded that the reason for delivery of extremely low-birth-weight infants does not have an impact on the immediate neonatal outcome.

A study from Queensland[20] has again shown no relationship between the primary cause for preterm delivery and outcome, in terms of survival and neurodevelopment.

MONITORING

The purpose of monitoring the fetal heart in labour is to detect fetal distress. Generally, this is detected by noting two abnormalities of the fetal heart-rate trace; that is, loss of variability and decelerations. The heart-rate variability of babies of very early gestation is extremely poor and, therefore, it is extremely difficult to interpret the abnormal from the normal. Decelerations have the same significance as they have for the term baby but the problem arises as to what to do if such decelerations are seen. The normal response of obstetricians in babies of greater gestational ages is to expedite delivery either by forceps or by caesarean section. However, at extremes of viability such a response is at least questionable. If the baby is delivered expeditiously, the likelihood is that such a delivery will produce a tiny baby in extremely poor condition and whose prognosis will be consequently extremely poor.

There is probably not a role for monitoring other than to provide information for the paediatrician about the likely clinical state of the baby. If monitoring is employed, it should be discrete to avoid concern by the parents and those using it must be able to resist the temptation to intervene suddenly unless the parents have indicated that all measures must be applied to try to save the baby's life.

MULTIPLE BIRTHS

Twin and higher-order births form a disproportionate number of preterm births, contributing to a large proportion of the work of a newborn nursery. Very preterm delivery in multiple pregnancy is extremely vexed and would appear to be becoming more frequent with the advent of assisted reproduction. The position is even more complicated by the emotional background to the pregnancy which may affect the obstetrician and will certainly affect the parents. Our experience suggests that the survival of multiple births at 23 and 24 weeks of gestation is poor. There is little information on this but there is some evidence which suggests that, provided an infant from a multiple pregnancy is of the same birthweight as a singleton at the same gestational age, survival is as good or better than a singleton pregnancy.[7] However, should the baby be smaller than expected, survival within a particular gestational age band will be reduced.

CAESAREAN SECTION

There would appear to be, at this time, no evidence to suggest that caesarean section is of benefit for babies being born extremely prematurely. A major concern is that caesarean section may result in a larger number of survivors but at the expense of handicap. A study in a large perinatal centre[21] showed that caesarean section below 800 g or less than 26 weeks of gestation was linked to increased survival but with twice the risk for serious long-term morbidity. It should also be recognised that caesarean section at these early gestations may be extremely difficult and is liable to be of the classical type leading to a vertical uterine scar. Obstetricians should be alert to vague feelings of 'doing something' and realise that they may do more harm than good by intervening.

THE ROLE OF THE PAEDIATRICIAN IN THE LABOUR WARD

It is useful if a paediatrician is present at the birth of babies from 22 weeks of gestation, just in case there has been an error in the estimation of gestational age or birthweight. The response of most paediatricians to the birth of extremely small babies is determined by the baby's condition at birth and by its size. There is limited information but it seems to be common sense that if a baby is born extremely small and in poor condition, the outcome will be much worse than for a larger baby born active and looking reasonably well. It may be valuable to weigh the baby in the delivery suite, as survival below 500 g is poor. Full cardiopulmonary resuscitation should not be given. Rennie[22] states that 'The outcome for very preterm infants after full cardiopulmonary resuscitation in the delivery suite is appalling'. For example, she cites the study of Sims[23] in Manchester where three of five babies of less than 28 weeks of gestation given adrenaline and bicarbonate died; the two survivors were handicapped.

We must bear in mind the wishes of the parents in these situations. If it is decided that the baby is to have no active treatment, it is imperative that the baby is swaddled up and given to the parents, when possible, to allow them time with their baby.

COST IMPLICATIONS

Very roughly, babies are discharged from neonatal nurseries when they have achieved a gestational age of approximately 34–35 weeks. In most places a baby born at 24 weeks of gestation will, if it survives, be looked after in a nursery for approximately ten weeks, of which about four weeks will be spent in intensive care. As a rule of thumb, intensive care costs roughly £1,000 per day, and high-dependency and special care between £300 and £500 per day, so it can be seen that the cost is not negligible. These figures should be added to the additional costs of the long-term effects of being born prematurely, which are significant. We would not advocate for a second that the cost of treatment should be the primary consideration in any doctor's mind, but we certainly cannot ignore the financial implications of our actions.

CONCLUSIONS

Care of babies at the extremes of viability is extremely difficult medically, ethically and financially. Survival of these babies in many cases may be achieved, but only at the cost of major risks in the long term to the baby. Each decision should be carefully considered by the parents, obstetricians and paediatricians prior to embarking on any heroic measures, and decisions should be made against the background of medical reality rather than a desire to do 'everything possible'. We should recognise that, at this point in time, our management of such patients is inadequate. We need to better understand the pathophysiological processes affecting these very tiny babies to devise better new means of treatment and, most of all, we need to prevent these occurrences of very premature birth.

References

1. Crosse, M. *The Premature Baby*. London: J. & A. Churchill; 1947
2. Hutton, J.L., Cooke, T., Pharoah, P.O. Life expectancy in children with cerebral palsy. *BMJ* 1994;**309**:431–5
3. Magowan, B.A., Bain, M., Juszczak, E., McInneny, K. Neonatal mortality amongst Scottish preterm singleton births (1985–1994). *Br J Obstet Gynaecol* 1998;**105**:1005–10
4. Kramer, W.B., Saade, G.R., Goodrum, L., Montgomery, L., Belfort, M., Moise, K.J. Neonatal outcome after active perinatal management of the very premature infant between 23 and 27 weeks' gestation. *J Perinatol* 1997;**17**:439–43
5. Oishi, M., Nishida, H., Sasaki, T. Japanese experience with micropremies weighing less than 600 grams born between 1984 to 1993. *Pediatrics* 1997;**99**:E7
6. Hussain, N., Galal, M., Ehrenkrantz, R.A., Herson, V.C., Rowe, J.C. Pre-discharge outcomes of 22–27 weeks gestational age infants born at tertiary care centers in Connecticut: implications for perinatal management. *Conn Med* 1998;**62**:131–7
7. Draper, E.S., Manktelow, B., Field, D.J., James, D. Prediction of survival for preterm births by weight and gestational age: retrospective population based study. *BMJ* 1999;**319**:1093–7
8. McGinn, M. Personal communication
9. Bohin, S., Draper, E.S., Field, D.J. Health status of a population of infants born before 26 weeks gestation derived from routine data collected between 21 and 27 months post-delivery. *Early Hum Dev* 1999;**55**:9–18
10. American Academy of Pediatrics. Perinatal care at the threshold of viability. *Pediatrics* 1995;**96**:974–6
11. International Neonatal Network, Scottish Neonatal Consultants, Nurses Collaborative Study Group. Risk adjusted and population based studies of the outcome for high risk infants in Scotland and Australia. *Arch Dis Child Fetal Neonatal Ed* 2000;**82**:F118–23
12. The Canadian Preterm Labor Investigators Group. Treatment of preterm labour with the beta-adrenergic agonist Ritodrine. *N Engl J Med* 1992;**327**:308–12
13. Liggins, B.C., Howie, R.N. A controlled trial of antepartum glucocorticoid treatment for prevention of respiratory distress syndrome in premature infants. *Paediatrics* 1972;**50**:515–25

14 Crowley, P. Corticosteroids prior to preterm delivery. In: Enkin, M.W., Keirse, M.J.N.C., Renfrew, M.J., Neilson, J.P., editors. Pregnancy and Childbirth Module of the Cochrane Database of Systematic Reviews. *The Cochrane Library*, Issue 1. Oxford: Update Software; 1996

15 Piper, J.M., Atkinson, M.W., Mitchell, E.F. Jr, Cliver, S.P., Snowden, M., Wilson, S.C. Improved outcomes for very low birth weight infants associated with the use of combined maternal corticosteroids and tocolytics. *J Reprod Med* 1996;**41**:692–8

16 Dunlop, S.A., Archer, M.A., Quinlivan, J.A., Newnham, J.P. Repeated prenatal corticosteroids delay myelination in the ovine central nervous system. *J Matern Fetal Med* 1997;**6**:309–13

17 Hagan, R., French, N., Evans, S. Repeated antenatal corticosteroids: growth and early childhood outcome. *Pediatr Res* 1997;**42**:405A

18 Wolf, E.J., Vintzileos, A.M., Rosenkrantz, T.S., Rodin, J.F., Saljia, C.M., Pezzullo, J.G. Do survival and morbidity of very-low-birth-weight infants vary according to the primary pregnancy complication that results in preterm delivery? *Am J Obstet Gynecol* 1993;**169**:1233–9

19 Iannucci, T.A., Tomich, P.G., Gianopoulos, J.G. Etiology and outcome of extremely low-birth-weight infants. *Am J Obstet Gynecol* 1996;**174**:1896–902

20 Gray, P.H., Hurley, T.M., Rogers, Y.M., O'Callaghan, M.J., Tudehope, D.I., Burns, Y.R. et al. Survival and neonatal and neurodevelopmental outcome of 24–29 week gestation infants according to primary cause of preterm delivery. *Aust N Z J Obstet Gynaecol* 1997;**37**:161–8

21 Bottoms, S.F., Paul, R.H., Iams, J.D., Mercer, B.M., Thom, E.A., Roberts, J.M. et al. Obstetric determinants of neonatal survival: influence of willingness to perform cesarean delivery on survival of extremely low-birth-weight infants. *Am J Obstet Gynecol* 1997;**176**:960–6

22 Rennie, J.M. Perinatal management at the lower margin of viability. *Arch Dis Child* 1996;**74**:F214–18

23 Sims, D.G., Heal, C.A., Bartle, S.M. Use of adrenaline and atropine in neonatal resuscitation. *Arch Dis Child* 1994;**70**:F3–9

28

Invasive diagnosis of fetal abnormalities and therapeutic methods

Deirdre J. Murphy and Peter W. Soothill

INTRODUCTION

Fetal medicine is developing rapidly with an ever-increasing range of invasive techniques for diagnosis, assessment and therapy. It is now possible to sample the fetus from 11 weeks of gestation to term in order to facilitate identification of chromosomal abnormalities, single-gene defects, metabolic disorders, intrauterine infection, anaemia, thrombocytopenia and some structural abnormalities. Invasive diagnostic tests often exclude an abnormality in high-risk cases where routine screening tests may be insufficient for adequate reassurance. Invasive methods carry a low but finite risk of pregnancy loss, so noninvasive genetic screening techniques are the focus of intense research. Isolating fetal nucleated red blood cells from maternal blood for genetic analysis is the least invasive method currently being investigated.[1] In addition, in some cases it has been possible to detect fetal aneuploidies using transcervical cell samples.[2] These methods are research tools at the present time. In current practice, amniocentesis, chorionic villus sampling (CVS) and fetal blood sampling are routinely used in the investigation or management of suspected fetal abnormalities and these invasive techniques are described in detail in this chapter.

In situations where a fetal abnormality or disease is confirmed it may be possible to institute therapy antenatally by invasive means; for example, transfusion for anaemia or thrombocytopenia, laser ablation for twin-to-twin transfusion syndrome, amniotic fluid drainage for polyhydramnios or pleuroamniotic shunting for pleural effusions. Fetal-medicine centres around the world are involved in the development of a wide range of additional specialised procedures including fetoscopy with micro-instruments, fetal surgery and intrapartum fetal therapy. Some of these advances are described briefly.

AMNIOCENTESIS

Amniocentesis is the aspiration of amniotic fluid containing fetal cells from the amniotic cavity. It is the most commonly used invasive test for prenatal diagnosis. The Royal College of Obstetricians and Gynaecologists has published guidelines for good practice which emphasise adequate training and supervision of practitioners who offer amniocentesis.[3] Recent advances in rapid culture and molecular biology techniques have added to its use across a wide range of gestational ages and for a wide range of indications. The procedure should only be performed under continuous ultrasound guidance and consideration should be given to referring multiple pregnancies that require amniocentesis to a tertiary centre.

Indications and methods

Fetal karyotyping is the most common indication for amniocentesis and may be offered for a positive biochemical screen for Down syndrome (cut-off level determined locally), ultrasound features suggestive of aneuploidy, advanced maternal age (traditionally over 35 years), parental balanced translocation or a previous fetal aneuploidy. The amniotic fluid contains cells from fetal skin, gastrointestinal, urogenital and respiratory tracts and from the amnion. The cells are cultured for two to three weeks to prepare for metaphase analysis, which then allows karyotyping. Approximately 0.5% of cultures fail and maternal contamination can lead to diagnostic difficulties in less than 0.2%. Culture of a second tissue is occasionally necessary due to fetal mosaicism (0.12–0.14%).[4]

Fluorescence *in situ* hybridisation (FISH) allows fast direct DNA probing of chromosomes in interphase or for a detectable monogenic disorder (for example haemophilia).[5,6] Polymerase chain reaction (PCR)-based primers can be applied to uncultured amniotic fluid cells to determine fetal rhesus status and Kell and platelet antigen type,[7-9] or for the rapid detection of trisomy 21 and other chromosome problems in extracted DNA. FISH and PCR are entering into mainstream clinical practice and in selected cases it may not be necessary to wait for confirmation by culture.[10]

Amniocentesis should no longer be performed at 16–20 weeks of gestation for the estimation of α-fetoprotein (α-FP) and acetylcholinesterase for diagnosis of open neural-tube defects. Indeed, the sensitivity of ultrasonography in skilled hands is such that the routine estimation of α-FP at amniocentesis, even when already performed for karyotyping, has been questioned.[11]

Amniocentesis can facilitate the diagnosis of fetal infection with toxoplasmosis and cytomegalovirus. PCR for gene sequences present in toxoplasma DNA extracted from amniotic fluid has several advantages over traditional mouse inoculation tests. A PCR test can be used in the first half of pregnancy and gives a result in a fraction of the time with greater sensitivities.[12,13] However, false-negative results occasionally occur if insufficient time has elapsed since the infection because they indicate the presence of the micro-organism rather than fetal infection. Fetal cytomegalovirus infection is reliably detected by culture of the virus in amniotic fluid as it is excreted in fetal urine.[14] PCR technology is also used with promising results from data that are currently available.[15,16]

Amniocentesis has been advocated in the assessment of premature rupture of the membranes and suspected chorioamnionitis on the basis of an association between amniotic fluid colonisation and preterm labour.[17] Successful amniocentesis has been described in up to 97% of patients with premature rupture of the membranes when performed under direct ultrasound guidance.[18] Amniotic fluid Gram's stain, microscopy, culture and assessment of pulmonary maturity can be performed. Those who advocate the procedure argue that it allows earlier diagnosis of intra-amniotic infection as well as identification of the responsible organism and its sensitivities.[19] However, there is currently a lack of data to support or refute this practice.

Amniocentesis has been used in the assessment of fetal lung maturity. However, improvements in neonatal care together with accurate ultrasound dating of pregnancy have led to a reduction in the need for confirmation of fetal lung maturity before delivery.[20]

Pregnancies with multiple gestations requiring amniocentesis present specific difficulties and should be ideally referred to a regional fetal medicine unit.[3] If the pregnancy is confirmed as monochorionic only one twin needs to be sampled. With dichorionic twins, a separate puncture as far away as possible from the intertwin septum is usually used for each twin. Alternatively, a single puncture technique can be used, passing the needle through the septum with the theoretical risk of contaminating the sample of one twin with that of the other.[21,22] Ultrasound guidance now renders dye labelling unnecessary in most patients. Furthermore, the previous use of dyes has led to aetiological concerns in relation to intestinal obstruction.[23] It is crucial, however, to record the septal and placental configurations to allow fetal identification if the results are discordant.

Procedure

Amniocentesis should no longer be performed without ultrasound imaging or as a separate procedure after identification of a pool of amniotic fluid and marking the overlying skin. Although historical reports on the value of ultrasound in enhancing the safety of amniocentesis have reported conflicting results, its continued use is so obviously an essential component of any invasive procedure that this requires no further study.

A 22-gauge, 7–10-cm sterile disposable needle is used, although occasionally a longer needle may be required because of the thickness of the maternal abdominal wall. After locating a suitable pool, an approach is chosen to avoid the fetus, placenta and cord. The needle guide technique uses a needle guide-channel attached to the transducer. Lines on the ultrasound screen indicate the path the needle will follow and this technique has the advantage of allowing thinner needles (22–26 gauge) to be used. However, this limits the operator's ability to adjust to difficulties during the procedure and allows guidance of only the needle tip rather than observation of its whole length. With the free-hand technique, the operator holds the ultrasound transducer in one hand and the needle in the other, directing the ultrasound beam across the planned needle path and allowing visualisation of the whole length of the needle. The advantages of this technique include the flexibility to make adjustments during the procedure and the same technique can be used for all ultrasound-guided invasive procedures. The needle is inserted and the first millilitre of fluid is discarded. The sample is aspirated and the syringe is removed prior to withdrawing the needle in order to prevent maternal contamination.

Timing

Prenatal diagnostic amniocentesis is traditionally performed between 15 and 17 weeks of gestation when the volume of amniotic fluid is 150–250 ml, which allows removal of 15–20 ml of fluid. Attention has focused on earlier amniocentesis, which would have the potential advantage of earlier diagnosis. Early amniocentesis at 12–14 weeks of gestation is technically easy, with only a 2% failure rate[24,25] and culture success rates well in excess of 95%.[26] However, randomised trials have shown significantly greater rates of loss, post-procedure fluid leakage and orthopaedic deformity among the early-amniocentesis group. Therefore, early amniocentesis (less than 15 weeks of gestation) should not be performed except in extraordinary circumstances.[27,28]

Complications

Most units quote a procedure-related additional risk of spontaneous abortion of 1%, which is based on the results of the only randomised controlled trial of low-risk women.[29] Perforation of the placenta was associated with a relative risk of 2.6 and a raised maternal serum α-FP with a relative risk for miscarriage of 8.3. Ideally, individual units should record and present their own results, which will more accurately reflect the case mix and the skills within the unit.

There have been inconsistent reports of an association between amniocentesis and neonatal respiratory morbidity.[29,30] Similarly, postural deformities, in particular talipes equinovarus, have been associated with amniocentesis.[30] The latter are probably the result of chronic leakage of fluid, which occurs occasionally.

Neonatal lesions such as fistulae, ileal atresia, corneal perforation and umbilical cord haematoma have been attributed to needle injury.[31] However, this risk is low and there were no cases of trauma in two large series where amniocentesis was performed by experienced operators under ultrasound guidance.[29,32]

The attributable risk of sensitisation of rhesus-negative women is approximately 1% above the background risk of 1.5%.[33] The use of small-gauge needles, avoiding a transplacental approach and administering anti-D immunoglobulin after the procedure will minimise this risk.

Therapy

Amniotic fluid drainage can relieve maternal symptoms of severe polyhydramnios and prolong gestation in both singleton and multiple pregnancies.[34,35] Criteria for amniotic fluid drainage are amniotic fluid index greater than 40 cm or the deepest single pool of greater than 12 cm but the decision is often best determined by maternal discomfort. Drainage of large volumes (3–5 litres) seems to result in better outcomes. A recent report suggests that the amniotic fluid index can be reduced by 1 cm for each 100 ml of amniotic fluid drained.[36] Potential complications include placental abruption, chorioamnionitis, preterm premature rupture of membranes and preterm labour.[37] It is impossible, however, to determine whether complications are due to the procedure or to the polyhydramnios itself.

A similar technique can be used to facilitate amnio-infusion. This is particularly useful in situations where marked oligohydramnios makes visualisation of the fetal structures difficult. Sterile warm saline can be infused through the needle into the amniotic cavity. The increased liquor improves the ultrasound image and allows visualisation of the fetal anatomy and, in particular, the fetal kidneys in situations where renal agenesis needs to be excluded. Similarly, fluid can be infused into the intraperitoneal cavity, which will further facilitate visualisation of the fetal kidneys.

CHORIONIC VILLUS SAMPLING AND PLACENTAL BIOPSY

Placental tissue can be sampled by catheter, needle aspiration or biopsy as an alternative to amniotic fluid and fetal blood can be sampled from the late first trimester onward. These procedures have the advantage of yielding a large amount of tissue and are, therefore, the method of choice where a large amount of DNA is required for the diagnosis of monogenic disorders. Early diagnostic testing offers parents the choice of termination of pregnancy prior to 13 weeks of gestation.

Indications and methods

Early prenatal diagnosis of a genetic disorder is the most common indication for placental sampling and is offered for advanced maternal age, previous fetal aneuploidy or monogenic disorder, parental balanced translocation and ultrasound features suggestive of aneuploidy. In addition, it is possible to detect chromosomal breakage syndromes such as fragile X syndrome and to perform rapid sexing for fetuses at risk of X-linked disorders. Biochemical testing of a chorionic villus sample is possible for almost all metabolic diseases that can be diagnosed from amniotic fluid cells. In the late second and third trimesters, placental sampling can be indicated for late ultrasound findings suggestive of aneuploidy, failed amniotic fluid cell cultures and late maternal serum screening results. However, in the Fetal Medicine Research Unit at St Michael's Hospital, Bristol, fetal blood sampling is preferred because of the superior cytogenetic banding quality.[38]

Direct chromosome preparations from the cytotrophoblast and rapid cell culture techniques using the mesenchymal core of the villi allow early and rapid karyotyping during the first trimester. Chorionic villi are an excellent source of DNA, supplying sufficient material for most molecular genetic techniques without prior culture. There is a steady increase in the number of diagnosable monogenic disorders due to rapid advances in molecular genetics and early genetic counselling is recommended.

Maternal contamination of chorionic cell cultures may cause a false-negative diagnosis and is particularly a problem in DNA diagnosis using PCR amplification and in some biochemical examinations. The risk of maternal cell contamination is closely related to the operator skill.[39] Diagnostic and counselling difficulties can arise with placental mosaicism. Where mosaicism is found it is often apparently confined to the placenta (1.9%)[40] with true mosaicism occurring in approximately 1% of samples. The simultaneous analysis of cultured cells reliably prevents diagnostic errors by raising the likelihood of detecting mosaicism in both the placenta and fetus. In mosaicism cases, it is important to consider confirmation of aneuploidy by examination of another tissue (usually fetal blood or amniotic fluid cells) before termination of pregnancy. Clearly, the presence of structural fetal abnormality on ultrasound examination makes aneuploidy on CVS less likely to be due to placental mosaicism.

Procedure

The transabdominal technique of CVS can be applied either as a free-hand, fine-needle aspiration or with a needle-guide ultrasound transducer as described for amniocentesis. In either case, continuous simultaneous ultrasound is vital. Some investigators use a 'double needle' technique where a guide needle is advanced through the uterine wall and an inner needle then placed for aspiration of villi. Others use a 'single needle' approach usually with a 17–20 gauge needle. A placental biopsy forceps may be used through an outer guide needle. With a single needle approach, the aspirated tissue needs to be carefully separated under a dissection microscope in order to exclude contamination with maternal cells. With a double needle system undertaken expertly entirely within the placenta, it is hard to imagine how maternal contamination could ever occur.

Complications

Various studies suggest that women would prefer an early rather than a late diagnosis, provided the risks of both procedures are equal.[41,42] In addition, the medical risks of pregnancy termination are considerably higher as gestational age advances. These factors would tend to favour CVS in the first trimester for the detection of genetic disorders rather than amniocentesis after 15 weeks of gestation. However, the issue of fetal loss is complex and critical to the debate on benefits and risks.

The pre-procedure risk of miscarriage for any invasive procedure is strongly influenced by the gestational age at which the procedure is performed, maternal age and the indication for sampling.[43,44] The additional procedure-related risk will be determined by the type of procedure performed, operator skill and technical difficulties encountered. It is important that these factors are taken into account when comparing procedures. There is also the theoretical argument that detecting aneuploidy early in pregnancy may lead to termination of a pregnancy that might have miscarried spontaneously had prenatal diagnosis been planned for a later stage. The difficulties in evaluating post-procedure loss rates have been clearly shown by the controversial results of several multicentre trials designed to compare safety and accuracy of CVS with other invasive techniques.[45–49] However, the Canadian,[46] American[47] and Danish[49] studies did not reveal a significant difference in fetal loss rates comparing first trimester CVS and mid-trimester amniocentesis. Most centres now quote a 1% additional procedure-related risk, above the individual pregnancy background risk, of miscarriage for CVS after 11 weeks of gestation.

Some concern has been raised that CVS may rarely cause severe limb deficiencies.[50,51] The World Health Organization initiated an international registration of post-CVS limb defects in 1992.[52] The cohort showed no differences from the background population in the overall frequency or pattern distribution of limb deficiencies. It is now reasonable to perform CVS at 11 weeks of gestation and beyond, with the understanding that there is no procedure-related increase in the risk of limb defects. CVS before 11 weeks of gestation is almost never indicated, so the possible association with earlier testing is unlikely to be studied further.

The safety and reliability of late placental biopsies have been established in several individual series,[53-55] as well as in a large international survey.[56] However, the superior cytogenetic banding quality of fetal blood will mean that fetal blood sampling will be the preferred procedure in units with expert cytogenetic facilities.[38]

FETAL BLOOD SAMPLING

Antenatal fetal blood sampling was first undertaken for the diagnosis of severe, inherited diseases with a view to pregnancy termination if the fetus was affected. With the development of a medical approach to fetal disease over the 1980s and 1990s, the role of fetal phlebotomy is now comparable with its place in postnatal medicine. Fetal blood sampling should only be performed by clinicians with extensive experience in the performance of the other ultrasound-guided needle procedures. Ideally, this should be within a centre with a considerable number of referrals for anomaly scanning and fetal medicine opinions.[57]

Diagnostic indications and methods

Fetal blood contains a high concentration of white blood cells, which divide rapidly allowing the preparation of a high-quality karyotype with good chromosome banding within 48–72 hours in most centres. The most common indication for a rapid karyotype is the presence of either a fetal malformation or severe early-onset fetal growth restriction on ultrasound assessment. Fetal blood sampling is performed less often for the prenatal diagnosis of single gene defects than in the past, as many can now be diagnosed earlier in gestation using the various DNA techniques described previously. This technique remains important for at-risk patients who book late in pregnancy, in families where DNA analysis is not possible and when faced with a mosaic result or culture failure by either amniocentesis or placental biopsy.

Although there are various indirect techniques to assess fetal anaemia, in particular Doppler ultrasonography,[58] the definitive test before and after birth is the measurement of haemoglobin concentration. This may be required in maternal red cell alloimmunisation[59] or some cases of non-immune hydrops.[60] Severe fetal thrombocytopenia may lead to cerebral haemorrhage before, during or after birth and subsequently to neurological impairment. In selected cases, the fetal platelet count can be measured to guide diagnosis and treatment.

Fetal acidaemia may be effectively ruled out by Doppler studies of the fetal vasculature. Suspected fetal hypoxia or acidaemia can be confirmed or refuted by fetal blood gas analysis.[61] This is increasingly important with emerging evidence that chronic fetal acidaemia is associated with poor long-term neurodevelopmental outcome.[62] However, there is no evidence that interventions such as preterm delivery based on the assessment of fetal acid/base status improve outcome. Fetal blood sampling for this indication should be considered when the potential benefit of changes in management outweigh the procedure-related risks, although such circumstances are likely to be rare due to the high sensitivity and specificity of Doppler studies.[63]

Fetal blood tests can investigate whether maternal infection has led to fetal infection. It is possible to test for infection-specific fetal IgM or specific genomic material by PCR or effects such as abnormal liver enzymes. As mentioned previously, it is not possible with these tests alone to differentiate between a fetus that is infected or affected by an infective organism. Fetal blood tests may prove to be unnecessary if the results of an amniotic fluid sample agree with ultrasound findings.[64]

Therapeutic indications and methods

Injection into the fetal circulation has provided dramatically effective therapy for some conditions and shows promise in others. Fetal anaemia of any cause can be treated by intravascular blood transfusion.[65] Platelet transfusion is controversial because the short half-life mandates frequent transfusion to maintain the fetal platelet count.[66,67] Thrombocytopenic fetuses have a greater chance of haemorrhage at the time of a blood sampling procedure and this must be balanced against the potential benefit of maintaining a normal fetal platelet count.

Fetal arrhythmias leading to hydrops fetalis and not responding to transplacental treatment can be corrected by injection of anti-arrhythmic drugs into the fetal circulation.[68] This is more likely to be of benefit at earlier gestations where there are considerable advantages in prolonging intrauterine life.

For selective feticide, intravascular injection of strong potassium solutions can be used when a handicapping abnormality is found in one fetus of a multiple pregnancy or when the number of fetuses is so great that survival of any is unlikely. It can also be used during late abortion of singleton pregnancies and for termination of viable fetuses with handicapping conditions in countries where this option is legal.

Procedure

Sampling site

Fetal blood sampling is now almost exclusively performed by ultrasound-guided cordocentesis, which can be performed without maternal sedation.[69] The placental umbilical cord insertion is usually the easiest site to puncture as the use of the fetal origin of the umbilical cord may be complicated by fetal movement after puncture. Although cordocentesis is usually done after 18 weeks of gestation, some groups have reported successful cordocentesis as early as 12 weeks but with a marked increase in fetal risk.[70]

The fetal heart is larger than the umbilical cord making ultrasound-guided needling relatively easy. Despite fear of structural damage, cardiac puncture is relatively safe.[71] It is a useful option if an emergency blood transfusion is required (for example to treat procedure-related bleeding) or for feticide.

Blood can be obtained from vessels within the substance of the liver.[72-74] Sampling is sometimes performed after fetal paralysis with intramuscular pancuronium.[75] Fetal hepatic necrosis within 24 hours of intrahepatic vein sampling has been reported[76] and most specialists would prefer to sample the heart in the few situations where cordocentesis is difficult and fetal blood sampling is vital.

Technique

As with the other techniques, fetal blood sampling can be performed either by the needle guide technique or the free-hand technique as described earlier. If the fetus is viable the procedure should be done where rapid access to an operative delivery room is possible. Consideration should be given to maternal administration of corticosteroids. A 12-cm needle is usually sufficient but the distance should be measured on the ultrasound screen at the outset. A transplacental approach is usually the easiest route to the placental cord insertion unless the placenta is entirely posterior. However, it is best to try to avoid the placenta in red-cell isoimmunised pregnancies. Many operators prefer the placental origin of the umbilical cord and because the blood obtained must be fetal the best site is about 1 cm from the placenta.

The needle is brought close to or even touching the cord, aiming for the umbilical vein, and then sharply advanced the remaining distance. After confirming that the needle tip is within the umbilical cord, a 1-ml syringe is applied and blood withdrawn. After 20 weeks of gestation, 3–5 ml may be removed but before 20 weeks of gestation the volume removed should be the bare minimum. If blood gas results are to be capable of interpretation, it is essential to identify the vessel and this can be by identification of the direction of turbulence produced after the rapid injection of up to 1 ml of normal saline.[69]

The heart is best entered through the anterior chest through the thick muscle of the ventricles to avoid damage to the valves or electrical conducting system and, theoretically, to reduce leakage of blood. If the intrahepatic vein is being sampled the abdomen is entered first, the direction checked and then the needle advanced into the sampling site as a separate movement.

After fetal blood sampling, a small sample should be sent for a haematology profile to check that the mean cell volume, haemoglobin concentration, white cell and platelet counts are normal.

Complications

Fetal blood sampling may be complicated by bleeding at the site of needling,[77] haematoma and obstruction to blood flow, fetal bradycardia (probably secondary to vasospasm, especially after puncture of the umbilical artery)[78,79] or intrauterine infection. Abruption shortly after cordocentesis has been reported.[80] Amniotic fluid leakage is rare, with a similar frequency to amniocentesis. There is a theoretical risk of carrying hepatitis or human immunodeficiency virus (HIV) from the mother's blood to the fetus. One study describes a four-fold increase in mother-to-child transmission of HIV-1 in association with third-trimester amniocentesis.[81] It is, therefore, advisable to avoid invasive procedures when a mother is known to be infected unless the indications warrant the additional risk.[82]

The use of the term 'procedure-related loss' to mean a fetal death within two weeks is misleading. The loss and complication rates are clearly related to the indication for sampling.[83] In common with other procedures, post-procedure loss rates are determined by the procedure-related risk added to the pre-procedure risk. In pregnancies of advanced gestation there may be a further reduction in loss related to emergency delivery of viable fetuses. Emergency delivery may prevent fetal death but could result in a death in the neonatal period or a child with permanent damage. Most units quote a 1–2% post-procedure pregnancy loss rate but transfusion carries a considerably higher procedure-related risk than blood sampling.

The main risk to the mother from fetal blood sampling is red-cell alloimmunisation. Anti-D immunoglobulin should be given to rhesus-negative women. Chorioamnionitis or emergency delivery pose additional risks to the mother. Needle injury to maternal intra-abdominal organs such as intestines or vessels may be quite common but significant morbidity as a result has not been reported after fetal blood sampling.

FURTHER THERAPIES

Pleuroamniotic shunt

Fluid collections can cause dilatation and damage to both the primary organ and the adjacent structures. Needling and aspiration using ultrasound-guided techniques, as described earlier, can provide temporary relief while awaiting a karyotype result. However, the fluid almost always reaccumulates. Pleuroamniotic shunting is an effective way of chronically draining fetal pleural effusions. This treatment can reverse fetal hydrops and correct polyhydramnios and thus reduce the risk of intrauterine death and preterm delivery. By allowing expansion of the lungs, pleuroamniotic shunting may also prevent pulmonary hypoplasia[84] and this is an especially dramatic and effective treatment for cases of chylothorax.

Vesico-amniotic shunting

The insertion of a double pig-tailed vesico-amniotic shunt is also a useful procedure in a few well-selected cases.[85] The main problem with vesico-amniotic shunting is that by the time the diagnosis of severe obstructive uropathy is made, renal function may already be severely and irreversibly damaged. The practical problems include unsatisfactory drainage owing to incorrect placement, occlusion or migration and infection or preterm labour after shunt insertion.[85]

Fetoscopy

Fetoscopy has been reintroduced in fetal diagnosis and therapy as a result of advances in microlaparoscopic technology. The high-resolution fibre optic equipment allows direct visualisation of the fetus and identification of surface anomalies beyond the scope of conventional ultrasound. Fetoscopic instrumentation has been used for the treatment of twin-to-twin transfusion syndrome, twin reversed arterial perfusion sequence, hydronephrosis, congenital diaphragmatic hernia, fetal tumours and myelomeningocele. Fetoscopy presents many potential advantages over open fetal surgery, in particular, a lower rate of preterm labour and fetal loss from preterm delivery. The main application of fetoscopy at present is the surgical treatment of complicated or abnormal monochorionic twin gestations. Though conceptually tempting, it has been recommended that further development of endoscopic fetal surgery should follow formal guidelines with prospective registration of world-wide experience.[86]

Laser ablation

Interruption of the vascular anastomosis between twin fetuses by fetoscopic laser ablation is a useful treatment in early-onset fetofetal transfusion syndrome when, if left untreated, the prognosis is poor indeed. The alternative is serial amniodrainage with a procedure-related risk at each drainage procedure and the continuing risk of cerebral damage in either fetus. In approximately one-third of cases treated by laser ablation both twins survive, in another third one twin survives and in the remaining third both twins die.[87,88] Laser ablation has also been used successfully to treat acardiac twin pregnancies by occluding the cord to the acardiac fetus or, in the unit at St Michael's Hospital, Bristol, by occlusion of the acardiac intra-abdominal vessels. These techniques may be appropriate in the management of vascular fetal tumours.

Open fetal surgery

Open fetal surgery has been successfully used in human pregnancies with a low acute maternal morbidity. However, preterm labour is common and the hysterotomy required always leads to the recommendation for caesarean section in current and future pregnancies. Open surgery has been undertaken for diaphragmatic hernia, urinary obstruction, cystic adenomatoid malformation of the lung, sacrococcygeal teratoma, twin-to-twin transfusion and congenital heart block.[89] The development of more effective tocolytic agents and the use of minimally invasive surgical techniques with miniaturised instruments will, it is hoped, cause less uterine irritability, giving better outcomes for fetal surgery.[89]

Ex utero intrapartum treatment

Ex utero intrapartum treatment describes a procedure for maintaining fetal gas exchange until adequate ventilation is achieved where there is life-threatening obstruction of the airway at birth. The procedure has been described in relation to the intrapartum airway management of giant fetal neck masses, such as lymphangiomas and cervical teratomas, and in a case of laryngeal atresia.[90-92] The rationale for performing the procedure is that a delay in adequately ventilating the neonate with airway obstruction can lead to hypoxia, acidosis, brain injury and death. The aim of the procedure is to maintain uteroplacental blood flow and fetal gas exchange until an airway is secured and adequate ventilation is achieved. The uteroplacental circulation is maintained by only partially delivering the fetus and maintaining complete uterine relaxation throughout the procedure. A successful case in the UK has recently been performed for a large anterior cervical teratoma.[93]

CONCLUSIONS

Amniocentesis, CVS and fetal blood sampling allow diagnosis, assessment and therapy for a large number of fetal abnormalities across a wide range of gestations. Early procedures may expedite diagnosis and decision making for parents but need to be balanced with the procedure-related risk of an adverse outcome and the possibility of terminating a pregnancy that may have miscarried spontaneously. Later procedures carry the risk of emergency delivery of a compromised fetus with the attendant risks to the mother and the possibility of neonatal death or subsequent handicap. Intrauterine transfusion in expert hands has revolutionised the management of fetal anaemia, particularly for rhesus isoimmunisation. The rapid progress in invasive, therapeutic and operative techniques within the specialty of fetal medicine is certain to result in a further increase in the range of options for the intrauterine management of fetal abnormalities.

References

1. Lamvu, G., Kuller, J.A. Prenatal diagnosis using fetal cells from the maternal circulation. *Obstet Gynecol Surv* 1997;**52**:433–7
2. Sherlock, J., Halder, A., Tutschek, B., Delhanty, J., Rodeck, C., Adinolfi, M. Prenatal detection of fetal aneuploidies using transcervical cell samples. *J Med Genet* 1997;**34**:302–5
3. Royal College of Obstetricians and Gynaecologists. *Amniocentesis.* London; 1996 (Guideline no. 8)
4. Worton, R.G., Stern, R.A. Canadian collaborative study of mosaicism in amniotic fluid cell cultures. *Prenat Diagn* 1984;**4**:131–44

5   Van Opstal, D., Van, H.J., Sachs, E.S. Fetal aneuploidy diagnosed by fluorescence *in situ* hybridisation within 24 hours after amniocentesis. *Lancet* 1993;**342**:802
6   Isada, N.B., Hume, R.J., Reichler, A., Johnson, M.P., Klinger, K.W., Evans, M.I. et al. Fluorescent *in situ* hybridization and second-trimester sonographic anomalies: uses and limitations. *Fetal Diagn Ther* 1994;**9**:367–70
7   Bennett, P.R., Le-Van-Kim, C., Colin, Y., Warwick, R.M., Cherif-Zahar, B., Fisk, N.M. et al. Prenatal determination of fetal RhD type by DNA amplification. *N Engl J Med* 1993;**329**:607–10
8   Bennett, P.R., Warwick, R., Vaughan, J., Chana, H., Lubenko, A., Fisk, N.M. Prenatal determination of human platelet antigen type using DNA amplification following amniocentesis. *Br J Obstet Gynaecol* 1994;**101**:246–9
9   Lighten, A.D., Overton, T.G., Sepulveda, W., Warwick, R.M., Fisk, N.M., Bennett, P.R. Accuracy of prenatal determination of RhD type status by polymerase chain reaction with amniotic cells. *Am J Obstet Gynecol* 1995;**173**:1182–5
10 Thein, A.T., Abdel-Fattah, S.A., Kyle, P.M., Soothill, P.W. An assessment of the use of interphase FISH with chromosome specific probes as an alternative to cytogenetics in prenatal diagnosis. *Prenat Diagn* 2000;**4**:275–80
11 Sepulveda, W., Donaldson, A., Johnson, R.D., Davies, G., Fisk, N.M. Are routine a-fetoprotein and acetylcholinesterase determinations still necessary at second-trimester amniocentesis? Impact of high-resolution ultrasonography. *Obstet Gynecol* 1995;**85**:107–12
12 Berrebi, A., Kobuch, W.E., Bessieres, M.H., Bloom, M.C., Rolland, M., Sarramon, M.F. et al. Termination of pregnancy for maternal toxoplasmosis. *Lancet* 1994;**344**:36–9
13 Hohlfield, P., Daffos, F., Costa, J.M., Thulliez, P., Forestier, F., Vidaud, M. Prenatal diagnosis of congenital toxoplasmosis with a polymerase-chain-reaction test on amniotic fluid. *N Engl J Med* 1994;**331**:695–9
14 Weiner, C.P., Grose, C. Prenatal diagnosis of congenital cytomegalovirus infection by virus isolation from amniotic fluid. *Am J Obstet Gynecol* 1990;**163**:1253–5
15 Borg, K.L., Nordbo, S.A., Winge, P., Dalen, A. Detection of cytomegalovirus using 'boosted' nested PCR. *Mol Cell Probes* 1995;**9**:251–7
16 Lazzarotto, T., Guerra, B., Spezzacatena, P., Varani, S., Gabrielli, L., Pradelli, P. et al. Prenatal diagnosis of congenital cytomegalovirus infection. *J Clin Microbiol* 1998;**36**:3540–4
17 Dodson, M.G., Fortunato, S.J. Microorganisms and premature labour. *J Reprod Med* 1988;**33**:87–96
18 Dudley, J., Malcolm, G., Ellwood, D. Amniocentesis in the management of preterm premature rupture of the membranes. *Aust N Z J Obstet Gynaecol* 1991;**31**:331–6
19 Morales, W.J., Angel, W.L., O'Brien, W.F., Knuppel, R.A., Finazzo, M. A randomised study of antibiotic therapy in idiopathic preterm labor. *Obstet Gynecol* 1988;**72**:829–33
20 James, D.K., Tindall, V.R., Richardson, T. Is the lecithin/sphingomyelin ratio outdated? *Br J Obstet Gynaecol* 1983;**90**:995–1000
21 Jeanty, P., Shah, D., Roussis, P. Single-needle insertion in twin amniocentesis. *J Ultrasound Med* 1990;**9**:511–17
22 Sebire, N.J., Noble, P.L., Odibo, A., Malligiannis, P., Nicolaides, K.H. Single uterine entry for genetic amniocentesis in twin pregnancies. *Ultrasound Obstet Gynecol* 1996;**7**:26–31
23 Nicolini, U., Monni, G. Intestinal obstruction in babies exposed *in utero* to methylene blue. *Lancet* 1990;**336**:1258–9
24 Johnson, A., Godmilow, L. Genetic amniocentesis at 14 weeks or less. *Clin Obstet Gynecol* 1988;**31**:345–52
25 Johnson, J.M., Wilson, R.D., Winsor, E.J., Singer, J., Dansereau, J., Kalousek, D.K. The early

amniocentesis study: a randomized clinical trial of early amniocentesis versus midtrimester amniocentesis. *Fetal Diagn Ther* 1996;**11**:85–93

26 Rebello, M.T., Gray, C.T., Rooney, D.E., Smith, J.H., Hackett, G.A., Loeffler, F.E. et al. Cytogenetic studies of amniotic fluid taken before the 15th week of pregnancy for earlier prenatal diagnosis: a report of 114 consecutive cases. *Prenat Diagn* 1991;**11**:35–40

27 Nicolaides, K.H., Brizot, M.L., Patel, F., Snijders, R. Comparison of chorion villus sampling and early amniocentesis for karyotyping in 1492 singleton pregnancies. *Fetal Diagn Ther* 1996;**11**:9–15

28 Canadian Early and Mid Trimester Amniocentesis Trial Group. Randomised trial to assess safety and fetal outcome of early and midtrimester amniocentesis. *Lancet* 1998;**351**:243–9

29 Tabor, A., Philip, J., Madsen, M., Bang, J., Obel, E.B., Norgaard-Pedersen, B. Randomised controlled trial of genetic amniocentesis in 4606 low-risk women. *Lancet* 1986;**i**:1287–93

30 Moessinger, A.C., Bassi, G.A., Ballantyne, G., Collins, M.H., James, L.S., Blanc, W.A. Experimental production of pulmonary hypoplasia following amniocentesis and oligohydramnios. *Early Hum Dev* 1983;**8**:343–50

31 Elias, S., Simpson, J.L. Amniocentesis. In: Milunsky, A., editor. *Genetic Disorders and the Fetus: Diagnosis, Prevention and Treatment*. New York: Plenum Press; 1986. p. 24–36

32 MRC Working Party on the Evaluation of Chorion Villus Sampling. Medical Research Council European trial of chorion villus sampling. *Lancet* 1991;**337**:1491–9

33 Murray, J.C., Karp, L.E., Williamson, R.A., Cheng, E.Y., Luthy, D.A. Rh-isoimmunisation related to amniocentesis. *Am J Med Genet* 1983;**16**:527–34

34 Mahoney, B.S., Petty, C.N., Nyberg, D.A., Luthy, D.A., Hickok, D.E., Hirsch, J.H. The 'stuck twin' phenomenon: ultrasonographic findings, pregnancy outcome and management with serial amniocenteses. *Am J Obstet Gynecol* 1990;**163**:1513–22

35 Saunders, N.J., Snijders, R.J., Nicolaides, K.H. Therapeutic amniocentesis in twin-twin transfusion syndrome appearing in the second trimester of pregnancy. *Am J Obstet Gynecol* 1992;**166**:820–4

36 Abdel-Fattah, S.A., Carroll, S.G., Kyle, P.M., Soothill, P.W. Amnioreduction: how much to drain? *Fetal Diagn Ther* 1999;**14**:279–82

37 Meagher, S.E., Fisk, N.M. Hydramnios, oligohydramnios. In: James, D.K., Steer, P.J., Weiner, B., Gonik, B., editors. *High Risk Pregnancy, Management Options*, 2nd ed. London: W.B. Saunders; 1999. p. 827–40

38 Carroll, S.G., Davies, T., Kyle, P.M., Abdel-Fattah, S., Soothill, P.W. Fetal karyotyping by chorionic villus sampling after the first trimester. *Br J Obstet Gynaecol* 1999;**106**:1035–40

39 Holzgreve, W., Miny, P. (1999) Chorionic villus sampling and placental biopsy. In: James, D.K., Steer, P.J., Weiner, B., Gonik, B., editors. *High Risk Pregnancy, Management Options*, 2nd ed. London: W.B. Saunders; 1999. p. 207–13

40 Holzgreve, W., Miny, P., Schloo, R. Late CVS. International registry compilation of data from 24 centres. *Prenat Diagn* 1990;**10**:159–67

41 Lippman, A., Perry, T.B., Mandel, S., Cartier, L. Chorionic villi sampling: women's attitudes. *Am J Med Genet* 1985;**22**:395–401

42 McGovern, M.M., Goldberg, J.D., Desnick, R.J. Acceptability of chorionic villi sampling for prenatal diagnosis. *Am J Obstet Gynecol* 1986;**155**:25–9

43 Ghidini, A., Sepulveda, W., Lockwood, C.J., Romero, R. Complications of fetal blood sampling. *Am J Obstet Gynecol* 1993;**168**:1339–43

44 Maxwell, D., Johnson, P., Hurley, P., Neales, K., Allan, L., Knott, P. Fetal blood sampling and pregnancy loss in relation to indication. *Br J Obstet Gynaecol* 1991;**98**:892–7

45 Rhoads, G.G., Jackson, L.G., Schlesselma, S.E., de la Cruz, F.F., Desnick, R.J., Golbus, M.M.

et al. The safety and efficacy of chorionic villus sampling for early prenatal diagnosis of cytogenetic abnormality. N Engl J Med 1989;320:609–14

46 Canadian Collaborative CVS-Amniocentesis Clinical Trial Group. Multicentre randomised clinical trial of chorion villus sampling and amniocentesis. Lancet 1989;i:1–6

47 MRC Working Party in the Evaluation of Chorionic Villous Sampling. Medical Research Council European trial of chorionic villous sampling. Lancet 1991;337:1491–9

48 Smidt-Jensen, S., Permin, M., Philip, J., Lundsteen, C., Gruning, L.K., Zachary, J.M. et al. Randomised comparison of amniocentesis and transabdominal and transcervical chorionic villous sampling. Lancet 1992;340:1237–44

49 Jackson, L.G., Zachary, J.M., Fowler, S.E., Desnick, R.J., Globus, M.S., Ledbetter, D.H. et al. A randomized comparison of transcervical and transabdominal chorionic-villus sampling. The US National Institute of Child Health and Human Development Chorionic-Villus Sampling and Amniocentesis Study Group. N Engl J Med 1992;327:594–8

50 Firth, H.V., Boyd, P.A., Chamberlain, P., MacKenzie, I.Z., Lindenbaum, R.H., Huson, S.M. Severe limb abnormalities after chorion villus sampling at 55–66 days' gestation. Lancet 1991;i:762–3

51 Schloo, R., Miny, P., Holzgreve, W., Horst, J., Lenz, W. Limb reduction defects following chorionic villus sampling. Am J Med Genet 1991;42:404–13

52 Froster, U.G., Jackson, L. Limb defects and chorionic limb sampling: results from an international registry, 1992–94. Lancet 1996;347:489–94

53 Nicolaides, K.H., Soothill, P.W., Rosevear, S. Transabdominal placental biopsy. Lancet 1987;ii:855–6

54 Hogdall, C.K., Doran, T.A., Shime, J., Wilson, S., Tashima, I. Transabdominal chorionic villus sampling in the second trimester. Am J Obstet Gynecol 1988;158:345–9

55 Chieri, P.R., Aldini, A.J.R. Feasibility of placental biopsy in the second trimester for fetal diagnosis. Am J Obstet Gynecol 1989;160:581–3

56 Holzgreve, W., Miny, P., Schloo, R. Late CVS. International registry compilation of data from 24 centres. Prenat Diagn 1990;10:159–67

57 Whittle, M. Safety of cordocentesis. Br J Hosp Med 1989;41:511

58 Mari, G., Deter, R.L., Carpenter, R.L., Rahman, F., Zimmerman, R., Moise, K.L. Jr et al. Noninvasive diagnosis by Doppler ultrasonography of fetal anaemia due to maternal red-cell alloimmunization. N Engl J Med 2000;342:9–14

59 Nicolaides, K.H., Soothill, P.W., Clewell, C.H., Rodeck, C.H., Mibasham, R. Fetal haemoglobin concentration to assess the severity of red cell iso-immunisation. Lancet 1988;i:1073–5

60 Soothill, P.W. Successful treatment of non-immune hydrops caused by parvovirus B19. Lancet 1990;336:121–2

61 Soothill, P.W. Cordocentesis: role in assessment of fetal condition. In: Manning, F., editor. Clinics in Perinatology. Philadelphia: W.B. Saunders; 1989. p. 755–69

62 Soothill, P.W., Ajayi, R.A., Campbell, S., Ross, E., Nicolaides, K.H. Fetal oxygenation at cordocentesis, maternal smoking and childhood neuro-development. Eur J Obstet Gynecol Reprod Biol 1995;59:21–4

63 Bobrow, C.S., Soothill, P.W. Causes and consequences of fetal acidosis. Arch Dis Child 1999;80:F246–9

64 Hohlfield, P., MacAleese, J., Capella-Pavlovski, M., Giovangrandi, Y., Thuliez, P., Forestier, F. Fetal toxoplasmosis: ultrasonographic signs. Ultrasound Obstet Gynecol 1991;1:241–4

65 Moise, K.J. Jr., Schumacher, B. Anaemia. In: Fisk, N.M., Moise, K.J. Jr, editors. Fetal Therapy: Invasive and Transplacental. Cambridge: Cambridge University Press; 1997. p. 141–63

66 Nicolini, U., Rodeck, C.H., Kochenour, N.K., Greco, P., Fisk, N.M., Letsky, E. et al. In utero platelet transfusion for alloimmune thrombocytopenia. Lancet 1988;ii:506

67 Murphy, M.F., Pullen, H.W., Metcalfe, P., Chapman, J.F., Jenkins, E., Waters, D.H. et al. Management of fetal allo-immune thrombocytopenia by weekly in utero platelet transfusions. Vox Sang 1990;58:45–9

68 Hansmann, M., Gembruch, U., Bald, R., Manz, M., Redel, A. Fetal tachyarrhythmias: transplacental and direct treatment of the fetus – a report of 60 cases. Ultrasound Obstet Gynecol 1991;1:162–70

69 Nicolaides, K.H., Soothill, P.W., Rodeck, C.H., Campbell, S. Ultrasound-guided sampling of umbilical cord and placental blood to assess fetal well-being. Lancet 1986;i:1065–7

70 Orlandi, F., Damiani, G., Jahil, C., Lairicella, S., Bertolini, O., Maggie, A. The risks of early cordocentesis (12–21 weeks): analysis of 500 cases. Prenat Diagn 1990;10:425–8

71 Westgren, M., Selbing, A., Stangenberg, M. Fetal intracardiac transfusions in patients with severe rhesus isoimmunisation. BMJ 1988;296:885–6

72 Bang, J., Bock, J.E., Trolle, D. Ultrasound-guided fetal intravascular transfusion for severe rhesus haemolytic disease. BMJ 1982;284:373–4

73 DeCrespigny, L.Ch., Robinson, H.P., Quinn, M., Doyle, L., Ross, A., Cauchi, M. Ultrasound guided fetal blood transfusions for severe red cell isoimmunisation. Obstet Gynecol 1985;66:529–32

74 Nicolini, U., Nicolaides, P., Fisk, N., Tannirandorn, Y., Rodeck, C.H. Fetal blood sampling from the intrahepatic vein: analysis of safety and clinical experience with 214 procedures. Obstet Gynecol 1990;76:47–53

75 DeCrespigny, L.Ch., Robinson, H.P., Ross, A.W., Quinn, M. Curarisation of fetus for intrauterine procedures. Lancet 1985;i:1164

76 Sturgiss, S.N., Wright, C., Davison, J.M., Robson, S.C. Fetal hepatic necrosis following blood sampling from the intrahepatic vein. Prenat Diagn 1996;16:866–9

77 Jaineaux, E., Douner, C., Simon, P., Vanesse, M., Hustin, J., Rodesch, F. Pathological aspects of the umbilical cord after percutaneous umbilical blood sampling. Obstet Gynecol 1989;73:215–18

78 Benacerraf, B., Barss, V.A., Salzmann, D.H., Greene, M.F., Penso, C.A., Frigoletto, F.D. Jr Acute fetal distress associated with percutaneous umbilical blood sampling. Am J Obstet Gynecol 1987;156:1218–20

79 Weiner, C.P. Cordocentesis for diagnostic indications: two years experience. Obstet Gynecol 1987;70:664–8

80 Feinkind, L., Nanda, D., Delke, I., Minkoff, H. Abruptio placentae after percutaneous umbilical cord sampling: a case report. Am J Obstet Gynecol 1990;162:1203–4

81 Tess, B.H., Rodrigues, L.C., Newell, M.L., Dunn, D.T., Lago, T.D. Breastfeeding, genetic, obstetric and other risk factors associated with mother-to-child transmission of HIV-1 in Sao Paulo State, Brazil. Sao Paulo Collaborative Study for Vertical Transmission of HIV-1. AIDS 1998;12:513–20

82 Workman, M.R., Philpott-Howard, J. Risk of fetal infection from invasive procedures. J Hosp Infect 1997;35:169–74

83 Wilson, R.D., Farquharson, D.F., Wittmann, B.K., Shaw, D. Cordocentesis: overall pregnancy loss rate as important as procedure loss rate. Fetal Diagn Ther 1994;9:142–8

84 Pettersen, H.N., Nicolaides, K.H. Pleural effusion. In: Fisk, N.M., Moise, K.J. Jr, editors. Fetal Therapy: Invasive and Transplacental. Cambridge: Cambridge University Press; 1997. p. 261–72

85 Merrill, D.C., Weiner, C.P. Urinary tract obstruction. In: Fisk, N.M., Moise, K.J. Jr, editors. Fetal Therapy: Invasive and Transplacental. Cambridge: Cambridge University Press; 1997. p. 273–86

86 Deprest, J.A., Lerut, T.E., Vandenberghe, K. Operative fetoscopy: new perspective in fetal therapy? *Prenat Diagn* 1997;**17**:1247–60
87 De Lia, J.E., Cruikshank, D.P., Keye, W.R. Fetoscopic neodymium:YAG laser occlusion of placental vessels in severe twin-twin transfusion syndrome. *Obstet Gynecol* 1990;**75**:1202–11
88 Ville, Y., Hyett, J., Hecher, K., Nicolaides, K.H. Preliminary experience with endoscopic laser surgery for severe twin-twin transfusion syndrome. *N Engl J Med* 1995;**332**:224–7
89 Rice, H.E., Harrison, M.R. Open fetal surgery. In: Fisk, N.M., Moise, K.J. Jr, editors. *Fetal Therapy: Invasive and Transplacental.* Cambridge: Cambridge University Press; 1997. p. 27–35
90 Mychaliska, G.B., Bealer, J.F., Graf, J.L., Rosen, M.A., Adzick, N.S., Harrison, M.R. Operating on placental support: the *ex utero* intrapartum treatment procedure. *J Pediatr Surg* 1997;**2**:227–30
91 Liechty, K.W., Crombleholme, T.M., Flake, A.W., Morgan, M.A., Kurth, C.D., Hubbard, A.M. et al. Intrapartum airway management for giant fetal neck masses: the EXIT (*ex utero* intrapartum treatment) procedure. *Am J Obstet Gynecol* 1997;**177**:870–4
92 DeCou, J.M., Jones, D.C., Jacobs, H.D., Touloukian, R.J. Successful *ex utero* intrapartum treatment (EXIT) procedure for congenital high airway obstruction syndrome (CHAOS) owing to laryngeal atresia. *J Pediatr Surg* 1998;**33**:1563–5
93 Murphy, D.J., Kyle, P.M., Cairns, P., Weir, P., Cusick, E., Soothill, P.W. Personal communication

29

Minimally invasive prenatal diagnosis: fantasy or reality?

Timothy G. Overton

INTRODUCTION

Prenatal diagnosis enables the identification of fetuses with a variety of genetic and nongenetic conditions. This information alerts parents and obstetricians to potential problems that the child may face. Since the first report of prenatal diagnosis of fetal malformation (anencephaly) by ultrasound with subsequent termination of pregnancy in 1972,[1] there have been great improvements in imaging techniques. In addition, the recent revolution in molecular biology now enables rapid definitive testing on minute samples of fetally derived genetic material. Physicians offering prenatal diagnosis bear a heavy responsibility. Diagnostic errors result in termination of normal pregnancies and the birth of handicapped children and the implementation of widespread and inappropriate testing can cause anxiety and miscarriage of normal pregnancies.

Prenatal diagnosis of genetic conditions currently involves the identification of high-risk pregnancies by widespread or selective screening followed by definitive diagnostic testing. Serum screening for Down syndrome is now commonplace and detection rates of up to 80% with a 5% false-positive rate are possible.[2] Recent interest has focused on using ultrasound technology to identify markers for fetal aneuploidy early in gestation. Using a combination of nuchal translucency, crown-rump length and maternal age, 77% of fetuses with Down syndrome can be detected if invasive testing is offered to 5% of the screened population.[3] However, definitive diagnosis relies on invasive tests such as amniocentesis, chorionic villus biopsy or cordocentesis. These tests are limited by the gestational age at which they can be performed, the safety of the test in relation to the continuing pregnancy and the skill of the operator. A test that reliably identifies a genetically abnormal fetus with minimal inconvenience to the woman and at no risk to the fetus is the 'holy grail' of current prenatal diagnosis research.

There are two possible routes from which fetal cells could be retrieved without threatening the pregnancy. Fetal cells have been known to exist at the lower pole of the uterus in early pregnancy since the early 1970s[4] and in the maternal circulation for over 100 years.[5] However, the success of isolating fetal cells from either of these places is hampered by one common problem: the target cells are present in extremely small numbers compared with an overwhelming background of maternal cells. It is the problem of hunting for a needle in a haystack. Until recently, the needle has been far too small to detect but the revolution in molecular biology and in particular the development of the polymerase chain reaction (PCR) and fluorescence *in situ* hybridisation (FISH) has provided the tools to dismantle the haystack making the search for the needle a reality.

TRANSCERVICAL CELL SAMPLING

After implantation, the cytotrophoblast and syncytiotrophoblast surround the inner cell mass. Initially, the chorionic villi are maintained on the outer surface but these are lost at about four

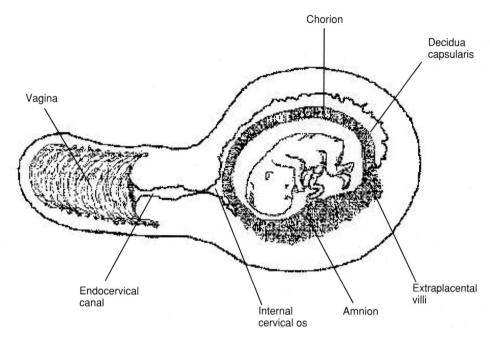

Figure 1 *Relationship of the placental membranes to the fetus at the end of the first trimester of pregnancy*

weeks when the smooth chorion laeve is formed (Figure 1). It was originally thought that these degenerating villi dropped off into the uterine cavity, some of which became trapped in the endocervical mucous plug. However, this did not take into account the fact that the villi in the wall of the gestation sac are covered by the decidua capsularis. Because the villi are not in direct contact with the uterine cavity, the chorion laeve is formed by a process of avascular necrosis and degeneration rather than exfoliation. Subsequent work has shown that trophoblast cells harvested transcervically are viable and have the ability to grow in culture.[6] It is now thought that these cells gain access to the uterine cavity directly by migrating through the decidua capsularis.[6]

In 1971, Shettles postulated that such cells could be used as a source of fetal DNA for prenatal diagnosis. Cotton swabs taken from the endocervix were analysed using Y-body fluorescence. The fetal gender was correctly typed in 6 of 18 male pregnancies and 4 of 12 female pregnancies.[4]

This study opened the floodgates for a series of reports where workers looked into the feasibility of using these cells for reliable prenatal diagnosis.[7–16] The cells were usually collected by simple smears or by rotating cotton-wool swabs in the endocervix but some workers designed more elaborate collecting devices such as the mucus extractor.[13] However, the common theme that emerged from all these preliminary experiments was their unreliability and irreproducibility. Enthusiasm for this technique was finally lost when it became apparent that the staining technique was fundamentally inaccurate.

With the development of PCR technology, transcervical sampling was resurrected in 1992 by Griffith-Jones *et al.*[17] The PCR detected male DNA on cotton wool swabs from the vaginal vault, endocervix and lower pole of the uterus in first trimester pregnancies. The presence of male DNA was ascribed to the presence of a male fetus. Accordingly, fetal gender was correctly predicted in

25 of 26 pregnancies. As before, this generated further interest as a possible approach to prenatal diagnosis. Morris and Williamson, using the same technique, correctly predicted the fetal gender in only 4 of 13 male pregnancies and found male 'contamination' in some of the female pregnancies.[18] The reports that followed were notable for two reasons. Firstly, there was considerable debate in the literature as to the usefulness of this approach.[19-23] Secondly, published papers generally had small numbers of subjects. It is important to appreciate that, in this type of study, only the male pregnancies are truly informative. Diagnosing a female pregnancy correctly using PCR may merely represent fortuitous detection of X-specific sequences from contaminating maternal cells.

In an attempt to resolve some of these issues, the fetal cell research group at Queen Charlotte's Hospital, London, conducted a large experiment to establish whether this is a feasible route for prenatal diagnosis.[24] Eighty-seven women were recruited in the first trimester prior to termination of pregnancy under a protocol approved by the local ethical committee (Figure 2). All samples were collected under ultrasound guidance prior to the termination of pregnancy (Figure 3). Fifty-one were analysed using PCR on genetic material extracted from endocervical swabs, endocervical flushes and lower pole swabs and 36 were analysed using dual FISH on cell preparations from endocervical swabs and flushes.

In the dual FISH experiments, female cells stained red whereas male cells stained red and green, enabling their distinction under the fluorescent microscope. For the swabs and flushes undergoing PCR, each sample was analysed using three different PCRs, two of which adopted a nested strategy. The first set of nested primers identified a region on the X chromosome coding for the amelogenin gene and a smaller homologous region on the Y chromosome. The second primers coded for a region specific to the Y chromosome and nested primers outside these Y specific ones were designed and which acted as the third set. After performing the termination of pregnancy, a

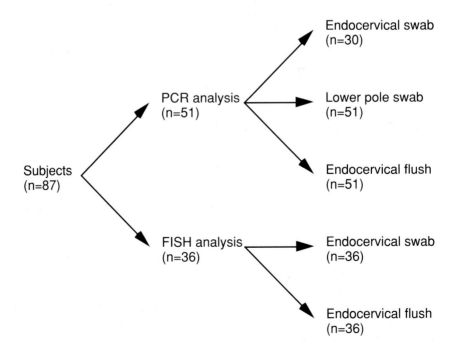

Figure 2 *Design of clinical trial to determine reliability of transcervical sampling*

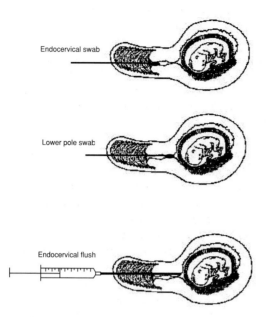

Figure 3 *Position of the sampling device in relation to cervix and conceptus*

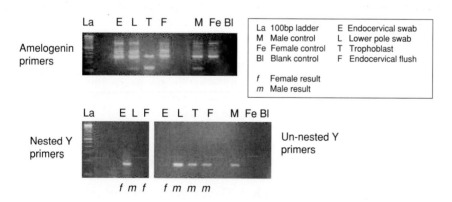

Figure 4 *Clinical sample tested with the three primer sets; the fetus is male as indicated by the trophoblast result with the un-nested Y-specific primers and amelogenin primers; male DNA has not been detected by the endocervical swabs analysed by all three primer sets and the endocervical flushes analysed by the amelogenin and nested Y-specific primers; Bl = blank control, E = endocervical swab; F = endocervical flush, f = female result, Fe = female control, L = lower pole swab, La, 100 bp bladder, M = male control, m = male result, T = trophoblast*

small fragment of fetal tissue was collected for definitive gender typing. A typical result from a clinical example is shown in Figure 4.

The results from the PCR experiments are summarised in Table 1. They were disappointing. Firstly, there was considerable variation in the ability of the primers and the harvesting technique to detect male DNA when the fetus was shown to be male. The lower pole swabs gave the best results probably because this was the most invasive technique and, therefore, most likely to collect fetal material. Of particular concern was the frequency with which male DNA was detected in

Table 1 *Success rates of gender prediction of harvesting techniques using three sets of polymerase chain reaction primers*

Method of cell collection	Un-nested Y-primers	Nested Y-primers	Amelogenin Primers
Lower pole swab ($n = 51$)			
Fetal gender			
Male	23 (0.79★★★)	22 (0.76★★)	18 (0.62)
Female	14 (0.64)	16 (0.73★)	12 (0.55)
Pooled success rate (95% CI)	0.72 (0.58–0.81)	0.74 (0.60–0.83)	0.58 (0.45–0.70)
Endocervical swab ($n = 30$)			
Male	11 (0.61)	12 (0.67)	5 (0.28)
Female	10 (0.83★)	9 (0.75)	8 (0.67)
Pooled success rate (95% CI)	0.72 (0.54–0.83)	0.71 (0.58–0.78)	0.47 (0.31–0.63)
Endocervical flush ($n = 51$)			
Male	19 (0.66)	16 (0.55)	17 (0.59)
Female	19 (0.86★★★)	18 (0.82★★)	18 (0.82★★)
Pooled success rate (95% CI)	0.76 (0.62–0.84)	0.69 (0.55–0.78)	0.70 (0.56–0.80)

Asterisks indicate *P* values of one-sided tests against 'null hypothesis' values of 0.5 for the success rate: ★ <0.05; ★★ <0.01; ★★★ <0.001

Table 2 *Numbers of samples where male DNA was detected with fluorescence* in situ *hybridisation (FISH)*

Method of cell collection	Fetal gender	Dual FISH with X and Y probes (%)
Endocervical swab ($n = 36$)	Male (15)	4/15 (27)
	Female (21)	2/21 (10)
Endocervical flush ($n = 36$)	Male (15)	6/15 (40)
	Female (21)	1/21 (5)

female pregnancies. This is a common finding with most studies of this nature and has often been attributed to the presence of sperm in the genital tract. Although sperm only remain viable for about seven days, the length of time the DNA contained within could act as a possible template for PCR is unknown. Laboratory contamination was also possible. The PCR experiments were all controlled with known female samples and 'blanks' (where no template DNA was added) to rule out contamination during the PCR experiment itself. However, this did not control for the possibility of contamination occurring during the collection of samples and transport to the laboratory.

The FISH results are summarised in Table 2. These experiments gave equally disappointing results. Male cells were detected less frequently than with the PCR. In cases where male cells were detected in female pregnancies this was not due to contamination with sperm; a 'male' sperm should only have a single male signal and the male cells detected in these experiment had both an X and a Y signal. Of greater concern was the fact that, in 73% of samples from endocervical swabs and 60% of samples from endocervical flushes, no fetal cells were detected.

So where does this leave transcervical sampling? Failure of detection of fetal cells by PCR or FISH may be due to their presence in such small numbers relative to the maternal cells or their absence altogether. With the former it may be possible to improve the detection rate by cell sorting with trophoblast-specific antibodies, which increases the purity of the fetal cell sample. Until recently, this approach has been limited by the difficulty in producing a specific antibody to trophoblast antigens. Micromanipulation techniques are also being employed to separate clumps of fetal syncytiotrophoblast nuclei from the maternal cells.[25] It may also be possible to selectively culture fetally-derived cells so as to increase the ratio of fetal to maternal cells. Some success has been achieved using this approach but the collection method employed was not ultrasound guided, preventing accurate monitoring of the invasiveness of the procedure.[26]

However, if fetal cells prove to be absent in a significant proportion of samples, the future of transcervical sampling for prenatal diagnosis will be less certain. An invasive procedure early in pregnancy that does not sample the target cell reliably would have little appeal to either the obstetrician or patient. One obvious way to improve the yield of fetal cells would be to increase the invasiveness of the sampling technique. The distinction between transcervical chorionic villus sampling (CVS) and sampling using swabs and flushes then becomes less clear, defeating the idea of minimally invasive prenatal diagnosis.

The safety of transcervical sampling itself has yet to be addressed fully. In one study, concern over the possibility that transcervical flushing might compromise the pregnancy by introducing infection into the uterus resulted in the abandonment of this procedure in favour of endocervical swabs and aspirates.[27] Reassuringly, in a study comparing 130 women who underwent endocervical aspiration immediately prior to transcervical CVS, with a control group undergoing CVS only, there was no detectable difference in pregnancy outcome.[6] The safety of transcervical sampling has yet to be fully evaluated. However, it would only be appropriate to perform such trials, which would require many thousands of patients, once the reliability of the technique had been established on cases prior to termination of pregnancy.

The needle in this particular haystack still remains elusive. Therefore, it is not surprising that researchers are looking at other haystacks where the needles may be more accessible.

FETAL CELLS IN THE MATERNAL CIRCULATION

The existence of fetal cells in the maternal circulation has been known about for over 100 years since Schmorl,[5] in 1893, identified trophoblastic cells trapped in the lungs of women who had died from eclampsia. In 1959, Douglas et al.[28] demonstrated the presence of trophoblasts in broad ligament veins and the inferior vena cavae of women suffering from eclampsia. A few years later a more extensive study of women dying during pregnancy, labour, or the immediate postpartum period, confirmed Schmorl's original findings.[29] Trophoblast cells were found in 96 of 220 lung sections and were more commonly seen when the woman had died during labour or shortly afterwards.

It was not until 1969, however, that the possibility of recovering these fetal cells for prenatal diagnosis was proposed. Walknowska et al. analysed unbanded metaphase spreads and detected male cells in the maternal circulation in 9 out of 22 women carrying a male fetus and in two out of eight with a female fetus.[30] Rather like transcervical sampling, this prompted a series of reports of a similar nature which suggested that such cells existed in rather large numbers, approximately 0.1–0.3%. However, it became clear that prenatal diagnosis by this route was not going to be straightforward when it was repeatedly observed that XY metaphases were present in women carrying female fetuses and absent in those carrying male fetuses, an observation now attributed to hybridisation artefact of the probes used.[31-33]

With the application of nested PCR technology, Lo et al.[34] rekindled interest in the possibility of prenatal diagnosis from fetal cells in the maternal circulation. DNA, prepared from blood samples taken from 19 pregnant women whose gestational ages varied from 9–41 weeks, was used as template for a nested PCR reaction specific for a Y chromosome repeat sequence. Male-specific DNA was detected in all 12 women carrying a male fetus but in none of the seven carrying a female.[34] They extended their work to the detection of a single Y-specific sequence, again using a nested PCR approach, on DNA extracted from peripheral blood. Of the 27 cases analysed, 13 gave a true-positive result and two gave a false-positive result.[35]

This early work also suggested that fetal cells were present in much smaller numbers than originally thought and that a more realistic ratio was in the region of one fetal cell for every million nucleated maternal cells. This inevitably meant that some form of enrichment procedure would be necessary for reliable prenatal diagnosis. There are currently two approaches whereby blood is centrifuged on a density gradient to retrieve nucleated cells and then separated by either fluorescent activated cell sorting (FACS) or magnetic activated cell sorting (MACS) using antibodies specific for receptors on the desired cells. FACS has the advantage of being able to use more than one antibody at a time, which may improve the yield of target cells slightly when compared with MACS. MACS, on the other hand, is significantly cheaper and easier to perform and may have the long-term advantage of convenience.

Of perhaps more importance is which fetal cell type to enrich for. Three sorts of cell have attracted most interest; the trophoblast, lymphocyte and nucleated red blood cell. Two problems exist with trophoblasts. Firstly, they are rapidly sequestered by the maternal lung, resulting in small numbers in the maternal peripheral circulation and, secondly, researchers have experienced some difficulty in raising specific antibodies to their placental antigens.[36] Fetal lymphocytes express the human leucocyte antigens and although specific antibodies can be produced, this requires a knowledge of the parental human leucocyte antigen status which is not always convenient. There is also the possibility that these cells can persist long after the antecedent pregnancy, causing inaccurate results in the future. The cell that has generated most interest is the nucleated red blood cell (nRBC). These comprise 10% of the red cell population of a ten-week fetus and 0.5% at 19 weeks, yet are relatively rare in peripheral adult blood.[37] It also seems unlikely that they persist for more than 90 days.[38] Fetal nRBC express the transferrin receptor (CD71) to which a specific antibody has been raised that is used for sorting in both MACS and FACS samples.

Despite Lo's initial success and a great deal of subsequent research aimed at detecting all three candidate cells by FISH or PCR, with or without prior enrichment with FACS or MACS, no one technique has been reliable in detecting fetal cells in a large series.

In a collaborative project with Wolfgang Holzgreve and Dorothee Gänshirt in Basle, the research group at Queen Charlotte's Hospital investigated the possibility of detecting fetal rhesus gene sequences in maternal blood in mothers who were RhD negative. This is analogous to detecting fetal Y sequences because RhD-negative individuals are missing a part of the RhD gene compared with their RhD-positive counterparts. RhD DNA could theoretically be detected in the maternal circulation of RhD-negative women carrying RhD-positive fetuses using PCR primers specific for the RhD gene. This situation also has direct clinical relevance in diagnosing the presence of a RhD-positive fetus in a potentially alloimmunised pregnancy. Conversely, the identification of a RhD-negative fetus would be reassuring for both the mother and obstetrician.

Twenty millilitres of maternal blood were taken from 41 RhD-negative women throughout gestation prior to any invasive procedure. From 20 samples, the DNA was extracted directly and tested in triplicate for the presence of RhD-positive DNA sequences using a nested RhD-specific PCR.[39] The remaining 21 were enriched for nRBC by triple density gradient centrifugation and MACS for the CD71 receptor. The DNA was extracted from the sorted cells and used as template for the nested RhD-positive PCR as before. The fetal RhD status was ascertained from DNA extracted following amniocentesis or cordocentesis or serologically following delivery. In a series of dilution experiments the nested PCR was shown to be able to detect down to a level of one RhD-positive cell in 5 µl of water or ten RhD-positive cells in 10 000 RhD-negative cells in 5 µl of water (Figure 5).

The results are shown in Tables 3 and 4. The success of other groups in detecting fetal RhD sequences in maternal blood was not matched. In the unsorted experiments, the technique was not sensitive enough to detect the fetal DNA and in the sorted samples false-positive amplification was noted. The sorted samples were being collected in the UK and transported to Basle for cell

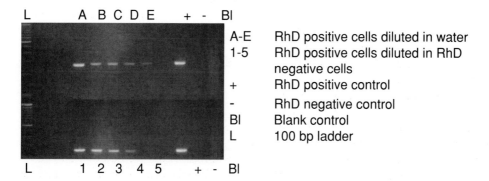

Figure 5 *Dilution series for the rhesus D (RhD) specific nested primers; one RhD-positive cell can be detected in 5 ml of water (E) or ten RhD-positive cells in 10 000 RhD negative cells in 5 ml of water (lane 4)*

sorting and DNA extraction. The DNA was subsequently analysed in the UK. Although contamination during the PCR itself was controlled for, it is possible that contamination was occurring during transport to and from Basle and in MACS sorting. The accuracy could theoretically be improved by performing MACS sorting in the UK or by increasing sensitivity without compromising specificity.

We addressed the latter by devising a system to detect RhD positive RNA rather than DNA. RNA has two important advantages over DNA in work of this kind. Firstly, it is an unstable molecule due to the abundance of RNAases. Contamination is unlikely to be a problem because extraneous RNA will be rapidly degraded. Provided that primers are designed to span intron–exon boundaries, contamination with DNA is easily recognised. Mature mRNA is essentially the same as DNA with the introns spliced out (Figure 6); primers that span intronic regions will generate products of different size for DNA and RNA enabling the ready detection of any contaminating DNA (Figure 7). In fact, if the primers span a sufficient number of introns and the introns and exons are of sufficient size it is possible that products will not be generated from DNA at all because they will be too large for effective PCR.

Table 3 *Results of rhesus D (RhD) testing on unsorted maternal blood samples*

Fetus	Results	
	Positive	Negative
RhD+ ($n = 14$)	1 (true)	13 (false)
RhD− ($n = 6$)	0 (false)	6 (true)

Table 4 *Results of rhesus D (RhD) testing on sorted maternal blood samples*

Fetus	Results	
	Positive	Negative
RhD+ ($n = 10$)	9 (true)	1 (false)
RhD− ($n = 11$)	7 (false)	4 (true)

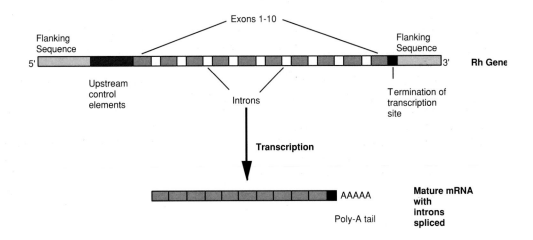

Figure 6 *Transcription from Rh gene to mRNA illustrating the essential differences between DNA and mRNA*

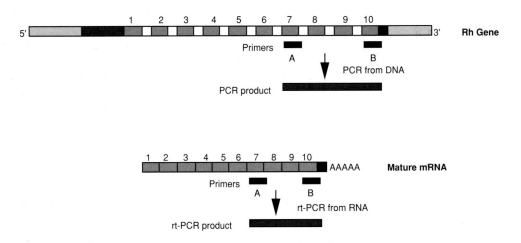

Figure 7 *Primers that span intron-exon boundaries will produce different sized polymerase chain reaction products from DNA and mRNA*

Secondly, another potential advantage in assaying for RNA is that there may be an increased copy number of the target sequence compared with DNA. In a nucleated red blood cell heterozygous for the RhD gene, there will only be one copy of the target RhD DNA sequence. In a cell that is actively expressing this gene there will be many mRNA transcripts produced. By five to six weeks of gestation, blood-borne pluripotent haemopoietic progenitors begin to colonise the fetal liver. These pluripotent stem cells form the colony-forming units that express the Rh antigens. Therefore, nucleated fetal red blood cells isolated early in pregnancy are likely to be a rich source of RhD RNA.

We have designed nested PCR primers that span introns 8–10 on the RhD gene. We used a RhD specific antisense primer for the initial reverse transcriptase step (Figure 6). In a series of dilution experiments we were able to detect as little as 0.05 fg of RhD-positive RNA diluted in 5 μl of water and 0.05 fg of RhD-positive RNA in 50 ng of RhD-negative RNA diluted in 5 μl of water – a considerable improvement in the sensitivity of detection of DNA.

This model system has now been used in a clinical study.[40] Fetal nRBC in peripheral blood, taken from 35 RhD-negative women throughout pregnancy, was enriched by triple-density gradient centrifugation and anti-CD71 magnetic sorting. Both DNA and RNA were then extracted and the accuracy of reverse-transcriptase-PCR (RT-PCR) and PCR for the prediction of fetal RhD genotype compared. RT-PCR was significantly more accurate ($P = 0.03$) than genomic-PCR, both overall (28/35 versus 22/35) and where the fetus was RhD positive (12/19 versus 6/19). This was the first study comparing the sensitivity of RT-PCR with genomic PCR although other groups have also recognised the potential advantages of this approach.[41] The success of this study was also notable for the absence of false-positive amplification with both RT-PCR and genomic PCR amplification.

CONCLUSIONS

So where does that leave us in the hunt for the needle in the haystack? Fetal cells undoubtedly exist at the lower pole of the uterus and in the maternal circulation. The main problem is their small number in relation to the large number of maternal cells. Studies addressing the feasibility of retrieving fetal cells from the lower pole of the uterus continue to show that fetal cells are not always collected and that misdiagnoses continue to occur. In one study, where 20 first-trimester pregnancies were sampled by endocervical aspiration, four samples failed to provide sufficient numbers of cells for analysis and only 10 of the 12 male pregnancies in the remaining 16 cases were accurately predicted.[42] Similarly, another study reported successful identification of syncytial fragments or cytotrophoblast in only 9/12 lavage samples and 4/10 aspirates.[43] Reports of the success of transcervical sampling continue to be based on small numbers (for example, five cases of successful detection of fetal aneuploidy)[44] and accurate prediction of haemoglobin mutations in four out of only six cases in one study[45] and six out of ten in another.[46] The safety of transcervical sampling has yet to be fully addressed and, in the absence of ultrasound guidance during sample collection, the difference between transcervical CVS and transcervical aspiration may well be small. For minimally invasive transcervical sampling to be accepted into clinical practice it needs to be as reliable but safer than CVS. There are no studies at the time of writing confirming either of these aspects.

The possibility of using fetal genetic material from the maternal circulation for prenatal diagnosis is more appealing since it will cause no threat to the pregnancy. Noninvasive prenatal diagnosis by message amplification techniques has potential application for detection of paternally inherited nucleic acid sequences, where the gene is expressed in early fetal cells. For the most common type of fetal cell sought in maternal blood, nucleated erythrocytes, this may include certain haematological disorders such as the haemoglobinopathies, especially when these are the result of mixed parental haplotypes (haemoglobin SC, sickle thalassaemia, etc.). Notwithstanding this, the difficulty in distinguishing true-negative diagnoses from false-negative amplification remains a significant barrier to clinical application of molecular rare-event amplification techniques that do not incorporate a step to confirm the presence of fetal cells in tested samples.

However, these approaches still remain hampered by the nonspecificity of the separation techniques, the absence of a specific fetal-cell marker and the difficulties in simultaneously identifying a fetal cell and making a diagnosis. One potential solution would be to use an anti-

RhD monoclonal antibody to separate fetal from maternal cells rather than the anti-CD71 antibody. This would be a truly fetal-specific antibody in RhD-negative women bearing a RhD-positive fetus. Cells separated by this process could then be analysed by RT-PCR for the epsilon globin mRNA to confirm fetal origin and then by FISH for prenatal diagnosis. This approach would also allow an accurate estimation of the number of fetal nucleated erythrocytes present in the maternal circulation. This would be important as it has been suggested that the majority of nRBC separated by conventional techniques are in fact of maternal origin.[47]

The need for a specific fetal-cell marker is vital. The demonstration that a cell is RhD-positive in an RhD-negative woman confirms its fetal origin. While accurate determination of fetal Rh type is important in the management of alloimmunised pregnancies, this fetal-cell identifier will only be applicable to 15% of pregnant women for general prenatal diagnostic tests. In addition, with the recent suggestion that the majority of nRBC in the maternal circulation are of maternal and not fetal origin, the importance of the development of a specific fetal-cell identifier is emphasised. As yet, there are no antibodies that are specific for fetal-cell surface antigens. There have been the reports as to the possibility of using intracytoplasmic antigens such as the embryonic haemoglobins as fetal-cell markers.[48] Fetal haemoglobin (HbF) is an obvious target, since it is the most abundant haemoglobin in fetal life, with production commencing at about eight weeks of pregnancy. However, HbF is also found in adult blood in 'F' cells, which contain from 14–25% HbF compared with in excess of 80% in fetal red blood cells. It is possible that this difference in concentration could be used to distinguish between fetal and maternal cells but there are situations where HbF levels in adult cells are much higher, such as hereditary persistence of HbF, myelofibrosis, familial HbF elevation and most anaemias. In addition, there remain significant technical problems combining antibody selection of nRBC and intracellular staining with FISH.[49] Other embryonic haemoglobins have also been considered. Zeta, epsilon, alpha and gamma chains are produced from as early as the fifth week of gestation and to date the epsilon chain has yet to be detected in adult blood. Fetal cells have been noted to express high intracellular levels of the DNA precursor pathway enzyme, thymidine kinase.[50] Since normal adult peripheral blood cells do not exhibit any thymidine kinase activity, this enzyme has the potential of being used as a marker both for detection and enrichment of fetal cells.

The small numbers of fetal cells obtained by the above techniques remains a significant limitation within this research field. If fetal cells could be selectively cultured, more material would be available for analysis. The haemopoietic stem/progenitor cells (HSC/P) are a potential target since they are present early in fetal life in abundance[51] and the fetal HSC/P possess higher proliferative potential than adult HSC/P. In addition, the earlier in ontogeny, the greater their proliferative and differentiation potential, the higher the number of cells in cell cycle and the greater the sensitivity to growth factors.[52-54] Although there have been only a few attempts to culture fetal HSC/P from maternal blood,[55-57] an editorial in 1997 concluded that this approach has great promise.[58]

The presence of fetal cells in the maternal circulation is no longer considered controversial. The refinement of molecular techniques, together with the identification of specific fetal cell markers and physiological characteristics, continues to bring the goal of non-invasive prenatal diagnosis closer.

Acknowledgements

I am indebted to my research supervisors, Professors Phillip Bennett and Nicholas Fisk at Queen Charlotte's and Chelsea Hospital, London. This work was funded by Action Research.

References

1. Campbell, S., Johnstone, F.D., Holt, E.M., May, P. Anencephaly: early ultrasonic diagnosis and active management. *Lancet* 1972;**2**:1226–7
2. Macri, J.N., Kasturi, R.V., Krantz, D.A., Cook, E.J., Moore, N.D., Young, J.A. et al. Maternal serum Down syndrome screening: free b-protein is a more effective marker than human chorionic gonadotropin. *Am J Obstet Gynecol* 1990;**163**:1248–53
3. Snijders, R.J., Noble, P., Sebire, N., Souka, A., Nicolaides, K.H. UK multicentre project on assessment of risk of trisomy 21 by maternal age and fetal nuchal-translucency thickness at 10–14 weeks of gestation. Fetal Medicine Foundation First Trimester Screening Group. *Lancet* 1998;**352**:343–6
4. Shettles, L.B. Use of the Y chromosome in prenatal sex determination. *Nature* 1971;**230**:52–3
5. Schmorl, G. *Pathologisch-anatomische Untersuchungen uber Puerperal-eklampsie*. Leipzig: F.C.W. Vogel; 1893
6. Rodeck, C., Tutschek, B., Sherlock, J., Kingdom, J. Methods for the transcervical collection of fetal cells during the first trimester of pregnancy. *Prenat Diagn* 1995;**15**:933–42
7. Bobrow, M., Lewis, B.V. Unreliability of fetal sexing using cervical material. *Lancet* 1971;**2**:486
8. Warren, R., Sanchez, L., Hammond, D., McLeod, A. Prenatal sex determination from exfoliated cells found in cervical mucus. *Am J Hum Genet* 1972;**24**:29a
9. Tsuji, K., Sasaki, M. Absence of Y-body in the cervical mucus of pregnant women. *Nature* 1973;**243**:539
10. Goldstein, A.I., Lukesh, R.C., Ketchum, M. Prenatal sex determination by fluorescent staining of the cervical smear for the presence of a Y chromosome: an evaluation. *Am J Obstet Gynecol* 1973;**115**:866
11. Manuel, M., Park, I.J., Jones, H.W. Prenatal sex determination by fluorescent staining of cells for the presence of Y chromatin. *Am J Obstet Gynecol* 1974;**119**:853–4
12. Rhine, S.A., Cain, J.L., Cleary, R.E., Palmer, C.G., Thompson, J.F. Prenatal sex detection with endocervical smears: successful results utilizing Y-body fluorescence. *Am J Obstet Gynecol* 1975;**122**:155–60
13. Rhine, S.A., Palmer, C.G., Thompson, J.F. A simple alternative to amniocentesis for first trimester prenatal diagnosis. *Birth Defects* 1977;**13**:231–47
14. Varner, R.E. Fluorescent Y bodies from endocervical smears for prenatal sex detection. *Alabama Journal of Medical Sciences* 1977;**14**:438
15. Goldberg, M.F., Chen, A.T.L., Ahn, Y.W., Reidy, J.A. First-trimester fetal chromosomal diagnosis using endocervical lavage: a negative evaluation. *Am J Obstet Gynecol* 1980;**138**:436–40
16. Coleman, D.V. Endocervical lavage in early pregnancy. *Am J Obstet Gynecol* 1982;**142**:118–19
17. Griffith-Jones, M.D., Miller, D., Lilford, R.J., Bulmer, J. Detection of fetal DNA in trans-cervical swabs from first trimester pregnancies by gene amplification: a new route to prenatal diagnosis? *Br J Obstet Gynaecol* 1992;**99**:508–11
18. Morris, N., Williamson, R. Non-invasive first trimester antenatal diagnosis. *Br J Obstet Gynaecol* 1992;**99**:446–8
19. Zimmermann, R., Huch, A., Bar, W. Detection of fetal DNA in trans-cervical swabs from first trimester pregnancy by gene amplification: a new route to prenatal diagnosis? *Br J Obstet Gynaecol* 1993;**100**:400

20. Zimmermann, R., Huch, A., Kratzer, A., Bar, W. First-trimester sex determination from fetal DNA in cervical swabs. *Ann NY Acad Sci* 1994;**731**:201–3
21. Chaouat, G., Lochu, P., Ville, Y. et al. Transcervical sampling: a preliminary prospective study. *Ann NY Acad Sci* 1994;**731**:197–200
22. Bahado-Singh, R.O., Kliman, H., Feng, T.Y., Hobbins, J., Copel, J.A., Mahoney, M.J. First-trimester endocervical irrigation: feasibility of obtaining trophoblast cells for prenatal diagnosis. *Obstet Gynecol* 1995;**85**:461–4
23. Kingdom, J., Sherlock, J., Rodeck, C., Adinolfi, M. Detection of trophoblast cells in transcervical samples collected by lavage or Cytobrush. *Obstet Gynecol* 1995;**86**:283–8
24. Overton, T.G., Lighten, A.D., Fisk, N.M., Bennett, P.R. First trimester transcervical sampling is unreliable for prenatal diagnosis. *Am J Obstet Gynecol* 1996;**175**:382–7
25. Tutschek, B., Sherlock, J., Halder, A., Delhanty, J., Rodeck, C., Adinolfi, M. Isolation of fetal cells from transcervical samples by micromanipulation: molecular confirmation of their fetal origin and diagnosis of fetal aneuploidy. *Prenat Diagn* 1995;**15**:951–60
26. Ishai, D., Diukman, R., Cogan, O., Lichtenstein, Z., Abramovici, H., Fejgin, M.D. Uterine cavity lavage: adding FISH to conventional cytogenetics for embryonic sexing and diagnosing common chromosomal aberrations. *Prenat Diagn* 1995;**15**:961–5
27. Briggs, J., Miller, D., Bulmer, J.N., Griffith, J.M., Rame, V., Lilford, R. Non-syncytial sources of fetal DNA in transcervically recovered cell populations. *Hum Reprod* 1995;**10**:749–54
28. Douglas, G.W., Thomas, L., Carr, M., Cullen, N.M., Morris R. Trophoblasts in the circulating blood during pregnancy. *Am J Obstet Gynecol* 1959;**58**:960–73
29. Attwood, H.D., Park, W.W. Embolism to the lungs by trophoblast. *J Obstet Gynaecol Br Cwlth* 1960;**68**:611–17
30. Walknowska, J., Conte, F.A., Grumbach, M.M. Practical and theoretical implications of fetal-maternal lymphocyte transfer. *Lancet* 1969;**i**:1119–22
31. Schröder, J., De la Chapelle, A. Fetal lymphocytes in the maternal blood. *Blood* 1972;**39**:153–62
32. Grosset, L., Barrelet, V., Odartchenko, N. Antenatal fetal sex determination from maternal blood during early pregnancy. *Am J Obstet Gynecol* 1974;**120**:60–3
33. Schröder, J., Tilikainen, A., Chapelle, A.D.L. Fetal leucocytes in the maternal circulation after delivery. *Transplantation* 1974;**17**:346–54
34. Lo, Y.M.D., Wainscoat, J.S., Gillmer, M.D.G., Patel, P., Sampietro, M., Fleming, K.A. Prenatal sex determination by DNA amplification from maternal peripheral blood. *Lancet* 1989;**334**:1363–5
35. Lo, Y.M., Patel, P., Sampietro, M., Gillmer, M.D., Fleming, K.A., Wainscoat, J.S. Detection of single-copy fetal DNA sequence from maternal blood. *Lancet* 1990;**335**:1463–4
36. Mueller, U.W., Hawes, C.S., Wright, A.E., Petropoulos, A., DeBoni, E., Firgaira, F.A. et al. Isolation of fetal trophoblast cells from peripheral blood of pregnant women. *Lancet* 1990;**336**:197–200
37. Simpson, J.L., Elias, S. Isolating fetal cells in maternal circulation for prenatal diagnosis. *Prenat Diagn* 1994;**14**:1229–42
38. Thomas, M.R., Tutschek, B., Frost, A., Rodeck, C.H., Yazdani, N., Craft, I. et al. The time of appearance and disappearance of fetal DNA from the maternal circulation. *Prenat Diagn* 1995;**15**:641–6
39. Overton, T.G. *Minimally Invasive Prenatal Diagnosis.* MD Thesis, University of London; 1998
40. Al-Mufti, R., Howard, C., Overton, T., Hulzgreve, W., Gaenshirt, D., Fisk, N.N. et al. Detection of fetal messenger ribonucleic acid in maternal blood to determine fetal RhD status as a strategy for noninvasive prenatal diagnosis. *Am J Obstet Gynecol* 1998;**179**:210–14

41 Hamlington, J., Cunningham, J., Mason, G., Mueller, R., Miller, D. Prenatal detection of rhesus D genotype. *Lancet* 1997;**349**:540

42 Daryani, Y., Penna, L.K., Patton, M.A. Detection of cells of fetal origin from transcervical irrigations. *Prenat Diagn* 1997;**17**:243–8

43 Bulmer, J.N., Rodeck, C., Adinolfi, M. Immunohistochemical characterisation of cells retrieved by transcervical sampling in early pregnancy. *Prenat Diagn* 1995;**15**:1143–53

44 Sherlock, J., Halder, A., Tutschek, B., Delhanty, J., Rodeck, C., Adinolfi, M. Prenatal detection of fetal aneuploidies using transcervical cells. *J Med Genet* 1997;**34**:302–5

45 Adinolfi, M., el-Hashemite, N., Sherlock, J., Ward, R.H., Petrou, M., Rodeck, C. Prenatal detection of Hb mutations using transcervical cells. *Prenat Diagn* 1997;**17**:539–43

46 Cirigliano, V., Sherlock, J., Petrou, M., Ward, R.H., Rodeck, C., Adinolfi, M. Transcervical cells and the prenatal diagnosis of haemoglobin (Hb) mutations. *Clin Genet* 1999;**56**:357–61

47 Slunga-Tallberg, A., El-Rifai, W., Keinnen, N., Ylinen, K., Kurki, T., Klinger, K. et al. Maternal origin of nucleated erythrocytes in peripheral venous blood of pregnant women. *Hum Genet* 1995;**96**:53–7

48 DeMaria, M.A., Zheng, Y.L., Zhen, D., Weinschenk, N.M., Vadnais, T.J., Bianchi, D.W. Improved fetal nucleated erythrocyte sorting purity using intracellular antifetal hemoglobin and Hoechst 33342. *Cytometry* 1996;**25**:37–45

49 Sant, R.A. *The Use of Anti-fetal Haemoglobin Antibodies for the Enrichment of Fetal Cells from the Maternal Circulation*. PhD Thesis, Universität Basel; 1996

50 Hengstschlager, M., Bernaschek, G. Fetal cells in the peripheral blood of pregnant women express thymidine kinase: a new marker for detection. *FEBS Lett* 1997;**404**:299–302

51 Campagnoli, C., Fisk, N., Overton, T., Bennett, P., Watts, T., Roberts, I. Circulating hematopoietic progenitor cells in first trimester fetal blood. *Blood* 2000;**95**:1967–72

52 Zauli, G., Valvassori, L., Capitani, S. Presence and characteristics of megakaryocyte progenitor cells in human fetal blood. *Blood* 1993;**81**:385–90

53 Zauli, G., Vitale, M., Visani, G., Marchisio, M., Milani, D., Capitani, S. *In vitro* growth of human fetal CD34+ cells in the presence of various combinations of recombinant cytokines under serum-free culture conditions. *Br J Haematol* 1994;**86**:461–7

54 Migliaccio, G., Baiocchi, M., Hamel, N., Eddleman, K., Migliaccio, A. Circulating progenitor cell in human ontogenesis; response to growth factors and replating potential. *J Hematother* 1996;**5**:161–70

55 Valerio, D., Aiello, R., Altieri, V., Malato, A.P., Fortunato, A., Canazio, A. Culture of fetal erythroid progenitor cells from maternal blood for non-invasive prenatal genetic diagnosis. *Prenat Diagn* 1996;**16**:1073–82

56 Little, M.T., Langlois, S., Wilson, R.D., Lansdorp, P.M. Frequency of fetal cells in sorted subpopulations of nucleated erythroid and CD34+ hematopoietic progenitor cells from maternal peripheral blood. *Blood* 1997;**89**:2347–58

57 Valerio, D., Aiello, R., Altieri, V. Isolation of fetal erythroid cells from maternal blood based on expression of erythropoietin receptors. *Mol Hum Reprod* 1997;**3**:451–5

58 Goldberg, J.D. Fetal cells in maternal circulation: progress in analysis of rare event. *Am J Med Genet* 1997;**61**:806–9

30

Shoulder dystocia

Eric Watson and Khaldoun Sharif

Shoulder dystocia is an obstetrician's nightmare, usually occurring unexpectedly, its resolution necessitating immediate action. There can be serious consequences for the mother, a fatal outcome for the fetus and, in this increasingly litigious age, significant repercussions for the *accoucheur*.

Shoulder dystocia occurs when the fetal shoulders impact at the pelvic inlet following delivery of the head, although strictly the term describes any difficulty in delivery of the shoulders. As this can obviously cover a wide range of 'difficulties', the decision as to whether or not shoulder dystocia has occurred is usually made subjectively by the *accoucheur* and, unfortunately, there is no standard accepted definition to help guide this decision.

The definition now most widely used in the literature specifies that shoulder dystocia has occurred when delivery of the shoulders requires special manoeuvres in addition to the standard technique of backward traction on the fetal head. This has been termed 'true' shoulder dystocia.[1,2] While this adds some objectivity to the definition, it relies upon the actions of the *accoucheur* as the defining point rather than what has happened to the fetal shoulders. It is easy to envisage two cases where the shoulders impact at the pelvic inlet, one where 'special manoeuvres' are employed to enable delivery, and the other where they are not: mechanically, both are shoulder dystocias, but only the former would be considered as 'true'.

Other definitions have been proposed which include: difficulty delivering the shoulders with the contraction subsequent to that which delivered the head;[3] prolonged head-to-body delivery interval[4] and grades of severity based upon the interventions required.[5]

INCIDENCE

The incidence of shoulder dystocia reported in the literature varies from at least 0.23% up to 2.1%.[2,6] The lack of consistency in defining the problem is partly responsible for this variation in reported incidence, as well as for differences in reports of its sequelae. Unfortunately, the situation is further confused by the use of differently defined populations as denominator in the incidence calculations: all births, all vaginal births, all vaginal births over a certain weight, and so on.

MECHANISM OF NORMAL DELIVERY AND SHOULDER DYSTOCIA

Recalling the mechanism of normal delivery is the key to understanding what occurs during shoulder dystocia. It is important to remember that, although the bisacromial diameter of a normally grown term fetus is larger than the biparietal diameter, the shoulders are mobile and compressible and the pelvic inlet is normally wider in the oblique diameter than the anteroposterior.

During labour, uterine contractions lead to flexion and engagement of the fetal head, if this has not preceded the onset of labour. The head enters the pelvic inlet in the occipitotransverse position, with the shoulders lying anteroposterior at this stage. Internal rotation of the head to the occipitoanterior position occurs as it reaches the level of the ischial spines, while the shoulders rotate to the oblique position. The fetal head then passes beneath the pubic symphysis, extending as it comes through the pelvic outlet and escapes the vaginal canal. As the head leaves the pelvis, the shoulders pass through the pelvic inlet in the oblique position. The posterior shoulder enters first, coming to rest in the sacral hollow or over the sacrosciatic notch, while the anterior shoulder follows it to lie over the obturator foramen. As further descent occurs, the anterior shoulder emerges from under the pubic ramus and the shoulder girdle rotates to allow delivery in the anterioposterior position, which is usually assisted by lateral flexion of the fetal body.

It is important to appreciate that, in shoulder dystocia, the point of obstruction occurs at the inlet of the pelvis. There is a relative disproportion between the fetal shoulders and the pelvic inlet, often due to a lack of rotation from the anterioposterior position, which prevents the shoulders from following the head into the pelvis. In view of the compressibility of the shoulders, this is only likely to happen if the bisacromial diameter is substantially larger than the diameter of the fetal head. Usually, the posterior shoulder enters the pelvis but the anterior shoulder, having failed to rotate to the oblique position, remains trapped behind the symphysis pubis. In more severe cases, both shoulders become impacted above the pelvic inlet, either in the unfavourable anterioposterior position or, sometimes, despite rotating to the more favourable oblique position. Once the shoulders impact at the pelvic inlet, the fetal head, which has already left the pelvis, often recoils tightly against the maternal perineum. This is termed the 'turtle sign' and may be the first indication that a shoulder dystocia is occurring.

FACTORS ASSOCIATED WITH SHOULDER DYSTOCIA

A number of antenatal and intrapartum factors are traditionally associated with the occurrence of shoulder dystocia. These have generally been identified using retrospective case analysis. Fetal macrosomia is the most important of these, which is logical when one considers the mechanism of shoulder dystocia. It is probable that the other antenatal 'risk factors' owe their association to a predisposition to the development of fetal macrosomia, while the intrapartum factors simply reflect the problem of the uterine powers being unable to propel a disproportionately large fetus down an inadequate passage.

Fetal macrosomia

Macrosomia is variously and arbitrarily defined as an actual birth weight of 4000 g or more, 4500 g or more, or more than the 90th centile for gestational age.[7,8] As birth weight increases so does the occurrence of shoulder dystocia; while only approximately 10% of infants have a birth weight of 4000 g or more,[9-11] up to 60% of cases of shoulder dystocia are seen in this group.[10,12,13] The incidence in the 4000–4499-g group is reported to be between 2% and 10%, rising to between 6% and 36% above 4500 g.[6,7,12,14-18] Macrosomia is also associated with an increased risk of fatal outcome; 75% of cases in the Confidential Enquiry into Stillbirths and Deaths in Infancy (CESDI) report weighed more than 4 kg compared with only 11% of the normal population.[19]

In strict terms, macrosomia describes disproportion between the fetal body and head, rather than absolute birth weight. It is logical that, irrespective of its weight, delivery of the shoulders of a fetus is more likely to occur if they are in proportion to the head than if they are enlarged relative to the head. Indeed, it has been shown that neonates who experienced shoulder dystocia have significantly greater shoulder-to-head disproportion than those of equivalent weight delivered without problem.[9] While this disproportion is probably more pronounced in larger infants, it can obviously occur at any weight, which explains why, despite a much lower overall incidence, approximately half of all shoulder dystocias occur during the delivery of infants weighing less than 4000 g.[18,20]

Maternal diabetes

The association between maternal diabetes and shoulder dystocia has long been recognised, with an incidence as high as 31% in vaginally delivered women with diabetes found in one study.[6] The infants of these women are theoretically at particular risk because the differences between their shoulder and head sizes are significant when compared with infants of similar weight resulting from pregnancies in women without diabetes;[9] this increased risk has been observed clinically.[6,12,17]

Maternal obesity

Obese mothers have an increased incidence of shoulder dystocia; a rate of 5.1% in women weighing 113.6 kg or more compared with 0.6% in women weighing less than 91 kg was reported by Johnson et al.[21] Those women who gain weight excessively during pregnancy also seem to be at risk.[11,22] The CESDI review of fatal shoulder dystocia[19] found that the mothers of cases were much more likely to be obese or very obese than the general population (42% compared with 10%) although the predictive value of maternal obesity was low. The association is probably because obesity has a positive influence on fetal weight itself, as well as predisposing to the development of gestational diabetes. Obese women also have a tendency towards prolonged pregnancy, which is again a reported factor,[11,13,15] although possibly only if the fetus is macrosomic.[6,12]

Maternal age and parity

While both maternal age and parity have been described as risk factors,[11,14] this would seem to be linked to increasing birth weights.[17]

Previous shoulder dystocia and macrosomia

A history of previous shoulder dystocia is often accorded great significance clinically as it seems logical that whatever factors acted to cause it previously are likely to act again. (Presumably for similar reasons an association with previous infants weighing more than 4000 g is also described.[20,23]) In fact, recurrent problems are not as common as might be expected, with rates of between 1% and 13% found in the literature.[15,24,25] These low recurrence rates may be in part due to those women who previously had severe dystocia subsequently having an elective caesarean section.

Male sex

As approximately 65% of macrosomic infants are male,[7,11,16,26,27] it is not surprising that male infants have also been noted to be more prone to shoulder dystocia.[28]

Prolonged pregnancy and induction of labour

Post-term pregnancy has been associated with shoulder dystocia,[6,29] although again this does not persist if allowance is made for macrosomia. The need for induction of labour has been noted,[12,28,30] although McFarland et al.[31] suggested that the association of induction may result from the cases in which it is used rather than anything inherent in induction itself.

Intrapartum delay

Slow progress during the first stage of labour, especially the decelerative phase, and prolonged second stage, leading to instrumental delivery, has been reported as strongly associated with shoulder dystocia, as has the resultant need for labour augmentation.[12,13,15,18,28,30,32] These associations tend to be much stronger with increasing fetal weight.[6,10,20,32] However, McFarland et al.[31] found no differences in labour abnormalities between pregnancies in which shoulder dystocia occurred and controls, although the study confirmed a higher rate of operative vaginal delivery. There is some evidence that the ventouse vacuum extractor may be associated with more problems than forceps.[28,32,33] The use of epidural anaesthesia has also been associated with shoulder dystocia in some reports.[13,30]

It is possible that delayed labour or abnormalities of labour indicate a 'protective' mechanism against fetopelvic disproportion.[34] If this is the case, the use of augmentation and induction are probably not factors contributing to the dystocia but simply indicate that there is an underlying problem. It is similarly difficult to envisage a mechanism by which epidural anaesthesia would cause impaction of the shoulders at the pelvic brim. An increased need for analgesia may conceivably result from prolonged labour and increased activity by a uterus trying to overcome resistance to the passage of a macrosomic fetus.

PREDICTION AND PREVENTION OF SHOULDER DYSTOCIA

It has been suggested that if factors associated with shoulder dystocia can be identified, those pregnancies in which it will occur can be predicted and subsequently managed to prevent the problem.[5,6,10,12,35] This assumes that:

(1) The factors are identifiable;

(2) They reliably predict the occurrence of shoulder dystocia;

(3) Interventions exist which will prevent shoulder dystocia;

(4) Preventing shoulder dystocia is advantageous.

As has already been discussed the factor most significantly associated with shoulder dystocia is macrosomia. Other factors either simply predispose to its development or are probably relevant only when it is present. Much research has, therefore, focused on the detection of fetuses weighing over 4000 g. The clinical estimation of fetal weight is unreliable[26] and, therefore, ultrasound biometry has been used to estimate both fetal weight and shoulder-to-head ratio in the belief that this should be more accurate. Unfortunately, at present the ultrasound detection of macrosomia is dependent on initial clinical suspicion of macrosomia. The option of performing biometry on all fetuses late in pregnancy might improve the detection rate for macrosomia but obviously has service implications. In practice, ultrasound diagnosis of macrosomia has not proved reliable, with high false-positive and false-negative rates reported[36-38] and average errors in estimating fetal weight of 15% or more of birth weight.[38,39] It has been found that clinical estimation of macrosomia is probably as accurate[40] and it is particularly sobering to note that maternal estimates of fetal weight are as reliable as clinical methods and more accurate than ultrasound.[41]

Even if fetuses weighing more than 4000 g could be accurately and reliably detected, this would not necessarily be of much help in the prediction of shoulder dystocia. As has already been discussed, around half of deliveries complicated by shoulder dystocia result in infants weighing less than 4000 g and the vast majority of macrosomic fetuses are delivered without problems.

An alternative approach to the problem has been the attempt to identify fetuses with shoulder-to-head disproportion using different surrogate ultrasound measurements, which, logically, should be more successful at predicting shoulder dystocia. Measuring humerospinous distance was not found to be useful[42] and bisacromial diameter would be a poor predictor of shoulder dystocia even if it could be measured reliably.[43] Cohen et al.[44,45] looked at the difference between the abdominal diameter and biparietal diameter in diabetics and this approach has shown some promise. Unfortunately, using such methods clinically would again entail performing late ultrasonography on the entire pregnant population.

It is generally accepted that, at present, the ability to predict shoulder dystocia is limited because, while factors may be present significantly in those pregnancies where the problem occurs, many more pregnancies will have these factors without the occurrence of shoulder dystocia.[6,18,20,46,47] For instance, Menticoglou et al.[35] reported that 75% of infants weighing 4500 g or more delivered vaginally with a dystocia rate of only 9.2%. In addition to this, many pregnancies complicated by shoulder dystocia will have had none of the associated factors.[6,15,48] Gross et al.[18] found that a birthweight greater than 4000 g plus prolonged second stage of labour retrospectively only predicted 16% of cases with trauma. They concluded that there is a major difference between a factor being statistically significant and its clinical use.

The preventative intervention most commonly advocated is caesarean section for macrosomia, especially if combined with labour abnormalities. This is proposed on the basis that abdominal delivery of every fetus weighing over a certain weight, or found to have disproportionately large shoulders, would greatly reduce the rate of shoulder dystocia.[5,7,9,16,17,32] This implies performing between 25 and 36 operations for fetuses weighing 4000 g or more in order to prevent one case of shoulder dystocia[37,46] and between nine and 12 for those weighing over 4500 g.[15,20,35] In practice, the overestimation of fetal weight would mean that many more operations would need to be performed to prevent a single case.[18] The use of caesarean section instead of midcavity forceps has also been suggested. Baskett and Allen[15] calculated that 35 abdominal deliveries would be required in order to prevent one shoulder dystocia associated with forceps.

The theory behind the abdominal delivery of any pregnancy, in which it has been predicted that shoulder dystocia will occur, is prevention of fetal injury. The number of caesarean sections that would be needed to prevent such injury is obviously even higher. Baskett and Allen[15] calculated that on fetal weight grounds, 54 operations would be needed to prevent one brachial palsy from occurring, while Sandmire and O'Halloin[49] estimated that this would rise to 978 in order to prevent a permanent palsy. It should be remembered that birth injuries could still occur, especially in macrosomic infants, despite delivery by caesarean section,[16,26] and increasing the caesarean rate for macrosomic infants has been shown not to improve the overall outcome.[11,50] It can therefore be argued that performing 'preventative' caesarean sections on the basis of fetal size is illogical in view of the low incidence of permanent injuries associated with shoulder dystocia.

Alternatively, the elective induction of labour has been proposed, with the aim of preventing further fetal growth and the risk of disproportion developing.[21,51] This has not been shown to reduce the fetal weight notably and as it is advised in cases already found to be 'macrosomic', it is likely to have little effect on the incidence of shoulder dystocia. In retrospective studies[52] of elective induction for macrosomia, the rate of dystocia was the same but the rate of caesarean sections increased. A single, prospective study[53] again showed no change in shoulder dystocia, but no difference in caesarean rate. As induction of labour itself is possibly a factor in some cases of shoulder dystocia, it may be that one problem is simply being exchanged for another.

Despite the evidence, once macrosomia has been detected there does seem to be a tendency to interfere with the pregnancy and labour. Several investigators have noted that, compared with non-identified macrosomia, there is an increased rate of induction and caesarean section in detected cases.[38,51,54]

In conclusion, the ability to predict and prevent shoulder dystocia is poor and the need for prevention is questionable. As most cases occur without warning and can be overcome without permanent fetal injury it is probably more appropriate to be able to manage the problem once it occurs than to attempt to predict it. If associated factors are noted, the possibility of shoulder dystocia should be clearly documented.[19] The literature suggests that uneventful vaginal delivery will be the most likely outcome in this situation and the pregnancy should be managed normally, with the exception that the most experienced staff available should be present at the time of delivery.

MANAGEMENT OF SHOULDER DYSTOCIA

The problem in shoulder dystocia is the failure of the fetal shoulders to enter the pelvic inlet. Manoeuvres to overcome shoulder dystocia should be performed with the intention of increasing the relative pelvic space, altering pelvic angles, reducing the bisacromial diameter or rotating the fetal shoulders. When the mechanics of shoulder delivery are considered there is no logic in continued traction on the fetal neck or applying fundal pressure, but there is potential danger to the fetus.

Summon assistance

Prior to embarking upon any manoeuvres to resolve the dystocia, the most experienced midwife and obstetrician available should be immediately summoned, together with paediatric and anaesthetic assistance. In many of the fatal cases reported by CESDI there was considerable delay in the arrival of such staff.[19]

Left lateral position

Positioning the patient in the left lateral position is frequently the first manoeuvre employed by midwives when shoulder dystocia occurs; it is often used when difficulties have been anticipated. It is probable that the position simply gives better access for traction posteriorly on the fetus, allowing mild degrees of dystocia to be overcome. The advantage is that the patient can be transferred to the position rapidly with minimal assistance while summoning help to perform more complicated manoeuvres if they are required.

McRoberts' manoeuvre

More significant degrees of dystocia will probably not deliver in the left lateral and therefore most authorities now recommend immediate use of the 'McRoberts' manoeuvre' to position the patient.[55] The patient lies in the supine position and her hips are flexed so that her thighs lie against the sides of her abdomen. This straightens the sacrum relative to the lumbar spine and rotates the symphysis pubis towards the patient's head, thereby reducing the angle of inclination of the pelvic inlet when compared with the lithotomy position. It has no effect upon the dimensions of the pelvis but the rotation of the symphysis pubis encourages the anterior shoulder to disimpact and pass under it. Maximum benefit comes from this manoeuvre if two assistants are used, one holding each maternal leg to produce hyperflexion of the hips. Gonik et al.[56] have shown that using this manoeuvre reduces the force required for fetal extraction and thus reduces stretching of the brachial plexus.

All-fours position

Popularised by Bruner et al.[57] the all-fours manoeuvre consists of moving the patient to her hands and knees. The exact mechanism whereby the dystocia is relieved is not clear, although both altered gravitational effect and increased pelvic diameters are proposed. Good results are claimed, with minimal morbidity for both mother and neonate, and most of the other manoeuvres are said to be possible in the all-fours position. While it would appear that moving the labouring woman to this position would be difficult, especially with epidural anaesthesia in place, its proponents claim otherwise, so it would certainly be worth attempting this manoeuvre in view of its apparent efficacy.

Suprapubic pressure

In order to dislodge the anterior shoulder from its place of impaction behind the symphysis pubis, suprapubic pressure can be applied by an assistant using a modification of the technique of 'rocking' the fetal shoulders described by Rubin.[58] Firm pressure is applied to the posterior aspect of the anterior shoulder through the maternal abdominal wall, in order to encourage rotation of the shoulder girdle to the oblique position and the anterior shoulder to slip under the symphysis. This technique will also tend to adduct the shoulders, thereby reducing the bisacromial diameter, which again aids delivery.

Episiotomy

The use of a generous episiotomy is usually recommended in the literature, both when shoulder dystocia is anticipated and when it has occurred. It should, however, be appreciated that as the obstruction to shoulder delivery is at the pelvic inlet, rather than the soft tissues of the perineum, episiotomy itself does not overcome shoulder dystocia.[7] The role of episiotomy is to allow access to the pelvic cavity by the accoucheur to facilitate intravaginal manipulations rather than to aid delivery of the shoulders. On this basis, it has been suggested that a shoulder dystocia that can be resolved by external manoeuvres probably does not require an episiotomy.[59] There is no evidence that the type of episiotomy performed is of importance.[48]

Woods' screw manoeuvre

First described in 1942, Woods and Westbury[60] compared the fetal shoulders to a screw and the maternal pelvis to a thread. In order for the screw to pass through the thread the shoulders need to rotate. Direct pulling will not release the fetus. The technique involves pushing on the anterior aspect of the posterior shoulder, thereby rotating it through 180 degrees, which should deliver the posterior shoulder out of the pelvis, and allow the anterior shoulder to enter the pelvis. The shoulder that was formerly anterior will now be lying in the sacral hollow; pushing on the anterior aspect of this and rotating the shoulders back through 180 degrees should deliver this shoulder out of the pelvis also.

One problem with Woods' screw manoeuvre is that the shoulders will tend to abduct thereby increasing the bisacromial diameter, which may be counterproductive.[58] Rubin[58] described an alternative which has come to be known as the 'reverse' Woods' manoeuvre. In this manoeuvre, a hand is inserted into the vagina behind the more easily accessible shoulder, which is usually the posterior, and this is then pushed towards the fetal chest. The intention is two-fold: reduction of the bisacromial diameter by adducting the shoulder, and rotation of the shoulders to the oblique position. Both of these outcomes may result in delivery of the shoulders; if they do not, the rotation of the shoulders can be continued through 180 degrees as before.

Delivery of the posterior arm

This manoeuvre reduces the bisacromial diameter and allows rotation of the shoulders by traction on the arm. This, by relieving the impaction, will allow the anterior shoulder to enter the pelvis.[23] If the fetus is lying with its back to the right, the *accoucheur's* right hand is inserted into the sacral hollow, and *vice versa*. The humerus is identified and followed to the elbow, which is then flexed and swept across the chest. The wrist is then grasped and the arm delivered. Unfortunately, the fetal humerus is often fractured using this technique.

Clavicular fracture and cleidotomy

The aim of these procedures is to reduce the bisacromial diameter. The clavicle often spontaneously fractures when there is shoulder dystocia, or as a result of manoeuvres to overcome it, but can be intentionally broken. Cleidotomy would normally only be employed on a dead fetus.

Cephalic replacement and symphysiotomy

Cephalic replacement is unusual in that, rather than attempting to complete vaginal delivery, the mechanism of normal delivery is reversed to replace the fetal head in the pelvis and the fetus is then delivered by caesarean section.[61,62] It has come to be known eponymously as the Zavanelli manoeuvre, after the obstetrician credited with its initial use.[61] The majority of reports of this technique suggest that the replacement of the head is generally easy, with minimal maternal or fetal trauma, and that once performed there is no great urgency to perform abdominal delivery.[5,61,63-65] There have been reports of difficulty achieving replacement of the head,[66-68] however, and the reported ease of the manoeuvre has been questioned.[68] Logic dictates that serious maternal trauma can be incurred and careful reading of the literature reveals that there is a significant occurrence of maternal complications, such as uterine rupture and lower segment lacerations, associated with the technique.[64]

Theoretically, symphysiotomy is a useful treatment option in severe shoulder dystocia, as it markedly increases pelvic capacity, especially the oblique diameters, possibly by as much as 25%.[63] The technique is also quick and therefore may be lifesaving for the fetus. The woman is placed in the lithotomy position with assistants supporting her legs to control the degree of abduction of the hips (to a maximum of 80 degrees) and restrict the separation of the pubic bones. Local anaesthetic is infiltrated into the symphysis pubis area, a urinary catheter passed so that the urethra can be displaced laterally and the fibrocartilage of the joint divided with a scalpel.[69]

The potential hazard of employing this technique is damage to the lower urinary tract and anterior vaginal wall. It is claimed that the risk of such complications can be minimised by limiting separation of the pubic bones to 2.5 cm and careful backwards displacement of the fetus.[70]

Both of these techniques are probably outside the experience of most obstetricians working in the UK. Cephalic replacement seems to have gained greater acceptance than symphysiotomy, in the literature at least, possibly because the morbidity associated with the former has been understated, while that associated with the latter has been exaggerated. The use of either technique can only be recommended for those cases where all other manoeuvres have failed.

As shoulder dystocia is usually a completely unexpected occurrence, it is important that all professionals involved in intrapartum care have a clear plan of action and are prepared to act promptly if it occurs. As the CESDI findings indicate, time is of the essence, as a relatively brief delay may be associated with poor outcome;[19] the option of waiting for someone else to deal with the problem does not exist. There is no consensus regarding which manoeuvres should be used or in which order to use them. It seems sensible to apply the most simple methods first, moving on to more complex invasive techniques if the shoulder dystocia is not overcome. Whatever manoeuvres are used they should be carried out swiftly in a predetermined and systematic manner, which must then be carefully documented. Morrison et al.[48] estimated that less than 5–10% of shoulder dystocias required 'major' interventions. Gherman et al.[71] found that the McRoberts' manoeuvre alone was successful in 42% of cases. Pearson[72] claimed that the majority of cases would be resolved by placing the patient into the McRoberts' position and applying lateral suprapubic pressure.

MATERNAL CONSEQUENCES

The effects of shoulder dystocia upon the mother are relatively neglected in the literature. Not surprisingly, those investigators who do address this point report a high incidence of soft tissue trauma in the lower genital tract and uterine atony. Rates of postpartum haemorrhage vary from 14.2% to 23%,[28,30] while those of vaginal tears vary from 12.5% to 19.3%.[12,28] The occurrence of uterine rupture following shoulder dystocia is also documented.[12,28] Genitourinary tract infection is another frequent consequence of shoulder dystocia with Johnstone[30] reporting a 27% rate.

The psychological effect of sustaining a shoulder dystocia upon the mother is mentioned[59] and personal experience suggests that it should not be underestimated.

FETAL CONSEQUENCES

Fetal morbidity following shoulder dystocia results from asphyxia and trauma to peripheral nerves or the skeleton. Rates of injury as high as 66% following shoulder dystocia are reported in the literature.[14]

The incidence of brachial plexus palsy varies from 7.9% to 13% after shoulder dystocia.[6,15] These injuries are usually transient, recovering in 80–100% of cases.[7,20,35,48,49] Gherman et al.[73] recently reported a permanent injury rate of 1.6%. The incidence of brachial nerve palsy, and the chances of it being permanent, increase with increasing fetal weight.[15,16,26,74,75]

Skeletal and peripheral nerve injuries, which occur during the process of delivering the impacted fetal shoulders, are frequently unavoidable and even exemplary management using appropriate manoeuvres can result in fetal injury. It follows that the more severe the dystocia and the more manoeuvres that are required to overcome it, the greater the potential for injury.[71]

Unfortunately, some neonatal morbidity associated with shoulder dystocia may result from the use of inappropriate interventions. For instance, strong traction on the fetal head may simply impact the anterior shoulder more firmly against the symphysis pubis, as may fundal pressure, which has been recommended in the past.[76] Gross et al.[2] found that these two manoeuvres were associated with all neonatal neurological and orthopaedic sequelae in their study, and Lipscomb et al.[7] postulated that the low rate of injury in their study was due to the avoidance of these manoeuvres.

It should be noted, however, that many of the injuries seen following shoulder dystocia can also occur following normal vaginal deliveries and even caesarean section.[16,20,29,50,77-82] These may, therefore, be due to factors other than the dystocia. Gherman et al.[73] reviewed the literature regarding brachial plexus injury and concluded that up to 50% may be *in utero* injuries and not traction mediated. Injury to the neonate will be iatrogenic in some cases but this does not automatically imply mismanagement; often it is the choice between 'death of the fetus ... and morbidity from successful delivery'.[48]

Earlier literature mentions neonatal deaths secondary to asphyxia resulting from shoulder dystocia[23] but this has not been a feature of most recent papers. However, CESDI reported on the findings in 56 cases of fatal shoulder dystocia occurring over a two-year period in England, Wales and Northern Ireland.[19] This confirms that, although rare, fatal shoulder dystocia does still occur with an approximate incidence of 0.04 per 1000 deliveries. A notable finding by CESDI was that many of the cases had a relatively short 'head-body delivery interval', being less than five minutes in 47% of those cases where this could be ascertained from the notes. Some of these cases may already have been compromised prior to delivery of the head while, in others, factors such as trauma may have contributed to the adverse outcome. However, this finding does tend to corroborate previously expressed views[83] that there is much less time to effect delivery of the body before severe asphyxia occurs than had been thought previously based upon animal studies and normal births.[84,85]

MEDICO-LEGAL ASPECTS SHOULDER DYSTOCIA

James[86] stated that shoulder dystocia 'is a common source of litigation since parents and their advisers find it difficult to accept that the problem could not have been predicted and circumvented'. Claims can be difficult to repudiate and can result in large awards for damages.[87] This is often due to the excessive significance which is given to associated factors with the benefit of hindsight. Most medical litigation is brought under tort law, which exists to compensate the victims of negligence. In the case of shoulder dystocia, legal action will usually only be initiated if there is a permanent brachial plexus injury to the infant.[73] In order to prove negligence in these cases it is necessary to show that the dystocia was predictable, that its management was not consistent with that of a reasonable body of others in the same circumstance or that injury could have been prevented by another course of action. The unpredictable nature of shoulder dystocia, the lack of consensus over its management and the fact that birth trauma may occur whatever course of action is followed, all should result in difficulty in proving negligence.

The key to minimising medico-legal problems is adequate documentation of decisions and actions, both antenatal and intrapartum. If shoulder dystocia has been anticipated, a plan of action for delivery should be clearly recorded and should be adhered to. When shoulder dystocia occurs, the manoeuvres used, and their order of usage, must be carefully recorded. This is simply standard good practice and while it will not eliminate claims for negligence (obviously decisions have to be logical and actions effective) it will make such claims easier to defend.

CONCLUSION

Shoulder dystocia is a rare but serious mechanical complication of vaginal delivery, which can be traumatic and at worst catastrophic. Certain factors may indicate the possibility of shoulder dystocia occurring but most cases are unanticipated. All midwives and obstetricians should have a logical plan of action for managing the problem when it occurs. Simple manoeuvres will resolve most cases rapidly while minimising the risk of fetal trauma. Unfortunately, injuries can be sustained by the neonate that are occasionally permanent; these often result in medico-legal action. Fatal outcome is rare.

References

1. Resnik, R. Management of shoulder girdle dystocia. *Clin Obstet Gynecol* 1980;**23**:559–64
2. Gross, S.J., Shime, J., Farine, D. Shoulder dystocia: predictors and outcome. *Am J Obstet Gynecol* 1987;**156**:334–6
3. Gibb, D. *A Practical Guide to Labour Management.* Oxford: Blackwell Scientific; 1988
4. Spong, C.Y., Beall, M., Rodrigues, D., Ross, M.G. An objective definition of shoulder dystocia: prolonged head-to-body delivery intervals and/or the use of ancillary obstetric maneuvers. *Obstet Gynecol* 1995;**86**:433–6
5. O'Leary, J.A., Leonetti, H.B. Shoulder dystocia: prevention and treatment. *Am J Obstet Gynecol* 1990;**162**:5–9
6. Acker, D.B., Sachs, B.P., Friedman, E.A. Risk factors for shoulder dystocia. *Obstet Gynecol* 1985;**66**:762–8
7. Lipscomb, K.R., Gregory, K., Shaw, K. The outcome of macrosomic infants weighing at least 4500 grams: Los Angeles County and University of Southern California experience. *Obstet Gynecol* 1995;**85**:558–64
8. Sanderson, D.A., Wilcox, M.A., Johnson, I.R. Relative macrosomia identified by the individualised birth weight ratio (IBR): a better method of identifying the at risk fetus. *Acta Obstet Gynecol Scand* 1994;**73**:246–9
9. Modanlou, H.D., Komatsu, G., Dorchester, W., Freeman, R.K., Bosu, S.K. Large-for-gestational age neonates: anthropometric reasons for shoulder dystocia. *Obstet Gynecol* 1982;**60**:417–23
10. Acker, D.B., Sachs, B.P., Friedman, E.A. Risk factors for shoulder dystocia in the average-weight infant. *Obstet Gynecol* 1986;**67**:614–18
11. Boyd, M.E., Usher, R.H., McLean, F.H. Fetal macrosomia: prediction, risks, proposed management. *Obstet Gynecol* 1983;**61**:715–22
12. Al-Najashi, S., Al-Suleiman, S.A., El-Yahia, A., Rahman, M.S., Rahman, J. Shoulder dystocia: a clinical study of 56 cases. *Aust N Z J Obstet Gynaecol* 1989;**29**:129–32
13. Hopwood, H.G. Jr. Shoulder dystocia: fifteen years' experience in a community hospital. *Am J Obstet Gynecol* 1982;**144**:162–6
14. Hassan, A.A. Shoulder dystocia: risk factors and prevention. *Aust N Z J Obstet Gynaecol* 1988;**28**:107–9
15. Baskett, T.F., Allen, A.C. Perinatal implications of shoulder dystocia. *Obstet Gynecol* 1995;**86**:14–17
16. Spellacy, W.N., Miller, S., Winegar, A., Peterson, P.Q. Macrosomia: maternal characteristics and infant complications. *Obstet Gynecol* 1985;**66**:158–61
17. Langer, O., Berkus, M.D., Huff, R.W., Samueloff, A. Shoulder dystocia: should the fetus weighing >4000 grams be delivered by Cesarean section? *Am J Obstet Gynecol* 1991;**165**:831–7
18. Gross, T.L., Sokol, R.J., Williams, T., Thompson, K. Shoulder dystocia: a fetal-physician risk. *Am J Obstet Gynecol* 1987;**156**:1408–18
19. Hope, P., Breslin, S., Lamont, L. et al. Fatal shoulder dystocia: a review of 56 cases reported to the Confidential Enquiry into Stillbirths and Deaths in Infancy. *Br J Obstet Gynaecol* 1998;**105**:1256–61
20. Nocon, J.J., McKenzie, D.K., Thomas, L.J., Hansell, R.S. Shoulder dystocia: an analysis of risks and obstetric maneuvers. *Am J Obstet Gynecol* 1993;**168**:1732–9

21 Johnson, S.R., Kolberg, B.H., Varner, M.W. Maternal obesity and pregnancy. *Surg Gynecol Obstet* 1987;**164**:431–7
22 Lewis, D.F., Edwards, M.S., Asrat, T., Adair, C.D., Brooks, G., London, S. Can shoulder dystocia be predicted? *J Reprod Med* 1998;**43**:654–8
23 Schwartz, B.C., Dixon, D.M. Shoulder dystocia. *Obstet Gynecol* 1958;**11**:468-71
24 Lewis, D.F., Raymond, R.C., Perkins, M.B., Brooks, G.G., Heymann, A.R. Recurrence rate of shoulder dystocia. *Am J Obstet Gynecol* 1995;**172**:1369–71
25 Smith, R.B., Lane, C., Pearson, J.F. Shoulder dystocia: what happens at the next delivery? *Br J Obstet Gynaecol* 1994;**101**:713–15
26 ACOG. Fetal macrosomia: Technical bulletin number 159: September 1991. *Int J Gynaecol Obstet* 1992;**39**:341–5
27 Parks, D.G., Ziel, H.K. Macrosomia: a proposed indication for primary cesarean section. *Obstet Gynecol* 1978;**52**:407–9
28 El Madany, A.A., Jallad, K.B., Radi, F.A., El Hamdan, H., O'deh, H.M. Shoulder dystocia: anticipation and outcome. *Int J Gynaecol Obstet* 1990;**34**:7–12
29 Jennett, R.J., Tarby, T.J., Kreinick. C.J. Brachial plexus palsy: an old problem revisited. *Am J Obstet Gynecol* 1992;**166**:1673–7
30 Johnstone, N.R. Shoulder dystocia: a study of 47 cases. *Aust N Z J Obstet Gynaecol* 1979;**19**:28–31
31 McFarland, M., Hod, M., Piper, J.M., Xenakis, E.M., Langer, O. Are labor abnormalities more common in shoulder dystocia? *Am J Obstet Gynecol* 1995;**173**:1211–14
32 Benedetti, T.J., Gabbe, S.G. Shoulder dystocia: a complication of fetal macrosomia and prolonged second stage of labour with midpelvic delivery. *Obstet Gynecol* 1978;**52**:526–9
33 Bofill, J.A., Rust, O.A., Devidas, M., Roberts, W.E., Morrison, J.C., Martin, J.N. Shoulder dystocia and operative vaginal delivery. *J Matern Fetal Med* 1997;**6**:220–4
34 Hernandez, C., Wendel, G.D. Shoulder dystocia. *Clin Obstet Gynecol* 1990;**33**:526–34
35 Menticoglou, S.M., Manning, F.A., Morrison, I., Harman, C.R. Must macrosomic fetuses be delivered by a caesarean section? A review of outcome for 786 babies (4500 g. *Aust N Z J Obstet Gynaecol* 1992; **2**:100–3
36 Pollack, R.N., Hauer-Pollack, G., Divon, M.Y. Macrosomia in post dates pregnancies: the accuracy of routine ultrasonographic screening. *Am J Obstet Gynecol* 1992;**167**:7–11
37 Delpapa, E.H., Mueller-Heubach, E. Pregnancy outcome following ultrasound diagnosis of macrosomia. *Obstet Gynecol* 1991;**78**:340–3
38 Levine, A.B., Lockwood, C.J., Brown, B., Lapinski, R., Berkowitz, R.L. Sonographic diagnosis of the large for gestational age fetus at term: does it make a difference? *Obstet Gynecol* 1992;**79**:55–8
39 Hadlock, F.P., Harrist, R.B., Fearneyhough, T.C., Deter, R.L., Park, S.K., Rossavik, I.K. Use of femur length/abdominal circumference ratio in detecting the macrosomic fetus. *Radiology* 1985;**154**:503–5
40 Johnstone, F.D., Prescott, R.J., Steel, J.M., Mao, J.H., Chambers, S., Muir, N. Clinical and ultrasound prediction of macrosomia in diabetic pregnancy. *Br J Obstet Gynaecol* 1996;**103**:747–54
41 Chauhan, S.P., Lutton, P.M., Bailey, K.J., Guerrierri, J.P., Morrison, J.C. Intrapartum clinical, sonographic, and parous patients' estimates of newborn birth weight. *Obstet Gynecol* 1992;**79**:956–8
42 Klaij, F.A.V., Geirsson, R.T., Nielsen, H., Hreinsdóttir, M., Haraldsdóttir, K.R. Humerospinous distance measurements: accuracy and usefulness for predicting shoulder dystocia in delivery at term. *Ultrasound Obstet Gynecol* 1998;**12**:115–19

43 Verspyck, E., Goffinet, F., Hellot, M.F., Milliez, J., Marpeau, L. Newborn shoulder width: a prospective study of 2222 consecutive measurements. *Br J Obstet Gynaecol* 1999;**106**:589–93

44 Cohen, B., Penning, S., Major, C., Ansley, D., Porto, M., Garite, T. Sonographic prediction of shoulder dystocia in infants of diabetic mothers. *Obstet Gynecol* 1996;**88**:10–13

45 Cohen, B.F., Penning, S., Ansley, D., Porto, M., Garite, T. The incidence and severity of shoulder dystocia correlates with a sonographic measurement of asymmetry in patients with diabetes. *Am J Perinatol* 1999;**16**:197–201

46 Geary, M., McParland, P., Johnson, H., Stronge, J. Shoulder dystocia: is it predictable? *Eur J Obstet Gynecol Reprod Biol* 1995;**62**:15–18

47 Naef, R.W., Martin, J.N. Emergent management of shoulder dystocia. *Obstet Gynecol Clin North Am* 1995;**22**:247–59

48 Morrison, J.C., Sanders, J.R., Magann, E.F., Wiser, W.L. The diagnosis and management of dystocia of the shoulder. *Surg Gynecol Obstet* 1992;**175**:515–22

49 Sandmire, H.F., O'Halloin, T.J. Shoulder dystocia: its incidence and associated risk factors. *Int J Gynaecol Obstet* 1988;**26**:65–73

50 Graham, E.M., Forouzan, I., Morgan, M.A. A retrospective analysis of Erb's palsy cases and their relation to birth weight and trauma at delivery. *J Matern Fetal Med* 1997;**6**:1–5

51 Combs, C.A., Singh, N.B., Khoury, J.C. Elective induction versus spontaneous labor after sonographic diagnosis of fetal macrosomia. *Obstet Gynecol* 1993;**81**:492–6

52 Leaphart, W.L., Meyer, M.C., Capeless, E.L. Labor induction with a prenatal diagnosis of fetal macrosomia. *J Matern Fetal Med* 1997;**6**:99–102

53 Gonen, O., Rosen, D.J.D., Dolfin, Z., Tepper, R., Markov, S., Fejgin, M.D. Induction of labor versus expectant management in macrosomia: a randomised study. *Obstet Gynecol* 1997;**89**:913–17

54 Weeks, J.W., Pitman, T., Spinnato, J.A. Fetal macrosomia: does antenatal prediction affect delivery route and birth outcome? *Am J Obstet Gynecol* 1995;**173**:1215–19

55 Gonik, B., Stringer, C.A., Held, B. An alternate maneuver for management of shoulder dystocia. *Am J Obstet Gynecol* 1983;**145**:882–4

56 Gonik, B., Allen, R., Sorab, J. Objective evaluation of the shoulder dystocia phenomenon: effect of maternal pelvic orientation on force reduction. *Obstet Gynecol* 1989;**74**:44–7

57 Bruner, J.P., Drummond, S.B., Meenan, A.L., Gaskin, I.M. All-fours maneuver for reducing shoulder dystocia during labour. *J Reprod Med* 1998;**43**:439–43

58 Rubin, A. Management of shoulder dystocia. *JAMA* 1964;**189**:835–37

59 Piper, D.M., McDonald, P. Management of anticipated and actual shoulder dystocia: interpreting the literature. *J Nurse Midwifery* 1994;**39**:91–105S

60 Woods, C.E., Westbury, N.Y. A principle of physics as applicable to shoulder delivery. *Am J Obstet Gynecol* 1943;**45**:796–804

61 Sandberg, E.C. The Zavanelli maneuver: a potentially revolutionary method for the resolution of shoulder dystocia. *Am J Obstet Gynecol* 1985;**152**:479–84

62 O'Leary, J.A., Gunn, D. Cephalic replacement for shoulder dystocia. *Am J Obstet Gynecol* 1985;**153**:592

63 Sandberg, E.C. The Zavanelli maneuver extended: progression of a revolutionary concept. *Am J Obstet Gynecol* 1988;**158**:1347–53

64 O'Leary, J.A. Cephalic replacement for shoulder dystocia: present status and future role of the Zavanelli maneuver. *Obstet Gynecol* 1993;**82**:847–50

65 Sandberg, E.C. The Zavanelli maneuver: 12 years of recorded experience. *Obstet Gynecol* 1999;**93**:312–17

66 O'Leary, J.A., Cuva, A. Abdominal rescue after failed cephalic replacement. *Obstet Gynecol* 1992;**80**:514–16

67 Dimitry, E.S. Cephalic replacement: a desperate solution for shoulder dystocia. *J Obstet Gynaecol* 1989;**10**:49–50
68 Graham, J.M., Blanco, J.D., Wen, T., Magee, K.P. The Zavanelli maneuver: a different perspective. *Obstet Gynecol* 1992;**79**:883–4
69 van Roosmalen, J. Symphysiotomy: a reappraisal for the developing world. In: Studd, J. (Ed.) *Progress in Obstetrics and Gynaecology* **9**. Edinburgh: Churchill Livingstone; 1991
70 Hartfield, V.J. Symphysiotomy for shoulder dystocia. *Am J Obstet Gynecol* 1986;**155**:228
71 Gherman, R.B., Goodwin, T.M., Souter, I., Neumann, K., Ouzounian, J.G., Paul, R.H. The McRoberts' maneuver for the alleviation of shoulder dystocia: how successful is it? *Am J Obstet Gynecol* 1997;**176**:656–61
72 Pearson, J.F. Shoulder dystocia. *Current Obstetrics and Gynaecology* 1996;**6**:30–4
73 Gherman, R.B., Ouzounian, J.G., Goodwin, T.M. Brachial plexus palsy: an *in utero* injury? *Am J Obstet Gynecol* 1999;**180**:1303–7
74 Ecker, J.L., Greenberg, J.A., Norwitz, E.R., Nadel, A.S., Repke, J.T. Birth weight as a predictor of brachial plexus injury. *Obstet Gynecol* 1997;**89**:643–7
75 Gilbert, W.M., Nesbitt, T.S., Danielsen, B. Associated factors in 1611 cases of brachial plexus injury *Obstet Gynecol* 1999;**93**:536–40
76 Hibbard, L.T. Shoulder dystocia. *Obstet Gynecol* 1969;**34**:424–9
77 Roberts, S.W., Hernandez, C., Maberry, M.C., Adams, M.D., Leveno, K.J., Wendel, G.D. Obstetric clavicular fracture: the enigma of normal birth. *Obstet Gynecol* 1995;**86**:978–81
78 Chez, R.A., Carlan, S., Greenberg, S.L., Spellacy, W.N. Fractured clavicle is an unavoidable event. *Am J Obstet Gynecol* 1994;**171**:797–8
79 Acker, D.B., Gregory, K.D., Sachs, B.P., Friedman, E.A. Risk factors for Erb-Duchenne palsy. *Obstet Gynecol* 1988;**71**:389–92
80 Jennett. R.J., Tarby, T.J. Brachial plexus palsy: an old problem revisited again. *Am J Obstet Gynecol* 1997;**176**:1354–7
81 Gherman, R.B., Goodwin, T.M., Ouzounian, J.G., Miller, D.A., Paul, R.H. Brachial plexus palsy associated with cesarean section: an *in utero* injury? *Am J Obstet Gynecol* 1997;**177**:1162–4
82 Peleg, D., Hasnin, J., Shalev, E. Fractured clavicle and Erb's palsy unrelated to birth trauma. *Am J Obstet Gynecol* 1997;**177**:1038–40
83 Beer, E., Folghera, M.G. Time for resolving shoulder dystocia. *Am J Obstet Gynecol* 1998;**179**:1376–7
84 Dawes, G.S., Jacobson, H.N., Mott, J.C., Shelley, H.J., Stafford, A. Treatment of asphyxia in newborn lambs and monkeys. *J Physiol (Lond)* 1963;**169**:167–84
85 Wood, C., Ng, K.H., Hounslow, D., Benning, H. Time: an important variable in normal delivery. *J Obstet Gynaecol Br Cwlth* 1973;**80**:295–300
86 James, C.E. Shoulder dystocia. *Current Obstetrics and Gynaecology* 1991;**1**:117–18
87 Leigh, T.H., James, C.E. Medicolegal commentary: shoulder dystocia. *Br J Obstet Gynaecol* 1998;**105**:815–17

31

Reducing teenage pregnancy

Kate Weaver and Anna Glasier

INTRODUCTION

The UK has the highest teenage pregnancy rate in Western Europe. In the whole of Europe, only Bulgaria, Romania and Hungary have higher teenage abortion rates. Most teenage conceptions are unplanned and unwanted, particularly those that occur among younger teenagers and those who are not married or cohabiting. Teenage conception is associated with high rates of abortion. There is no doubt that teenage pregnancies incur considerable costs both to the individuals involved and to society as a whole. Globally, teenage births remain common, at 15 million per year, accounting for more than 10% of all births.[1] The UK Government signalled its concern in *The Health of the Nation*,[2] published in 1992, in which it set the ambitious target of halving teenage conceptions by 2010.

STATISTICS

England, Scotland and Northern Ireland all had live-birth rates of approximately 30 per 1000 teenage women in 1997 and in Wales the rate was 37 per 1000. In England and Wales in 1998, there were 3.56 legal abortions per 1000 women under the age of 15 years, and 27 per 1000 women aged 16–19 years. The abortion rate was highest among the younger teenagers; around 50% of conceptions in under 16s ended in abortion. Overall, roughly three-fifths of all teenage conceptions resulted in a live birth.[3] Breaking down teenage conception rates by age, in Scotland in 1998, the conception rate in those under 16 years was 8.4 per 1000 women and, in 16–19 year-olds, 67.6 per 1000.[4] In Scotland in 1998, approximately 50% of pregnancies in those under 16 years ended in abortion. Among Scottish 16–19-year-olds, the abortion rate is steadily rising and abortion was the outcome of 43% of all teenage conceptions in 1998.[4]

TRENDS AND COMPARISONS IN PREGNANCY RATES

Such statistics are alarming but need to be seen in the context of long-term trends and international comparisons to be usefully interpreted. Trends in pregnancy rates show apparent correlations with legislative changes and media 'pill scares', for example. Comparisons between countries can suggest the importance of social, behavioural, legislative and economic factors in explaining teenage pregnancy rates.

Trends in the UK over time

UK teenage birth rates peaked in 1971 and then declined sharply until the late 1980s, when they levelled off. These changes have all occurred against the background of rapidly rising teenage sexual activity initiated at ever-younger ages. More widespread contraceptive use has prevented dramatic rises in teenage pregnancy. Only 30% of women born in 1931 had experienced sexual intercourse before the age of 20 years, compared with almost 90% of women born in 1971.[5] For women born before 1950, a steady rise in sexual activity was mirrored by a rise in teenage births. For women born after 1950, the increase in sexual activity was accompanied by a parallel increase in contraceptive use at first intercourse. The teenage birth rate per sexually active teenager declined among women born after 1950. This is consistent with reports of more widespread contraceptive use and more reliable methods of contraception being employed by teenagers in recent decades.[5] It is worth noting that teenage sexual activity has continued to increase over recent decades, despite whatever discouraging influences society and parents have brought to bear. Even in the early 1990s, the Health Behaviours of Scottish Schoolchildren Survey[6] found a significant increase in sexual activity among 15-year-old boys and girls. In samples of more than 4000 Scottish schoolchildren, 26% of both boys and girls aged 15 years reported sexual intercourse in 1990 compared with 37% of 15-year-olds sampled in 1994.

The overall decline in teenage pregnancy in the 1970s followed the extension of contraceptive services to unmarried women and the availability of contraception free of charge under the NHS. Similar falls in teenage births have been seen across Europe as contraception and abortion services have been made more widely available.

The levelling off in teenage conception rates seen in the UK in the 1980s, after the dramatic falls of the 1970s, is often ascribed to a climate of hostility to teenage contraception and sexuality, making teenagers reluctant to visit clinics and surgeries for advice. After the liberalising of sexual health provision in the 1970s, there were few large-scale interventions of significance in the 1980s. Instead, it seemed to become more difficult for teenagers to obtain contraception. In the early 1980s, Victoria Gillick attempted to prevent her local health authority providing contraception and advice to her teenage daughters. Although she lost her case in the House of Lords, the publicity surrounding the case must have affected many teenagers' willingness to request contraceptive services.[7]

Since the late 1980s, both live-birth and abortion rates have fluctuated within narrow limits. Small increases in pregnancy and abortion rates have followed 'pill scares' in 1976, 1983 and 1995.[7,8] Pregnancy rates fell in the early 1990s after the publication of *The Health of the Nation*[2] signalled renewed Government commitment to teenagers' sexual health and led to the opening of many new sexual health clinics targeted at young people. Figure 1 relates major events to changes in teenage birth and abortion rates from 1990 to 1996.

While the number of teenage births was declining in the 1970s, recorded abortion rates were climbing dramatically after the legalisation of abortion in 1967. From the mid-1980s onwards, patterns of teenage abortion rates have broadly mirrored live-birth rates, with abortion as the outcome of roughly one-third of all teenage conceptions.[7]

European comparisons

In devising strategies to reduce teenage pregnancy, it is helpful to look at patterns in other countries, particularly those in which unintended teenage pregnancies have been successfully reduced. Kane and Wellings[7] collected data on teenage pregnancy and abortion from across Europe and looked at factors associated with teenage pregnancy rates. They also examined trends in conception rates in relation to societal and legislative changes affecting teenage sexuality in several European countries.

Across Europe, there are enormous variations in teenage pregnancy rates. In 1996, Bulgaria had the highest live-birth rate to teenagers, at 51.2 per 1000 women. This was more than ten times the figure for Switzerland, which had the lowest incidence at 4 per 1000 teenage women. Within this

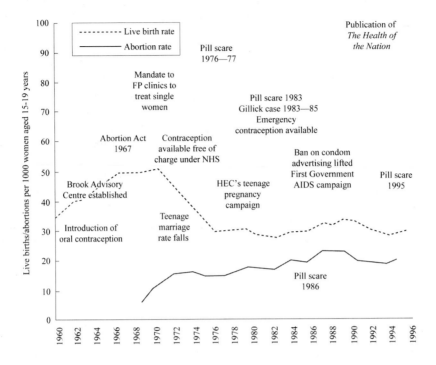

Figure 1 *Live births and abortions per 1000 women aged 15–19 years and associated events, England and Wales, 1960-96 (reproduced with permission from Kane and Wellings[7])*

range, the UK ranked relatively high at 29.7 live births per 1000 teenage women, the highest in Western Europe and exceeded only by Bulgaria, Romania and Yugoslavia. The rate of teenage births in the UK is twice that of Germany, three times that of France and six times higher than in the Netherlands. The statistics for abortion show an even greater spread, but with the UK still ranking fourth in Europe and first in Western Europe. Of the countries with low live-birth rates, some, like Denmark and Sweden, achieve this at the expense of a relatively high abortion rate. Others, like the Netherlands, Belgium, Finland, France and Italy, combine low abortion rates with low live-birth rates. The Netherlands and Belgium have always had relatively low teenage pregnancy rates, whereas other countries, like France, Italy and Finland have seen dramatic falls in teenage pregnancy after liberalisation of contraceptive services and sex education, as in the UK.[7]

Comparing pregnancy rates within and between countries allows the assessment of factors correlated with teenage pregnancy. Difficult though it may be to interpret such comparisons reliably, some factors are consistently associated with higher teenage pregnancy rates. These are discussed below.

Deprivation is linked with a higher incidence of teenage pregnancy in many studies.[7,9,10] Teenagers in socially deprived areas are more likely to conceive and more likely to proceed with a pregnancy, perpetuating a cycle of deprivation. Smith reviewed case notes of teenagers from Tayside attending NHS hospitals for abortion, live- or stillbirth between 1980 and 1990.[10] Deprivation categories were assigned using postal code and local government district. Teenage conception was up to eight times more frequent in the most deprived areas compared with the most affluent. Only one-quarter of teenage conceptions ended in therapeutic abortion in the most deprived areas while two-thirds of teenage pregnancies were terminated in the most affluent areas.[10] Daughters of teenage mothers and single parents are at particularly high risk of teenage pregnancy themselves.[9] Inequalities in wealth distribution appear as important as absolute poverty[1] and the UK has marked socio-economic inequality compared with other Western countries.[1,11]

It is popularly assumed that many teenagers get pregnant in order to get a council house and financial support. However in European comparisons, higher spending on maternity and family protection benefits did not correlate with higher teenage pregnancy rates.[7] The Social Exclusion Unit's 1999 report[12] on teenage pregnancy acknowledges that the prospect of benefits does not motivate teenagers to become parents but rather that many young people 'can see no reason not to get pregnant'.

Education and employment appear to be significant protective factors, offering teenagers realistic alternative goals and aspirations to young motherhood. As shown in worldwide surveys,[1] young people who spend more years in education have lower teenage pregnancy rates. Moreover, better-educated teenagers are more likely to choose to terminate an unplanned pregnancy.[7] Similarly, where more young women are in employment, more teenagers elect to terminate unplanned pregnancies.[7]

Broader societal aspects such as marriage patterns appear to relate to teenage pregnancy. Countries where women tend to marry at a younger age generally have higher live-birth and abortion rates among teenagers.[7]

Religious factors are harder to interpret. Religious sanctions against pre-marital sex and promiscuity are sometimes seen as a solution. However, comparison between European countries shows no obvious relationship between active religious membership and teenage pregnancy rates.[7]

General attitudes to sexuality, and to teenage sexuality in particular, are hard to measure and analyse but there is a strong suggestion that the open, pragmatic attitudes prevalent in countries like Denmark contribute to their low teenage conception rates.[7]

CONSEQUENCES

The personal consequences of any teenage pregnancy are far-reaching. Of course some teenagers will be happy to be pregnant, will have good family support and antenatal care and will find the role of mother fulfilling. Many are less fortunate and the UK has the highest live-birth rate to unmarried teenagers in the Western world.[7] While it is true that more young people are cohabiting instead of marrying, the UK does seem to have a high rate of single and unsupported mothers. This country combines a relatively low cohabitation rate with a high teenage pregnancy rate, compared with other European countries.[7]

Worldwide, teenage pregnancy is associated with increased risk of complications during pregnancy and delivery, as well as higher perinatal mortality.[1] In developed countries this is not necessarily the case. Improved nutrition and earlier menarche mean that most UK teenagers are physically mature enough to experience uneventful pregnancy and delivery (although many will struggle emotionally and mentally to cope with the demands of parenthood). Konje et al.[13] compared case records for 3576 pregnant women in their twenties with 1660 pregnant teenagers in Hull hospitals. The teenagers were more likely to be anaemic, but no more likely to experience proteinuric hypertension or other pregnancy complications. Teenagers had half the caesarean section rate but forceps deliveries were twice as common. Perinatal mortality rates were marginally lower for the teenage group. Uptake of antenatal care was high among these teenagers and the authors suggest that poor obstetric outcome for teenage pregnancies in other studies is more likely to be due to teenagers receiving poor (or no) antenatal care, for complex social reasons. Similarly, social factors probably account for much of the increased risk of adverse health outcomes in the offspring of teenage parents, including the higher incidence of sudden infant death syndrome, accidental injury and abuse.[9]

Socio-economically, teenage parents and their offspring can face bleak prospects. Teenage parents have reduced employment opportunities, are more likely to rely on state welfare and live with poor nutrition and housing, compared with older parents.[9]

Education often suffers as well. Many teenage mothers leave school early and have fewer educational opportunities thereafter. Young children of teenage parents are more likely to display developmental delays.[9] It is clear that teenage birth can frequently result in educational and socio-economic disadvantage as well as poor health for both mother and child.

For those who decide to terminate the pregnancy, there are likely to be emotional consequences, although there is no evidence of an increase in psychiatric problems. Physical adverse effects are rare but around 1% of women experience post-termination pelvic infection and up to 5% may require repeat uterine evacuation for retained products of conception.

INTERVENTIONS

Some of the factors that appear to correlate with higher chances of teenage pregnancy are not amenable to health-oriented interventions. Areas with high socio-economic deprivation have higher teenage pregnancy rates. It seems clear that poverty, poor education and poor employment prospects can make teenagers view pregnancy and child-rearing less negatively. Improved socio-economic status would perhaps discourage many teenagers from conceiving or from continuing with unintended pregnancy. However, this is a largely political issue and not directly amenable to medical intervention.

In other areas, health professionals may play a role in interventions that are not strictly medical. Promoting sex education and more consistent, supportive attitudes towards teenage sexuality are important areas where health professionals, particularly public health specialists, can be influential. Sex education and contraceptive provision are widely shown to reduce unwanted teenage pregnancy[7,9,14,15] yet efforts to introduce and improve such services are often hampered by objections that young people will be encouraged into greater promiscuity and sexual activity at a younger age. There is little evidence that this is the case. Grunseit[16] systematically reviewed the research literature on the impact of sexual health education and HIV/AIDS education on young people's sexual behaviour. Out of 53 interventional studies, 27 reported no change in sexual activity, pregnancy and sexually transmitted diseases (STDs). More encouragingly, 22 studies reported delayed coitarche or fewer sexual partners or reductions in unplanned pregnancy and STDs. Only three studies showed increases in sexual activity, or its unwanted outcomes, after educational programmes.[16] Different types of intervention are considered in more detail below.

Discouraging teenagers from having sex

It is a simplistic but common assumption that teenagers can be persuaded not to have sex, thereby reducing the teenage pregnancy rates. So-called abstinence programmes aim to encourage young people to delay sexual activity by developing decision-making and refusal skills, but have not been shown to have any effect on age of coitarche or on teenage pregnancy rates. A review of 42 evaluations of different educational approaches to preventing teenage pregnancy found that abstinence programmes were no better at delaying onset of sex or reducing pregnancy rates than the usual sex education programmes.[9]

Promoting more open attitudes to teenage sexuality

As mentioned above, teenage sexual activity has been rapidly rising over recent decades, despite societal disapproval and efforts to discourage early sexual intercourse, as well as widespread publicity about the dangers of HIV. It seems only sensible to accept that many teenagers are sexually active and to acknowledge the pleasures of a healthy sex life while helping them to cope with its demands and dangers.

Young people are bombarded with conflicting and confusing messages about sex by the media, school, family and peers. In Kane and Welling's[7] European comparisons, countries like Denmark and the Netherlands with an open, positive approach to teenage sexuality were those with lower teenage pregnancy rates. Teenagers in these countries receive clearer, more harmonious messages about their sexuality from sex education, in the media and at home. Their contraceptive needs were more likely to be recognised and met.

Conversely, the experience of the UK in the 1980s suggests that a negative atmosphere and conflicting messages about teenage sexuality can be harmful. Media reports on the Gillick case focused attention on parental disapproval and doubt was raised about the confidentiality teenagers could expect from doctors. At the same time, efforts to promote contraceptive use and safe sex continued. Over these years, falls in teenage conception were reversed as sexual activity continued to rise but contraceptive use fell.[5,7]

The role of the media in promoting teenage sexual health has been mixed. Teen magazines and television programmes can disseminate positive, helpful messages. On the other hand, exaggerated concerns and scare stories in the media about the safety of the contraception following the latest 'pill scare' seem to have contributed to the upturn in unwanted teenage pregnancy in 1995.[7] The British Pregnancy Advisory Service estimates that it saw an 11% rise in abortion requests over the following months, with 61% of those requesting abortion admitting that they had stopped oral contraceptive pills mid-way through a packet, after being alarmed by the media reports.[8]

Making contraception available

In terms of broad trends, many European countries recorded dramatic reductions in teenage pregnancy following legislative interventions liberalising contraceptive provision to young people in the 1960s and 1970s.[7] In Denmark, for example, teenage birth rates fell from 49.6 per 1000 women in 1966 to 8.3 per 1000 in 1995.[7] Figure 2 shows the falling teenage fertility rates in Denmark and the dates of key changes to contraceptive and abortion services. Large surveys of the population of Finnish teenagers between 1981 and 1991 showed a tripling in the use of oral contraceptives which coincided with decreasing conception and abortion rates.[15] The increase in oral contraceptive use came with the availability of new lower dose pills, which Finnish medical journals recommended as suitable for teenage women. Finnish doctors, working in an increasingly liberal climate, were therefore well-disposed to prescribe oral contraceptive pills to those young women who requested contraceptive advice and the results of increased oral contraceptive use were encouraging (Figure 3).

The cost of contraception may be a discouraging factor for some young people. In one municipality of Sweden, teenage abortion rates were halved after a research project heavily subsidised the cost of contraceptive pills for young women.[17] In a 1994 survey of 1373 Scottish schoolchildren aged 13-16 years, questions were asked about use of contraception on the most recent occasion of sexual intercourse. Only 71% reported using contraception of any kind and only 58% of the young people questioned had used a condom during their last sexual intercourse. Nearly 20% of the sample agreed that 'condoms are too expensive to use regularly'.[6] It is highly

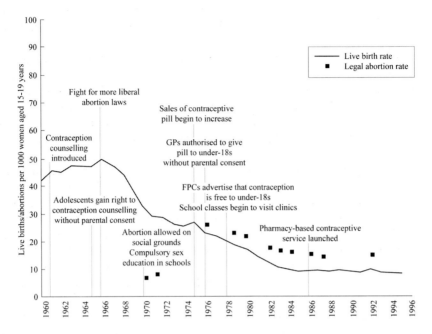

Figure 2 *Live births and abortions per 1000 women aged 15–19 years and associated events, Denmark, 1960-96 (reproduced with permission from Kane and Wellings[7])*

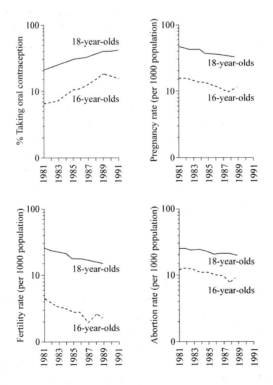

Figure 3 *Percentage of women taking oral contraceptives and pregnancy, fertility and abortion rates per 1000 Finnish women aged 16 and 18 years, 1981–91 (reproduced with permission from Rimpela et al.[15])*

regrettable if the personal cost of condoms is preventing more young people benefiting from their use. Condoms are available free of charge through family planning clinics but not through GP surgeries. Most young people say they feel more comfortable obtaining condoms from anonymous sources like shops and pharmacies.[18] Some local distribution schemes like the C-card system in Edinburgh are heavily used, with young people collecting free condoms at community outlets such as youth clubs and student unions. Family planning services overall are highly cost-effective; in a recent UK analysis, contraceptive provision to teenagers saved the NHS £400 per unwanted pregnancy avoided.[9] It therefore appears that more imaginative schemes for free or subsidised condom distribution to young people could be highly beneficial, both in financial and wider social terms.

It is particularly important that emergency contraception is readily available, since many teenagers are knowledgeable about contraception but are not always organised in advance. Timely use of hormonal emergency contraception can reduce the risk of unwanted pregnancy by around 75%, yet many young people do not know where to get it or are unable to get an appointment with their GP within the time limit. Visiting the doctor to request emergency contraception can seem daunting to many teenagers. In a questionnaire survey in ten schools in Lothian, 93% of 14-16-year-olds had heard of emergency contraception and 76% knew that they could get it from their own GP. Only 31% of sexually active girls had used emergency contraceptive pills and knowledge of time limits was poor.[19] Again, a combination of education and better provision is required before emergency contraception can become more widely used. Trials in which emergency contraceptive pills are made more easily available have been encouraging. In a large randomised controlled trial, 553 women kept emergency contraceptive pills at home and 530 obtained emergency contraception, as needed, from the doctor.[20] Comparing the two groups, self-administration was safe and did not lead to overuse or risk-taking. There was also a (nonsignificant) reduction in unwanted pregnancies in the self-administering group. Larger trials are under way in Lothian[21] and Manchester. The Lothian Family Planning Service is running a two-year trial in which Lothian's GPs can offer women supplies of emergency contraceptive pills to keep at home. The Manchester, Trafford and Salford Health Action Zone has been running a scheme to allow pharmacists to supply emergency contraception according to a strict protocol.

It is to be hoped that emergency contraception will become available over the counter in this country in the near future. The new progesterone-only formulations are more likely to be acceptable in this respect and studies suggest they have similar efficacy to the Yuzpe regimen.[22] An all-party group of Members of Parliament meeting in February 2000 recommended that hormonal emergency contraception should be available, without prescription, through community pharmacies.[23] This has been the situation in France since June 1999. In addition, French school nurses are now able to dispense levonorgestrel emergency contraceptive pills without a prescription.[24]

Dedicated sexual health services for young people

In the UK, contraception has been available to unmarried women since the late 1960s and free of charge since the mid-1970s, from GPs and family planning clinics. Nevertheless, many teenagers are still deterred from requesting contraception from the GP or mainstream family planning clinic by fears about moralising or lack of anonymity and confidentiality. In addition, simple practicalities like the timing and location of clinics can make it impossible for school pupils to attend. The NHS Centre for Reviews and Dissemination[9] undertook a systematic review of research evidence and concluded that there is good evidence that youth-oriented clinics are more effective than general family planning clinics in reducing pregnancy rates. This should not be surprising given the different needs and emotional and mental maturity of teenagers compared with older users of family planning clinics. There is a proven association between lower teenage conception rates and local availability of specialist youth-oriented family planning clinics.[14] The study by Clements et al.[14] analysed teenage conception data for Wessex between 1991 and 1994 and looked at census wards within the whole of the Regional Health Authority area of Wessex, containing more than 120 000 teenage females in total. Teenage conception rates were directly correlated with greater distance from a specialist young people's clinic, so that easier access to specialist provision did seem to be associated with lower teenage pregnancy in local areas.[14]

Accessibility of clinics

To be successful, youth clinics need to be accessible to teenagers but young people should not feel embarrassed about entering the premises. Once through the doors of the clinic, young people need to feel assured of sensitive treatment and confidentiality. General Medical Council rulings on this issue mean that doctors can feel comfortable guaranteeing confidentiality under almost all circumstances.[25] Opening times of clinics must take account of young people's schedules. Such services need to be widely and appropriately advertised and their details included in sex education classes in local schools. Combining accessibility with confidentiality and anonymity is not always easy, yet in the USA some schools offer contraceptive clinic services either within the school or at nearby premises. Despite parental opposition, some of these school-based clinics are used by a high proportion of pupils and have achieved higher rates of contraceptive use among their pupils. Longer-running programmes have been able to demonstrate falling pregnancy rates compared with schools without such clinics. Encouraging reports on several such clinics were reviewed and summarised in Graham's[26] review of adolescent contraceptive clinics for the International Planned Parenthood Foundation.[26]

Services for young men

Young men are often neglected in efforts to improve sexual health. In surveys, teenage boys say their sex education is inadequate and, perhaps as a consequence, rates of safe sex practices and condom use were disappointingly low in one survey of US college students.[27] This represents a failure to support young men at a difficult time of life and also has clear repercussions for their health and safety and that of their partners. Youth-oriented clinics need to cater for the needs of young men as well as women, particularly in provision of free condoms and in supporting them in the initial anxiety and potential difficulties of condom use, which may create lasting aversion to condoms.[27]

Sex education

To reduce teenage pregnancy rates, increased contraceptive provision needs to be complemented by heightened awareness of sexual issues, for example by education programmes. Isolated increases in youth-oriented clinics have not always proven effective in encouraging contraceptive use and reducing unwanted pregnancy.[9] Successful programmes integrate school sex education with youth clinics by clinic personnel coming into the school or by arranging for pupils to visit the local clinic.[9]

The 1993 Education Act made sex education compulsory in all secondary schools but did not stipulate the content or structure, leaving these for school governors to decide. As a result, provision of sex education remains extremely variable.

Good sex education helps young people achieve sexual health, including emotional well-being and freedom from sexually transmitted infection and unwanted pregnancy. Effective sex education needs to be targeted at the needs of the relevant group. Young people who have already initiated sexual activity are unlikely to change their sexual and contraceptive behaviour.[9] Hence timing is important, so that sex education is age-appropriate and starts as young as possible,[28] progressing from teaching of simple concepts to discussion of complex issues in the realms of ethics, values and morals. Young people need to discuss and rehearse the personal skills needed to put knowledge into practice in relationships. The involvement of peers is another facet of some successful programmes.

The evidence from Europe suggests that teenage conceptions are further reduced when education programmes provide integrated sexual health messages concerning protection against unwanted pregnancy, reduction of STDs and personal sexual wellbeing.[7]

SUMMARY

Unwanted teenage conception remains a major problem worldwide, with far-reaching consequences for individuals and for society as a whole. UK teenage pregnancy rates compare poorly with those in Europe but are now relatively steady after falling from much higher levels in the 1960s. There is plenty of evidence that teenage pregnancy rates reflect socio-economic and societal factors, which are slow to change and difficult or impossible for the medical profession to influence. However, sex education and sexual health clinic services can make an impact on the sexual well-being of teenagers, especially against a background of accepting, consistent advice about teenage sexuality.

References

1. The Alan Guttmacher Institute. *Into A New World; Young Women's Sexual and Reproductive Lives.* New York: The Alan Guttmacher Institute; 1998
2. Department of Health. *Health of the Nation: A Strategy for Health in England.* London: HMSO; 1992 (Cm 1986)
3. Office for National Statistics. *Conceptions in England and Wales 1997.* London: The Stationery Office; 1999
4. NHS in Scotland Information and Statistics Division. *Teenage Pregnancy in Scotland 1988–1998.* Edinburgh; 1999 (Health Briefing No. 99)
5. Johnson, A.M., Wadsworth, J., Wellings, K., Field, J. *Sexual Attitudes and Lifestyles.* London: Blackwell Scientific; 1994
6. Currie, C., Todd, J., Thomson, C. *Health Behaviours of Scottish Schoolchildren, Report No. 6. Sex Education, Personal Relationships, Sexual Behaviour and HIV/AIDS Knowledge and Attitudes in 1990 and 1994.* Edinburgh: Health Education Board for Scotland; 1997
7. Kane, R., Wellings, K. *Reducing the Rate of Teenage Conceptions. An International Review of the Evidence: Data from Europe.* London: Health Education Authority; 1999
8. Furedi, F., Furedi, A. *The International Impact of a Pill Panic in the UK.* London: Birth Control Trust; 1996
9. NHS Centre for Reviews and Dissemination. Preventing and Reducing the Adverse Effects of Unintended Teenage Pregnancies. *Effective Health Care* 1997;**3**
10. Smith, T. Influence of socio-economic factors on attaining targets for reducing teenage pregnancies. *BMJ*;**306**:1232–5

11 Moore, P. UK young people's health affected by relative poverty. *Lancet* 1997;**349**:1152
12 Mawer, C. (1999) Preventing teenage pregnancies, supporting teenage mothers. BMJ 1999;**318**:1713–14
13 Konje, J.C., Palmer, A., Watson, A., Hay, D., Imrie, A. Early teenage pregnancies in Hull. *Br J Obstet Gynaecol* 1992;**99**:969–73
14 Clements, S., Stone, N., Diamond, I., Ingham, R. Modelling the spatial distribution of teenage conception rates within Wessex. *Br J Fam Plann* 1998;**24**:61–71
15 Rimpela, A.H., Rimpela, M.K., Kosunen, E.A.L. Use of oral contraceptives by teenagers and its consequences in Finland 1981–91. *BMJ* 1992;**305**:1053–7
16 Grunseit, A. *Impact of HIV and Sexual Health Education on the Sexual Behaviour of Young People: a Review Update.* Geneva: Joint United Nations Programme on HIV/AIDS; 1997
17 Csillag, C. Abortions among teenagers halved. *Lancet* 1993;**341**:1084
18 Harden, A., Ogden, J. Sixteen to nineteen year olds' use of, and beliefs about, contraceptive services. *Br J Fam Plann* 1999;**24**:141–4
19 Graham, A., Green, L., Glasier, A. Teenagers' knowledge of emergency contraception: questionnaire survey in south east Scotland. *BMJ* 1996;**123**:1567–9
20 Glasier, A., Baird, D. The effects of self-administering emergency contraception. *N Engl J Med* 1998;**339**:1–4
21 Christie, B. Project makes emergency pill more available. *BMJ* 1999;**319**:661
22 Task Force on Postovulatory Methods of Fertility Regulation. Randomised controlled trial of levonorgestrel versus Yuzpe regimen of combined oral contraceptives for emergency contraception. *Lancet* 1998;**352**:428–33
23 All Party Pharmacy Group. *The Supply of Emergency Contraception through Community Pharmacies. A Report to Health Ministers.* London: The Stationery Office; 2000
24 Daley, S. France provides morning-after pill to schoolgirls. *New York Times* 8 February 2000
25 *Confidentiality and People Under 16.* London: British Medical Association; 1993 (Guidance issued jointly by the BMA, GMSC, HEA, Brook Advisory Centres, FPA and RCGP)
26 Graham, A. Contraceptive clinics for adolescents. *IPPF Medical Bulletin* 1998;**32**:3–4
27 Yamey, G. Sexual and reproductive health: what about the boys and men? *BMJ* 1999;**319**:1315–16
28 Thomson, R. Sexual health starts at school. *Primary Health Care* 1993;**3**:8–11

32

Maternal death and anaesthesia – a perspective

Sheila M. Willatts

A maternal death is a tragedy for the whole family, which has major repercussions for many people. It is a tribute to doctors providing obstetric anaesthesia that deaths directly due to anaesthesia are falling. Nevertheless, the complications of pregnancy and patient co-morbidities dictate that anaesthetists are involved in resuscitation, surgery and intensive care of patients who develop critical illness or die during pregnancy and childbirth and play a major role in efforts to reduce mortality.

The Confidential Enquiries into Maternal Deaths in England and Wales began in 1952 and in 1985 combined with Enquiries of Scotland and Northern Ireland. Reports from the joint Enquiries are now published triennially as a report covering the whole of the UK. It has become the most comprehensive and influential clinical self-audit in the world.

The most recent report was the fourth combined report. It showed overall maternal mortality at 12.2 per 100 000 maternities in 1994–96. This apparent increase from 9.9 per 100 000 for 1991-93 is due to increased case ascertainment.[1] Contrast this with international estimates of maternal mortality which indicate that, globally, there are some 585 000 maternal deaths each year, 99% of them in developing countries. There are about 80 000 more deaths than earlier estimates which indicates a substantial underestimation of maternal mortality in the past.[2] Reduction of maternal mortality is one of the common goals of the World Health Organization and UNICEF but the objective of reducing maternal mortality by 50% by the year 2000 was not achieved in parts of Africa such as Nigeria.[3] These new estimates show that, in developing countries as a whole, maternal mortality ranges from 190 per 100 000 live births to 870 per 100 000 live births, with extremely high ratios of over 1000 per 100 000 live births in sub-Saharan Africa.[4-6] In some countries, maternal mortality continues to rise despite improved obstetric services due to the increase in malaria and AIDS-associated tuberculosis.[7]

One of the problems in assessing maternal mortality is the requirement for knowledge of the cause of death in women of reproductive age and whether or not the woman was pregnant at the time of death or had recently been so. Few countries count births and deaths and even fewer register the causes of death. Thus, in the long term, accurate information about maternal mortality will depend on improvement in vital registration systems and their incorporation into all national health information systems.

The UK Enquiries are based on individual anonymised case reports of all known maternal deaths and are initiated by regional directors of public health or chief administrative medical officers. Completion of the case reports is not a statutory requirement but nevertheless is considered to be 96–98% complete. *A First Class Service – Quality in the New NHS*,[8] published in 1998, states that all doctors are required to participate in the work of public enquires; any health care professional who is aware of a maternal death is required to report it either direct to the Enquiries or to their director of public health. After completion of the report form, each case is

Table 1 *Definitions of maternal deaths*

Classification	Definition
Maternal deaths[a]	Deaths of women while pregnant or within 42 days of termination of pregnancy, from any cause related to or aggravated by the pregnancy or its management, but not from accidental causes
Direct[a]	Deaths resulting from obstetric complications of the pregnant state (pregnancy, labour and puerperium), from interventions, omissions, incorrect treatment, or from a chain of events resulting from any of the above
Indirect[a]	Deaths resulting from previous existing disease, or disease that developed during pregnancy and which was not due to direct obstetric causes, but which was aggravated by the physiologic effects of pregnancy
Late[b]	Deaths occurring between 42 days and one year after abortion, miscarriage or delivery that are due to direct or indirect maternal causes
Fortuitous[a]	Deaths from unrelated causes which happen to occur in pregnancy or the puerperium

[a] International Classification of Diseases definition[9]; [b] International Classification of Diseases definition[11]

Table 2 *Deaths directly associated with anaesthesia (excluding indirect and late deaths), estimated rate per 1 000 000 maternities and percentage of direct maternal deaths, UK 1985-96*

Triennium	Deaths directly associated with anaesthesia (n)	Death rate per million maternities	% of maternal deaths
1985–87	6	2.6	4.3
1988–90	4	1.7	2.7
1991–93	8	3.5	6.5
1994–96	1	0.5	0.8

assessed by a local assessor in obstetrics, anaesthetics, pathology and midwifery, looking for evidence of substandard care. Recommendations are prepared and published with the expectation that they will be followed to improve practice.[9]

Deaths are classified according to the categories shown in Table 1.[1] The major causes of direct maternal deaths in the UK remain thrombosis and thromboembolism, hypertensive disorders of pregnancy, amniotic fluid embolus and haemorrhage. Deaths due to sepsis are increasing and a substantial proportion of indirect deaths are related to cardiac disease. The number of deaths directly attributable to anaesthesia continues to fall (Table 2).[1] This should be compared with the total number of deaths reported to the Registrars General and to the Enquiries for a similar time period but bearing in mind the increased case ascertainment for the last triennium (Table 3).[1]

Despite the increase in reported maternal deaths for the triennium 1994–96, there is only one death directly attributable to anaesthesia, compared with eight in the previous report. The

Table 3 *Maternal deaths and mortality rates per 100 000 reported to the Registrars General and the Confidential Enquiries into Maternal Deaths, UK 1985–96*

Years	Total maternities	Direct deaths[a]	Indirect deaths[a]	Total[a]
1985–87	2 268 766	137 (6)	86 (3.8)	223 (9.9)
1988–90	2 360 300	145 (6.1)	93 (3.9)	238 (10.1)
1991–93	2 315 204	128 (5.6)	100 (4.2)	228 (9.9)
1994–96	2 197 640	134 (6.1)	134 (6.1)	268 (12.2)

[a] Number (rate)

remainder of deaths are those in which the death was associated with an anaesthetic being given (20 deaths) or where the anaesthetist was involved only in resuscitation. This is a significant improvement on the last report and a tribute to those responsible for the provision of obstetric anaesthetic services despite the difficulties that are still encountered.

DEATH DIRECTLY ATTRIBUTABLE TO ANAESTHESIA

This one death was associated with combined spinal/epidural anaesthesia. The woman was short and was due to undergo an elective caesarean section as she was thought to have a big baby and had undergone a previous caesarean section for failure to progress in labour. The anaesthetist had several attempts to administer a combined spinal and epidural anaesthetic. This consisted of spinal injection of 2.25 ml heavy bupivacaine, 125 µg alfentanil and 150 µg clonidine and 15 ml 0.375% bupivacaine into the epidural space. Shortly afterwards, she complained of a headache, shooting pains down her legs and difficulty with breathing. It was thought that the spinal might have been a little high so oxygen was given. Her blood pressure fell despite 2.5 litres of fluid and ephedrine and oxygen saturation deteriorated despite breathing 100% oxygen. She complained of tightness in her chest and increasing difficulty with breathing and a decision was taken to intubate and ventilate her, during which she experienced florid pulmonary oedema and it was decided that she should be transferred to a larger hospital for ventilation. Diuretics and glyceryl trinitrate were given, intravenous fluids stopped, central and arterial lines inserted and adrenaline was given with midazolam and ketamine for sedation. While waiting for the ambulance she deteriorated, suffered a cardiac arrest and was given adrenaline and isoprenaline and external cardiac pacing but could not be resuscitated.

The anaesthetic technique used in this case was not common. The spinal anaesthetic used excessive doses and, coupled with a large volume of local anaesthetic injected into the epidural at the same time, led to hypotension due to extensive sympathetic block. The use of clonidine, which is still controversial, would worsen hypotension, especially at high doses. Resuscitation was also unconventional, particularly in relation to the use of isoprenaline. Administration of 2.5 litres of intravenous fluids probably had no adverse effect in this case. Care was substandard and death entirely avoidable.

DEATHS ASSOCIATED WITH ANAESTHESIA

In many cases of maternal death the patient had been anaesthetised without incident but there were twenty cases in this triennium of women who were anaesthetised and died from associated conditions (Table 4).

Table 4 *Deaths associated with anaesthesia*

Cause of death	Number
Pulmonary hypertension and cardiac failure	4
Amniotic fluid embolism	5
Eclampsia/pregnancy induced hypertension	2
Haemorrhage	4
Sepsis	1
Phaeochromocytoma	2
Mitral valve disease	1
Fortuitous	1

Examples of these circumstances include a woman with a known case of pulmonary hypertension in which the risks of pregnancy and need for contraception were inadequately appreciated. She underwent a termination of pregnancy under general anaesthesia (GA) but no anticoagulant was prescribed because the risk of bleeding was thought to exceed that of thromboembolic complications. She was readmitted as an emergency eight days later, when thromboembolism was diagnosed and heparin advised. However, during the next day she suffered a cardiac arrest and resuscitation was unsuccessful.

Between the two deaths from eclampsia in this triennium, one woman was admitted unconscious to an accident and emergency department with sluggish pupillary reactions, having been normotensive 11 days previously at an antenatal clinic visit. She had proteinuria and a blood pressure of 160/115 mmHg at admission, was assumed to have had an eclamptic fit and was delivered by caesarean section under GA for fetal distress. She was managed in the intensive care unit appropriately for two days but without improvement until brain-stem death was diagnosed. The second woman died two days after delivery with fulminant hepatic failure consequent to severe pregnancy-induced hypertension.

Among the deaths due to haemorrhage, one patient developed eclampsia while awaiting transfer to a regional centre for further care and delivery. She was treated with diazepam and antihypertensive agents and transferred by ambulance. During the journey intrauterine death occurred and on arrival she had severe coagulopathy precluding abdominal delivery. Vaginal delivery was followed by profuse bleeding and an emergency laparotomy was performed under GA. Intraperitoneal bleeding could not be controlled so the patient was stabilised with intra-abdominal packing and transferred to the intensive care unit where she died. Autopsy showed a ruptured necrotic liver.

A patient who had mitral valve disease with pulmonary hypertension was advised not to become pregnant by both consultant cardiologist and obstetrician. She was admitted with an antepartum haemorrhage, cough and tachycardia. Echocardiography showed the mitral valve to be thrombosed or stenosed. By this time she was in cardiogenic shock so her transfer for cardiac surgery was arranged. She was accompanied by an anaesthetist and a nurse but died a few minutes after arrival at the receiving hospital.

DEATHS IN WHICH ANAESTHETISTS WERE INVOLVED IN RESUSCITATION

In this category in this triennium there were three patients with amniotic fluid embolus, two of whom sustained cardiac arrest in the accident and emergency department and one in the labour ward. All had caesarean sections during the resuscitation. There were eight deaths in which resuscitation was required for massive haemorrhage in which the main factors were:

(1) Delay in recognition of bleeding;

(2) Misdiagnosis;

(3) Inadequate fluid therapy;

(4) Delay in institution of invasive monitoring;

(5) Failure of postoperative monitoring to detect continuing bleeding.

In many cases pulmonary embolus presented as cardiovascular collapse and death occurred before an anaesthetist could be involved with the resuscitation. Cases of ruptured uterus, eclampsia, phaeochromocytoma and right ventricular failure from progressive pulmonary hypertension also presented with the requirement for resuscitation only.

COMMENTS AND RECOMMENDATIONS ON THE FINDINGS FROM ALL DEATHS IN 1991–96

(1) Obstetric units which are isolated from main hospitals should always keep a large stock of group O rhesus-negative blood and, ideally, these units should be provided with their own blood transfusion laboratory to expedite delivery of blood and blood products.

(2) Monitoring of central venous, systemic and pulmonary artery pressure is not always well performed on an obstetric unit.

(3) Until patients can be transferred to an intensive care unit there should be good quality high-dependency care on the delivery suite or in the labour ward theatre.

(4) Failed forceps delivery often leads to an immediate caesarean section for which the anaesthetist must be prepared either by good epidural top-up or by safe GA, recognising the increased risk of hypotension.

(5) In cases where the dose of thiopental was thought to contribute to the outcome by producing relatively long-lasting hypotension it is tempting to recommend a shorter acting drug but (especially in small doses) this alternative has the potential problem of awareness.

(6) Obstetric patients should have a high priority where there are limited intensive-care facilities.

(7) The anaesthetist plays a key role in the multidisciplinary team for the benefit of patients who develop life-threatening complications of pregnancy.

(8) Improvement is needed in keeping records and ensuring their availability to assessors in strict confidence.

(9) Full implementation of previous recommendations is required for dedicated obstetric and anaesthetic consultant sessions for delivery unit supervision.

(10) Improvement is required in the quality of information provided to women.

(11) Identification of a lead consultant and clear guidelines are needed for management of hypertensive disorders in pregnancy, including eclampsia, and ready access to a regional advisory service lead by a consultant with special expertise is also essential.

(12) The guidance for management of severe haemorrhage and further guidance for the management of women who refuse blood transfusion should be implemented.

(13) Adoption of the recommendations of the Working Party of the Royal College of Obstetricians and Gynaecologists on prophylaxis of thromboembolism is essential.[10]

(14) Early involvement of consultant anaesthetists should be usual in high-risk cases, with ready access to all appropriate monitoring equipment and high-care areas.

In those cases associated with substandard care the key factors can be summarised as:

(1) Failure of communication and wise decision making;

(2) A lack of consultant availability;

(3) Failure of trainee doctors to recognise severity of illness;

(4) Delay in providing adequate resuscitation;

(5) Delay in obtaining blood products;

(6) Split site working contributing to slow laboratory input, access to medical staff and other emergency facilities (usually the obstetric unit is separate from and often some distance from the main hospital);

(7) Difficulty with transporting patients to acute hospitals and delay or inadequate access to intensive and high-dependency facilities.

Lack of teamwork and failure of consultants to attend (or delegate appropriately) remain significant causes of substandard care. Consultant involvement coupled with regular staff training has the potential to reduce death and morbidity. Early antenatal identification of potential problems should be routine and obstetric anaesthetists should be aware of expected difficulties. Coexisting medical diseases, such as heart disease and epilepsy, require particular care and a high level of suspicion is needed for the diagnosis of deep-vein thrombosis and pulmonary embolus. The value of peri-operative antibiotics for patients undergoing caesarean section is now proven. When a mother becomes septic, repeated bacteriological specimens should be evaluated urgently and in some cases parenteral antibiotics must be given before the diagnosis is confirmed.

By comparison with the UK, anaesthesia-related deaths in the USA were reviewed from 1979–90 and a reduction from 43 (1979–81) to 17 (1988–90) per 100 000 live births was found.[11] The number of deaths associated with GA had remained stable but the number of regional anaesthesia-associated deaths had decreased. Most maternal deaths due to complications of anaesthesia occurred during GA for caesarean section. Risks associated with regional anaesthesia were related to toxicity of local anaesthetics and excessive high regional blocks. Findings from the Netherlands show that birth by caesarean section is seven times more hazardous than vaginal birth but it is not clear how this relates to anaesthesia.[12]

DEATHS INVOLVING INTENSIVE CARE

There were 74 maternal deaths recorded in the 1991–93 report where there was a need for intensive care and 107 deaths, including seven fortuitous and six late in the 1994–96 triennium. These are shown in Table 5. Due to incomplete forms for some cases it is likely that the total number is actually higher. Intensive care services were required for a range of reasons from resuscitation for a few hours only to over 40 days of treatment for multiple organ failure often, following acute respiratory distress syndrome (ARDS).

There is a discrepancy between the types of condition causing mortality and those causing admission to an intensive care unit. This is because fatal conditions may cause rapid death before admission to the unit and because late maternal deaths are often not reported to the Confidential Enquiry. In addition, some specific disorders are cared for on specialist units and medical disorders are often managed on medical wards.

For direct deaths, 75% of the women who suffered a haemorrhage required intensive care and 50% of those with sepsis; 35% of women with pregnancy-induced hypertension and 35% of those with amniotic fluid embolism survived long enough to be transferred to an intensive care unit. Not surprisingly, given the speed of collapse following pulmonary embolism, only 19% of these women were admitted to an intensive care unit. Half the women who died in early pregnancy also required such support. Late deaths from indirect causes, including neoplastic disease, fortuitous deaths, such as myocardial infarction and cystic fibrosis, are extremely difficult to identify as in many cases the medical attendants have forgotten that the patient had been pregnant within the time defined for late deaths. Substance abuse and suicide are unfortunately causes of death which appear to be increasing.

Table 5 Number of direct and indirect cases admitted to intensive care units in the UK 1994–96

Principal disorder	Number[a]	Cases receiving intensive care (%)	Duration of stay (days)
Thrombosis and thromboembolism	9 (48)	19	0.4–20
Hypertensive disease of pregnancy	7 (20)	35	1–19
Haemorrhage	9 (12)	75	0.5–33
Amniotic fluid embolism	6 (17)	35	0.5–5
Early pregnancy deaths[b]	7 (15)	47	0.5–41
Sepsis	7 (14)	50	0.2–42
Other direct			
Genital tract trauma	3 (5)	60	1–23
Other	0 (2)		
Anaesthetic	1 (1)	100	0
Cardiac	9 (39)	23	3–42
Psychiatric	1 (9)	10	12
Other indirect	32 (86)	37	1–34
Total direct and indirect	94		

[a] Total number of cases with disorder are given in parenthesis; [b] ectopic, spontaneous miscarriage, legal termination

Acute respiratory distress syndrome and respiratory conditions

ARDS in pregnancy is now better recognised by pathologists and its incidence may be increasing as patients are kept alive for longer as organ support defers death and ARDS becomes established. The major causes are haemorrhage and sepsis, but hypertensive disorders of pregnancy, inhalation of gastric contents, dead fetus and amniotic fluid embolus are all aetiological factors and the use of β-adrenergic agents for patients in premature labour contributes. ARDS is frequently the prelude to development of multiple organ failure.

In patients who survive the initial collapse caused by amniotic fluid embolus, acute right heart failure occurs, often associated with left ventricular failure.[13,14] About 75% of those who survive the original collapse develop increased alveolar-capillary permeability and ARDS. This is a condition with a high mortality (80%) which makes considerable demands upon intensive-care facilities. The initial hypoxia may be sufficient to produce severe neurological damage and even brain-stem death.

Asthma is associated with prematurity, low birth weight and increased perinatal mortality, probably due to poor asthma control, but pregnancy is not a contraindication to steroid treatment.[15]

Tocolytic-induced pulmonary oedema is due to administration of β-adrenergic agents, especially terbutaline and ritodrine, which are used to inhibit uterine contractions. Their use may be associated with hypokalaemia, hyperglycaemia, tachyarrhythmia and sodium retention as well as pulmonary oedema in pregnancy.

Cardiovascular conditions

About half the patients admitted with cardiovascular problems had underlying cardiac disease. While patients with pre-existing cardiac disease may be expected to have complications during pregnancy and delivery, most of the patients in this group had unpredictable requirements for intensive therapy. Congenital heart disease is usually diagnosed and recognised to be a problem in pregnancy, but ischaemic heart disease is becoming more prevalent.

Intensive care requirements for pregnant patients

Previous reports have highlighted the additional risk that pregnancy and childbirth present to a mother with co-existent disease. However, even identification of the risk factors does not eliminate the need for intensive therapy for unexpected emergencies.[16] Pregnant patients may develop critical illness as a direct result of their pregnancy or coincidentally.[17] Pregnancy predisposes to infection, for example pneumonia due to viruses such as varicella and herpes simplex, and increases its severity. The lack of readily available intensive-care facilities contributed to death in seven cases in the latest triennial report and, in the 1991–93 triennium, five patients had to be transferred to another hospital for intensive therapy; four others had their admission to the intensive care unit delayed because of the lack of an available bed. It is clear that intensive care and high-dependency facilities must be readily available for obstetric patients in the same hospital as the maternity unit. Most authorities believe that critical illness should be managed on a general intensive therapy unit in the same way as other patients with similar conditions.[17] Good liaison between intensive care specialists, obstetricians and physicians, together with easy access to fetal monitoring, is essential.[18] There is emerging evidence that provision of intensive and high-dependency care reduces morbidity and mortality and that the best chance of success occurs when patients are treated early in their illness.[17,19]

The requirement for, or availability of, intensive care world-wide for obstetric patients has been variously reported as 1–9 per 1000 deliveries.[20,21] In a five-year review of 39 parturient patients admitted to a general intensive care unit, it was suggested that a fall in maternal mortality reflected an improvement in organ support in the unit but as a result there was an increase in the number of deaths from ARDS.[22] In that study, the majority of patients were admitted to the unit either as a direct result of pregnancy or by a medical or surgical problem which was aggravated by the physiological problems of pregnancy.

In a study of 435 obstetric patients[23] in which the frequency of severe diseases was 36 per 100 000 live births, the mortality was lower with scheduled delivery in a teaching hospital. The authors concluded that most obstetric patients with serious diseases were referred for suitable care but those who were not had a higher mortality.

Obstetric admissions to an intensive care unit in a deprived inner city area were reviewed to see whether admission could have been predicted.[24] Sixty-seven percent of patients had no previous medical or obstetric history. As in other series, the major reasons for admission were hypertensive disorders of pregnancy (66%) and haemorrhage (19%); 79% followed caesarean section and 40% required ventilatory support. The perinatal mortality was 6% and there were three maternal deaths. The need for admission was unpredictable in two-thirds of cases. The authors agreed that only a small proportion of women who develop complications of pregnancy (0.1–0.9%) require admission to an intensive care unit. However, a policy of early intervention and treatment on a multidisciplinary basis, which may involve intubation, ventilation, invasive monitoring and vasoactive drugs, should be used preventatively. This approach to management by early involvement of all relevant specialties to provide optimal care, can alleviate the progression to multiple organ failure and improve prognosis. High-dependency care may be just as effective for patients who are conscious and have single-organ dysfunction.

Hospital records of obstetric patients admitted to an intensive care unit for respiratory support after an anaesthetic complication were reviewed.[25] In a ten-year period, there were 126 obstetric admissions to the unit from 61 435 deliveries, of which 16 were due to anaesthetic complications, 12 followed general and 4 regional anaesthesia. One-third of deliveries had required some form of anaesthesia, of which one-third was given as general anaesthesia and the remainder as regional anaesthesia. Complications included anaphylaxis, high spinal block and failure of endotracheal intubation. The incidence of major complication after general anaesthesia causing admission to an intensive care unit was 1/932 and for regional anaesthesia 1/4177. If a complication requiring admission to the intensive care unit and mechanical ventilation is used as the criterion of safety, it appears that regional anaesthesia is safer than general anaesthesia for delivery.

Severe maternal morbidity is easy to underestimate because pregnant women are usually healthy, recover quickly and are discharged with relatively little follow-up. A recent review identified a small but sick group of pregnant women with high rates of medical intervention, many of whom did not go home with their babies or with their fertility intact.[26] The end-point for a near-miss in this case was admission to an intensive care unit. High-risk features included hypertension, age over 35 years, pre-existing medical problems, twin pregnancy, weight greater than 100 kg and parity greater than four. Nearly half these near misses were related to haemorrhage.

Availability of facilities

A postal survey has been undertaken of all UK obstetric units concerning provision of recovery, high-dependency and intensive-care facilities in consultant obstetric units. The response rate was 89%; 62% had a designated staffed recovery unit and 41% had specific high-dependency beds. There were a number of units without consultant anaesthetic sessions or trained anaesthetic assistants available 24 hours a day.[27] Purchasers of health care have been encouraged to ensure that national standards and recommendations of the Confidential Enquiries are implemented.[28]

Outcome

One study of the outcome of obstetric patients requiring intensive care found a low standardised mortality rate (SMR) of 0.416, indicating that these patients did better than predicted.[29] There are various explanations, age alone having been excluded in the analysis. Firstly, the subgroup itself may be uniquely different or there may be better care for this subgroup and, therefore, a better outcome. The physiological range of variables considered by the Acute Physiology and Chronic Health Evaluation (APACHE II) score and the weighting for deviation from the norm is for a normal, non-pregnant, population and there are changes in physiological variables for the pregnant state (for example tachycardia or pH changes).[30] Secondly, APACHE II does take into account the more serious changes of disease in pregnancy such as deranged liver function, uric acid and platelets. However, other workers have found that APACHE II and other severity scores assess the intensive-care outcome of critically ill obstetric patients as accurately as non-obstetric patients.[31] The high emergency caesarean section rate, with its significant weighting in the risk equation, may have contributed to the low SMR.

THE FUTURE

It would be helpful to have international comparisons of maternal mortality based on uniformity of data collection, verification and analysis. At present there are differences in interpretation of definitions and, from a survey of European countries, evidence of under-reporting.[32] An audit of previous recommendations from these reports[33] provides anecdotal evidence for improvement in facilities but action is still required by purchasers and providers to address the shortfall in previous recommendations. With the publication in the UK of the Cumberlege report[34] on changing childbirth, it is likely that most antenatal and intranatal care in the UK will be carried out by midwives who will not have had an extensive training in general nursing. One suggestion is that obstetric anaesthetists should be involved in teaching programmes for all labour ward staff and in provision of information to mothers.[35]

Epidemiological data suggest a likely increase in maternal mortality until 2005.[36] These data suggest that the decline in maternal mortality in the UK has stopped. In France maternal mortality is higher than in most European countries and has been increasing since 1990. Based on population projections published by Eurostat,[36] maternal mortality predictions have been made and a rise in maternal mortality of more than 0.5 per 100 000 births is expected by 2005 for both France and the UK. This rise is expected to be due to increasing maternal age and the greater proportion of births to women over the age of 30 years.

It is important to keep the contribution of anaesthesia to overall maternal deaths in perspective. Contrast the one death due directly to anaesthesia in the last triennial report with the international picture. Maternal mortality due to violence against pregnant women, including suicide, homicide and road traffic accidents, is a growing problem in developing countries.[37] In northern Nigeria, maternal mortality is greater than 1000 deaths per 100 000 live births. Important factors contributing to this are:

(1) The Islamic culture, which undervalues women;

(2) A perceived social need for a woman's reproductive capacity to be under strict male control;

(3) The practice of purdah, which restricts women's access to medical care;

(4) Almost universal female illiteracy;

(5) Early pregnancy before pelvic growth is complete;

(6) Harmful traditional medical practices;

(7) Inadequate facilities for obstetric emergencies;

(8) A poor economy;

(9) A political culture marked by rampant inefficiency.[38]

However, we must not be complacent; vigilance, competence and good communications must continue to try to prevent all deaths of mothers. Although some studies are in progress,[39,40] the UK Confidential Enquiries do not address near-miss scenarios and maternal morbidity. It would be possible to review intensive care admissions related to obstetrics by collaboration with the Intensive Care National Audit and Research Centre for identification of cases and review of their outcome.

The Confidential Enquiries will continue and the 1997–99 report will mark 50 years of the Confidential Enquiry by a special issue looking backwards as well as forwards. By this time we should see the advance of information technology, the ability to compare international data and perhaps have a mechanism in place to look at the near misses and thereby learn how to reduce mortality.

References

1 Department of Health. *Why Mothers Die. Report on Confidential Enquiries into Maternal Deaths in the United Kingdom 1994–96.* London: The Stationery Office; 1998

2 World Health Organization. *Revised 1990 Estimates of Maternal Mortality. A New Approach by*

WHO and UNICEF. Geneva: WHO; 1996
3 Ujah, I.A., Uguru, V.E., Aisien, A.O., Sagay, A.S., Otubu, J.A. How safe is motherhood in Nigeria? The trend of maternal mortality in a tertiary health institution. *East Afr Med J* 1999;**76**:436–9
4 AbouZahr, C., Wardlaw, T., Stanton, C., Hill, K. Maternal mortality. *World Health Stat Q* 1996;**49**:77–87
5 Prual, A. Pregnancy and delivery in western Africa: high risk motherhood. *Santé Publique* 1999;**11**:155–65
6 Vork, F.C., Kyanamina, S., van Roosmalen, J. Maternal mortality in rural Zambia. *Acta Obstet Gynecol Scand* 1997;**76**:646–50
7 Ahmed, Y., Mwaba, P., Chintu, C., Grange, J.M., Ustianowski, A., Zumla, A. A study of maternal mortality at the University Teaching Hospital, Lusaka, Zambia: the emergence of tuberculosis as a major non-obstetric cause of maternal death. *Int J Tuberc Lung Dis* 1999;**3**:675–80
8 Department of Health. *A First Class Service – Quality in the New NHS.* London; 1998
9 Hibbard, B., Milner, D. Auditing the audit – the way forward for the Confidential Enquiries into Maternal Deaths in the United Kingdom. *Contemp Rev Obstet Gynaecol* 1995;**7**:97–100
10 Royal College of Obstetricians and Gynaecologists. *Report of the RCOG Working Party on Prophylaxis Against Thromboembolism in Gynaecology and Obstetrics.* London; 1995
11 Hawkins, J.L., Koonin, L.M., Palmer, S.K., Gibbs, C.P. Anaesthesia related deaths during obstetric delivery in the United States 1979–1990. *Anesthesiology* 1997;**86**:277–84
12 Schuitemaker, N., van Roosmalen, J., Dekker, G., van Dongen, P., van Geijn, H., Gravenhorst, J.B. Maternal mortality after cesarean section in the Netherlands. *Acta Obstet Gynecol Scand* 1997;**76**:332–34
13 Vanmaele, L., Noppen, M., Vincken, W., DeCatte, L., Huyghens, L. Transient left heart failure in amniotic fluid embolism. *Intensive Care Med* 1990;**16**:269–71
14 Clark, S.L. New concepts of amniotic fluid embolism: a review. *Obstet Gynecol Surv* 1990;**45**:360–8
15 Lapinsky, S.E. Respiratory care of the critically ill pregnant patient. *Current Opinion in Critical Care* 1996;**3**:1–6
16 Lapinsky, S.E. Critical care management of the obstetric patient. *Can J Anaesth* 1997;**44**:325–9
17 Hinds, C., Watson, D. Obstetric intensive care. *Intensive Care: a Concise Handbook,* 2nd ed. London: W.B. Saunders; 1995. p. 395–406
18 Phelan, J.P. Critical care obstetrics: management of the fetus. *Crit Care Clin* 1991;**7**:917–28
19 Franklin, C.M., Rackow, E.C., Mandani, B. Decreases in mortality on a large urban medical service by facilitating access to critical care. *Arch Intern Med* 1993;**148**:1403–5
20 Kilpatrick, S.J., Matthay, M.A. Obstetric patients requiring critical care: a five year review. *Chest* 1992;**101**:1407–12
21 Lapinsky, S.E., Kruczynski, K., Slutsky, A.S. Critical care in the pregnant patient. *Am J Respir Crit Care Med* 1995;**152**:427–55
22 Umo-Etuk, J., Lumley, J., Holdcroft, A. Critically ill parturient women and admission to intensive care: a 5 year review. *International Journal of Obstetric Anaesthesia* 1996;**5**:79–84
23 Bouvier-Colle, M-H., Salanave, B., Ancel, P-Y., Varnoux, N., Fernandez, H., Papiernik, E. Obstetric patients treated in intensive care units and mortality. *Eur J Obstet Gynecol Reprod Biol* 1996;**65**:121–5
24 Wheatley, E., Farkas, A., Watson, D. Obstetric admissions to an intensive therapy unit. *International Journal of Obstetric Anaesthesia* 1995;**5**:221–4

25 Stephens, I.D. ICU admissions from an obstetric hospital. *Can J Anaesth* 1991;**38**:677–81
26 Bewley, S., Creighton, S. 'Near-miss' obstetric enquiry. *Journal of Obstetrics and Gynaecology* 1997;**17**:26–9
27 Cordingley, J.J., Rubin, A.P. A survey of facilities for high risk women in consultant obstetric units. *International Journal of Obstetric Anaesthesia* 1997;**6**:56–160
28 Royal College of Anaesthetists. *Purchasers Guidelines for Obstetric Anaesthetic and Intensive Care Facilitates*, rev. ed. London; 1998
29 Lewinsohn, G., Herman, A., Leonov, Y., Klinowski, E. Critically ill obstetrical patients: Outcome and predictability. *Crit Care Med* 1994;**22**:1412–14
30 Scarpinato, L., Gerber, D. Critically ill obstetrical patients: outcome and predictability. *Crit Care Med* 1995;**23**:1449–50
31 El-Solh, A.A., Grant, B.J.B. A comparison of severity of illness scoring systems for critically ill obstetric patients. *Chest* 1996;**110**:1299–304
32 Hibbard, B.M., Milner, D. Maternal mortality in Europe. *Eur J Obstet Gynecol Reprod Biol* 1994;**56**:37–41
33 Hibbard, B.M., Milner, D. Reports on Confidential Enquiries into Maternal Deaths: an audit of previous recommendations. *Health Trends* 1994;**26**:26–8
34 Department of Health. *Changing Childbirth: Report of the Expert Maternity Group* (Chairman: Baroness Cumberlege). London: HMSO; 1993
35 May, A.E. The Confidential Enquiry into Maternal deaths 1988–1990. *Br J Anaesth* 1994;**73**:129–31
36 Salanave, B., Bouvier-Colle, M.H. The likely increase in maternal mortality rates in the United Kingdom and in France until 2005. *Paediatr Perinat Epidemiol* 1996;**10**:418–22
37 Rizzi, R.G., Cordoba, R.R., Maguna, J.J. Maternal mortality due to violence. *Int J Gynaecol Obstet* 1998;**61** Suppl 1:S19–24
38 Wall, L.L. Dead mothers and injured wives: the social context of maternal morbidity and mortality among the Hausa of northern Nigeria. *Stud Fam Plann* 1998;**29**:341–59
39 Clark, S.L., Hankins, G.D., Dudley, D.A., Dildy, G.A., Porter, T.F. Amniotic fluid embolus: analysis of the National Registry. *Am J Obstet Gynecol* 1995;**172**:1158–69
40 British Eclampsia Survey Team. BEST Report: eclampsia in the United Kingdom. *BMJ* 1994;**309**:1395–9

Index

abdominal approach, vault prolapse surgery 220–1
abdominal cystocele repair 65
abdominal paravaginal repair of lateral wall defects 65
   results 65–6
abdominoperineal procedure for anterior vaginal wall defects 67
abortion (spontaneous) *see* miscarriage
abortion (therapeutic termination) 301
   maternal suicide 272
   teenage
      consequences 342
      European data 340, 343, 344
accouchement forcé 2-3
acidaemia, fetal, diagnosis 300
actinomycin D *see* vincristine–actinomycin D–cyclophosphamide
Acute Physiology and Chronic Health Evaluation II score in obstetrics 357
acute respiratory distress syndrome and maternal death 355
adenocarcinoma
   cervical
      cervical intraepithelial glandular neoplasia as precursor of 123
      clear-cell variant *see* clear-cell adenocarcinoma
      paediatric 160–3
   vaginal clear-cell *see* clear-cell adenocarcinoma
adenocarcinoma *in situ*
   cervical, treatment 127–30
   vulval 139
adenomyomas, rectovaginal 226–7, 234
adolescents
   gynaecological cancer 157–69
   pregnancy 328–48
      consequences 341–2
      epidemiology/statistics 338–9
      interventions 342–7
      suicide in/after 272
adrenal hyperplasia, congenital 147, 153-4
β-adrenergic agonists *see* tocolytics
adult (acute) respiratory distress syndrome and maternal death 355
aerobics in pregnancy 256, 259
age
   gestational, estimation 290
   maternal, and shoulder dystocia 326
airway management, *ex utero* intrapartum 304
akinesia, fetal 284

all-fours position, in shoulder dystocia 320
alveolar bone loss and HRT 198
amenorrhoea, achievement in period-free HRT 98-103
amniocentesis 295–8
amnio-infusion 298
amniotic fluid drainage 298
anabolic steroids and pregnancy 257
anaemia, fetal, treatment 301
anaesthesia and maternal death 349–60
anaesthetists involved in resuscitation, maternal deaths with 352
anal canal, lumps protruding from 177
anal incontinence (faecal incontinence) 170–87
   causes 172–5
      obstetric *see* childbirth
   clinical features 176–7
anal manometry 178
anal sphincters
   abnormalities causing incontinence 173–5
      management 179–80, 181–3, 184
      obstetric trauma 31, 32, 174, 180, 181–3
   anatomy/physiology 170, 171
   biofeedback exercises 179
androgen insensitivity syndromes 147, 154
annual appraisal 48
anorectum 25–34
   anatomy/physiology 170–1
   cancer, causing incontinence 174
      see also colorectal cancer
   congenital anomalies
      associated genital tract anomalies 150–1
      treatment affecting sexual function 148–9
   sensation 178
   see also references under anus
anovulation, treatment 84
antenatal booking, psychiatric aspects 273–4
antenatal diagnosis 295–302, 310–23
   congenital adrenal hyperplasia 147–8
   invasive (= fetal cell sampling) 295–302
   minimally 310–23
anus *see* anorectum *and entries under* anus
APACHE II score in obstetrics 357
appraisal, annual 48
arm, posterior, delivery in shoulder dystocia 331
arrhythmias, fetal 301
   hydrops and 278, 283
artificial (intrauterine) insemination 80

361

before IVF 81
assisted reproduction *see* infertility, treatment
asthma and maternal death 355
athletes, pregnant *see* exercise
audit (for implementing and monitoring change) 51
   infertility treatment 83

Barnes, Robert 4–5
Beckwith–Wiedemann syndrome 158
beech extraction in placenta praevia 5–6
benefits (in economic analysis), infertility and 72
   see also cost benefit analysis
beta-adrenergic agonists *see* tocolytics
biofeedback exercises, anal sphincters/pelvic floor 179
biopsy
   cervical intraepithelial glandular neoplasia 126
   placental 298–300
bipolar disorder and maternal suicide 273
bipolar version, Braxton Hicks' 5–6
birthweight of 4000 g or more *see* macrosomia
bladder
   development 145
   developmental anomalies 145
      exstrophy 146, 150
      presenting as incontinence 147
      surgery and its obstetric complications 147, 148
   herniation into vagina *see* cystocele
   support mechanisms 62
   see also vesico-amniotic shunt *and entries under* cysto-
bladder neck surgery
   for congenital anomalies, and its obstetric complications 147, 148
   for stress incontinence 190
bleeding in period-free HRT
   causes 102
   patterns 98–103
   see also haemorrhage
bleomycin *see* cisplatin–etoposide–bleomycin; cisplatin–vincristine–bleomycin
blood (fetal)
   sampling 300–2
   tests in hydrops 281
blood (maternal)
   fetal cells in, recovery 315–19, 319–20
   tests in fetal hydrops 281
   volume in pregnancy and exercise 251
blood transfusion *see* transfusion
BMA and surrogacy 240–1
bone anchor fixation for bladder neck support 147–8
bone loss/density decrease
   HRT and 107–9, 198
   pregnancy and exercise and 257–8
botryoid sarcoma, paediatric genital 157–9
bowel
   cancer *see* cancer
   as cause of faecal incontinence 173
   endometriosis *see* rectovaginal endometriosis
   fistula *see* fistula
   function, questionnaire 176
   see also specific parts
brachial plexus injury, shoulder dystocia 332, 333
brachytherapy, rhabdomyosarcoma, paediatric genital 160
brain and HRT 199–200

Braxton Hicks' bipolar version 5–6
BRCA1/2 and ovarian cancer 91–2
breast cancer and HRT 201
   period-free HRT risk 109
   previous cancer contraindicating HRT 110
British Medical Association and surrogacy 240–1
Burch colposuspension 188
   laparoscopic 189–90

caesarean section
   elite athlete 258
   macrosomia 328
   in placenta praevia, history 7–8
   rates, NCT concerns 57
   vaginal delivery after *see* childbirth
   very preterm babies 292
cancer (gynaecological) 89–97, 137–43, 157–69
   breast *see* breast cancer
   cervical *see* cervical cancer
   childhood/adolescence 157–69
   endometrial, HRT and 201–2
      period-free HRT risk 104
      previous cancer and HRT use 110, 199
   ovarian *see* ovarian cancer
   uterine, embolisation 213
   vaginal, hormones and 139
   vulval, hormones and 138–9, 160
cancer (non-gynaecological), bowel
   anorectal cancer causing incontinence 174
   colorectal cancer and HRT 199
carcinoma *see specific tissue/organs and histological type*
Cardiovascular Health Study in Australia 198
cardiovascular system
   disease (fetal), hydrops associated with 278, 283
   disease (maternal)
      deaths and 355
      HRT and risk of 106–7, 197
   in pregnancy 250
      and exercise 251
central venous pressure and fetal hydrops 277, 281
cephalic replacement in shoulder dystocia 331–2
cerebrovascular disease and HRT 197–8
cervical cancer (carcinoma) 137–8, 160–3
   cervical intraepithelial glandular neoplasia as precursor of adenocarcinoma 123
   hormones and 137–8
   paediatric 160–3
cervical conisation *see* conisation
cervical intraepithelial glandular neoplasia 119–36
   aetiology 123
   detection 123–7
   differential diagnosis 122
   histopathology 119–22
   as precursor of adenocarcinoma 123
   treatment/follow-up 127–31
cervical intraepithelial neoplasia
   adolescent 162–3
   colposcopy 125–6
cervical swabs/flushes, fetal cell sampling from 310–15, 319
change, audit of *see* audit
Changing Childbirth 54–5, 58
chemotherapy (gynaecological cancer)
   childhood cancer

ovarian cancer 164–5
rhabdomyosarcoma 159, 160
ovarian cancer
neoadjuvant 95
paediatric 164–5
childbirth (incl. vaginal delivery)
anogenital trauma 31–2, 174, 181–3
faecal incontinence with (and its management) 31, 32, 174, 180, 181–3
prevention 184
with caesarean section in previous pregnancy 263–9
decision analysis 264
outcome of attempted vaginal delivery 263
predicting likelihood of vaginal delivery 264–5
predicting scar integrity 265
risk management 266
safeguarding scar integrity 265–6
counselling in early preterm labour 289
elite athlete and 258
ex utero treatment during 304
induction *see* induction
mechanism of normal delivery vs. shoulder dystocia 324–5
see also labour
Childlessness Overcome Through Surrogacy (COTS) 243, 244
children, gynaecological cancer 157–69
see also adolescents; neonates
Chlamydia infection, population screening 81
chorionic villus sampling 298–300
transabdominal technique 299
transcervical, vs transcervical swabs and flushes 315, 319
chromosomal disorders
antenatal diagnosis (incl. karyotyping)
amniocentesis 296
blood samples 300
chorionic villus/placental biopsy 298–9, 300
fetal hydrops and 278, 283–4
cisplatin–etoposide–bleomycin (PEB), paediatric ovarian cancer 164, 165
cisplatin–vincristine–bleomycin (PVB), paediatric ovarian cancer 164, 165
clavicular fracture in shoulder dystocia 331
clear-cell adenocarcinoma
cervical 160–2
paediatric 160–2
vaginal 160–2
diethylstilboestrol and 139, 160, 161
paediatric 160–2
cleidotomy in shoulder dystocia 331
clinical effectiveness 51–2
clinical guidelines 49–50
infertility care 82–3
cloaca, development 145–6
anomalies/malformations 146, 150
clomiphene 84
controversies 80
ovarian cancer and 140
cognitive function and HRT 199–200
colon (in faecal incontinence)
causes relating to 173
management 178–9
transit studies 178

colonoscopy in incontinence 178
colorectal cancer and HRT 199
see also anorectum, cancer
colorectal specialist, faecal incontinence and referral to 183–4
colpocleisis 28–9
colporrhaphy, anterior 64
urinary function after 68
colposcopy, cervical intraepithelial neoplasia and intraepithelial glandular neoplasia 125–6
colposuspension
in stress incontinence 188–90
in vaginal vault prolapse 220
conception rates, teenage 339
condoms, teenagers 343–5
Confidential Enquiries into Maternal Deaths (CEMD) 349
suicide and 270, 273, 274
Confidential Enquiries into Stillbirth and Deaths in Infancy (CESDI)
macrosomia and 325
shoulder dystocia and 333
management of 332
maternal obesity and 326
congenital adrenal hyperplasia 147, 153–4
congenital hydrothorax 283
congenital urogenital anomalies 144–56
conisation, cervical 128–9
cytological follow-up 130–1
constipation
causes 175
investigation/treatment 183
consultant, in consultant-based service 36
advantages/disadvantages 39–40
input 42–3
timetable/workload 36–7
consultant-based service (Hinchingbrooke Hospital) 36–44
advantages/disadvantages 37–41
history 35–6
protocols 40–1
staffing structure 36
consumer's right, evidence-based health care 52–60
continence
faecal
loss *see* anal incontinence
normal 171–2
urinary, loss, *see* urinary incontinence
continuing medical education 47
continuing professional development 47–8
contraception
oral *see* oral contraceptives
teenage 343–5
cordocentesis
sampling site 301
technique 301–2
coronary heart disease and HRT 106–7, 197
corticosteroids and preterm delivery 290–1
cost(s)
bleeding in 'no-bleed' HRT 103
infertility 71
very preterm babies 292–3
cost benefit analysis, infertility 73, 75
cost consequence analysis, infertility 74
cost effectiveness analysis, infertility 74, 75, 83–5

cost minimisation, infertility 72–3
cost needed to treat, infertility 74–5
cost utility analysis, infertility 73
COTS (Childlessness Overcome Through Surrogacy) 243, 244
counselling
　early preterm labour 289
　fetal hydrops 280, 282
　surrogate pregnancy 243–4
Crohn's disease 25–6
culdoplasty 218–19, 222
cycling in pregnancy 256
cyclophosphamide *see* vincristine–actinomycin D–cyclophosphamide
cystocele, surgery 65
　historical aspect 61
cystopexy 221
cystoplasty, obstetric implications 148
cytogenetics *see* chromosomal disorders
cytology, cervical intraepithelial glandular neoplasia 124–5
　in follow-up after treatment 130–1
cytoreductive surgery, ovarian cancer 94

death *see* mortality
debulking surgery, ovarian cancer 94-5
decision analysis, infertility 74
defaecation, normal 171–2
　see also anal incontinence
Delancey, JOL 62
dementia and HRT 199
depression and maternal suicide
　chronic 270
　postnatal 273
deprivation and teenage pregnancy 340–1
descending perineum syndrome 175
dexamethasone, fetal therapy in congenital adrenal hyperplasia 147–8
diabetes, maternal, shoulder dystocia and 326
diet and exercise in pregnancy 259
diethylstilboestrol
　cervical cancer and 160, 161
　vaginal cancer and 139, 160, 161
DNA tests, antenatal
　amniocentesis 296
　blood samples
　　fetal 300
　　maternal 315–17, 319
　chorionic villus sampling 299
　transcervical samples 311–14
doctors
　in consultant-based service 36
　mentoring and support of 48
　see also general practitioners
droloxifene 203
drugs
　deliberate overdose in pregnancy 271–2
　very preterm labour/birth 290–1
dysgerminoma, paediatric 163
dystocia *see* shoulder dystocia

eclampsia, maternal death 352
economics, health, infertility 71–88
　see also cost; socioeconomic aspects

education (professionals), continuing medical 47
education (public) and teenage pregnancy
　consequences of pregnancy for education 342
　influence of education on pregnancy rates 341
　sex education 346–7
Effective Care in Pregnancy 55
embolisation, uterine artery 209–14
embryo transfer, surrogacy 244
embryonal carcinoma 163
emergency contraception, teenage 345
employment and teenage pregnancy rates 341
endoanal ultrasound in incontinence 178
endocervical curettage, cervical intraepithelial glandular neoplasia 126–7
endocervical swabs/flushes, fetal cell sampling from 310–15, 319
endocrine investigations, infertility 84
endodermal sinus (yolk sac) tumours, paediatric
　ovarian 163
　vaginal 165
endometriosis 226–38
　HRT and history of 110
　rectovaginal 226–38
　treatment 84, 232–6
endometrium in HRT 199
　cancer *see* cancer
　in period-free HRT
　　bleeding from atrophic endometrium 103
　　histology 103-5
endopelvic fascia and anterior vaginal prolapse 62–3
enterocele 215
　aetiology 218
epidural/spinal combined anaesthesia, deaths 351
epigastric vessels, laparoscopic injury 232
episiotomy 31–2, 183, 184
　in shoulder dystocia 320
epispadias, female 147
erythroleukaemia 283
ethical issues, surrogate pregnancy 239–40
ethnicity and maternal suicide 272
Europe, teenage pregnancy statistics 339–41
European Organization for Research and Treatment of Cancer (EORTC), ovarian cancer
　debulking surgery 94–5
　neoadjuvant chemotherapy 95
European Women's International Study of Long Duration Oestrogen after Menopause (WISDOM) 197, 201
European Working Hours Directive and consultant-based services 41–2
evidence-based clinical guidelines, national 50
evidence-based health care, consumer's right 52–60
ex utero intrapartum treatment 304
exercise in pregnancy (incl. sport/athletics) 247–62
　advice/management
　　American College of Obstetricians and Gynaecologists guidelines 259
　　elite athletes 257–8
　　specific sports 255–6
　benefits 252–3
　discontinuation and contraindications 254–5
　history of 248–9
　legal aspects 258–9
　outcome of pregnancy and effects of 253

physiological changes 250–2
postpartum exercise 258
prevention of disease and 253
psychological effects 253, 257
safety considerations 252–3, 253–5
eye, HRT effects 200

faecal incontinence *see* anal incontinence
fallopian tubes (in infertility)
patency assessment 84
treatment of disease 84
familial ovarian cancer, prophylactic oophorectomy 91–2
fascia, endopelvic, in vault prolapse
in anterior vaginal wall prolapse 62–3
in pelvic floor repair 218–19
females, external genital development 146
anomalies 147
fertility
fibroid embolisation
efficacy regarding fertility 211, 213
preservation of fertility 209
problems *see* infertility
teenage fertility rates 343, 344
fetofetal transfusion syndrome 303
fetomaternal haemorrhage causing hydrops 282–3
fetoscopy 303
fetus
age or size estimation 290
diagnosis of disorders (incl. cell sampling) *see* antenatal diagnosis
heart *see* heart
hydrops *see* hydrops
loss/death *see* abortion; miscarriage; mortality; stillbirth
shoulder dystocia effects 332–3
as tampon in placenta praevia 5–6
therapies (incl. surgery) 298, 301, 303–4
viability limits *see* preterm infant
fibroid embolisation 209–14
FISH *see* fluorescence in situ hybridisation
fistula, intestinal–gynaecological 26-8, 32
faecal incontinence 174
sexual function and treatment of 149
fluorescence in situ hybridisation (FISH), antenatal 296
maternal blood samples 316
transcervical samples 312–14
fluorescent activated cell sorting, fetal cells in maternal blood 316
folate (in pregnancy) 15–24
dietary requirements 19–21
recommended daily allowance (RDA) 18, 20, 21, 22
historical perspectives 16–17
metabolism 16
defects 17–18
neural tube defects and 17–18
structure 15–16
forceps, scalp, Willet's 6–7
forceps delivery, perineal trauma 182–3

General Medical Council (GMC), professional regulations and 47–8
general practitioners, consultant-based service

advantages/disadvantages for 37–8
genetic metabolic disease and fetal hydrops 279
see also chromosomal disorders
genitourinary system, development 144–7
anomalies 144–56
germ-cell tumours, paediatric 163
treatment 165
gestational age or size estimation 290
gestational surrogacy *see in vitro* fertilisation
Giffard, William 2
glucocorticoids and preterm delivery 290–1
glucose-6-phosphate dehydrogenase deficiency 283
gonadal development 144
gonadotrophins and ovarian cancer 139, 140
government (UK) and surrogate pregnancy 241–2
grafts, anterior vaginal wall prolapse 65
granulosa cell tumours, paediatric 163
gynaecologist, role in faecal incontinence 183–4

haemodynamics in pregnancy and exercise 251
haemoglobin (in fetus)
concentration 300
embryonic, as fetal cell markers 320
haemopoietic stem/progenitor cells, fetal, growth/culture 320
haemorrhage
fetomaternal, causing hydrops 282–3
maternal, causing death 352
see also bleeding
head–body disproportion, fetal *see* macrosomia
health economics, infertility 71–88
health services, sexual, young people 345–6
heart (fetal)
blood samples from 301, 302
disease, hydrops associated with 278, 283
rate, monitoring in very preterm labour 291
heart (women)
disease (women), HRT and 106–7, 197
output, in pregnancy 250
and exercise 251
Heart and Estrogen/Progestin Replacement Study (HERS) 197
hepatic tissue *see* liver
hermaphroditism, true 154
high density lipoprotein (HDL) HRT 106–7
high uterosacral ligament suspension 218, 222
Hinchingbrooke Hospital *see* consultant-based service
historical perspectives
anterior vaginal wall prolapse 61–2
consultant-based service 35–6
folate in pregnancy 16–17
placenta praevia management 1–14
rectovaginal endometriosis 226
sport and women 247–8
and pregnancy 248–9
homocysteine, toxicity 18–19
hormonal emergency contraception, teenagers 345
hormone(s), gynaecological cancer and 137–43
hormone replacement therapy (HRT) 98–118, 196–208
adverse effects/risks 105–6, 109–10, 201–2
cervical neoplasia 138
ovarian neoplasia 140–1
benefits 106–9, 197–201

future prospects 202–3
long-term 196–208
period-free/continuous combined 98–118
   alternatives to 110
   bleeding *see* bleeding
   bone conservation 107–9
   clinical scenarios 110
   discontinuation 105–6
   endometrial histology 103–4
   metabolic effects 106–7
   symptom control 105
hospital, consultant-based service
   advantages/disadvantages for 38–9
host surrogacy *see in vitro* fertilisation
Human and Fertilisation and Embryology Act (1990) and surrogacy 241–2
Human Fertilisation and Embryology Authority 243
human papillomavirus (HPV) and cervical neoplasia 123
   hormones and 137
hydrops, fetal 277–87
   definition/aetiology 277
   diagnosis 280
   incidence 277
   management 280–4
   pathophysiology 277
   risks
      for fetus 277–8
      for mother 280
hydrothorax, congenital 283
hymen, imperforate 152
hyperhomocysteinaemia 18–19
hyperplasia
   congenital adrenal 147, 153
   endometrial, HRT and 103–4, 201–2
hypertension, pulmonary, maternal death 352
hypoxia, fetal, diagnosis 300
hysterectomy
   abdominal, cystocele repair at time of 65
   cervical intraepithelial glandular lesions 127–8
   fibroid embolisation leading to 211
   vault prolapse after *see* vagina, vault prolapse

ileopectineal ligament, ipsilateral, in laparoscopic colposuspension 189
ileovaginal fistula 26
iliac artery, internal, in sacrospinous fixation 219
immune fetal hydrops 277, 278
in situ hybdridisation, fluorescence *see* fluorescence in situ hybridisation
in vitro fertilisation (IVF) 80
   artificial insemination before 81
   monitoring of 83
   surrogacy involving (host/gestational/full surrogacy) 240
      guidelines 243
      outcomes 244, 245
      procedure 244
incontinence *see* anal incontinence; urinary incontinence
incremental cost effectiveness ratio (cost effectiveness analysis), infertility 74, 75
induction of labour in shoulder dystocia
   elective, in prevention of dystocia 328

   as risk factor for dystocia 326–7
infection (fetal)
   blood tests in diagnosis of 303
   hydrops due to 279, 284
      diagnosis of infection 280–1
infection (women)
   fibroid embolisation and risk of 211, 212
   maternal, leading to fetal infection, diagnosis 301
infertility 71–88
   diagnostic tests 83–4
   dropout rates 80
   economic analysis 71–88
   outcome
      evaluating 79–80
      measures, determining 78–9
   surrogacy in 242–3
   treatments (assisted reproduction) 84–5, 242–3
      impact of new technologies 77–8
      ovarian cancer risk 139–40
      over treatment 81
      perinatal costs of 85
   type of clinic offering services 81
   unexplained 84–5
information, evidence-based, consumer access to 57–8
inherited disease *see* chromosomal disorders; genetic metabolic disease
injury *see* trauma
inspection
   anal incontinence 176–7, 184
   rectovaginal endometriosis 230
instrumental delivery, perineal trauma 182–3
   prevention 184
intensive care, maternal deaths involving 354–7
International Olympic Committee 248
intersex 153–4
intestine *see* bowel
intracytoplasmic sperm injection (ICSI), cost utility analysis 72
intraepithelial neoplasia of cervix *see* cervical intraepithelial glandular neoplasia; cervical intraepithelial neoplasia
intrauterine devices containing progestogen (in HRT) 202
intrauterine insemination *see* artificial insemination
invasive antenatal diagnosis *see* antenatal diagnosis
IUDs containing progestogen (in HRT) 202
IVF *see in vitro* fertilisation

jogging in pregnancy 256
joint disease and HRT 200

karyotyping *see* chromosomal disorders
keratoconjunctivitis sicca and HRT 200
Kerr, Munro 8
kidney, development 144
   anomalies 147
      fetal hydrops and 278
Kitzinger, Shirley 249

labour
   early preterm
      counselling 289
      delaying 290
      fetal heart rate monitoring 291

induced *see* induction
  prolonged/delayed, shoulder dystocia risk 327
labour ward, paediatrician role with very preterm babies 292
laparoscopy
  diagnostic, rectovaginal endometriosis 231–2
  therapeutic *see* minimally invasive surgery
laparotomy, rectovaginal endometriosis 233
large loop excision of transformation zone 129–30
laser ablation of vascular anastomoses between twin fetuses 303
law *see* legal issues
left lateral position in shoulder dystocia 329
legal issues
  exercise and pregnancy 258–9
  shoulder dystocia 333
  surrogate pregnancy 241–2, 243–4
leiomyomas (fibroids), embolisation 209–14
Leisure World Cohort 198
Leydig cells in development 144
Li–Fraumeni syndrome 158
limb deficiency, chorionic villus sampling causing 300
lipid profiles and HRT 106–7
liver, fetal
  blood sampling 301
  hydrops and disorders of 279
LLETZ (large loop excision of transformation zone) 129–30
low density lipoprotein (LDL) HRT 106–7
lung function/disease *see* respiratory system
lymphadenectomy (in gynaecological cancer)
  cervical clear-cell adenocarcinoma 162
  ovarian cancer, laparoscopic 93

Macafee, Charles 8–9
McCall's culdoplasty 218–19, 222
McRobert's manoeuvre 329–30, 332
macrosomia, fetal 325–6, 327–9
  detection 327–8
  previous, as risk factor for shoulder dystocia 326
magnetic activated cell sorting, fetal cells in maternal blood 316, 317
magnetic resonance imaging, fibroid embolisation 211
male
  external genitalia, development 146
  fetus, shoulder dystocia risk 326
  infertility, diagnostic tests 82–3
  sexual health services for young men 346
malignant tumours *see* cancer
manic–depressive illness and maternal suicide 273
manometry, anal 178
Markov's model 74
maternal matters *see* mother
maternity services, consumer's right to evidence-based care 52–60
Mauriceau, François 3
Mayer-Rokitansky-Küster-Hauser syndrome 153
media and teenage sexuality 343
medico-legal issues *see* legal issues
medroxyprogesterone acetate (MPA) in period-free HRT 99
melanoma and HRT 199
menopausal symptom control, period-free HRT 105
mental disorder *see* psychiatric disorder

mentoring of doctors 48
mesonephric duct 144, 145
metabolic disease, genetic, fetal hydrops and 279
metabolic effects
  HRT (oestrogen and progestogen) 106–7
  oestrogen deficiency 197
metastases, laparoscopic ovarian cancer surgery and risk of 90–1
methionine synthase and neural tube defects 18
methylenetetrahydrofolate reductase (MTHFR) 16
  defects in 10, 18–19
midwives
  in consultant-based service 36
  psychiatry and 274
minimally invasive antenatal diagnosis 310–23
minimally invasive surgery
  ovarian cancer 89–97
  rectovaginal endometriosis 233–5
  stress incontinence 188–95
  vaginal vault prolapse 219, 221, 222
miscarriage (fetal loss)
  maternal suicide 272
  parvovirus B19 and 284
  procedural risk
    amniocentesis 297
    blood sampling 302
    chorionic villus sampling 299–300
mitral valve disease and maternal death 352
Mitrofanoff procedure 148
monoclonal antibody, rhesus D 320
mortality/death (maternal)
  anaesthesia and 349-60
  definitions 350
  suicide 270–6
mortality/death (perinatal)
  shoulder dystocia and 326, 333
  vaginal delivery following caesarean section 266
  very preterm infant 288–9
mother
  death *see* mortality
  fetal cells in maternal circulation, recovery 315–19, 319–20
  fetal hydrops and
    maternal blood tests 281
    maternal causation 279
    maternal outlook 280
  in shoulder dystocia
    consequences for mother 332
    disorders causing dystocia 326
mother-and-baby inpatient units 274–5
Müllerian (paramesonephric) duct development 145, 146
  anomalies 146, 152, 153
Mülleriosis 329
multiple pregnancy
  amniocentesis 296–7
  laser ablation of vascular anastomoses 303
  very preterm delivery 292
musculoskeletal system
  injury in shoulder dystocia 332
  pregnancy and exercise-related alterations 252
myogenic faecal incontinence 174
  treatment 180

National Childbirth Trust
   caesarean section rates and 57
   Changing Childbirth and 54
National Health and Nutrition Examination Study 198
National Health Service, infertility services 81
needles (in invasive fetal procedures)
   amniocentesis 297
      twin pregnancy 296
   blood sampling 302
   chorionic villus sampling 299
negligence and exercise in pregnancy 258
neoadjuvant chemotherapy, ovarian cancer 95
neonates
   amniocentesis complications affecting 297–8
   mortality in vaginal delivery following caesarean section 266
   urogenital sinus persistence 152
   very preterm *see* preterm infant, very
neoplasms *see* cancer; tumours
nerve damage in shoulder dystocia 332–3
neural tube defects and folate 17–18
neurogenic faecal incontinence 173–4
   management 180
neurological damage in shoulder dystocia 332–3
neurological function and HRT 199–200
NHS, infertility services 81
Nigeria, maternal mortality 358
norethisterone acetate (NETA) in period-free HRT 99, 100
   dose effects 101
      adverse reactions 106
      bone conservation 107–9
      symptom control 105
number needed to treat, cost needed to treat derived from 74–5

obesity, maternal, and shoulder dystocia 326
obstetrician, faecal incontinence prevention 184–5
ocular effects of HRT 200
oedema, pulmonary, tocolytic-induced 355
oestrogen deficiency, metabolic effects 197
oestrogen in period free HRT (incl. oestradiol) 99
   dose/dose effects
      adverse effects/risks 106, 109
      bone conservation 107
      metabolic effects 106
      reduction 101
      symptom control 105
oestrogen receptor modulators, selective 202–3
oophorectomy
   bilateral, HRT following 141
   laparoscopic prophylactic 91–2
   radical 30–1, 32
ophthalmological effects of HRT 200
oral contraceptives
   cervical neoplasia risk 137
   teenagers 343, 344
      emergency pills 345
osteoporosis
   HRT and 107–9, 198
   pregnancy and exercise and 257–8
ovarian cancer
   hormones and 139–40
   paediatric 163–5

surgery 30–1, 32
   minimal access 89–97
ovarian endometriosis, bowel involvement 227
ovarian failure in fibroid embolisation 211
ovarian tumours, paediatric benign 163
ovariectomy *see* oophorectomy
overdose, antenatal, deliberate 271–2
ovulation induction therapy and ovarian cancer 139–40
oxytocin in labour, caesarean scar and 266

$p53$, HPV and cervical neoplasia and 123
paediatrician role with very preterm babies 292
paediatrics, *see* adolescents; children; neonates
Paget's disease of vulva 139
palpation
   anal incontinence 177
   rectovaginal endometriosis 231
para-aortic lymphadenectomy, laparoscopic 93
paramesonephric duct *see* Müllerian (paramesonephric) duct
Paré, Ambrose 3
parity and shoulder dystocia 326
parvovirus B19 284
patient in consultant-based service, advantages/disadvantages 37–8
PEB (cisplatin–etoposide–bleomycin), paediatric ovarian cancer 164, 165
pelvic examination
   anal incontinence 176–7, 184
   rectovaginal endometriosis 230
pelvic fascia *see* fascia, endopelvic
pelvic floor
   anatomy/physiology 170–1
   biofeedback exercises 179
   deficiency, total 29
   repair, post-hysterectomy vault prolapse 218–22
pelvic-floor clinic 185
pelvic inlet, shoulder dystocia and 325
pelvic lymphadenectomy, cervical clear-cell adenocarcinoma 162
Pelvic Organ Prolapse Quantitation system 216
Pereyra procedure 190, 221
performance appraisal, annual 48
perinatal mortality, vaginal delivery following caesarean section 266
perineal body 31
perineum
   descending (syndrome) 175
   obstetric trauma/tears 31, 32
      classification 182
      instrumental delivery 182–3
      prevention 184
   single orifice in cloacal anomaly 150, 151
peripheral nerve damage in shoulder dystocia 332–3
peritoneal endometriosis, pathogenesis 229
physical exercise in pregnancy *see* exercise
physiological changes, pregnancy and exercise 250–2
phyto-oestrogens 203
placenta
   abruption, folate and 16
   biopsy 298-300
   fetal hydrops related to 279
   localisation 9–10

placenta praevia 1–14
  current controversies 10
  evolution of management 1–14
  pathophysiology 2
plasma volume in pregnancy and exercise 251
platelet transfusion, fetal 301
platinum-based regimens, paediatric ovarian cancer 164, 165
pleural effusions and fetal hydrops 281
pleuroamniotic shunt 303
poisoning, antenatal, deliberate 271–2
polymerase chain reaction, antenatal
  amniocentesis 296
  infection diagnosis 280–1
  maternal blood samples 315, 319
  transcervical sampling 311–14
population (in infertility)
  pregnancy rates assessment by technique vs. 80
  screening for *Chlamydia* infection 81
port site metastases, laparoscopic ovarian cancer surgery 91
Portal, Paul 2
post-anal repair 180
postpartum period
  exercise in 258
    elite athlete 258
  psychiatric illness and suicide risk 270–1, 274
post-term pregnancy, shoulder dystocia risk 326–7
pouch of Douglas
  rectal prolapse and vaginal pulsion and 29
  in rectovaginal endometriosis
    in diagnostic laparoscopy 232
    palpation 231
poverty (deprivation) and teenage pregnancy 340–1
pregnancy
  cervical neoplasia risk 137
  consumer's right to evidence-based health care 52–60
  costs after successful infertility treatment 85
  exercise in *see* exercise
  folate in *see* folate
  following fibroid embolisation 211, 213
  loss *see* abortion; miscarriage; stillbirth
  lower urinary tract reconstruction and 148
  multiple/twin *see* multiple pregnancy
  prolonged, shoulder dystocia risk 326–7
  rates in infertility treatment
    assessment by population vs. technique 80
    background rates 79–80
  suicide in 272–3
  surrogate *see* surrogate pregnancy
  teenage *see* adolescents
premature infant *see* preterm infant
prenatal diagnosis *see* antenatal diagnosis
preterm infant, very 288–94
  cost implications 292–3
  counselling 289–90
  gestational age or size 290
  management/outcome 290–2
  place of birth 290
  survival rates 288–9, 291
preterm labour, early *see* labour
proctogram 178
proctoscopy, anal incontinence 177

professional development, continuing 47–8
professional regulations 47
progestogen (in HRT)
  dose effect (in period-free HRT) 101
    adverse reactions/risks 106, 109
    bone conservation 107–9
    metabolic effects 106
    symptom control 105
  intrauterine devices containing 202
  in period-free HRT 99
    dose effects 101
Prolene tape 191–2
prostheses, anterior vaginal wall prolapse 65
psychiatric disorder/illness and suicide risk
  chronic 270
  postnatal 270–1, 274
  recommendations regarding 273–5
psychological effects
  exercise in pregnancy 253, 256
  shoulder dystocia upon mother 332
pubo-urethral ligament plication 221
pudendal nerve terminal motor latency 178
pulmonary function/disease *see* respiratory system
pulmonary hypertension, maternal death 352
punch biopsy, cervical intraepithelial glandular neoplasia 126
PVB (cisplatin–vincristine–bleomycin), paediatric ovarian cancer 164, 165

quality of life
  HRT and 200
  infertility and 72

race/ethnicity and maternal suicide 272
radiologist, fibroid embolisation 210
radiotherapy, rhabdomyosarcoma, paediatric genital 160
raloxifene 202–3
Raz procedure 190
Read, Dick 249
rectocele 30, 175
rectopexy 29, 30, 179
rectovaginal endometriosis 226–38
  clinical features 229–30
  clinical literature 226–7
  differential diagnosis 229
  examination 220–1
  history 226
  investigations 231–2
  pathogenesis 228–9
  pathology 227–8
rectum 25–34
  lumps protruding from anus 177
  prolapse 174
    surgery 29, 30, 179
  see also anorectum; colorectal specialist *and entries under* procto-
regulations, professional 47
religion and teenage pregnancy rates 341
renal system *see* kidney
Report on Confidential Enquiries into Maternal Deaths (CEMD), suicide and 270, 273, 274
respiratory distress syndrome, acute, maternal death and 355
respiratory system (lungs etc.)

fetal
  gas exchange, *ex utero* intrapartum treatment
    maintaining 304
      hydrops and disorders of 278, 283
  maternal
    death and disorders of 355
    in pregnancy and exercise 251
resuscitation, maternal deaths with anaesthetists involved in 352
retroperitoneal approach, ovarian cancer surgery 30–1, 32
revalidation 49
reverse transcriptase-PCR, fetal RhD genotype prediction 319
rhabdomyosarcoma, paediatric genital 157–9
rhesus D
  isoimmunisation risk with amniocentesis 298
  in prenatal diagnosis 320
    fetal genotype prediction from maternal blood samples 316–19
rheumatic disease and HRT 200
Rigby, Edward 3-4
RNA, Rhesus D, detection from maternal blood samples 317–19
Royal College of Obstetricians and Gynaecologists
  annual appraisal and 48
  clinical guidelines and 49-50
    infertility care 83
  mentoring and 48
  professional regulations and 48
  revalidation and 49
running (jogging) in pregnancy 256

sacrocolpopexy 30, 220–1, 222
sacrospinous ligament fixation
  vaginal hysterectomy 218
  vaginal vault prolapse 219, 222
sacrouterine fold (uterosacral ligament) suspension, high 218, 222
sarcoma, uterine, embolisation 213
sarcoma botryoides, paediatric genital 157–9
screening
  ovarian cancer 92
  population, *Chlamydia* infection 81
selective oestrogen receptor modulators 202–3
self-harm, women
  antenatal 271–2
  postnatal 270–1
semen analysis 82–3
senior house officers in consultant-based service 36
  advantages/disadvantages 39
sensation, anorectal 178
Sertoli cells in development 144
sex (gender), fetal, shoulder dystocia risk 326
sex-cord stromal tumours, paediatric 163
  treatment 165
sex duct development 144
sex education 346–7
sex steroids, cervical neoplasia risk 137
sexual activity, teenage
  conflicting/confusing messages about 343
  delaying/discouraging 342
sexual ambiguity 153–4
sexual function

congenital anorectal anomalies and 148–9
HRT and 200–1
sexual health services, young people 345–6
sexuality, teenage, teenage attitudes
  pregnancy rates and 341
  promoting more open attitudes 343
shift systems, consultant-based service 42
shoulder dystocia 324–37
  associated factors 325–7
    previous dystocia 326
  definition 324
  fetal consequences 332–3
  incidence 324
  management 329-32
  maternal consequences 332
  mechanism of normal delivery and 324–5
  medico-legal aspects 333
  prediction/prevention 327–8, 327–9
sigmoidoscopy, anal incontinence 177
Simpson, James Young 2
Sims' speculum, anterior vaginal wall examination 63
skeletal system *see* musculoskeletal system
social services and surrogacy 242
socioeconomic aspects in teenage pregnancy
  consequences of pregnancy 342
  as factor in pregnancy rates 340–1
sonography *see* ultrasound
soy phyto-oestrogens 203
specialist training 44
sperm (in infertility treatment)
  assessment 84
  dysfunction, treatment 84
  intracytoplasmic injection (ICSI), cost utility analysis 72
sphincters, anal *see* anal sphincters
spinal/epidural combined anaesthesia, deaths 351
sport in pregnancy *see* exercise
squamous cells (cervical) of unknown significance, atypical (ASCUS), adolescent 162–3
SRY 144
staging
  ovarian cancer, laparoscopic 92–3
  rhabdomyosarcoma, child 158, 159
Stamey procedure 190
stem cells, fetal haemopoietic, growth/culture 320
steroids *see* anabolic steroids; corticosteroids
stillbirths, maternal suicide 272
stress incontinence 188–95
  HRT and 200
  surgery 221
    minimal access 188–95
  in vault prolapse 221
stroke and HRT 197–8
suicide, maternal 270–6
supine position, pregnancy and exercise in 259
suprapubic pressure in shoulder dystocia 320
surrogate pregnancy 239–46
  counselling 243–4
  ethical issues 239–40
  full surrogacy *see in vitro* fertilisation
  indications 242–3
  law and 241–2
  medical procedures 244
  medical profession and 240–1

outcomes 244–5
terminology 240
suture material, vaginal surgery 221
swimming in pregnancy 256–7
symphysiotomy in shoulder dystocia 331–2

Tait, Robert Lawson 7–8
tamponade, in placenta praevia
  fetus for 5–6
  vaginal and uterine 4–5
teenagers *see* adolescents
tension-free vaginal tape 191–2
teratoma, immature, paediatric 163
tetrahydrofolate (THF) 16
thalassaemia and fetal hydrops 282
thermoregulation in pregnancy and exercise 251–2
  swimming and 256
thrombocytopenic fetuses, blood sampling/transfusion 301
thromboembolic disease *see* venous thromboembolism
thrombophilias 19
tibolone in period-free HRT 99, 100
tocolytics (β-tocolytics)
  pulmonary oedema with 255
  very preterm labour delay 290
tooth loss and HRT 198
training
  obstetric trauma prevention 184
  specialist 44
  see also education
transcervical cell sampling 310–15, 319
transformation zone, large loop excision 129–30
transfusion (blood/blood products), fetal
  in hydrops 282
  platelets 301
  see also fetofetal transfusion syndrome
transvaginal bladder-neck needle suspension 190
trauma/injury
  anogenital (and associated faecal incontinence) 174
    obstetric trauma *see* childbirth
    see also self-harm
  infant, in shoulder dystocia 332–3
tubal pathology *see* fallopian tubes
tumours
  benign ovarian, paediatric 163
  fetal, surgery 283
  malignant *see* cancer
twin-twin transfusion syndrome 303
  see also multiple pregnancy

ultrasound
  endoanal, in incontinence 178
  fetal, macrosomia detection 328
  IVF monitoring 83
ultrasound-guided fetal blood sampling 301
umbilical cord blood sampling *see* cordocentesis
umbilical venous pressure, fetal hydrops 277, 281, 283, 284
ureter
  ectopic 147
  in vaginal hysterectomy, position 217
ureteric buds 144
  double/additional 144
urethra, congenitally short 147

urge incontinence (faecal) 178–9
urinary bladder *see* bladder
urinary function with anterior vaginal repair 68
urinary incontinence 188–95
  congenital anomalies presenting in later life as 147
  HRT and 200
  stress *see* stress incontinence
urinary tract development
  anomalies
    with associated genital tract anomalies 150–1
    fetal hydrops and 278
    presenting as incontinence in later life 147
  lower 145–6
  upper 144
urinary tract reconstruction, lower, with congenital
  anomalies 147
  obstetric implications 148
urogenital sinus 146
  persistent (neonatal) 152
urogenital system *see* genitourinary system
urogynaecology, minimal access 188–95
USA
  anaesthesia-related maternal deaths 354
  surrogacy 245
uterine activity, augmentation, caesarean scar and 266
uterine artery embolisation 209–14
uterosacral ligament suspension, high 218, 222
uterus (cervix)
  didelphys 152
  fibroids, embolisation 209–14
  infertility relating to 84
  prolapse, rectal prolapse and 174
  sarcoma, embolisation 213
  support mechanisms 62
  tamponade, for placenta praevia 4–5
uterus (neck) *see entries under* cervical

VAC *see* vincristine–actinomycin D–cyclophosphamide
vacuum delivery, perineal trauma 182–3, 184
vagina
  anterior wall prolapse 61–70
    anatomical aspects 62–3
    diagnosis of defects and examination 63–4
    historical aspects 61–2
    surgical approaches 64–7
    surgical complications 68
  cancer (carcinoma)
    hormones and 139, 160
    paediatric 160–2, 165–6
  developmental anomalies 146
    agenesis 153
    double/duplicated vagina 152, 153
  endometriosis *see* rectovaginal endometriosis
  proctological fistula involving 26–8
  sexual function and treatment of 149
  pulsion, rectal prolapse ad 29
  tamponade, placenta praevia 4–5
  vault prolapse (post-hysterectomy)
    assessment and documentation 216
    epidemiology/aetiology 216
    investigations 216–17
    prevention 217–18
    treatment 217, 218–22
  vault support at hysterectomy 217–18

vaginal approaches
    hysterectomy, vault prolapse prevention 217–18
    vault prolapse 218–20
vaginal paravaginal repair of lateral wall defects 65
vaginal tape, tension-free 191–2
vaginoplasty 153
vascular anastomoses between twin fetuses, laser
    ablation 303
venous pressure, central, fetal hydrops and 277, 281
venous thromboembolism
    homocysteine and 19
    HRT risk 109–10, 202
vesico-amniotic shunt 303
vestibule of vagina, proctological fistula involving,
    sexual function and treatment of 149
vincristine–actinomycin D–cyclophosphamide (VAC)
    ovarian cancer 164
    rhabdomyosarcoma 160
vincristine–cisplatin–bleomycin, paediatric ovarian
    cancer 164, 165
virilisation 147, 153–4
vulval cancer and hormones 138–9

waiting times
    consultant-based service 42
    infertility treatment 79

weight gain
    HRT 202
    pregnancy, exercise effects 252
    see also obesity
White, GR 61
Willet's scalp forceps 6–7
Williams, John Whitridge 8
WISDOM 197, 201
wolffian (mesonephric) duct 144, 145
Women's Health Initiative 197, 201
Women's International Study of Long Duration
    Oestrogen after Menopause (WISDOM) 197, 201
Wood's screw manoeuvre 320–1
workload in consultant-based service 42
    consultant 36–7
    night-time 44–5

Y chromosome, gonadal development and 144
yolk sac tumours *see* endodermal sinus tumours

Zavanelli manoeuvre 331–2